PARKINSON'S
DISEASE

PARKINSON'S DISEASE

GENETICS AND PATHOGENESIS

Edited By

Ted M. Dawson

Johns Hopkins University School of Medicine
Baltimore, Maryland, USA

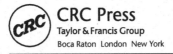

CRC Press
Taylor & Francis Group
Boca Raton London New York

CRC Press is an imprint of the
Taylor & Francis Group, an **informa** business

CRC Press
Taylor & Francis Group
6000 Broken Sound Parkway NW, Suite 300
Boca Raton, FL 33487-2742

First issued in paperback 2019

© 2007 by Taylor & Francis Group, LLC
CRC Press is an imprint of Taylor & Francis Group, an Informa business

No claim to original U.S. Government works

ISBN-13: 978-0-8493-3697-3 (hbk)
ISBN-13: 978-0-367-38915-4 (pbk)

This book contains information obtained from authentic and highly regarded sources. While all reasonable efforts have been made to publish reliable data and information, neither the author[s] nor the publisher can accept any legal responsibility or liability for any errors or omissions that may be made. The publishers wish to make clear that any views or opinions expressed in this book by individual editors, authors or contributors are personal to them and do not necessarily reflect the views/opinions of the publishers. The information or guidance contained in this book is intended for use by medical, scientific or health-care professionals and is provided strictly as a supplement to the medical or other professional's own judgement, their knowledge of the patient's medical history, relevant manufacturer's instructions and the appropriate best practice guidelines. Because of the rapid advances in medical science, any information or advice on dosages, procedures or diagnoses should be independently verified. The reader is strongly urged to consult the relevant national drug formulary and the drug companies' and device or material manufacturers' printed instructions, and their websites, before administering or utilizing any of the drugs, devices or materials mentioned in this book. This book does not indicate whether a particular treatment is appropriate or suitable for a particular individual. Ultimately it is the sole responsibility of the medical professional to make his or her own professional judgements, so as to advise and treat patients appropriately. The authors and publishers have also attempted to trace the copyright holders of all material reproduced in this publication and apologize to copyright holders if permission to publish in this form has not been obtained. If any copyright material has not been acknowledged please write and let us know so we may rectify in any future reprint.

Visit the Taylor & Francis Web site at
http://www.taylorandfrancis.com

and the CRC Press Web site at
http://www.crcpress.com

NEUROLOGICAL DISEASE AND THERAPY

Advisory Board

Preface

Parkinson's disease is the most common neurodegenerative movement disorder. A number of advances in genetics, epidemiology, neuropathology, and the development of new experimental models of Parkinson's disease are providing important new insights into the pathogenesis of Parkinson's disease. Combined, they have brought spectacular advances and created a renaissance in understanding the molecular mechanisms of neurodegeneration in Parkinson's disease. Many of these advances hold particular promise for mechanistic-based treatments that will slow or halt the progression of Parkinson's disease. Currently, there is no text that covers all the emerging aspects of Parkinson's disease and for this reason I felt that a volume dedicated to these topics was timely.

The authors are all leading scientists and clinicians working in the field of Parkinson's disease who come from different perspectives. In particular, the authors have expertise in clinical neurology, genetics, molecular neuroscience, epidemiology, pathology, and animal models of neurodegenerative diseases. I have tried to draw together a comprehensive view of the recent major advances in our understanding of Parkinson's disease. The first four chapters serve as an introduction to Parkinson's disease, they review the major aspects of the disease including neuropathology, genetics, epidemiology, clinical features and therapy. This is followed by a comprehensive review of the genetics of Parkinson's disease, which leads into chapters on the major pathogenic hypotheses of Parkinson's disease, including alpha-synuclein, *PARKIN*, *DJ-1*, *PINK-1*, *LRRK2*, mitochondrial dysfunction, and ubiquitin proteasomal dysfunction. Each chapter reviews advances and how these discoveries may lead to new therapeutic opportunities. The last section discusses animal models and summarizes the emerging new targets for therapeutics.

I hope that this book is a useful resource for clinicians, researchers, as well as experts and students alike who have an interest in Parkinson's disease. Ultimately, I hope it helps in our efforts to improve the care and ultimately cure the victims of Parkinson's disease.

Ted M. Dawson

Contents

Contributors

Patrick M. Abou-Sleiman Department of Molecular Neuroscience, Institute of Neurology, London, U.K.

M. Flint Beal Department of Neurology and Neuroscience, Weill Medical College of Cornell University and New York Presbyterian Hospital, New York, New York, U.S.A.

Ranjita Betarbet Center for Neurodegenerative Diseases, Emory University, Atlanta, Georgia, U.S.A.

Alexis Brice Neurology and Experimental Therapeutics, INSERM U679, Université Pierre and Marie Curie and Fédération des Maladies du Système Nerveux and Department de Génétique, Cytogénétique, Groupe Hospitalier Pitié-Salpetriere, Paris, France

Anabel Chade Department of Clinical Research, The Parkinson's Institute, Sunnyvale, California, U.S.A.

Jordi Clarimón Alzheimer's Laboratory, Sant Pau Hospital, Barcelona, Spain

Mark R. Cookson Cell Biology and Gene Expression Unit, Laboratory of Neurogenetics, National Institute on Aging, Bethesda, Maryland, U.S.A.

Marc Cruts Department of Molecular Genetics, Neurodegenerative Brain Diseases Group, Laboratory of Neurogenetics, Institute Born-Bunge, University of Antwerp, Antwerpen, Belgium

Ted M. Dawson Institute for Cell Engineering, Department of Neurology and Neuroscience, Johns Hopkins University School of Medicine, Baltimore, Maryland, U.S.A.

Valina L. Dawson Institute for Cell Engineering, Department of Neurology, Neuroscience, and Physiology, Johns Hopkins University School of Medicine, Baltimore, Maryland, U.S.A.

Dennis W. Dickson Departments of Neuroscience and Pathology (Neuropathology), Mayo Clinic Jacksonville, Jacksonville, Florida, U.S.A.

Alexandra Durr Neurology and Experimental Therapeutics, INSERM U679, Université Pierre and Marie Curie and Department de Génétique, Cytogénétique, Groupe Hospitalier, Pitié-Salpetriere, Paris, France

Stanley Fahn Neurological Institute, Columbia University, New York, New York, U.S.A.

Matt Farrer Neurogenetics, Department of Neuroscience, Mayo Clinic Jacksonville, Jacksonville, Florida, U.S.A.

Matthew S. Goldberg Center for Neurologic Diseases, Brigham and Women's Hospital, Harvard Medical School, Boston, Massachusetts, U.S.A.

J. Timothy Greenamyre Pittsburgh Institute for Neurodegenerative Diseases, University of Pittsburgh, Pittsburgh, Pennsylvania, U.S.A.

Peter Heutink Section of Medical Genomics, Department of Human Genetics, VU University Medical Center, Amsterdam, The Netherlands

Meike Kasten Department of Clinical Research, The Parkinson's Institute, Sunnyvale, California, U.S.A.

Michael K. Lee Department of Pathology, Johns Hopkins University School of Medicine, Baltimore, Maryland, U.S.A.

Virginia M.-Y. Lee Center for Neurodegenerative Disease Research, Department of Pathology and Laboratory Medicine, Institute on Aging, University of Pennsylvania, Philadelphia, Pennsylvania, U.S.A.

Ebba Lohmann Neurology and Experimental Therapeutics, INSERM U679, Université Pierre and Marie Curie and Fédération des Maladies du Système Nerveux and Department de Génétique, Cytogénétique, Groupe Hospitalier Pitié-Salpetriere, Paris, France

Miratul M. K. Muqit Department of Molecular Neuroscience, Institute of Neurology, London, U.K.

Sofia A. Oliveira Instituto Gulbenkian de Ciência, Oeiras, Portugal

Leo J. Pallanck Department of Genome Sciences, University of Washington, Seattle, Washington, U.S.A.

Serge Przedborski Department of Neurology, Pathology, and Cell Biology and Center for Motor Neuron Biology and Disease, Columbia University, New York, New York, U.S.A.

Rosa Rademakers Department of Molecular Genetics, Neurodegenerative Brain Diseases Group, Laboratory of Neurogenetics, Institute Born-Bunge, University of Antwerp, Antwerpen, Belgium

Ian J. Reynolds Neuroscience Drug Discovery, Merck Research Laboratories, West Point, Pennsylvania, U.S.A.

Merle Ruberg Neurology and Experimental Therapeutics, INSERM U679, Université Pierre and Marie Curie, Paris, France

Daniel S. Sa Department of Neurology and Neuroscience, Weill Medical College of Cornell University and New York Presbyterian Hospital, New York, New York, U.S.A.

Jie Shen Center for Neurologic Diseases, Brigham and Women's Hospital, Harvard Medical School, Boston, Massachusetts, U.S.A.

Andrew B. Singleton Laboratory of Neurogenetics, National Institute of Aging, National Institutes of Health, Bethesda, Maryland, U.S.A.

Daniel M. Skovronsky Avid Radiopharmaceuticals, Inc., Philadelphia, Pennsylvania, U.S.A.

James H. Soper Center for Neurodegenerative Disease Research, Department of Pathology and Laboratory Medicine, Institute on Aging, University of Pennsylvania, Philadelphia, Pennsylvania, U.S.A.

Leonidas Stefanis Section of Basic Neurosciences, Foundation for Biomedical Research of the Academy of Athens, Athens, Greece

Caroline M. Tanner Department of Clinical Research, The Parkinson's Institute, Sunnyvale, California, U.S.A.

John Q. Trojanowski   Center for Neurodegenerative Disease Research, Department of Pathology and Laboratory Medicine, Institute on Aging, University of Pennsylvania, Philadelphia, Pennsylvania, U.S.A.

Christine van Broeckhoven   Department of Molecular Genetics, Neurodegenerative Brain Diseases Group, Laboratory of Neurogenetics, Institute Born-Bunge, University of Antwerp, Antwerpen, Belgium

Jeffery M. Vance   Division of Human Genetics, Center for Molecular Genetics and Genomic Medicine, Miami Institute for Human Genomics, University of Miami, Miami, Florida, U.S.A.

Tatyana V. Votyakova   Division of Immunogenetics, Department of Pediatrics, University of Pittsburgh, Pittsburgh, Pennsylvania, U.S.A.

Andrew B. West   Institute for Cell Engineering, Department of Neurology, Johns Hopkins University School of Medicine, Baltimore, Maryland, U.S.A.

Andrew Whittle   Neurogenetics, Department of Neuroscience, Mayo Clinic Jacksonville, Jacksonville, Florida, U.S.A.

Alexander J. Whitworth   Department of Biomedical Sciences, University of Sheffield, Sheffield, U.K.

Garry Wong   Department of Neurobiology, A.I. Virtanen Institute and Department of Biochemistry, Kuopio University, Kuopio, Finland

Nicholas W. Wood   Department of Molecular Neuroscience, Institute of Neurology, London, U.K.

Section I: Overview

1 Neuropathology and Staging of Parkinson's Disease

Dennis W. Dickson
Departments of Neuroscience and Pathology (Neuropathology), Mayo Clinic Jacksonville, Jacksonville, Florida, U.S.A.

INTRODUCTION

In the present discussion, Parkinson's disease (PD) is considered to be a term for an extrapyramidal motor syndrome characterized by bradykinesia, rigidity, postural instability, and tremor, while Lewy body disease (LBD) is a pathologic term for a disorder characterized by neuronal lesions [i.e., Lewy bodies (LBs)] composed of α-synuclein (SNCA). Autopsy studies have shown that LBD is the most common substrate for PD, but other disorders, most notably progressive supranuclear palsy (PSP) and multiple system atrophy (MSA), can produce a similar extrapyramidal syndrome. Complicating this discussion is the fact that nonmotor manifestations are common in PD, and it is possible that the earliest clinical features of PD may not be those of an extrapyramidal motor dysfunction, but rather a syndrome characterized by autonomic dysfunction, anosmia, or a sleep disturbance. Clinical features of advanced PD may be overwhelmingly cognitive or psychiatric in nature, rather than motor. Moreover, LBD is also the pathologic substrate of non-PD clinical syndromes, including focal dystonias, pure autonomic failure, rapid eye movement behavior disorder (RBD) and some cases of essential tremor as well as dementia, with fluctuations and psychotic features referred to as dementia with Lewy bodies (DLB).

Genetics has offered clues to the molecular basis of PD, and many, but not all, of the genetically determined parkinsonian disorders are associated with LBs (Table 1). Some are associated with nonspecific neuronal loss in the substantia nigra, while others are characterized by neuronal inclusions composed of proteins other than α-synuclein. This review focuses on the neuropathology and staging of sporadic and familial parkinsonian disorders.

SPORADIC PARKINSON'S DISEASE

There are surprisingly few published studies that address the postmortem pathologic substrate of PD (1–4). In most cases it is assumed that PD is synonymous with LBD, but LBD is found in only 75% to 90% of PD cases (1,2). The ability to predict typical LBD in PD increases to over 90% in cases followed longitudinally by movement disorder specialists (3). Accuracy is lowest for archival, retrospective diagnoses based on the chart review, where the proportion of PD cases with LBD approaches only 60% (4). The pathologically confirmed disorders most often mistaken for PD in both the retrospective and prospective studies are PSP and MSA, which are briefly reviewed with a focus on the clinical and pathologic differential diagnoses of PD.

1

TABLE 1 Neuropathology of Genetic Forms of Parkinson's Disease

Chromosome	Gene	Name	Neuropathology
4q21	*SNCA* (α-synuclein)	*PARK 1*	LBs
6q25.2–27	*PARKIN*	*PARK 2*	Nonspecific nigral degeneration (tau positive lesions; LBs in some compound heterozygous cases)
2p13	Unknown	*PARK 3*	LBs
4q21 (initially linked to 4p15)	*SNCA*	*PARK 4*	LBs
4p14–15	*UCHL-1*	*PARK 5*	Not described (giant axonal dystrophy in mouse UCHL1 mutants)
1q35–36	*PINK*	*PARK 6*	Not described
1p36	*DJ-1*	*PARK 7*	Not described (LBs in heterozygous individuals)
12p11.2–q13.1	*LRRK2*	*PARK 8*	Variable pathology (nonspecific nigral degeneration; LBs; NFTs)
1p36	Unknown	*PARK 9*	Not described (pallidal-pyramidal degeneration on imaging)
1p32	Unknown	*PARK 10*	Not described
2q36–37	Unknown	*PARK 11*	Not described

Abbreviations: LB, Lewy body; NFT, neurofibrillary tangles.

Lewy Body Disease

As mentioned previously, the most common pathologic substrate of PD is LBD. LBs are granulofilamentous intraneuronal inclusions composed of α-synuclein and other proteins (5) (Figs. 1A and 2A). Typical LBs are easily recognized, round cytoplasmic inclusions, but more subtle lesions are also found, the so-called cortical LBs (Figs. 1D and 2D). Neurons with LBs are susceptible to cell death and phagocytosis by microglia, a process referred to as neuronophagia (Fig. 1B). Inclusions similar to LBs are also found within neuronal processes as intraneuritic LBs (Figs. 1C and 2C). In addition to these lesions, which are readily detected with routine histologic methods, there are also more subtle neuritic lesions that contain abnormal aggregates of α-synuclein, known as Lewy neurites (LNs) (Fig. 2D). LNs are only visible with immunohistochemical methods, while intraneuritic LBs can be detected with routine histologic methods (Fig. 1C). While originally described in the hippocampus (6) and later the amygdala (7), LNs are now known to be more widely distributed than originally suspected and may be the most abundant type of pathologic lesion in any given region affected by the disease process. They may also be the earliest cytologic alteration in affected neurons (8), and they may precede LB formation in perikarya or axons (9). The contribution of neuritic degeneration to the clinical phenotype is increasingly recognized (10).

The vulnerability of selected populations of neurons to LBs has been known for many years [(11–13); reviewed in (14)] and is the focus of increasing interest. Neurons that are most vulnerable to LBs include the monoaminergic neurons of the substantia nigra, locus ceruleus, and raphe nuclei (Fig. 3), as well as the cholinergic neurons of the basal forebrain. Due to the neuronal loss of pigmented neurons in the substantia nigra and locus ceruleus, these nuclei show loss of neuromelanin pigmentation on gross examination (Fig. 3). This neuronal loss corresponds to decrease in dopaminergic terminals in the striatum as detected by tyrosine hydroxylase immunohistochemistry, the rate-limiting enzyme in dopamine synthesis (Fig. 4).

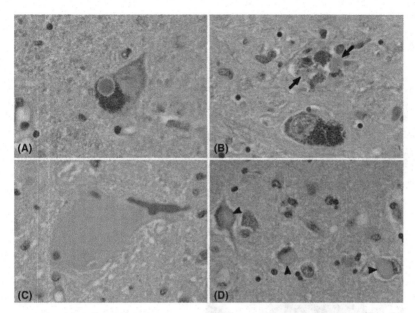

FIGURE 1   An LB within the cytoplasm of a neuromelanin-containing neuron of the pars compacta of the substantia nigra (**A**). A neuron with extracellular LBs (*arrows*) and neuromelanin undergoing phagocytosis by microglia (**B**). A swollen dystrophic axon in the dorsal motor nucleus of the vagus has intraneuritic LBs (**C**). Several neurons in the amygdala have cortical-type LBs (*arrowheads*) (**D**). *Abbreviation*: LB, Lewy body.

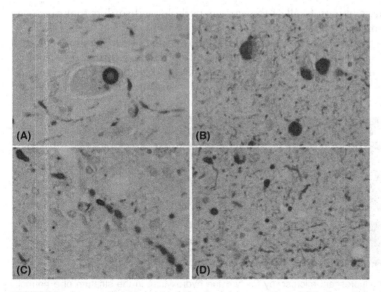

FIGURE 2   Immunohistochemistry for α-synuclein reveals an LB in the substantia nigra (**A**), cortical type LBs in the amygdala (**B**), intraneuritic LBs in the basal nucleus of Meynert (**C**), and Lewy neutrites in the amygdala (**D**) in a case of Lewy body disease. *Abbreviation*: LB, Lewy body.

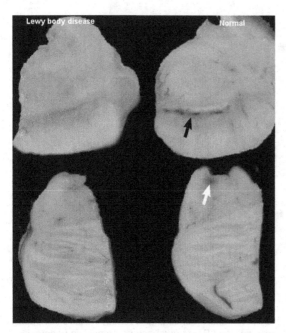

FIGURE 3 Gross cross sections of the midbrain (*upper two images*) and rostral pons (*lower two images*) in a case of LBD (*left*) and an age-matched normal (*right*). Note the black arrow pigment in the pars compacta of the normal that is nearly completely absent in LBD. Similarly, white arrow pigment in the locus ceruleus is visible in the normal, but not in LBD. *Abbreviation*: LBD, Lewy body disease.

These features are common to all of the various pathologic disorders that produce clinical parkinsonism.

In addition to brainstem monoaminergic neurons, neurons in the dorsal motor nucleus of the vagus and the medullary and pontine reticular formation are also vulnerable. LBs are uncommon in the basal ganglia, but LNs are often detected in the striatum (15). The neurons of the thalamus are resistant, but LBs are common

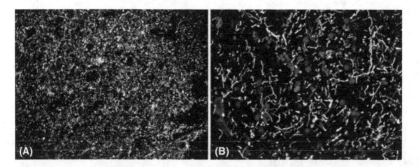

FIGURE 4 Immunofluorescent microscopy for tyrosine hydroxylase in the striatum of a normal individual (**A**) and a person with PD (**B**). Note fewer neurites and the more coarse and tortuous nature of the neurites in PD compared to the dense and fine punctate neuritic staining in the normal. *Abbreviation*: PD, Parkinson's disease.

in the hypothalamus, especially the posterior and lateral hypothalamus. The oculomotor nuclear complex is also vulnerable, particularly the parasympathetic Edinger-Westphal nucleus. In the pons, the subpeduncular and pedunculopontine nuclei are often affected, but neurons of the pontine base are not affected. LBs have not been described in the cerebellar cortex or the cerebellar deep nuclei. In the spinal cord, the neurons of the intermediolateral cell column are most vulnerable, but LNs are more widespread. LBs can be found in the autonomic ganglia, including submucosal ganglia of the lower esophagus (16). Neurons in the anterior olfactory nucleus in the olfactory bulb are also vulnerable (17). Cortical neurons are less often affected in PD, with limbic cortices and multimodal-association cortices of the temporal and frontal lobe most vulnerable. The neurons of the parietal and occipital cortices, as well as the primary motor and sensory cortices, are resistant to LBs.

Neuropathologic Staging of Parkinson's Disease

Recently, Braak and coworkers proposed a pathologic staging system for PD (18). In this staging system, nigral pathology occurs at mid-stage disease, whereas involvement of medulla and pontine tegmentum occurs earlier. The anterior olfactory nucleus is also affected early in the disease course. In the endstage, LBs involve cortical areas, and at this stage many patients with PD are expected to have significant cognitive problems. The pathology at this stage is similar to that found in diffuse LBD, an increasingly recognized late-life dementing disorder (19). The cortical stages proposed by Braak are similar to those originally described by Kosaka et al. (20) and adopted by the Consortium for Dementia with LBs (21) (Table 2). The major change proposed by Braak was to extend the staging system to brainstem regions. Several studies suggest that the most common cause of later-developing dementia in patients who initially had typical PD is in fact diffuse LBD (22,23). The staging system addresses neuronal loss only superficially, but suggests that α-synuclein pathology precedes neuronal loss by one or more stages. That being the case, by the time an individual presents with extrapyramidal symptoms, which reflect significant neuronal loss in the substantia nigra, it is likely that LB pathology has spread far beyond the midbrain. This hypothesis remains to be verified in autopsy studies of normal controls and PD patients with various disease durations.

The general principles of the proposed staging system have been confirmed in several studies of PD, but it does not appear to fit with cases of LBD with a different clinical presentation, most notably clinical syndromes presenting with dementia or

TABLE 2 Neuropathologic Staging of Parkinson's Disease

Anatomical region	Braak PD stage	Kosaka LBD types
Anterior olfactory nucleus	1	(Not assessed)
Dorsal motor nucleus of vagus		
Locus ceruleus	2	Brainstem
Substantia nigra	3	
Basal nucleus of Meynert		
Amygdala	4	Transitional
Parahippocampal and cingulate limbic cortices		
Multimodal association cortices of temporal, frontal and parietal lobes	5	Diffuse
Primary motor and visual cortices	6	

Abbreviations: LBD, Lewy body disease; PD, Parkinson's disease.

psychosis. A large cross-sectional study of 904 brains by Parkkinen and coworkers, (24) who used α-synuclein immunohistochemistry to study the frequency and distribution of LBs, largely concurred with the Braak staging scheme; however, they also described several cases in which LBs were only found in the substantia nigra without involvement of the medulla. A study by Jellinger also found exceptions (25). The stage at which autonomic ganglia are affected is unknown, but involvement of the spinal cord intermediolateral column has been addressed in a recent study, which suggests that spinal cord involvement occurs after the medulla, but before the midbrain (26).

It is increasingly recognized that LBs are frequent in the setting of advanced Alzheimer's disease (AD) (27) and that the most common location for LBs in AD is the amygdala (28,29). In a cross-sectional study of AD, LBs were almost completely limited to the amygdala in about 15% to 20% of the cases (30). Most of these cases did not have brainstem pathology, including the dorsal motor nucleus of the vagus and surrounding areas, which is the earliest stage in the scheme proposed by Braak and coworkers. Thus, LBs in advanced AD begin de novo in the amygdala without progressing through the several brainstem stages that have been described for PD. The stage at which the basal ganglia are affected has not been addressed systematically, but it is probably a late manifestation. It is also clear that brainstem involvement is often minimal in some cases of diffuse LBD, particularly patients who present with dementia and minimal or no parkinsonism (31). This form of LBD also appears to have a different pattern of disease progression than that described for PD.

Clinical Features of Various Stages of Parkinson's Disease

If the staging scheme proposed by Braak is correct, nonmotor, nondopaminergic symptoms should precede motor symptoms. In particular, one might predict that early PD may be characterized by autonomic dysfunction, olfactory dysfunction, sleep disorder, and depression, given the role that lower brainstem monoaminergic nuclei, as well as spinal and enteric ganglia have in these processes. It is of interest that epidemiologic studies indicate that autonomic symptoms may precede clinical PD by as much as 12 years (32). One might speculate that the pathology responsible for this syndrome is LBs in autonomic nuclei of the lower brainstem and spinal cord, as well as the enteric plexus. Several studies suggest that a history of anxiety and depression or both may precede PD (33). While the anatomic substrate for depression is unknown, some studies have implicated norepinephrine, which is the major neurotransmitter of the locus ceruleus (34). Another clinical syndrome that may be a harbinger of PD is RBD, a condition that appears a number of years before PD (35). The RBD syndrome appears to have its anatomic origins within lower brainstem nuclei (36) that are consistently affected in LBD. Olfactory dysfunction is common in PD (37), and it may precede overt motor symptoms (38). The later stages of PD are associated with involvement of limbic cortices and multimodal association and, finally, unimodal association and primary cortices. These latter stages may be characterized largely by cognitive and psychiatric features similar to those found in DLB (39).

MULTIPLE SYSTEM ATROPHY

MSA is a nonheritable neurodegenerative disease characterized by parkinsonism, cerebellar ataxia, and idiopathic orthostatic hypotension (40). The concept of MSA unifies three separate entities, namely olivopontocerebellar atrophy, Shy-Drager syndrome, and striatonigral degeneration. In an individual, the predominant signs and symptoms depend on neuronal systems predominantly affected—those with predominant degeneration in cerebellar circuitry have ataxia (MSA-C), while those with degeneration in the basal ganglia have a DOPA-nonresponsive parkinsonism (MSA-P). While the clinical presentation is often sufficiently distinctive to differentiate MSA from idiopathic PD, it remains one of the pathologic processes most often mistaken for PD in autopsy series, particularly cases with MSA-P (2,4). Autonomic dysfunction is virtually always present in MSA and it is also common in many cases of PD.

The MSA-P brain shows atrophy and discoloration of the posterolateral putamen and loss of pigment in the ventrolateral substantia nigra (Fig. 5), with neuronal loss and gliosis in the substantia nigra (Fig. 6A) and striatum. In the later location, there is often prominent accumulation of brown granular (hemosiderin-like) pigment (Fig. 6B). There may or may not be concurrent atrophy of the pontine base, inferior olive, and cerebellum. In MSA-P olivopontocerebellar involvement is often only detected with histologic methods. The histopathologic findings include neuronal loss, gliosis, and microvacuolation involving the putamen and substantia nigra. Lantos first described glial (oligodendroglial) cytoplasmic inclusions (GCI) in MSA (41). GCI can be detected with silver stains, in particular the Gallyas silver stain, but are best seen with antibodies to α-synuclein and ubiquitin, where they appear as flame- or sickle-shaped inclusions in oligodendrocytes (Fig. 6D). At the

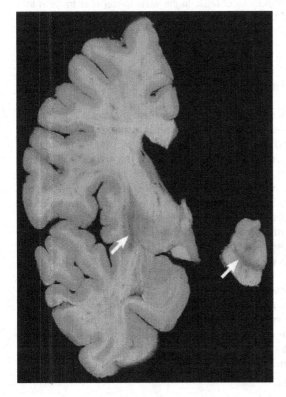

FIGURE 5 Gross evaluation of MSA-P reveals atrophy and brown pigmentation of the lateral putamen (*left arrow*) and loss of neuromelanin pigment in the substantia nigra (especially the lateral part; *right arrow*) of the midbrain. *Abbreviation*: MSA, multiple system atrophy.

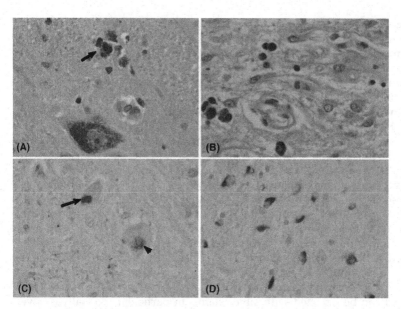

FIGURE 6   Microscopic findings in MSA reveal neuronal loss, with neuromelanin-laden macrophages in the substantia nigra (**A**) and severe neuronal loss and astrocytic gliosis in the putamen (**B**). Note also the presence of coarsely granular hemosiderin pigment (*left side* of figure). Immunohistochemistry for α-synuclein reveals neuronal cytoplasmic inclusions (*arrow*) and intranuclear filaments (*arrowhead*) (**C**) in neurons of the inferior olivary nucleus of MSA. In the white matter fiber tracts in the pontine base numerous GCI are evident (**D**). *Abbreviation*: MSA, multiple system atrophy.

ultrastructural level, GCI are nonmembrane-bound cytoplasmic inclusions composed of 10 to 20 nm diameter coated filaments (42,43), which are similar to the filaments in LBs.

While most cellular inclusions in MSA are in oligodendroglial cells, some neuronal inclusions and neuritic processes are also detected, and occasional neurons also have synuclein-immunoreactive fibrils within their nuclei (Fig. 6C) (44–46). Some of the neuronal inclusions in MSA superficially resemble LBs, but the anatomical distribution of the neuronal inclusions in MSA is distinct from LBD. In MSA, neuronal inclusions are most often found in the pontine base, inferior olive, and putamen, regions that rarely, if ever, have LBs in LBD. Interestingly, α-synuclein-immunoreactive glial lesions have also been reported in LBD, mostly in brainstem nuclei (47). Glial pathology may be particularly striking in early onset familial PD (48), suggesting that MSA and LBD are part of a pathologic spectrum. On the other hand, glial lesions in sporadic LBD are sparse and their presence is unlikely to lead to difficulties in differential diagnosis. Biochemical studies of α-synuclein in brain homogenates from MSA and LBD show similar changes in the properties of α-synuclein. In both conditions, α-synuclein is abundant in detergent and formic acid extractable fractions, whereas in normal controls it is largely confined to the buffer soluble fractions (49). High molecular-weight forms that may represent post-translationally modified or aggregated forms of synuclein are detected in both. In some of the high molecular weight aggregates, there is evidence of ubiquitination. There is also evidence for truncation of α-synuclein in LBD (50).

PROGRESSIVE SUPRANUCLEAR PALSY

Progressive supranuclear palsy (PSP) is one of the major causes of levodopa-nonresponsive parkinsonism (51). Given the fact that it is associated with additional clinical features not typical of PD, it is considered one of the "parkinsonism-plus" syndromes. One of the earliest clinical features of PSP is unexplained falls. While falls occur in PD, they more often occur later in the disease course than in PSP. Whereas the initial presentation of PSP often suggests PD, when patients fail to respond to I-DOPA and begin to develop characteristic features of postural instability, vertical gaze paresis, nuchal and axial rigidity, and dysarthria (52), the diagnosis becomes more evident. Eye movement abnormalities are the hallmark of PSP (53) and are characterized initially by impairment of down-gaze, followed later by difficulties with up-gaze and even horizontal gaze, but they are not detected in all cases. Other clinical features include dysarthria and dysphagia, which are not specific and can also be detected to some degree in PD. Despite many differences in clinical presentation, it is not uncommon for an individual to carry a diagnosis of PD for years before a correct diagnosis of PSP is made (50,52). It has been suggested that only with longitudinal evaluation is it possible to accurately differentiate PD from other parkinsonian disorders (54). Recently, it has been suggested that a subset of cases of pathologically confirmed PSP have parkinsonism with many similarities to PD, the so-called PSP-P, throughout the course of their illness (55).

The brain in PSP usually has mild frontal and more marked midbrain atrophy (56). The latter is uncommon in LBD. The substantia nigra invariably shows depigmentation and the subthalamic nucleus is smaller than expected (Figs. 7 and 8). The latter does not occur in LBD. The superior cerebellar peduncle (Fig. 7) and the hilus of the cerebellar dentate nucleus are often attenuated due to myelinated fiber loss.

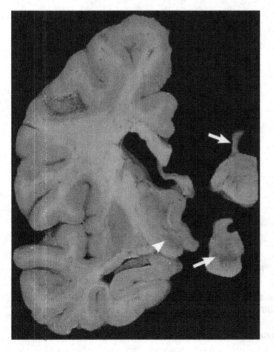

FIGURE 7 Gross findings in progressive supranuclear palsy include atrophy of the subthalamic nucleus (*arrowhead*), atrophy of the superior cerebellar peduncle (*top arrow*), and loss of neuromelanin pigment in the substantia nigra (especially the lateral part (*arrow*).

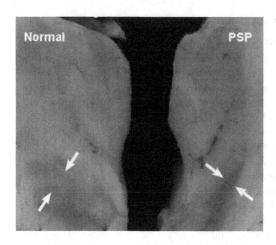

FIGURE 8 Subthalamic nucleus atrophy in PSP (*right*) compared to an age-matched normal individual (*left*). *Abbreviation*: PSP, progressive supranuclear palsy.

These are also useful in the differential diagnosis. Microscopic findings include neuronal loss and fibrillary gliosis affecting globus pallidus, subthalamic nucleus, and substantia nigra. As in all parkinsonian disorders, neuronal loss in the substantia nigra is usually greatest in the ventrolateral tier. Other regions that are affected include striatum, diencephalon, and brainstem. Silver stains or immunostaining for tau reveal neurofibrillary tangles and glial lesions (Fig. 9), in contrast to LBs and

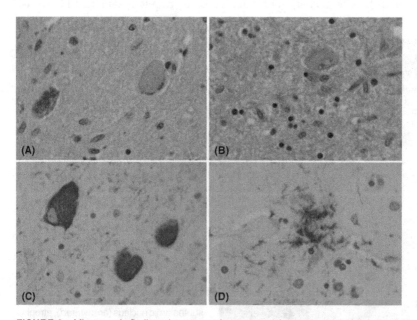

FIGURE 9 Microscopic findings in progressive supranuclear palsy include globose neurofibrillary tangles in the substantia nigra (**A**) and subthalamic nucleus (**B**), which also has severe astrocytic gliosis. Neuronal lesions (neurofibrillary tangles and pretangles in the substantia nigra) (**C**), and glial lesions (tufted astrocytes in the caudate nucleus) (**D**) are visible with tau immunohistochemistry.

LNs. The distribution of pathology is highly characteristic of PSP and permits differentiation from other tauopathies (56). The brainstem regions that are affected include the superior colliculus, periaqueductal gray matter, oculomotor nuclei, locus ceruleus, pontine nuclei, pontine tegmentum, vestibular nuclei, medullary tegmentum, and inferior olives. The cerebellar dentate nucleus is frequently affected. Spinal cord involvement is common, where neuronal inclusions can be found in anterior horn and intermediolateral cells.

In addition to NFT, which often have a rounded or globose appearance, PSP is also characterized by lesions in both astrocytes (the so-called "tufted astrocytes") and oligodendroglia (the so-called "coiled bodies") (57,58). These glial lesions are distinct from the GCI of MSA and the sparse glial lesions detected in LBD, based not only upon their immunoreactivity with tau, but also on their morphology.

FAMILIAL PARKINSON'S DISEASE
Genetics of Parkinsonism
The first mutations discovered in familial PD were those in the gene for α-synuclein (*SNCA*) (59). This discovery, in fact, preceded recognition that α-synuclein was the major structural component of LBs (60). At present, 11 genetic assignments have been proposed for familial PD (Table 2) (61). *PARK1* and *PARK4* are autosomal dominant forms of early-onset PD due to mutations in *SNCA* (59,62). *PARK2* and *PARK 7* are autosomal recessive early-onset PD due to mutations in *PARKIN* (63) and *DJ-1* (64), respectively. The most common genetic basis of typical late-onset autosomal dominant PD, assigned to *PARK8*, is the gene *LRRK2* (65,66). Genes for the other familial PD assignments remain unknown or controversial at present. Mutations in the tau gene (*MAPT*) have been discovered in some forms of frontotemporal dementia (67), and some of these kindreds have prominent parkinsonism (68), most often with features similar to PSP or corticobasal degeneration (CBD). The accepted term for this disorder is FTDP-17 (69). For this reason, *MAPT* is sometimes included among the genes responsible for parkinsonism. Some forms of spinocerebellar ataxia (SCA), particularly SCA2 and SCA3 (70,71), may also have prominent parkinsonism and might also be added to the list of familial PD genes. The following is a brief description of the pathologic findings in familial PD.

PARK1/4 (SNCA)
Several mutations have been discovered in *SNCA*, including the A53T mutation originally reported in the Contursi kindred (57). Two other coding mutations have been reported (A30P and E46K) (72,73), but to date there are no reports of postmortem pathology in any individual with these mutations. A final type of *SCNA* mutation is multiplication of the gene, with duplications and triplications reported (62,74). The pathology of cases with *SNCA* mutations, both A53T and triplication mutations, is consistently that of LBD, and at autopsy most of the reported cases have had widespread diffuse LBD with extensive involvement of cortical areas (48,74,75). Limbic system pathology is particularly severe, and hippocampal neuritic pathology and neuronal loss in CA2 sector is often marked (48,74).

PARK2 (PARKIN)
Neuropathologic studies are sparse or absent in most of the familial PD assignments. Even the most common of the familial PD, autosomal recessive juvenile-onset PD

(ARJP) due to *PARKIN* mutations, has been the subject of only a limited number of autopsy studies (76). The available autopsy studies of ARJP have shown substantia nigra degeneration with no specific histopathologic lesions. In some compound heterozygous patients, who are predicted to have decreased, but not total absence of, *PARKIN* function, LBs have been described (77,78). There is also report of tau pathology in some cases (79), but it remains to be determined if this is greater than expected for the age of the individual, since most cases have long-duration disease and die in late adulthood.

PARK3 (Unknown)
The genetic basis for PARK3 remains to be determined, but patients with this assignment on chromosome 2p have a typical clinical presentation of PD, with late age of onset and I-DOPA responsive parkinsonism. Cases that have come to autopsy also have had typical LB pathology with the brunt of the pathology in brainstem and basal forebrain nuclei and minimal involvement of limbic and association cortices (80).

PARK5 (UCHL-1)
The PARK5 locus has been assigned to a German kindred for which no autopsy studies are available (81). The gene implicated, *UCHL-1*, plays a role in the ubiquitin proteasome pathway. Variants in the gene may be risk factors for PD (82) that show typical LB pathology (4).

PARK6 (PINK1)
Like PARK2, this assignment is associated with early-onset PD (83). The clinical and genetic features of PARK6 are similar to those of PARK2 and include features that are not typical of PD, including juvenile age of onset, hyperreflexia, dystonia, and sleep benefit. The disease progression is typically slow. Given the relatively benign nature of the disease, most reported cases have had long disease duration. To date there have been no autopsies of patients carrying homozygous mutation in the *PINK1* gene.

PARK7 (DJ-1)
The clinical syndrome in PARK7, which is due to mutation in the *DJ-1* gene (64), is early-onset parkinsonism. Except for the early age of onset, the other clinical features are typical of PD (84). Autopsy findings have not been reported, but several cases of otherwise typical LB parkinsonism have been found to harbor heterozygous *DJ-1* mutations (85).

PARK8 (LRRK2)
The most common genetic basis for PD appears to be PARK8, which is associated with mutation in the *LRRK2* gene. The phenotype in most cases is indistinguishable from typical sporadic PD, with late age of disease onset, as well as presence of resting tremor, asymmetry, levodopa responsiveness, and potential for motor complications (86). The most common mutation is G2019S (87–89) and autopsy studies suggest that the most common pathology in affected with this mutation is LBD (90). There are rare individuals that have PSP-like tau pathology. The largest kindred

with *LRRK2* mutation is Family D, which is associated with an R1441C mutation (65). The pathology in this kindred is heterogeneous. Some individuals have LBD, while others have PSP-like tau pathology or only nonspecific neuronal loss and gliosis in the substantia nigra (91). In other kindreds (Family A), there is only nonspecific neuronal loss and gliosis in the substantia nigra (65).

Other Familial Parkinson's Disease
There are several other familial PD assignments (*PARK9, PARK10, PARK11*), but none of these kindreds has autopsy confirmation. Recently, mutation in the gene for Gaucher's disease, glucocerebrosidase, has been implicated in PD in Ashkenazi Jews and perhaps other populations (92). The few available autopsies have revealed LBD (93). Some families, particularly among ethnic minorities or the Chinese, that carry mutations in genes that cause spinocerebellar ataxia (SCA2 and SCA3) have predominantly a parkinsonian clinical phenotype (70,71). While no autopsies have been reported in these kindreds, in unrelated individuals, the pathology is that of nonspecific neuronal loss and gliosis in the substantia nigra. The most distinctive histologic hallmark of these trinucleotide-repeat disorders is the presence of neuronal intranuclear inclusions. It remains to be seen if this is the pathologic substrate of parkinsonism in SCA.

REFERENCES
1. Jellinger K. Pathology of Parkinson's syndrome. In: Handbook of Experimental Pharmacology, Vol. 88. Calne DB, Ed. Springer-Verlag: Berlin, 1989; pp. 47–112.
2. Hughes AJ, Daniel SE, Kilford L, et al. Accuracy of clinical diagnosis of idiopathic Parkinson's disease: a clinicopathologic study of 100 cases. J Neurol Neurosurg Psychiatry 1992; 55:181–184.
3. Hughes AJ, Daniel SE, Ben-Shlomo Y, et al. The accuracy of diagnosis of parkinsonian syndromes in a specialist movement disorder service. Brain 2002; 25:861–870.
4. Bower JH, Dickson DW, Taylor L, et al. Clinical correlates of the pathology underlying parkinsonism: a population perspective. Mov Disord 2002; 17:910–916.
5. Pollanen MS, Dickson DW, Bergeron C. Pathology and biology of the Lewy body. J Neuropathol Exp Neurol 1993; 52:183–191.
6. Dickson DW, Ruan D, Crystal H, et al. Hippocampal degeneration differentiates diffuse Lewy body disease (DLBD) from Alzheimer's disease: light and electron microscopic immunocytochemistry of CA2-3 neurites specific to DLBD. Neurology 1991; 41:1402–1409.
7. Braak H, Braak E, Yilmazer D, et al. Amygdala pathology in Parkinson's disease. Acta Neuropathol (Berl) 1994; 88:493–500.
8. Braak E, Sandmann-Keil D, Rub U, et al. Alpha-synuclein immunopositive Parkinson's disease-related inclusion bodies in lower brain stem nuclei. Acta Neuropathol (Berl) 2001; 101:195–201.
9. Kuusisto E, Parkkinen L, Alafuzoff I. Morphogenesis of Lewy bodies: dissimilar incorporation of alpha-synuclein, ubiquitin, and p62. J Neuropathol Exp Neurol 2003; 62:1241–1253.
10. Churchyard A, Lees AJ. The relationship between dementia and direct involvement of the hippocampus and amygdala in Parkinson's disease. Neurology 1997; 49:1570–1576.
11. den Hartog Jager WA, Bethlem J. The distribution of Lewy bodies in the central and autonomic nervous systems in idiopathic paralysis agitans. J Neurol Neurosurg Psychiatry 1960; 23:283–290.
12. Ohama E, Ikuta F. Parkinson's disease: distribution of Lewy bodies and monoamine neuron system. Acta Neuropathol (Berl) 1976; 34:311–319.
13. Forno LS. The Lewy body in Parkinson's disease. Adv Neurol 1987; 45:35–43.

14. Jellinger KA, Mizuno J. Parkinson's disease. In: Dickson DW, ed. Neurodegeneration: The Molecular Pathology of Dementia and Movement Disorders. Basel: ISN Neuropath Press, 2003:159–187.
15. Duda JE, Giasson BI, Mabon ME, et al. Novel antibodies to synuclein show abundant striatal pathology in Lewy body diseases. Ann Neurol 2002; 52:205–210.
16. Wakabayashi K, Takahashi H, Takeda S, et al. Lewy bodies in the enteric nervous system in Parkinson's disease. Arch Histol Cytol 1989; 52:191–194.
17. Pearce RK, Hawkes CH, Daniel SE. The anterior olfactory nucleus in Parkinson's disease. Mov Disord 1995; 10:283–287.
18. Braak H, Del Tredici K, Rub U, et al. Staging of brain pathology related to sporadic Parkinson's disease. Neurobiol Aging 2003; 24:197–211.
19. McKeith I, Mintzer J, Aarsland D, et al. Dementia with Lewy bodies. Lancet Neurol 2004; 3:19–28.
20. Kosaka K, Yoshimura M, Ikeda K, et al. Diffuse type of Lewy body disease: progressive dementia with abundant cortical Lewy bodies and senile changes of varying degree—a new disease? Clin Neuropathol 1984; 3:185–192.
21. McKeith IG, Galasko D, Kosaka K, et al. Clinical and pathological diagnosis of dementia with Lewy bodies (DLB): report of the consortium on dementia with Lewy bodies international workshop. Neurology 1996; 47:1113–1124.
22. Apaydin H, Ahlskog JE, Parisi JE, et al. Parkinson's disease neuropathology: later-developing dementia and loss of the levodopa response. Arch Neurol 2002; 59:102–112.
23. Hurtig HI, Trojanowski JQ, Galvin J, et al. Alpha-synuclein cortical Lewy bodies correlate with dementia in Parkinson's disease. Neurology 2000; 54:1916–1921.
24. Parkkinen L, Soininen H, Alafuzoff I. Regional distribution of alpha-synuclein pathology in unimpaired aging and Alzheimer's disease. J Neuropathol Exp Neurol 2003; 62:363–367.
25. Jellinger KA. Alpha-synuclein pathology in Parkinson's and Alzheimer's disease brain: incidence and topographic distribution—a pilot study. Acta Neuropathol (Berl) 2003; 106:191–201.
26. Klos KJ, Ahlskog JE, Josephs KA, et al. Alpha-synuclein pathology in the spinal cord of neurologically asymptomatic aged individuals. Neurology 2006; 66:1100–1111.
27. Hamilton RL. Lewy bodies in Alzheimer's disease: a neuropathological review of 145 cases using alpha-synuclein immunohistochemistry. Brain Pathol 2000; 10:378–384.
28. Lippa CF, Schmidt ML, Lee VM, et al. Alpha-synuclein in familial Alzheimer's disease: epitope mapping parallels dementia with Lewy bodies and Parkinson disease. Arch Neurol 2001; 58:1817–1820.
29. Dickson DW, Corral A, Lin W, et al. Alzheimer's disease with amygdaloid Lewy bodies: a form of Lewy body disease distinct from AD and diffuse Lewy body disease. Neurology 2000; 54(suppl 3):451.
30. DeLucia MW, Cookson N, Dickson DW. Synuclein-immunoreactive Lewy bodies are detected in the amygdala in less than 20% of Alzheimer (AD) cases. J Neuropathol Exp Neurol 2002; 61:454.
31. Tsuboi Y, Dickson DW. Dementia with Lewy bodies and Parkinson's disease with dementia: are they different? Parkinsonism Relat Disord 2005; 11(suppl 1):S47–S51.
32. Abbott RD, Petrovitch H, White LR, et al. Frequency of bowel movements and the future risk of Parkinson's disease. Neurology 2001; 57:456–462.
33. Shiba M, Bower JH, Maraganore DM, et al. Anxiety disorders and depressive disorders preceding Parkinson's disease: a case-control study. Mov Disord 2000, 15:669–677.
34. Ressler KJ, Nemeroff CB. Role of norepinephrine in the pathophysiology and treatment of mood disorders. Biol Psychiatry 1999; 46:1219–1233.
35. Schenck CH, Bundlie SR, Mahowald MW. Delayed emergence of a parkinsonian disorder in 38% of 29 older men initially diagnosed with idiopathic rapid eye movement sleep behaviour disorder. Neurology 1996; 46:388–393.
36. Kayama Y, Koyama Y. Control of sleep and wakefulness by brainstem monoaminergic and cholinergic neurons. Acta Neurochir Suppl 2003; 87:3–6.
37. Hawkes CH, Shephard BC, Daniel SE. Olfactory dysfunction in Parkinson's disease. J Neurol Neurosurg Psychiatry 1997; 62:436–446.

38. Berendse HW, Booij J, Francot CM, et al. Subclinical dopaminergic dysfunction in symptomatic Parkinson's disease patients' relatives with a decreased sense of smell. Ann Neurol 2001; 50:34–41.
39. Aarsland D, Ballard C, Larsen JP, et al. A comparative study of psychiatric symptoms in dementia with Lewy bodies and Parkinson's disease with and without dementia. Int J Geriatr Psychiatry 2001; 16:528–536.
40. Wenning GK, Tison F, Ben Shlomo Y, et al. Multiple system atrophy: a review of 203 pathologically proven cases. Mov Disord 1997; 12:133–147.
41. Lantos PL. The definition of multiple system atrophy: a review of recent developments. J Neuropathol Exp Neurol 1998; 57:1099–1111.
42. Arima K, Murayama S, Mukoyama M, et al. Immunocytochemical and ultrastructural studies of neuronal and oligodendroglial cytoplasmic inclusions in multiple system atrophy. 1 Neuronal cytoplasmic inclusions. Acta Neuropathol (Berl) 1992; 83:453–460.
43. Dickson DW, Lin W, Liu WK, et al. Multiple system atrophy: a sporadic synucleinopathy. Brain Pathol 1999; 9:721–732.
44. Kato S, Nakamura H. Cytoplasmic argyrophilic inclusions in neurons of pontine nuclei in patients with olivopontocerebellar atrophy: immunohistochemical and ultrastructural studies. Acta Neuropathol (Berl) 1990; 79:584–594.
45. Arima K, Ueda K, Sunohara N, et al. NACP/-synuclein immunoreactivity in fibrillary components of neuronal and oligodendroglial cytoplasmic inclusions in the pontine nuclei in multiple system atrophy. Acta Neuropathol (Berl) 1998; 96:439–444.
46. Lin W, DeLucia MW, Dickson DW. Alpha-synuclein immunoreactivity in neuronal nuclear inclusions and neurites in multiple system atrophy. Neurosci Lett 2004; 354:99–102.
47. Wakabayashi K, Takahashi H. Gallyas-positive, tau-negative glial inclusions in Parkinson's disease midbrain. Neurosci Lett 1996; 217:133–136.
48. Gwinn-Hardy K, Mehta ND, Farrer M, et al. Distinctive neuropathology revealed by α-synuclein antibodies in hereditary parkinsonism and dementia linked to chromosome 4p. Acta Neuropathol (Berl) 2000; 99:663–672.
49. Dickson DW, Liu WK, Hardy J, et al. Widespread alterations of alpha-synuclein in multiple system atrophy. Am J Pathol 1999; 155:1241–1251.
50. Li W, West N, Colla E, et al. Aggregation promoting C-terminal truncation of alpha-synuclein is a normal cellular process and is enhanced by the familial Parkinson's disease-linked mutations. Proc Natl Acad Sci USA 2005; 102:2162–2167.
51. Rajput AH, Offor KP, Beard CM, et al. Epidemiology of parkinsonism: incidence, classification, and mortality. Ann Neurol 1984; 16:278–282.
52. Tolosa E, Valldeoriola F, Pastor P. Progressive supranuclear palsy. In: Jankovic JJ, Tolosa E, Eds. Parkinson's Disease & Movement Disorders, 4th edn. Philadelphia: Lippincott Williams & Wilkins, 2002:152–169.
53. Steele JC, Richardson JC, Olszewski J. Progressive supranuclear palsy: a heterogenous degeneration involving the brainstem, basal ganglia and cerebellum with vertical gaze and pseudobulbar palsy, nuchal dystonia, and dementia. Arch Neurol 1964; 10:333–339.
54. Rajput AH, Rozdilsky B, Rajput A. Accuracy of clinical diagnosis in parkinsonism—a prospective study. Can J Neurol Sci 1991; 18:275–278.
55. Williams DR, de Silva R, Paviour DC, et al. Characteristics of two distinct clinical phenotypes in pathologically proven progressive supranuclear palsy: Richardson's syndrome and PSP-parkinsonism. Brain 2005; 128:1247–1258.
56. Dickson DW. Sporadic tauopathies: Pick's disease, corticobasal degeneration, progressive supranuclear palsy and argyrophilic grain disease. In: Esiri MM, Lee VMY, Trojanowski JQ, eds. *The Neuropathology of Dementia*, 2nd ed. New York: Cambridge University Press, 2004:227–256.
57. Yamada T, Calne DB, Akiyama H, et al. Further observations on tau-positive glia in the brains with progressive supranuclear palsy. Acta Neuropathol (Berl) 1993; 85:308–315.
58. Komori T, Arai N, Oda M, et al. Astrocytic plaques and tufts of abnormal fibers do not coexist in corticobasal degeneration and progressive supranuclear palsy. Acta Neuropathol (Berl) 1998; 96:401–408.
59. Polymeropoulos MH, Lavedan C, Leroy E, et al. Mutation in the alpha-synuclein gene identified in families with Parkinson's disease. Science 1997; 276:2045–2047.

60. Spillantini MG, Schmidt ML, Lee VM, et al. Alpha-synuclein in Lewy bodies. Nature 1997; 388:839–840.

61. McInerney-Leo A, Hadley DW, Gwinn-Hardy K, et al. Genetic testing in Parkinson's disease. Mov Disord 2005; 20:1–10.

62. Singleton AB, Farrer M, Johnson J, et al. Alpha-synuclein locus triplication causes Parkinson's disease. Science 2003; 302:841.

63. Kitada T, Asakawa S, Hattori N, et al. Mutations in the parkin gene cause autosomal recessive juvenile parkinsonism. Nature 1998; 392:605–608.

64. Bonifati V, Rizzu P, van Baren MJ, et al. Mutations in the DJ-1 gene associated with autosomal recessive early-onset parkinsonism. Science 2003, 299:256–259.

65. Zimprich A, Biskup S, Leitner P, et al. Mutations in LRRK2 cause autosomal-dominant parkinsonism with pleomorphic pathology. Neuron 2004; 44:601–607.

66. Paisan-Ruiz C, Jain S, Evans EW, et al. Cloning of the gene containing mutations that cause PARK8-linked Parkinson's disease. Neuron 2004; 44:595–600.

67. Hutton M, Lendon CL, Rizzu P, et al. Association of missense and 5'-splice-site mutations in tau with the inherited dementia (FTDP-17). Nature 1998; 393:702–705.

68. Wszolek ZK, Tsuboi Y, Farrer M, et al. Hereditary tauopathies and parkinsonism. Adv Neurol 2003; 91:153–163.

69. Foster NL, Wilhelmsen K, Sima AAF, et al. Frontotemporal dementia and parkinsonism linked to chromosome 17: a consensus conference. Ann Neurol 1997; 41:706–715.

70. Gwinn-Hardy K, Singleton A, O'Suilleabhain P, et al. Spinocerebellar ataxia type 3 phenotypically resembling Parkinson's disease in a black family. Arch Neurol 2001; 58:296–299.

71. Gwinn-Hardy K, Chen JY, Liu HC, et al. Spinocerebellar ataxia type 2 with parkinsonism in ethnic Chinese. Neurology 2000; 55:800–805.

72. Kruger R, Kuhn W, Muller T, et al. Ala30Pro mutation in the gene encoding alpha-synuclein in Parkinson's disease. Nat Genet 1998; 18:106–108.

73. Zarranz JJ, Alegre J, Gomez-Esteban JC, et al. The new mutation, E46K, of alpha-synuclein causes Parkinson and Lewy body dementia. Ann Neurol 2004; 55:164–173.

74. Farrer M, Kachergus J, Forno L, et al. Comparison of kindreds with parkinsonism and alpha-synuclein genomic multiplications. Ann Neurol 2004; 55:174–179.

75. Duda JE, Giasson BI, Mabon ME, et al. Concurrence of alpha-synuclein and tau brain pathology in the Contursi kindred. Acta Neuropathol (Berl) 2002; 104:7–11

76. Hayashi S, Wakabayashi K, Ishikawa A, et al. An autopsy case of autosomal-recessive juvenile parkinsonism with a homozygous exon 4 deletion in the parkin gene. Mov Disord 2000; 15:884–888.

77. Farrer M, Chan P, Chen R, et al. Lewy bodies and parkinsonism in families with *Parkin* mutations. Ann Neurol 2001; 50:293–300.

78. Pramstaller PP, Schlossmacher MG, Jacques TS, et al. Lewy body Parkinson's disease in a large pedigree with 77 *Parkin* mutation carriers. Ann Neurol 2005; 58:411–422.

79. Tsuboi Y, Espinoza M, Davies P, et al. Epitope mapping of tau lesions in the frontal cortex of autosomal recessive juvenile Parkinsonism with parkin mutations. Mov Disord 2002; 17:S1106.

80. Wszolek ZK, Gwinn-Hardy K, Wszolek EK, et al. Neuropathology of two members of a German-American kindred (Family C) with late onset parkinsonism. Acta Neuropathol (Berl) 2002; 103:344–350.

81. Leroy E, Boyer R, Auburger G, et al. The ubiquitin pathway in Parkinson's disease. Nature 1998; 395:451–452.

82. Facheris M, Strain KJ, Lesnick TG, et al. UCHL1 is associated with Parkinson's disease: a case-unaffected sibling and case-unrelated control study. Neurosci Lett 2005; 381:131–134.

83. Valente EM, Abou-Sleiman PM, Caputo V, et al. Hereditary early-onset Parkinson's disease caused by mutations in PINK1. Science 2004; 304:1158–1160.

84. Albanese A, Valente EM, Romito LM, et al. The PINK1 phenotype can be indistinguishable from idiopathic Parkinson disease. Neurology 2005; 64:1958–1960.

85. Abou-Sleiman PM, Healy DG, Quinn N, et al. The role of pathogenic DJ-1 mutations in Parkinson's disease. Ann Neurol 2003; 54:283–286.

86. Aasly JO, Toft M, Fernandez-Mata I, et al. Clinical features of LRRK2-associated Parkinson's disease in central Norway. Ann Neurol 2005; 57:762–765.
87. Nichols WC, Pankratz N, Hernandez D, et al. Genetic screening for a single common LRRK2 mutation in familial Parkinson's disease. Lancet 2005; 365:410–412.
88. Di Fonzo A, Rohe CF, Ferreira J, et al. A frequent LRRK2 gene mutation associated with autosomal dominant Parkinson's disease. Lancet 2005; 365:412–415.
89. Gilks WP, Abou-Sleiman PM, Gandhi S, et al. A common LRRK2 mutation in idiopathic Parkinson's disease. Lancet 2005; 365:415–416.
90. Ross OA, Toft Ml, Whittle AJ, et al. Lrrk2 and Lewy body disease. Ann Neurol 2006; 59:388–393.
91. Wszolek ZK, Pfeiffer RF, Tsuboi Y, et al. Autosomal dominant parkinsonism associated with variable synuclein and tau pathology. Neurology 2004; 62:1619–1622.
92. Aharon-Peretz J, Rosenbaum H, Gershoni-Baruch R. Mutations in the glucocerebrosidase gene and Parkinson's disease in Ashkenazi Jews. N Engl J Med 2004; 351: 1972–1977.
93. Lwin A, Orvisky E, Goker-Alpan O, et al. Glucocerebrosidase mutations in subjects with parkinsonism. Mol Genet Metab 2004; 81:70–73.

2

Genetics of Parkinson's Disease

Andrew B. Singleton
Laboratory of Neurogenetics, National Institute of Aging, National Institutes of Health, Bethesda, Maryland, U.S.A.

Jordi Clarimón
Alzheimer's Laboratory, Sant Pau Hospital, Barcelona, Spain

HEREDITY AND GENETICS IN PARKINSON'S DISEASE

Eighty years after James Parkinson wrote his "Essay On the Shaking Palsy," Gowers (1) suggested that genetics may play a substantial role in Parkinson's disease (PD), a view shared by Charcot's student Leroux, who stated, "A true cause of *paralysis agitans*, and perhaps the only true one, is heredity." The past two decades have witnessed the field attempting to characterize the nature of this genetic influence and to identify genes that underlie and contribute to disease. While a role for genetics in PD has been established, the weight and mode of this contribution is still largely unknown. Here, we discuss the genetic advances in parkinsonism and the potential for further research in this area.

Up to 20 years ago, much of the field's general appreciation of the role genetics played in PD was based on the lack of familiality noted in most patient histories. The first attempts to test this largely anecdotal observation were made using structured epidemiologic studies. Two main approaches have been utilized in this effort—case-control and twin studies. A case-control methodology involves the analysis of disease occurrence among relatives of index patients compared to incidence of disease in relatives of neurologically normal subjects. Case-control studies have consistently indicated a genetic component to PD, with 10% to 15% of patients reporting a first-degree relative suffering from the same movement disorder (2). Recurrence risks for first degree relatives of PD patients range from 2.3% to 14.6% (3–8), and this empiric risk appears to be higher in relatives of young-onset PD patients, compared to those of typical late-onset PD subjects, suggesting a more readily apparent role of genetics in young-onset cases (9,10). A similar, although more complex, approach has been utilized by researchers at DeCode in Iceland; using the extensive genealogic and medical records of the inhabitants of this island, the researchers have shown that PD patients are more closely related to one another than non-PD patients are. This study has lent considerable weight to the argument that genetics plays a role in PD, and, as discussed later, this research group is currently attempting to localize genes for PD within the Icelandic population.

Twin studies are employed to test the concordance rate of a trait in monozygotic (MZ) and dizygotic (DZ) twins. Because MZ twins share 100% of their genome and DZ twins only 50%, an excess of disease concordance among MZ twins compared to DZ twins suggests a genetic contribution. In contrast to the data described earlier, several twin studies have shown similar rates of concordance in MZ and DZ twin pairs, suggesting that genetic predisposition plays, at best, a minor role in disease (11–16). Many of the twin studies have been criticized because they were performed using a cross-sectional survey, where individuals are observed at only

TABLE 1   *PARK* Loci

Designation	Location	Age at onset	MOI	Official Gene Symbol	Year of linkage (gene)	
PARK1	4q21	~45	AD	*SNCA*	1996	(1997)
PARK2	6q25.2–q27	7–60	AR	*PARK2*	1997	(1998)
PARK3	2p13	59	AD	–	1998	–
PARK4	4q21	30–60	AD	*SNCA*	1999	(2003)
PARK5	4p14	30–60	AD	*UCHL-1*	–	(1998)
PARK6	1p36	36–60	AR	*PINK1*	2001	(2004)
PARK7	1p36	27–40	AR	*PARK7*	2001	(2003)
PARK8	12q12	38–79	AD	*LRRK2*	2002	(2004)
PARK9	1p36	Teens	AR	–	2001	–
PARK10	1p	Late	AD	–	2002	–
PARK11	2q36–q37	58±12	AD	–	2002	–

one point in time. Therefore, this study design does not exclude the possibility that, in twins discordant for disease, the unaffected twin may develop PD at a later date. There is recent evidence, based on positron emission tomography (PET) studies, indicating that there may be decreased dopamiregic nigral function even in the absence of manifest parkinsonian symptoms and signs in the asymptomatic cotwins (17,18). This is consistent with data showing a characteristic reduction of striatal tracer uptake in clinically unaffected members of PD kindreds (19). Notably, Piccini and coworkers (1997) (19) reported a three times higher concordance rate of decreased ^{18}F-fluorodopa uptake for MZ twins compared to DZ pairs (58% vs. 18%, respectively). These data suggest that the initial twin concordance studies may have underestimated the role of genetics in PD. However, these data also indicate that genetics is not the sole determinant of disease. It is likely that the majority of typical PD cases are a result of a complex interplay between genetic variability, environmental exposures, and chance events (at the molecular level). Later, we will briefly discuss some of the research aimed at teasing out risk genes for typical, apparently nonfamilial PD; however, at this point in time, most of our current understanding of the role genetics plays in PD etiology and pathogenesis has arisen directly and indirectly from the study of rare, familial forms of parkinsonism (Table 1). The following sections of this chapter will deal with this research.

GENES CAUSING PARKINSONISM
SNCA (α-synuclein; Locus ID *PARK1*; Chr4q21–23)
Golbe and his colleagues first reported a large family with an autosomal dominant form of parkinsonism in 1990 (20). Beginning with patients living in New Jersey, United States. the ancestry of this family was traced to a single couple in the village of Contursi, in the Campania region near Salerno in the south of Italy. Members of this family had immigrated to the United States around the turn of the 20th century and more than 60 family members over five generations had been diagnosed with disease. The disease described in this family ranged from a relatively typical PD to a disorder more reminiscent of diffuse Lewy body disease. The mean age at onset is early (mean: 45.6, SD: 13–48) and patients often develop dementia (21).

In 1996, Polymeropoulos and collaborators (22) identified linkage of disease in this family to an interval within the long arm of chromosome 4 (position 4q21–q23). The following year, a mutation within the first candidate gene assessed, α-synuclein, named for its apparent localization to the synapse and nucleus, was identified. This mutation, a G-to-A transition at nucleotide 209, resulted in an alanine to threonine (A53T) substitution in this protein (23). The same mutation segregated with a similar disease in an additional three Greek kindreds examined by the authors. Subsequently, two other missense mutations within *SNCA* have been identified, an A30P mutation, described in a German family (24) and an E46K mutation described in a family from Spain (25). Missense mutation of *SNCA* appears to be an extremely rare cause of familial PD (26–29). While mutations in the α-synuclein gene are rare, they have been informative. The disconnect between rare, most often extremely aggressive, atypical familial forms of PD and typical, sporadic PD, was often argued to be a fatal flaw in the idea that identifying a gene in the former disease would lead to understanding the latter. The discovery of the A53T *SNCA* mutation was followed almost immediately by data showing that α-synuclein is a significant component of the hallmark lesion of PD, the Lewy body. These two findings tied the familial and sporadic diseases together elegantly and suggested that understanding the genetics of PD is a tractable problem.

In 2003, our group identified a genomic triplication of the *SNCA* locus, including the entire α-synculein gene and 1.5 megabases of flanking genomic sequence, segregating with disease in a large family called the Iowan kindred (30). Similar to the kindreds described with A53T mutation, the phenotype in these families ranged clinically and pathologically from PD to dementia with Lewy bodies. Subsequently, additional families were identified with disease caused by *SNCA* triplication and duplication (31,32). In these families, the α-synuclein gene is normal in sequence but abnormal in dose. Disease caused by genomic duplication of the *SNCA* locus more closely resembles sporadic PD than that caused by triplication, with a lack of prominent dementia and more typical signs and symptoms. The phenotypic differences between duplication and triplication patients may be largely attributed to dose. Clinically and pathologically, the associated disease is more severe in patients with triplication of *SNCA* compared to those with duplication. These data immediately implied that overexpression of wild type α-synuclein is sufficient to cause disease and that this occurs in a dose-dependent manner. Less explicitly, they also suggest that α-synuclein dose may be a common theme to all PD; that is, smaller increases in the level of α-synuclein, either due to increased expression or decreased clearance, may contribute to typical PD. The genetic evidence supporting this idea is intriguing and will be discussed later in this chapter.

PARKIN (*PARKIN*; Locus ID *PARK2*; CHR6Q5.5–Q27)

In 1998, the second locus for parkinsonism (*PARK2*) was mapped to the long arm of chromosome 6 (6q5.2–q27) (33). In April of the same year, a deletion of exon 4 in the *PARKIN* gene was found to cause an autosomal recessive juvenile parkinsonism (ARJP) occurring in a consanguineous Japanese family (34). *PARKIN* is encoded by 12 exons spanning more than 500 kb, encoding a protein 465 amino acids in size. *PARKIN* is a ubiquitin E3 ligase, although this may not be *PARKIN'S* only function, the role of this protein in this system, which facilitates the removal of waste proteins, is intriguing in a disease of protein deposition and degeneration. In the past six years, a wide variety of disease-causing *PARKIN* mutations have been identified in nearly all populations studied, regardless of ethnic origin (35–42). These mutations include exon rearrangements, single base pair substitutions, and small deletions or insertions of one or several base pairs. Two European screenings in early-onset PD patients with a positive family history described a frequency of

PARKIN mutation ranging from 32% to 42% (43,44). An overall mutation rate of 9.0% was identified in a German series of young-onset patients, collected irrespective of family history (45). Mutations that obviously destroy or dramatically alter *PARKIN* appear to be unequivocally linked to disease when present as homozygous or compound heterozygous alterations; however, recently much attention has been focused on the role of single heterozygous mutations in disease. The current data suggest that possession of a single *PARKIN* mutation is not sufficient to cause disease but that this type of mutation contributes to lifetime disease risk. The genetic evidence for this is supported by fDOPA positron emission tomography (PET) scanning of heterozygous carriers of *PARKIN* mutations, which shows a marked deficit in these subjects. The relative frequency of *PARKIN* disease and the availability of genetic testing for this gene mean that pathogenicity of *PARKIN* mutation is an key issue to resolve.

UCHL-1 (Locus ID *PARK5*; Chr4p14)

Ubiquitin carboxy-terminal hydrolase L-1 (*UCHL-1*, PARK5) was the next gene suggested to contain mutations that cause PD (46). After sequencing the *UCHL-1* gene in probands from 72 families with PD, a heterozygous missense mutation was identified that changed the normal and evolutionary conserved isoleucine at position 93 to a methionine (I93M). This mutation was identified in two brothers with PD from Germany and absent from 250 control individuals with different ethnic backgrounds. It has been suggested that this mutation will reduce the catalytic activity of this enzyme, and, given the role of *PARKIN* in the ubiquitin proteasome system, *UCHL-1* is a strong candidate for a PD gene. However, the primary genetic evidence for mutation of this gene as a cause of PD is extremely weak, and, to date, no other kindreds have been described with disease caused by this or other mutations within *UCHL-1*. In the absence of further genetic evidence, this gene should not be considered a cause of familial PD (47,48).

DJ-1 (Locus ID *PARK7*; Chr1p36)

In 2001, van Duijn and his colleagues identified a novel locus for early onset recessive parkinsonism located on the short arm of chromosome 1, and this locus was given the designation PARK7 (49). This finding was replicated in an independent set of families a year later. In 2003, Bonifati and collaborators identified mutations in a gene called *DJ-1* that cosegregated with early-onset PD in two of the consanguineous families from these studies, from the Netherlands and Italy (50). Patients from the Dutch kindred possessed a 14 kb homozygous deletion that removed the first 4 kb of *DJ-1*. The deletion was absent in 400 chromosomes from individuals living in regions closely surrounding the genetic isolate, suggesting that this mutation was most probably confined to this specific region of the Netherlands. Disease in the Italian kindred segregated with a homozygous point mutation, resulting in the substitution of the highly conserved leucine at position 166 with a proline (L166P). Structural analysis of the mutated protein using a modeling approach revealed that this mutation could easily destabilize the terminal helix of the *DJ-1* protein, and subsequent in vitro work shows that this mutation results in a rapid degradation and turnover of *DJ-1* (51). Mutation screenings of *DJ-1* have revealed additional mutations. Screening of 185 unrelated early-onset PD patients, revealed a homozygous A-to-G change in exon 2 of the *DJ-1* gene, which resulted in a substitution of the highly conserved methionine at position 26 to isoleucine (M26I) (52). Other heterozygous mutations and homozygous substitutions have also been found (52–55) but mutation of this gene appears to be a rare cause of familial parkinsonism (56,57). To date, the majority of unequivocally causal mutations appear to be acting in a true recessive manner, that is, resulting in a lack of functional protein, either by major structural alteration of the protein or through increasing degradation of *DJ-1*.

PINK1 (Locus ID *PARK6*; Chr1p36)

In 2001 a novel locus for autosomal recessive early-onset parkinsonism, *PARK6*, was mapped to chromosome 1p36 through linkage analysis in a large Italian family from Sicilia (the Marsala kindred), which presented a high frequency of consanguineous marriages (58). Subsequent analysis of 28 European families with ARJP negative for *PARKIN* mutation, provided additional evidence of linkage to *PARK6* and lead to the refinement of the critical interval (59). Sequence analysis of candidate genes resulted in the identification of two homozygous mutations in the PTEN-induced putative kinase 1 (*PINK1*) gene (60). One of the mutations was a G-to-A transition in exon 7, and resulted in the change of the triptophan at position 437 to a STOP codon (W437X), thus truncating the last 145 amino acids of the protein. This homozygous mutation was present in the Marsala kindred as well as another family from Italy. A glycine to aspartic acid mutation in codon 309 (G309D) was found in one Spanish family. Although mutations in *PINK1* were described only recently, numerous screening reports have identified mutations within this gene as a cause of autosomal recessive parkinsonism (61,62). Like *PARKIN*, *PINK1* mutations are not restricted to the European population, and it appears that mutation of this locus is a relatively frequent cause of early-onset autosomal recessive parkinsonism. Although *PINK1* has only recently been identified as a gene for parkinsonism, it appears that the disease-causing mutation in this gene is considerably more frequent than mutations in *DJ-1*, but less than in *PARKIN*. Screening for *PINK1* mutation in a cohort of Italian early-onset PD patients revealed two sporadic patients with homozygous and compound heterozygous mutations (A168P and C92F/R464H, respectively) in *PINK1*, and five other sporadic cases with heterozygous point mutations (60). These results suggest that heterozygous *PINK1* mutations may represent a risk factor for PD development, much in the same way that single *PARKIN* mutation is suggested to. Again, similar to parallel data in *PARKIN* mutation carriers, PET studies demonstrate a reduction of striatal ^{18}F-dopa uptake directly proportional to the number of mutated alleles in *PINK1* (63). While this finding adds weight to the idea that possession of a single *PINK1* mutation may contribute to disease, the paucity of data relating to population frequency of *PINK1* mutation means that there is some way to go before the field should reach this conclusion.

LRRK2 (Dardarin; Locus ID *PARK8*; Chr12)

In 2002, a whole genome-linkage scan in a family from Sagamihara City (Japan) with autosomal dominant PD mapped the *PARK8* locus to chromosome 12 (12p11.2–q13.1) (64). Unlike disease caused by mutation of *SNCA*, *PARKIN*, *DJ-1*, and *PINK1*, disease in the Sagamihara kindred presented with an onset and course closely resembling typical PD (mean age of onset: 51 ± 6 years). Subsequent to the identification of this linkage, several groups identified additional families with disease segregating to this locus (65,66).

Late in 2004, our group and an additional team identified the gene, Leucine-rich repeat kinase 2 (*LRRK2*) that contained mutations underlying *PARK8* disease. Both reports followed a standard positional cloning approach; the work performed by Zimprich et al. described five, possibly six, mutations segregating with disease, and our data showed two mutations segregating with disease in four Basque families and one British family with PD.

LRRK2 is a large, 51-exon gene spanning 140 kb on the long arm pericentromeric of chromosome 12. We named the protein, which is 2527 amino acids in size, dardarin, derived from the Basque word for tremor, a predominant symptom of PD. The protein is of unknown function but contains a leucine-rich repeat, a RAS domain, a WD40 domain, and a kinase domain.

Subsequent to the identification of *LRRK2* mutation as a cause of familial PD, it has become apparent that this gene also plays a role in apparently sporadic disease. Screening of a series of PD patients from the Basque region revealed that the mutation, originally identified by us in the four Basque families, also caused disease in 8% of typical nonfamilial disease. While this mutation has not been reported to occur at an appreciable frequency in other populations, an additional mutation, G2019S has been identified that occurs in many populations (67–69). The G2019S mutation alters an amino acid that is part of the consensus sequence for the activation loop of a kinase. This mutation has been identified in North American and European series ranging in prevalence from 1% to 8%, as such this is the most common mutation causing PD to date.

Although dardarin mutation has been linked to clinically and neuropathologically typical PD, mutations in this gene may also lead to other disparate clinical and pathologic phenotypes. While clinical presentation was relatively normal in the Sagamihara kindred, pathologically, the patients showed pure nigral degeneration in the absence of Lewy bodies. Furthermore, two families found to contain mutations by Zimprich et al showed striking heterogeneity, presenting with disease that ranged clinically through PD, dementia, and amyotrophy, and, neuropathologically, that showed varying degrees of ubiquitin, tau and α-synuclein deposition and neuronal degeneration. These preliminary data suggest that *LRRK2* mutation may have a remarkably wide range of pathology and may shed light on the complex genotype-phenotype relationship in neurodegenerative disorders.

EXTANT LOCI IN PARKINSON'S DISEASE

There are currently four different *PARK* loci where a chromosomal region has been identified, but at the time of writing, the underlying genetic lesions remain unknown.

PARK3

In 1998, Gasser and collaborators mapped the third PD locus (*PARK3*) to the long arm of chromosome 2 (2p13) by linkage analysis performed in a group of families of European origin (70). Due to the incomplete penetrance (estimated to be below 40%) and late age of onset, a possible role of this locus in both familial and sporadic forms of PD was proposed. A traditional, positional, cloning approach has as yet failed to identify the gene-bearing mutations at this locus (71). An additional project which undertook genotyping of 23 single nucleotide polymorphisms (SNP) spanning a 2.2 Mb region of the *PARK3* locus in 527 patients with familial PD, revealed a significant association between a polymorphism located in the promoter region of the sepiapterin reductase (*SPR*) gene and the age of PD onset (72). A haplotype involving three SNPs, spanning a region of 16 kb, and including the same *SPR* polymorphism, significantly increased the age-related association, thus indicating that *PARK3* could influence onset age for PD (73). Evidence of *PARK3* influencing PD onset was also found by an independent analysis (74). While the absence of mutations in *SPR* segregating with disease in the original linked families suggest that this gene is unlikely to be the cause of disease, the identification of association lends some, albeit limited, support to this as a genuine locus for PD.

PARK9

PARK9-linked disease was originally reported as a very young onset (between 11 and 16 years of age) neurodegenerative disorder with an autosomal recessive pattern of inheritance in a consanguineous Jordanian family (75). Clinical features of this disease include parkinsonism without intention tremor in addition to spasticity, supranuclear upgaze paralysis, and the development of dementia. The syndrome, named Kufor-Rakeb (*PARK9*) was mapped to the short arm of chromosome 1 (1p36) by whole genome-linkage analysis in 2001 (76). To date no gene has been identified.

PARK10

Following on from the work suggesting that PD in Iceland had a substantial genetic component, researchers at DeCode performed a genomewide linkage study in which 117 PD patients from Iceland from 51 different families, were analyzed (77). A susceptibility locus for late-onset PD was localized to chromosome 1 (1p32) within a critical interval of 9 Mb. Proof of linkage awaits gene identification and convincing independent replication. However, this locus is intriguing in that it is linked to PD absolutely typical in nature.

PARK11

In 2002 Pankratz et al. (78) used a sib-pair approach to identify susceptibility loci for PD. The authors reported linkage of disease to chr2q. A year later, the authors (79) used a sample of 150 families which met the strictest clinical diagnostic definition of Parkinson disease to confirm this linkage, the authors further restricted this group to include only those with the strongest family history of disease. Linkage analyses at this locus supported the existence of a PD susceptibility gene, with the small set of pure PD families generating a lod score of 5.1. However, while these results are intriguing, proof positive of the existence of a gene for PD at this locus awaits independent confirmation.

GENETIC VARIANTS WHERE PARKINSONISM IS PART OF THE CLINICAL SPECTRUM

There are other genetic variants where parkinsonism is part of the clinical spectrum but where detailed clinical evaluation may preclude PD as a diagnosis. Although it would be distracting to describe all diseases where parkinsonism may be a feature, we have chosen four to discuss briefly.

Spinocerebellar Ataxias 2 and 3

Spinocerebellar ataxias (SCAs) represent a family of genetically heterogeneous, dominant, neurodegenerative disorders that are mainly characterized by progressive ataxia resulting from the degeneration of cerebellar and spinal systems. In SCA-1, -2, -3, -6, -7, and -17, causal mutations have been characterized as expanded CAG repeats, which are translated into poly glutamine tracts within the protein product. L-dopa-responsive parkinsonism with minimal cerebellar deficits has been described in several of the SCAs, particularly SCA2 and SCA3 (also known as Machado-Joseph disease) (80–85).

In 2000, a Taiwanese family was described with SCA2 expansion ranging from 33 to 43 repeats (normal 17 to 31 repeats) segregating with disease (80). Two of the four affected family members fit clinical criteria for typical PD, one of the patients matched the criteria of probable progressive supranuclear palsy, and the fourth presented with ataxia. In an additional study, screening of 19 Taiwanesse families with a family history of PD revealed two individuals with 36 and 37 repeats in SCA2 (86) both presenting with levodopa-responsive parkinsonism. PET scanning in these patients revealed decreased ^{18}F-dopa distribution in the bilateral striatum, indicating that the nigorstriatal dopaminergic system was involved. Parkinsonism is a presentation of SCA2 expansion not only in Asian patients but also in other populations. Screening of 136 unrelated patients with familial parkinsonism (most of them Caucasian) revealed two patients with expanded SCA2 repeats (33 and 35 repeats) with good response to L-dopa (83), and an Indian family with homozygous carriers of SCA2-expansion mutations presented early-onset dopa-responsive parkinsonism (87). It is as yet unclear what drives the clinical heterogeneity of SCA2 patients; however, it is of note that most parkinsonian SCA2 patients have relatively small pathogenic expansions at the SCA2 locus and, probably in the presence or absence of other genetic variabilities or environmental exposures, this may present with a markedly different phenotype, without cerebellar signs or symptoms, compared to larger pathogenic expansions that drive a clinically more typical SCA disease.

In 2002, SCA3 expansion from 67 to 75 repeats (normal 13 to 36 repeats) was reported in a family of Sub-Saharan African descent living in Antigua, the United States, and England. These individuals presented with clinical characteristics resembling PD, including good response to levodopa, bradykinesia, resting tremor, and no cerebellar signs (82). An analysis of eight different African American families with SCA3 disease revealed that the phenotype ranged from ataxia with parkinsonian signs to a syndrome clinically almost indistinguishable from idiopathic, levodopa responsivene PD (88). The fact that parkinsonian symptoms appear less common in European families with SCA3 expansions, where ataxia is the predominant feature and parkinsonian signs are on the edge of the phenotype spectrum, suggested that differences in genetic background may alter the clinical phenotype of Machado-Joseph disease. A common founder for SCA3 mutation among the families of African descent was ruled out, suggesting that other *trans*-acting genetic variation or shared environmental exposures may drive the disease preferentially toward parkinsonism rather than pure ataxia.

Lubag

X-linked recessive dystonia-parkinsonism (XDP) (also known as "Lubag") is a severe progressive disorder restricted to males predominantly from the Filipino Island of Panay. First described by Johnston and McKusick as a sex-linked recessively inherited spastic paraplegia and parkinsonism (89), and later renamed by Lee and collaborators in 1976 (90), it is characterized by a progressive dystonia often in conjunction with parkinsonism, which is predominantly a later element of the disease seen in approximately one-third of XDP patients. The range of onset ranges from 12 to 48 years (91). Because of overlapping features between dystonia and parkinsonism and the existence of patients with pure parkinsonism preceding, or even overshadowing, the dystonic symptoms (92,93), Lubag can be misdiagnosed as PD, PD-plus syndrome, or essential tremor. The genetic defect responsible for XDP has been localized to the long arm of chromosome X at Xq13.1, within a 350 kb interval (94). Sequencing of a substantial portion of this critical interval revealed a multiple-transcript system within the region and suggests a base change within exon 4 of this gene is causing disease (95). To date, this finding has not been replicated in any non-Filipino patients with a similar disorder, and although this variant segregates with disease, independent confirmation is required to prove pathogenicity.

Frontotemporal Dementia with Parkinsonism Linked To Chromosome 17

Frontotemporal dementia with parkinsonism linked to chromosome 17 (FTDP-17) is an autosomal dominant disease, characterized initially by behavioral and motor disturbances that, in the latter stage of the disease, are associated with cognitive impairment. This disorder was linked to chromosome 17q21 in several nonrelated families, and termed frontotemporal dementia with parkinsonism linked to chromosome 17 (96–98). In 1998, exonic and intronic mutations in the gene *MAPT* were reported to segregate with FTDP-17 (99,100). Subsequent to this discovery, in excess of 60 separate families carrying more than 25 different mutations in *MAPT* have been identified (101,102). The vast majority of *MAPT* mutations are missense, deletion, or silent mutations in the coding region (most of them within exon 10), or mutations located close to the splice-donor site of the intron that follows alternatively-spliced exon 10. Clinical presentation can differ not only between mutations, but also within a single mutation and even within individual families. This allelic and clinical heterogeneity suggests that the genotypic background of an individual might also affect the phenotype observed with a particular *MAPT* mutation.

Parkinsonism features seem to be more frequently present in families with mutations that alter tau splicing, whereas Pick's disease without motor dysfunctions has been diagnosed in individuals with different missense mutations in exon 9 and exon 13 (103–105). Beneficial response to levodopa therapy has also been observed in some families with FTDP-17; however, this response was shown to be temporary and occurred only in the initial stages of the disease (106–108).

IDENTIFYING COMMON RISK-FACTOR GENES FOR PARKINSON'S DISEASE

As described earlier, the hunt for genes causing parkinsonism in rare families has been particularly successful over the past eight years. Less successful, both in PD and in other complex genetic disorders, are attempts at understanding the role common variability in genes plays in the disease process. While it seems clear that genetic variability influences disease pathogenesis, course, and endpoint, it is also evident that these aspects of disease are also modulated by factors extrinsic to the genome.

The probable interplay between genetics and environment makes risk-gene identification difficult. In the past 15 years, more than 150 case-control candidate-gene association studies have been performed that aim to test genes for association with disease. These reports, which are often positive, are largely unsubstantiated or subsequently refuted. The problem of assessing a single gene from the compliment of ~30,000 and choosing the correct variant to genotype, mean that these approaches are largely explorative endeavors. Where this field has found some success is in the more focused assessment of genes involved in monogenic forms of disease as risk-factor loci. Most notably, common variation within the α-synuclein gene appears to be a risk factor for PD (109,110). A large amount of this research has focused on a polymorphic repeat within the promoter of SNCA, and risk variants of this polymorphism have been shown to increase α-synuclein expression in vitro (111–113). These data are consistent with the SNCA duplication and triplication mutations described earlier and suggest that increased α-synuclein levels are central to the etiology of PD. Likewise, similar analysis has been performed for the gene encoding tau, which contains mutations causing FTDP-17. While much of the published data suggest a role for MAPT polymorphism as a risk factor for neurodegenerative diseases, the data relating to PD are still relatively preliminary and should be interpreted with caution (114,115).

Case-control genetic-association analyses have received a hard press over the previous five years, many were performed with a poor study design that captured little genetic variability and tested hypotheses in underpowered sample series. Sample size remains an issue, but the development of more sophisticated methodologies, such as haplotype tagging and whole genome association, in combination with the availability of increasing numbers of sample series, including a publicly available cohort, suggests that this approach may be fruitful in the near future.

In summary, the previous decade has been an incredibly successful one for geneticists working on PD. Numerous genes and chromosomal loci have been identified, and it is hoped that these will provide a key into the pathogenesis and etiology of PD. Identifying risk factor loci for PD will likely present a considerable challenge, but technologic advances suggest that, provided the necessary resources are available, this is a tractable problem.

REFERENCES

1. Gowers W. Diseases of the nervous system. Vlakiston, Son, 1888.
2. Vieregge P. Genetic factors in the etiology of idiopathic Parkinson's disease. J Neural Transm Park Dis Dement Sect 1994; 8(1–2):1–37.
3. Marder K, Tang MX, Mejia H, et al. Risk of Parkinson's disease among first-degree relatives: A community-based study. Neurology 1996; 47(1):155–160.
4. Semchuk KM, Love EJ, Lee RG. Parkinson's disease: a test of the multifactorial etiologic hypothesis. Neurology 1993; 43(6):1173–1180.
5. Morano A, Jimenez-Jimenez FJ, Molina JA, et al. Risk-factors for Parkinson's disease: case-control study in the province of Caceres, Spain. Acta Neurol Scand 1994; 89(3):164–170.
6. Payami H, Larsen K, Bernard S, et al. Increased risk of Parkinson's disease in parents and siblings of patients. Ann Neurol 1994; 36(4):659–661.
7. Bonifati V, Fabrizio E, Vanacore N, et al. Familial Parkinson's disease: a clinical genetic analysis. Can J Neurol Sci 1995; 22(4):272–279.
8. De Michele G, Filla A, Volpe G, et al. Environmental and genetic risk factors in Parkinson's disease: a case-control study in southern Italy. Mov Disord 1996; 11(1):17–23.
9. Elbaz A, Grigoletto F, Baldereschi M, et al. Familial aggregation of Parkinson's disease: a population-based case-control study in Europe. EUROPARKINSON Study Group. Neurology 1999; 52(9):1876–1882.

10. Marder K, Levy G, Louis ED, et al. Familial aggregation of early- and late-onset Parkinson's disease. Ann Neurol 2003; 54(4):507–513.
11. Duvoisin RC, Eldridge R, Williams A, et al. Twin study of Parkinson disease. Neurology 1981; 31(1):77–80.
12. Ward CD, Duvoisin RC, Ince SE, et al. Parkinson's disease in 65 pairs of twins and in a set of quadruplets. Neurology 1983; 33(7):815–824.
13. Marsden CD. Parkinson's disease in twins. J Neurol Neurosurg Psychiatry 1987; 50(1):105–106.
14. Marttila RJ, Kaprio J, Koskenvuo M, et al. Parkinson's disease in a nationwide twin cohort. Neurology 1988; 38(8):1217–1219.
15. Vieregge P, Schiffke KA, Friedrich HJ, et al. Parkinson's disease in twins. Neurology 1992; 42(8):1453–1461.
16. Tanner CM, Ottman R, Goldman SM, et al. Parkinson disease in twins: an etiologic study. Jama 1999; 281(4):341–346.
17. Burn DJ, Mark MH, Playford ED, et al. Parkinson's disease in twins studied with 18F-dopa and positron emission tomography. Neurology 1992; 42(10):1894–1900.
18. Holthoff VA, Vieregge P, Kessler J, et al. Discordant twins with Parkinson's disease: positron emission tomography and early signs of impaired cognitive circuits. Ann Neurol 1994; 36(2):176–182.
19. Piccini P, Morrish PK, Turjanski N, et al. Dopaminergic function in familial Parkinson's disease: a clinical and 18F-dopa positron emission tomography study. Ann Neurol 1997; 41(2):222–229.
20. Golbe LI, Di Iorio G, Bonavita V, et al. A large kindred with autosomal dominant Parkinson's disease. Ann Neurol 1990; 27(3):276–282.
21. Spira PJ, Sharpe DM, Halliday G, et al. Clinical and pathological features of a Parkinsonian syndrome in a family with an Ala53Thr alpha-synuclein mutation. Ann Neurol 2001; 49(3):313–319.
22. Polymeropoulos MH, Higgins JJ, Golbe LI, et al. Mapping of a gene for Parkinson's disease to chromosome 4q21–q23. Science 1996; 274(5290):1197–1199.
23. Polymeropoulos MH, Lavedan C, Leroy E, et al. Mutation in the alpha-synuclein gene identified in families with Parkinson's disease. Science 1997; 276(5321):2045–2047.
24. Kruger R, Kuhn W, Muller T, et al. Ala30Pro mutation in the gene encoding alpha-synuclein in Parkinson's disease. Nat Genet 1998; 18(2):106–108.
25. Zarranz JJ, Alegre J, Gomez-Esteban JC, et al. The new mutation, E46K, of alpha-synuclein causes Parkinson and Lewy body dementia. Ann Neurol 2004; 55(2):164–173.
26. Vaughan J, Durr A, Tassin J, et al. The alpha-synuclein Ala53Thr mutation is not a common cause of familial Parkinson's disease: a study of 230 European cases. European Consortium on Genetic Susceptibility in Parkinson's Disease. Ann Neurol 1998; 44(2): 270–273.
27. Vaughan JR, Farrer MJ, Wszolek ZK, et al. Sequencing of the alpha-synuclein gene in a large series of cases of familial Parkinson's disease fails to reveal any further mutations. The European Consortium on Genetic Susceptibility in Parkinson's Disease (GSPD). Hum Mol Genet 1998; 7(4):751–753.
28. Farrer M, Wavrant-De Vrieze F, Crook R, et al. Low frequency of alpha-synuclein mutations in familial Parkinson's disease. Ann Neurol 1998; 43(3):394–397.
29. Chan DK, Mellick G, Cai H, et al. The alpha-synuclein gene and Parkinson disease in a Chinese population. Arch Neurol 2000; 57(4):501–503.
30. Singleton AB, Farrer M, Johnson J, et al. alpha-Synuclein locus triplication causes Parkinson's disease. Science 2003; 302(5646):841.
31. Farrer M, Kachergus J, Forno L, et al. Comparison of kindreds with parkinsonism and alpha-synuclein genomic multiplications. Ann Neurol 2004; 55(2):174–179.
32. Chartier-Harlin MC, Kachergus J, Roumier C, et al. Alpha-synuclein locus duplication as a cause of familial Parkinson's disease. Lancet 2004; 364(9440):1167–1169.
33. Matsumine H, Yamamura Y, Kobayashi T, et al. Early onset parkinsonism with diurnal fluctuation maps to a locus for juvenile parkinsonism. Neurology 1998; 50(5): 1340–1345.
34. Kitada T, Asakawa S, Hattori N, et al. Mutations in the parkin gene cause autosomal recessive juvenile parkinsonism. Nature 1998; 392(6676):605–608.

35. Dogu O, Johnson J, Hernandez D, et al. A consanguineous Turkish family with early-onset Parkinson's disease and an exon 4 parkin deletion. Mov Disord 2004; 19(7):812–816.

36. Illarioshkin SN, Periquet M, Rawal N, et al. Mutation analysis of the parkin gene in Russian families with autosomal recessive juvenile parkinsonism. Mov Disord 2003; 18(8):914–919.

37. Gouider-Khouja N, Larnaout A, Amouri R, et al. Autosomal recessive parkinsonism linked to parkin gene in a Tunisian family. Clinical, genetic and pathological study. Parkinsonism Relat Disord 2003; 9(5):247–251.

38. Khan NL, Graham E, Critchley P, et al. Parkin disease: a phenotypic study of a large case series. Brain 2003; 126(Pt 6):1279–1292.

39. Kim JS, Lee KS, Kim YI, et al. Homozygous exon 4 deletion in parkin gene in a Korean family with autosomal recessive early onset parkinsonism. Yonsei Med J 2003; 44(2): 336–339.

40. Rawal N, Periquet M, Lohmann E, et al. New parkin mutations and atypical phenotypes in families with autosomal recessive parkinsonism. Neurology 2003; 60(8):1378–1381.

41. Hoenicka J, Vidal L, Morales B, et al. Molecular findings in familial Parkinson disease in Spain. Arch Neurol 2002; 59(6):966–970.

42. Hedrich K, Marder K, Harris J, et al. Evaluation of 50 probands with early-onset Parkinson's disease for Parkin mutations. Neurology 2002; 58(8):1239–1246.

43. Abbas N, Lucking CB, Ricard S, et al. A wide variety of mutations in the parkin gene are responsible for autosomal recessive parkinsonism in Europe. French Parkinson's Disease Genetics Study Group and the European Consortium on Genetic Susceptibility in Parkinson's Disease. Hum Mol Genet 1999; 8(4):567–574.

44. Lucking CB, Durr A, Bonifati V, et al. Association between early-onset Parkinson's disease and mutations in the parkin gene. French Parkinson's Disease Genetics Study Group. N Engl J Med 2000; 342(21):1560–1567.

45. Kann M, Jacobs H, Mohrmann K, et al. Role of parkin mutations in 111 community-based patients with early-onset parkinsonism. Ann Neurol 2002; 51(5):621–625.

46. Leroy E, Boyer R, Auburger G, et al. The ubiquitin pathway in Parkinson's disease. Nature 1998; 395(6701):451–452.

47. Harhangi BS, Farrer MJ, Lincoln S, et al. The Ile93Met mutation in the ubiquitin carboxy-terminal-hydrolase-L1 gene is not observed in European cases with familial Parkinson's disease. Neurosci Lett 1999; 270(1):1–4.

48. Lincoln S, Vaughan J, Wood N, et al. Low frequency of pathogenic mutations in the ubiquitin carboxy-terminal hydrolase gene in familial Parkinson's disease. Neuroreport 1999; 10(2):427–429.

49. van Duijn CM, Dekker MC, Bonifati V, et al. Park7, a novel locus for autosomal recessive early-onset parkinsonism, on chromosome 1p36. Am J Hum Genet 2001; 69(3):629–634.

50. Bonifati V, Rizzu P, Squitieri F, et al. DJ-1(PARK7):a novel gene for autosomal recessive, early onset parkinsonism. Neurol Sci 2003; 24(3):159–160.

51. Miller DW, Ahmad R, Hague S, et al. L166P mutant DJ-1, causative for recessive Parkinson's disease, is degraded through the ubiquitin-proteasome system. J Biol Chem 2003; 278(38):36588–36595.

52. Abou-Sleiman PM, Healy DG, Quinn N, et al. The role of pathogenic DJ-1 mutations in Parkinson's disease. Ann Neurol 2003; 54(3):283–286.

53. Clark LN, Afridi S, Mejia-Santana H, et al. Analysis of an early-onset Parkinson's disease cohort for DJ-1 mutations. Mov Disord 2004; 19(7):796–800.

54. Hering R, Strauss KM, Tao X, et al. Novel homozygous p.E64D mutation in DJ1 in early onset Parkinson disease (PARK7). Hum Mutat 2004; 24(4):321–329.

55. Hague S, Rogaeva E, Hernandez D, et al. Early-onset Parkinson's disease caused by a compound heterozygous DJ-1 mutation. Ann Neurol 2003; 54(2):271–274.

56. Ibanez P, De Michele G, Bonifati V, et al. Screening for DJ-1 mutations in early onset autosomal recessive parkinsonism. Neurology 2003; 61(10):1429–1431.

57. Healy DG, Abou-Sleiman PM, Valente EM, et al. DJ-1 mutations in Parkinson's disease. J Neurol Neurosurg Psychiatry 2004; 75(1):144–145.

58. Valente EM, Bentivoglio AR, Dixon PH, et al. Localization of a novel locus for autosomal recessive early-onset parkinsonism, PARK6, on human chromosome 1p35-p36. Am J Hum Genet 2001; 68(4):895–900.

59. Valente EM, Brancati F, Ferraris A, et al. PARK6-linked parkinsonism occurs in several European families. Ann Neurol 2002; 51(1):14–18.
60. Valente EM, Salvi S, Ialongo T, et al. PINK1 mutations are associated with sporadic early-onset parkinsonism. Ann Neurol 2004; 56(3):336–341.
61. Rohe CF, Montagna P, Breedveld G, et al. Homozygous PINK1 C-terminus mutation causing early-onset parkinsonism. Ann Neurol 2004; 56(3):427–431.
62. Hatano Y, Li Y, Sato K, et al. Novel PINK1 mutations in early-onset parkinsonism. Ann Neurol 2004; 56(3):424–427.
63. Khan NL, Brooks DJ, Pavese N, et al. Progression of nigrostriatal dysfunction in a parkin kindred: an [18F]dopa PET and clinical study. Brain 2002; 125(Pt 10):2248–2256.
64. Funayama M, Hasegawa K, Kowa H, et al. A new locus for Parkinson's disease (PARK8) maps to chromosome 12p11.2–q13.1. Ann Neurol 2002; 51(3):296–301.
65. Paisan-Ruiz C, Jain S, Evans EW, et al. Cloning of the gene containing mutations that cause PARK8-linked Parkinson's disease. Neuron 2004; 44(4):595–600.
66. Zimprich A, Biskup S, Leitner P, et al. Mutations in LRRK2 cause autosomal-dominant parkinsonism with pleomorphic pathology. Neuron 2004; 44(4):601–607.
67. Di Fonzo A, Rohe CF, Ferreira J, et al. A frequent LRRK2 gene mutation associated with autosomal dominant Parkinson's disease. Lancet 2005; 365(9457):412–415.
68. Nichols WC, Pankratz N, Hernandez D, et al. Genetic screening for a single common LRRK2 mutation in familial Parkinson's disease. Lancet 2005; 365(9457):410–412.
69. Kachergus J, Mata IF, Hulihan M, et al. Identification of a Novel LRRK2 Mutation Linked to Autosomal Dominant Parkinsonism: Evidence of a Common Founder across European Populations. Am J Hum Genet 2005; 76(4):672–680.
70. Gasser T, Muller-Myhsok B, Wszolek ZK, et al. A susceptibility locus for Parkinson's disease maps to chromosome 2p13. Nat Genet 1998; 18(3):262–265.
71. West AB, Zimprich A, Lockhart PJ, et al. Refinement of the PARK3 locus on chromosome 2p13 and the analysis of 14 candidate genes. Eur J Hum Genet 2001; 9(9):659–666.
72. Karamohamed S, DeStefano AL, Wilk JB, et al. A haplotype at the PARK3 locus influences onset age for Parkinson's disease: the GenePD study. Neurology 2003; 61(11):1557–1561.
73. DeStefano AL, Lew MF, Golbe LI, et al. PARK3 influences age at onset in Parkinson disease: a genome scan in the GenePD study. Am J Hum Genet 2002; 70(5):1089–1095.
74. Pankratz N, Uniacke SK, Halter CA, et al. Genes influencing Parkinson disease onset: replication of PARK3 and identification of novel loci. Neurology 2004; 62(9):1616–1618.
75. Najim al-Din AS, Wriekat A, Mubaidin A, et al. Pallido-pyramidal degeneration, supranuclear upgaze paresis and dementia: Kufor-Rakeb syndrome. Acta Neurol Scand 1994; 89(5):347–352.
76. Hampshire DJ, Roberts E, Crow Y, et al. Kufor-Rakeb syndrome, pallido-pyramidal degeneration with supranuclear upgaze paresis and dementia, maps to 1p36. J Med Genet 2001; 38(10):680–682.
77. Hicks AA, Petursson H, Jonsson T, et al. A susceptibility gene for late-onset idiopathic Parkinson's disease. Ann Neurol 2002; 52(5):549–555.
78. Pankratz N, Nichols WC, Uniacke SK, et al. Genome screen to identify susceptibility genes for Parkinson disease in a sample without parkin mutations. Am J Hum Genet 2002; 71(1):124–135.
79. Pankratz N, Nichols WC, Uniacke SK, et al. Significant linkage of Parkinson disease to chromosome 2q36–37. Am J Hum Genet 2003; 72(4):1053–1057.
80. Gwinn-Hardy K, Chen JY, Liu HC, et al. Spinocerebellar ataxia type 2 with parkinsonism in ethnic Chinese. Neurology 2000; 55(6):800–805.
81. Sasaki H, Fukazawa T, Wakisaka A, et al. Central phenotype and related varieties of spinocerebellar ataxia 2 (SCA2): a clinical and genetic study with a pedigree in the Japanese. J Neurol Sci 1996; 144(1–2):176–181.
82. Gwinn-Hardy K, Singleton A, O'Suilleabhain P, et al. Spinocerebellar ataxia type 3 phenotypically resembling parkinson disease in a black family. Arch Neurol 2001; 58(2):296–299.
83. Payami H, Nutt J, Gancher S, et al. SCA2 may present as levodopa-responsive parkinsonism. Mov Disord 2003; 18(4):425–429.

84. Tuite PJ, Rogaeva EA, St George-Hyslop PH, et al. Dopa-responsive parkinsonism phenotype of Machado-Joseph disease: confirmation of 14q CAG expansion. Ann Neurol 1995; 38(4):684–687.

85. Wilkins A, Brown JM, Barker RA. SCA2 presenting as levodopa-responsive parkinsonism in a young patient from the United Kingdom: a case report. Mov Disord 2004; 19(5):593–595.

86. Shan DE, Soong BW, Sun CM, et al. Spinocerebellar ataxia type 2 presenting as familial levodopa-responsive parkinsonism. Ann Neurol 2001; 50(6):812–815.

87. Ragothaman M, Sarangmath N, Chaudhary S, et al. Complex phenotypes in an Indian family with homozygous SCA2 mutations. Ann Neurol 2004; 55(1):130–133.

88. Subramony SH, Hernandez D, Adam A, et al. Ethnic differences in the expression of neurodegenerative disease: Machado-Joseph disease in Africans and Caucasians. Mov Disord 2002; 17(5):1068–1071.

89. Johnston A, McKusick VA, Sex-linked recessive inheritance in spastic paraplegia and parkinsonism. In Proc Second Int Cong Hum Genet, 1963:1652–1654.

90. Lee LV, Pascasio FM, Fuentes FD, et al. Torsion dystonia in Panay, Philippines. Adv Neurol 1976; 14:137–151.

91. Lee LV, Kupke KG, Caballar-Gonzaga F, et al. The phenotype of the X-linked dystonia-parkinsonism syndrome. An assessment of 42 cases in the Philippines. Medicine (Baltimore) 1991; 70(3):179–187.

92. Evidente VG, Gwinn-Hardy K, Hardy J, et al. X-linked dystonia ("Lubag") presenting predominantly with parkinsonism: a more benign phenotype? Mov Disord 2002; 17(1):200–202.

93. Wilhelmsen KC, Weeks DE, Nygaard TG, et al. Genetic mapping of "Lubag"(X-linked dystonia-parkinsonism) in a Filipino kindred to the pericentromeric region of the X chromosome. Ann Neurol 1991; 29(2):124–131.

94. Nemeth AH, Nolte D, Dunne E, et al. Refined linkage disequilibrium and physical mapping of the gene locus for X-linked dystonia-parkinsonism (DYT3). Genomics 1999; 60(3):320–329.

95. Nolte D, Niemann S, Muller U. Specific sequence changes in multiple transcript system DYT3 are associated with X-linked dystonia parkinsonism. Proc Natl Acad Sci USA 2003; 100(18):10347–10352.

96. Wilhelmsen KC, Lynch T, Pavlou E, et al. Localization of disinhibition-dementia-parkinsonism-amyotrophy complex to 17q21–22. Am J Hum Genet 1994; 55(6):1159–1165.

97. Foster NL, Wilhelmsen K, Sima AA, et al. Frontotemporal dementia and parkinsonism linked to chromosome 17: a consensus conference. Conference Participants. Ann Neurol 1997; 41(6):706–715.

98. Wijker M, Wszolek ZK, Wolters EC, et al. Localization of the gene for rapidly progressive autosomal dominant parkinsonism and dementia with pallido-ponto-nigral degeneration to chromosome 17q21. Hum Mol Genet 1996; 5(1):151–154.

99. Hutton M, Lendon CL, Rizzu P, et al. Association of missense and 5′-splice-site mutations in tau with the inherited dementia FTDP-17. Nature 1998; 393(6686):702–705.

100. Spillantini MG, Murrell JR, Goedert M, et al. Mutation in the tau gene in familial multiple system tauopathy with presenile dementia. Proc Natl Acad Sci USA 1998; 95(13): 7737–7741.

101. van Slegtenhorst M, Lewis J, Hutton M. The molecular genetics of the tauopathies. Exp Gerontol 2000; 35(4):461–471.

102. Ingram EM, Spillantini MG. Tau gene mutations: dissecting the pathogenesis of FTDP-17. Trends Mol Med 2002; 8(12):555–562.

103. Murrell JR, Spillantini MG, Zolo P, et al. Tau gene mutation G389R causes a tauopathy with abundant pick body-like inclusions and axonal deposits. J Neuropathol Exp Neurol 1999; 58(12):1207–1226.

104. Rizzini C, Goedert M, Hodges JR, et al. Tau gene mutation K257T causes a tauopathy similar to Pick's disease. J Neuropathol Exp Neurol 2000; 59(11):990–1001.

105. Heutink P, Stevens M, Rizzu P, et al. Hereditary frontotemporal dementia is linked to chromosome 17q21–q22: a genetic and clinicopathological study of three Dutch families. Ann Neurol 1997; 41(2):150–159.

106. Wszolek ZK, Tsuboi Y, Uitti RJ, et al. Two brothers with frontotemporal dementia and parkinsonism with an N279K mutation of the tau gene. Neurology 2000; 55(12):1939.
107. Tsuboi Y, Baker M, Hutton ML, et al. Clinical and genetic studies of families with the tau N279K mutation (FTDP-17). Neurology 2002; 59(11):1791–1793.
108. Arima K, Kowalska A, Hasegawa M, et al. Two brothers with frontotemporal dementia and parkinsonism with an N279K mutation of the tau gene. Neurology 2000; 54(9):1787–1795.
109. Farrer M, Maraganore DM, Lockhart P, et al. alpha-Synuclein gene haplotypes are associated with Parkinson's disease. Hum Mol Genet 2001; 10(17):1847–1851.
110. Tan EK, Chai A, Teo YY, et al. Alpha-synuclein haplotypes implicated in risk of Parkinson's disease. Neurology 2004; 62(1):128–131.
111. Chiba-Falek O, Nussbaum RL. Effect of allelic variation at the NACP-Rep1 repeat upstream of the alpha-synuclein gene (SNCA) on transcription in a cell culture luciferase reporter system. Hum Mol Genet 2001; 10(26):3101–3109.
112. Kruger R, Vieira-Saecker AM, Kuhn W, et al. Increased susceptibility to sporadic Parkinson's disease by a certain combined alpha-synuclein/apolipoprotein E genotype. Ann Neurol 1999; 45(5):611–617.
113. Tan EK, Matsuura T, Nagamitsu S, et al. Polymorphism of NACP-Rep1 in Parkinson's disease: an etiologic link with essential tremor? Neurology 2000; 54(5):1195–1198.
114. Skipper L, Wilkes K, Toft M, et al. Linkage disequilibrium and association of MAPT H1 in Parkinson disease. Am J Hum Genet 2004; 75(4):669–677.
115. Kwok JB, Teber ET, Loy C, et al. Tau haplotypes regulate transcription and are associated with Parkinson's disease. Ann Neurol 2004; 55(3):329–334.

3 Epidemiology of Parkinson's Disease

Anabel Chade, Meike Kasten, and Caroline M. Tanner
Department of Clinical Research, The Parkinson's Institute, Sunnyvale, California, U.S.A.

INTRODUCTION

Epidemiology is the investigation of the distribution and determinants of a disease or condition in a population. In this chapter, we present a literature overview of Parkinson's disease (PD) and factors influencing its distribution. Information collected in epidemiologic studies can provide clues regarding the causes of disease, as well as critical information for public health planning and health care delivery.

DESCRIPTIVE EPIDEMIOLOGY
Incidence
Incidence is the number of new cases of a disease occurring in a population during a specific duration of time, usually a year. The incidence rate is the number of such individuals in relation to a unit of population, and it is the most useful measure of disease frequency because survival and migration do not affect it. However, the age and gender distributions of a population influence its incidence rate, so these crude rates can be adjusted for certain populations to compare groups. Since PD is a relatively rare disorder, a very large number of people must be studied to obtain reliable estimates of incidence. For PD, reported crude incidence rates range from five to 20 new cases per 100,000 individuals per year (Table 1) (1–19). This fourfold discrepancy may, in part, reflect age distribution differences among these populations, as well as variation in case definition and diagnostic criteria, rather than a true difference in disease frequency. Some studies used medical records alone to diagnose parkinsonism (3) and, therefore, may have included persons with other disorders. For example, a study performed in Finland initially identified 775 patients as having PD after a review of their medical records, but, when examined, 201 of these individuals were diagnosed with essential tremor (8). For studies that include only cases of PD, the estimated incidence rates are more similar but can still vary significantly with minor alterations in diagnostic criteria (20). Incidence for the very old and among different racial and ethnic groups remains particularly uncertain.

Prevalence
Prevalence is a measurement of the total number of individuals in a population who have a disease at a fixed point in time, that is, how widespread a disease is in a population. Estimates of crude prevalence often yield very discrepant values. In a review of worldwide epidemiologic studies published through 1991 (21), the authors found that the crude prevalence of PD ranged from 10/100,000 in Igbo-Ora, Nigeria, to 405/100,000 in Montevideo, Uruguay. While age adjustment reduces this 40-fold difference across populations, the range of estimated PD prevalence remains broad.

TABLE 1   Incidence of Parkinson's Disease: Selected Worldwide Studies

Reference	Country	Population/number of cases	Incidence (crude/100,000/yr)
Ashok et al., 1986 (11)	Libya	518,745/58	4.5
Bower et al., 1999 (10)	U.S.A.	95,000/154	11
Brewis et al., 1966 (3)	U.K.	69,400/60	12
Chen et al., 1996 (18)	Taiwan	75,579/15	10
Fall et al., 1996 (14)	Sweden	147,777/49	11
Granieri et al., 1991 (7)	Italy	187,381/394	10
Gudmundsson 1967 (2)	Iceland	171,500/272	16
Harada et al., 1983 (9)	Japan	121,812/62	10
Hofman et al., 1989 (12)	The Netherlands	163,577/51	11.5
Jenkins 1966 (4)	Australia	83,001/35	7
Kusumi et al., 1996 (17)	Japan	131,704/79	15
Mayeux et al., 1995 (16)	U.S.A.	213,000/83	13
Marttila et al., 1976 (8)	Finland	402,988/179	15
Morens et al., 1996 (5)	U.S.A.	8,006/92	11
Nobrega et al., 1969 (1)	U.S.A.	33,400/125	12
Rajput et al., 1984 (6)	U.S.A.	53,885/138	20
Sutcliffe et al., 1995 (15)	U.K.	298,985/175	12
Vines et al., 1999 (19)	Spain	523,563/86	8.2
Wender et al., 1989 (13)	Poland	1,308,000/163	13

This may likely reflect variations in subject ascertainment and diagnostic criteria. However, real differences in prevalence may be due to shortened survival in some populations (22). A clear geographic pattern does not emerge because the studies vary so much in their case ascertainment methods.

Door-to-door prevalence studies generally screen populations using a set of questions designed to identify all individuals who may have the disease, even those who have not received medical attention (23–25). After the initial screening process, individuals suspected of having the disease are asked to have a careful evaluation performed by a neurologist and, possibly, may undergo ancillary diagnostic tests. For reasons of convenience and economy, medical record- and community-based surveys are usually confined to small, geographically circumscribed populations. Ethnic homogeneity of the area limits generalization to other populations. Descriptive epidemiology conducted in an ethnically diverse location may be more easily generalized to other areas. Optimal areas have little emigration or immigration, an educated population to maximize the interest in assisting a scientific inquiry, and good healthcare access to increase the likelihood that subjects with symptoms will have medical records of diagnostic value available. Particularly for medical record-based studies, it is important that the population has universal access to high-quality medical care. Studies based on the Mayo Clinic medical records linkage system (10) and Kaiser Permanente (26) typifies this approach.

Indirect measures of prevalence are often less costly, but the accuracy of these estimates is less certain. The most common such approach used for studying parkinsonism is to determine the number of levodopa prescriptions or sales, to use as a surrogate measure for PD prevalence. However, many individuals with PD do not require, benefit from, or tolerate levodopa; others have not received medical attention. Such investigations are most effective in countries with universal access to medical care and centralized pharmacy records (27–29).

Mortality

Mortality associated with PD is not easily studied because PD is typically not the direct cause of death and not often noted on the death certificate. Compared to controls of the same age and gender, mortality is increased approximately two-fold among individuals with PD (5,30–32). A diminishing north-south gradient of PD mortality has been described, but this may be an artifact of differential access to medical care or death-certificate-completion inconsistencies among physicians (33). Studies that compare mortality figures, such as assessments of temporal and geographic differences, mitigate this concern. In a national population-based survey, the authors suggested that death certificate-based investigations of PD should be interpreted with extreme caution, particularly when the study involved factors associated with, or influenced by, socioeconomic status (34).

Geographic Variation

Estimates of PD prevalence vary widely, from 31 per 100,000 persons in Libya (35) to 328 per 100,000 among the Parsi community in Bombay, India (36). Although differences in population age distributions, diagnostic criteria, and ascertainment methods may explain some of this variation, even after adjusting for many of these inconsistencies, there are still international differences in PD frequency (21). In some countries twelves and colleagues' (37) adjusted reported rates for PD were more than twice those of others (22), ranging from 8 per 100,000 in Italy to 18 per 100,000 in the U.K.

Several North American studies have also described significant regional prevalence differences, and suggested northwest to southeast gradients in Canada and the United States (38–40). Since prevalence is also a function of duration, this geographic pattern may reflect a more rapid fatal course or less access to healthcare in areas with lower prevalence. Alternately, different distributions of causal risk factors across populations may contribute to this variation in disease frequency. These factors may include genetic differences in exposure to causative and protective influences or susceptibility (41).

Temporal Changes

A number of studies have investigated changes in PD frequency and attempted to identify patterns that provide important evidence about risk factors for the disease. For example, if an increasing PD incidence rate correlates with the industrialization of a region, exposures associated with the industrialization or related lifestyle changes may be the causal factors. Similarly, periodic fluctuation of incidence rates may suggest an infectious causation.

Zhang and Roman (21) reviewed studies published through 1991, and after adjusting the results for age and gender, they did not find that prevalence rates changed over the past 50 years in Europe and the U.S. In general, studies of PD show slightly increasing or stable incidence and prevalence (42). An important caveat to this statement is that few have made comparisons within the same populations and those conducted have been over relatively short periods of time and been based on very few cases. PD incidence was assessed in Olmsted County, Minnesota during 1935–1988. A single neurologist classified each case using existing diagnostic criteria to minimize variability in research design (43). Estimated incidence increased from 9.2 per 100,000 annually from 1935–1944, to 16.3 per 100,000 from 1975–1984

(44). Using similar methods, a comparison of age-adjusted prevalence rates in Finland from 1971–1992 showed an increased overall prevalence (139 to 166) (45). A significant rise in the prevalence among men could reflect changes in risk factors or better diagnosis or survival. Since incidence rates followed the same trend, differential survival is less likely as an explanation. In an Australian door-to-door survey, there was at least a 42.5% higher prevalence in 2001 than was estimated in 1996, even when methodologic differences between the studies were taken into account (46). Another investigation in Northampton, England used comparable methods to identify cases through their general practitioners and found a moderate increase in prevalence (108–121 per 100,000) from 1982–1990 (15). In China, a recent study found prevalence in Chinese cities to be similar to that of western populations, many times increased compared to prevalence in the same cities decades before (47). An increasing awareness of PD symptoms, as well as changing diagnostic attitudes and criteria could explain these results. Alternatively, changes in risk factors in these populations could cause such an increase.

Gender
Since the distribution of men and women differ among populations, crude estimates cannot be compared directly, and age-adjusted or age-specific prevalence rates are more useful for understanding potential causes of PD (22). Most prevalence (14,16,45,48,49) and incidence (10,16,26,45,49) studies have found a preponderance of PD among males. A few studies conducted in Japan are exceptions to this trend and observed a higher prevalence of PD among females (50,51). This may reflect longer survival among Japanese women, differential access to healthcare, an ascertainment bias against male cases, or actual differences in risk factors for disease.

Age
The risk of PD increases with advancing age (16,18,52–53). Before the age of 50, the disease is rare; incidence and prevalence rise steadily until approximately the ninth decade for incidence or the tenth decade for prevalence, when rates seem to decline. This apparent decline among the most elderly likely reflects incomplete ascertainment of PD among this age group, particularly for individuals with comorbid conditions. The small numbers of people with PD in the oldest age groups result in imprecise estimates of incidence and prevalence. Comparisons of disease frequency among populations must adjust for differing age distributions (21).

Race Distribution
For many decades, there has been controversy about whether PD frequency varies by race or ethnicity. Almost all prior reports on PD frequency have considered only a single race or ethnic group (5,10). An exception is a study that investigated incidence among blacks, whites and "other" racial groups in Manhattan, New York (16). This study found a higher incidence rate of PD among blacks compared to whites and did not identify any cases of PD among young white men. The results contradict most other studies of PD prevalence, which estimate a lower prevalence rate among blacks than among whites (33,39,54–56). A more recent study has also estimated PD incidence (Fig. 1) among blacks and whites in Northern California (Figs. 2–3) (26). The overall incidence rate for black men in this study was lower

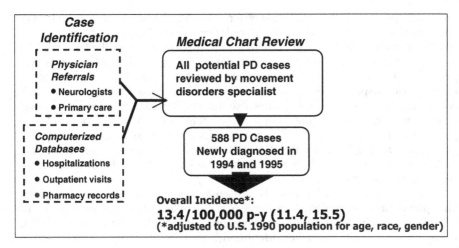

FIGURE 1 Case identification: Parkinson's disease incidence, Northern California Kaiser Permanente. *Abbreviation*: PD, Parkinson's disease. *Source*: From Ref. 26.

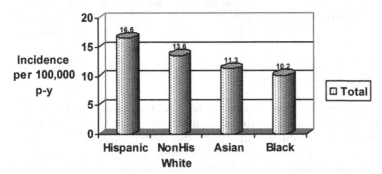

FIGURE 2 Age- and gender-adjusted Parkinson's disease incidence according to race/ethnricity, Northern California Kaiser Permanente. *Note*: Age-adjusted to the 1990 U.S. population. *Source*: From Ref. 26.

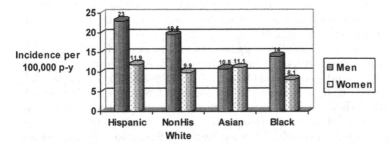

FIGURE 3 Age-adjusted Parkinson's disease incidence according to gender and race/ethnicity, Northern California Kaiser Permanente. *Note*: Age-adjusted to the 1990 U.S. population. *Source*: From Ref. 26.

than for whites (Fig. 2), about half that observed in Manhattan. Variations in host or environmental exposures between the populations-studied exposures, case-finding methods, as well as underascertainment of minority members in the base population may explain some or all of the differences. The overall incidence rate was highest for Hispanics in the Northern California study; incidence was higher in Hispanic, non-Hispanic white, and black men as compared to women in each of those groups (Fig. 3). The investigators also found, after adjusting for age, a lower incidence among Asian/Pacific Islanders than that found in the Honolulu Asian Aging Study of incident PD (5). This may be due, in part, to ancestral differences between the groups. The category of Asian/Pacific Islander in the California study was largely Chinese and Filipino (26), while the Honolulu study was composed solely of Japanese American men.

Importantly, the incidence studies discussed here were conducted in multi-ethnic populations within the U.S., and may not reflect incidence in these racial or ethnic groups in other countries. Also, precision of the estimates is poor, as relatively few nonwhite cases were identified.

ANALYTICAL EPIDEMIOLOGY

The study of PD presents special challenges for risk-factor assessment. There is likely a long period of time when neurons are already damaged, but symptoms are not yet apparent. The length of this "silent period" may vary among individuals. For this reason, it is difficult to estimate the optimal time frame for queries about past exposures.

Risk Factors for Parkinson's Disease
Chemicals
Interest and results in the search for environmental risk factors associated with the development of PD have increased steadily since the discovery of MPTP (1-methyl-4-phenyl-1,2,3,6-tetrahydropyridine) in the early 1980s. MPTP is a relatively simple pyridine compound that induces a parkinsonian syndrome very similar to PD in humans and in animal models (57–62). MPTP itself is rare, and exposure is unlikely, but several chemically-similar compounds are more common. For instance, the herbicide paraquat is a structural analogue to MPTP. Paraquat can induce dopaminergic neuron loss in rats (63) and exposure to paraquat has been associated with an increased risk of PD in humans (64–66). It has been suggested that repeated exposure or combined exposure to paraquat and the fungicide, Maneb, increases toxicity (67,68). Also, exposure to low doses of Maneb not leading to cell death may lead to increased susceptibility to oxidative stress, so that a second exposure even in a low dose may cause substantial damage (69).

In general, case-control studies suggest exposure to pesticides increases risk for PD (Table 2). A meta-analysis of 19 such studies from Asia, Europe, and North America up to 1999 found a combined OR of 1.94 (CI 1.49–2.53) for PD in pesticide users (70). Nevertheless, little is known about the association of specific pesticide agents with PD risk. There are a variety of chemicals in use as pesticides, fungicides and herbicides, and their broad and often poorly characterized actions, make it difficult to identify the mechanisms that increase the risk of PD. Among the classes and agents studied so far, organochlorines (71), alkylated phosphates (71), carbamates (71,72), paraquat (65), and dieldrin (73) have been implicated as increasing the risk of PD. In addition to pesticides, the drinking of well water (74–76) and rural living

TABLE 2 Factors Associated with the Risk of Parkinson's Disease

Factors associated with increased risk

Demographic factors	Environmental exposures	Infections/inflammation
Increasing age	MPTP and alike compounds	Encephalitis
Male gender	Pesticides	Nocardia asteroides
White race	Industrial agents	Inflammation (chronic)
Family history of PD	Carbon monoxide	
Diet	Metals	
Head trauma	Drinking well water	
Physical and emotional stress	Pulp mills	
	Farming	
Personality traits	Rural residence	
	Occupation	

Factors associated with decreased risk

Smoking
Caffeine intake
NSAID use
Alcohol (?)

Abbreviations: MPTP, 1-methyl-4-phenyl-1,2,3,6-tetrahydropyridine; NSAID, nonsteroidal anti-inflammatory drug; PD, Parkinson's disease.

(74,76) also showed an association with increased risk of PD, but this may be due to their co-occurrence with pesticide exposure or other unidentified factors.

In addition to pesticide use, the exposure to "any chemicals" (77,78), industrial settings (79,80), solvents (71,78), wood preservatives (71), glues, paints or lacquers (71), carbon monoxide (71) and general anesthesia (71) have been implicated in the development of PD. Not every individual exposed to pesticides develops PD. Differences in the ability to metabolize pesticides may alter the effects of exposure. For example, pesticide exposure increased PD risk in only those with the "poor metabolizer" phenotype of cytochrome P450 2D6 in one study (81).

Metals
Exposure to metals may alter many metabolic processes, possibly causing neuronal injury. For example, iron is increased in brain samples from PD patients and may increase oxidative stress (82,83) Manganese is known to cause a parkinsonian syndrome after high exposure (84). To date, studies show conflicting results regarding the impact of exposures to metals (27,80).

Combined high dietary intake of iron and manganese may result in an increased risk for PD (85). Dietary intake of manganese alone does not seem to have toxic effects, except in individuals with liver failure (86). Further complicating the study of metals as risk factors is the finding that certain exposure combinations may be associated with increased risk, while each single exposure at a similar level is not.

Head Trauma and Inflammation
The role of head trauma remains controversial, although it has been addressed in many case-control studies (12,71,72,75,87–90). Several studies report a positive association (71,72,87,88), while others have found no relation between head trauma and PD risk (12,75,89,90). Head injury may be involved in triggering, or predisposing to,

processes leading to the loss of nigral neurons. One possible pathway may be the activation of inflammatory processes after a head injury. Chronic inflammation is associated with a broad range of neurodegenerative diseases, one of them PD (91). It has also been hypothesized that the higher risk for PD seen in teachers and health care workers (92) is associated with higher exposure to infections in these occupations (93,94). However, to date, an infectious agent has never been shown to cause typical PD. The soil pathogen, *Nocardia asteroides*, causes a levodopa-responsive movement disorder and nigral degeneration in mice (95) but a serologic case-control study did not support its role in human PD (96).

Dietary Factors

The assessment of diet is, in general, a difficult task, and may yield unreliable results if information about diet in early life or over a long period of time is queried. An additional challenge is the number of components in single food items and the fact that each component may be the factor of interest. However, total fat intake (97,98)—in particular animal fat (97,99)—has been related to an increased risk of PD. This may be due to oxidative stress, as lipids are a source of oxygen radicals through peroxidation. A recent study reported intake of >16 ounces of milk per day (vs. no milk) increased risk of PD. The relative risk (RR) for milk drinkers was 2.3 (CI 1.3–4.1) and was independent of calcium intake (100). A second study had similar findings (101). Although a biologic explanation for this association is not known, toxicants proposed to be associated with PD may be concentrated in milk (102).

Other Associations

Several factors related to life experiences have been associated with the occurrence of PD. Emotional stress, which may cause increased dopamine turnover resulting in increased oxidative stress (103,104) has been associated with an increased risk for PD in two studies of persons surviving extreme emotional and physical hardship (105–107).

Several studies, including twin studies have identified a particular personality type as more common before the onset of PD than among controls (108). This personality is described as shy, cautious, inflexible, punctual, and depressive. It is not known if there is an association between this personality type and risk of PD, or if it represents early "premotor" features of the neurochemical changes due to the disease. Similar possible "premotor" associations include constipation (109), midlife adiposity (109,110) altered olfaction (111) and certain cardiac changes (112).

Genetic and Familial Factors

Over the last years, much progress has been made in the study of genetic aspects of PD, and these advances are discussed comprehensively elsewhere in this book. The results of epidemiologic research may, however, provide important information about the influence of genetic factors in the development of PD.

In case-control studies, those with PD consistently report more affected family members than do the controls. The odds ratios (ORs) for a positive family history in cases versus controls range from 3.5–14.6 for cases identified at specialty clinics (75,77,90,113–119). Community studies have confirmed this increased risk, but at a lower magnitude, with ORs ranging from 2.3–3.7 (72,120). However, recall bias has been found to contribute to this phenomenon in at least one study that reported histories verified by examinations (121). One prospective community-based study

(122) assessed the risk of developing PD in persons with one or two affected relatives. After a follow-up period of two years, the RR for persons with one affected first-degree relative was 2.5 compared to persons with no known relatives with PD. For those with at least two affected relatives, the RR was 10.4, but the confidence interval (CI) was wide (1.2–89.2).

Twin studies offer important clues to the relative contribution of genetic factors in disease development. In a disease with primarily genetic causes, monozygotic (MZ) twins would be more likely to be either both affected or both unaffected, while dizygotic (DZ) twins would be as likely to be affected as discordant siblings. To date, twin studies have shown similar concordance rates for MZ and DZ twins (123–129). But one large twin study (129) showed significantly higher concordance rates for MZ twins when symptoms began before age 50. The same study reported discrepancies of up to 28 years in age at onset between MZ twins. In a late life disorder with a potentially long presymptomatic period, it is possible that cross-sectional studies underestimate twin concordance by failing to identify presymptomatic individuals and those who died before developing disease.

A large population-based, case-control study in Iceland assessed how closely persons with and without PD were related (130). Iceland provides unique means for this investigation because genealogic information is available for 610,920 people over the past 11 centuries. Relatedness was determined for 772 cases (including a subgroup of 560 patients with onset of PD at >50 years of age) and in as many matched controls. PD cases were significantly more related in the whole group and in the old-onset group and extended beyond the nuclear family. The calculated RRs are 6.7 (CI 4.3–9.6) for siblings; 3.2 (CI 1.2–7.8) for offspring; and 2.7 (CI 1.6–3.9) for nephews and nieces of persons with late-onset PD. Whether this information can be generalized to other populations is unknown, as the Icelandic population is a relative genetic isolate.

Factors Associated with Decreased Risk for Parkinson's Disease
Smoking
An inverse association of cigarette smoking and PD has been seen in both case-control and cohort studies (65,71,78,89,131–135), with multiple studies confirming an inverse dose-response pattern with regard to cumulative lifetime dose (134–36). But not all studies have confirmed this association (137,138), and the biologic pathways are not yet fully understood. Therefore, it is not known if smoking is protective. An alternative explanation is the hypothesis that PD patients show differences in certain personality traits and in the dopaminergic reward system (139,140) long before any other disease symptoms, and that these characteristics make them less likely to start smoking. This hypothesis is unproven and remains controversial, and the dopaminergic influence on the described personality characteristics remains elusive (141).

The component(s) of cigarettes and cigarette smoke that may protect against PD are not known. Smoking may reduce the monoamineoxidase B (MAO-B) activity in the animal and human brain (142,143). MAO-B activates 1-methyl-4-phenyl-1,2,3,6-tetrahydropyridine (MPTP), and MAO-B inhibitors may offer neuroprotection in PD (57,144), although this has not yet been proven, even for stronger MAO-B inhibitors like selegiline. Another hypothesis is that nicotine is neuroprotective (132), perhaps because it has antioxidant properties (145). Nicotine has also been shown to be neuroprotective in several animal models of neurodegeneration, including those for PD and Alzheimer's disease (146). Furthermore, nicotinic receptors are functionally linked with motor behavior, and their numbers are decreased in brains affected by PD; activation can improve parkinsonian symptoms (147).

Caffeine and Alcohol

Coffee drinking or caffeine intake is inversely associated with the risk of PD (133,135,148,149). In one large prospective cohort of men, a dose-response was observed (133). But other results indicate that caffeine may not affect all persons similarly. Among women within the Nurses' Health Study, caffeine seemed to reduce the risk for PD among women not using postmenopausal hormones, but to increase risk among hormone users (150). As a result, there was not a clear overall relationship between caffeine intake and PD in this cohort. These observations suggest a potential interaction between estrogen exposure and caffeine consumption in development of PD. In laboratory studies, the biologic effects of caffeine are mediated in part through its antagonist action on the adenosine A2 receptor, which in turn modulates dopaminergic neurotransmission (151,152) and protects against striatal dopamine loss caused by MPTP (153–155).

Several studies have also reported an inverse association of alcohol and PD (149,156,157), although the associations were of borderline significance. The variability across these studies is great, and the evidence for concluding that there is an inverse association of alcohol intake and risk of PD is weak at this time.

Nonsteroidal Anti-inflammatory Drugs

As discussed previously, inflammation may contribute to the etiology of PD. Studies of Alzheimer's disease have shown that the regular use of NSAIDs may reduce the risk of Alzheimer's in humans (158–161). The similarities in the pathogenetic background of PD and Alzheimer's disease and animal data suggesting that anti-inflammatory drugs may protect against PD (162–165) have encouraged investigation of the association between NSAID use and PD risk in humans. The regular use of nonaspirin NSAIDs was associated with a 45% lower risk of PD in one such prospective study, suggesting neuroprotective effects of the drugs (166). Important goals for future studies will be to identify the specific compounds and mechanisms that may mediate the protective effects of smoking, caffeine intake and NSAID use and determine whether or not there are common factors among these behaviors.

CONCLUSIONS

Epidemiologic studies can contribute clues to the etiology of PD. Multiple risk and protective factors and interactions between genetic and environmental factors have already been suggested. The challenge over the coming years will be to discern which associations are etiologically relevant and to identify their biologic mechanisms. This warrants strong collaboration between clinical and basic research. It will be crucial and fruitful to take epidemiologic findings to the laboratory to try to identify their biologic mechanisms. Likewise, biologically founded hypotheses from the laboratory will also be valuable in designing epidemiologic studies to test effects in humans.

ACKNOWLEDGMENTS

The authors wish to acknowledge Jennifer Wright for editorial assistance, support from the Michael J. Fox Foundation Fellowship (Drs. Chade and Kasten), and grants R01 NS40467, R01 ES10803, and U54 ES12077 (Dr. Tanner).

REFERENCES

1. Nobrega F, Glattre E, Kurland LT, Okazaki H. Comments on the epidemiology of parkinsonism including prevalence and incidence statistics for Rochester, Minnesota, 1935–1966. In Brunette JR, Barbeau JR, eds. Progress in Neurogenetics. Amsterdam: Excerpta Medica, 1969:474–485.
2. Gudmundsson KR. A clinical survey of parkinsonism in Iceland. Acta Neurol Scand 1967; 43(suppl 33):9–61.
3. Brewis M, Proskanzer DC, Rolland C, Miller H. Neurological diseases in an English city. Acta Neurol Scand 1966; 42(suppl 24):1–89.
4. Jenkins AC. Epidemiology of parkinsonism in Victoria. Med J Aust 1966; 2:496–502.
5. Morens D, Davis J, Grandinetti A, et al. Epidemiologic observations on Parkinson's disease: incidence and mortality in a prospective study of middle-aged men. Neurology 1996; 46(4):1044–1050.
6. Rajput AH, Offord KP, Beard CM, Kurland LT. Epidemiology of parkinsonism: incidence, classification, and mortality. Ann Neurol 1984; 16:278–282.
7. Granieri E, Carreras M, Casetta I, et al. Parkinson's disease in Ferrara, Italy, 1967 through 1987. Arch Neurol 1991; 48:854–857.
8. Marttila RJ, Rinne UK. Epidemiology of Parkinson's disease in Finland. Acta Neurol Scand 1976; 53:81–102.
9. Harada H, Nishikawa S, Takahashi K. Epidemiology of Parkinson's disease in a Japanese city. Arch Neurol 1983; 40:151–154.
10. Bower JH, Maraganore DM, McDonnell SK, Rocca WA. Incidence and distribution of parkinsonism in Olmsted County, Minnesota, 1976–1990. Neurology 1999; 52:1214–1220.
11. Ashok PP, Radhakrishnan K, Sridharan R, Mousa ME. Epidemiology of Parkinson's disease in Benghazi, North-East Libya. Clin Neurol Neurosurg 1986; 88:109–113.
12. Hofman A, Collette HJ, Bartelds AI. Incidence and risk factors of Parkinson's disease in The Netherlands. Neuroepidemiology 1989; 8(6):296–299.
13. Wender M, Pruchnik D, Kowal P, Florczak J, Zalejski M. [Epidemiology of Parkinson's disease in the Poznan province] (Polish). Przegl Epidemiol 1989; 43:150–155.
14. Fall P, Axelson O, Fredrikson M, et al. Age-standardized incidence and prevalence of Parkinson's disease in a Swedish community. J Clin Epidemiol 1996; 49(6):637–641.
15. Sutcliffe RL, Meara JR. Parkinson's disease epidemiology in the Northampton District, England, 1992. Acta Neurol Scand 1995; 92(6):443–450.
16. Mayeux R, Marder K, Cote LJ, et al. The frequency of idiopathic Parkinson's disease by age, ethnic group, and sex in northern Manhattan, 1988–1993. Am J Epidemiol 1995; 142(8):820–827.
17. Kusumi M, Nakashima K, Haranda M, et al. Epidemiology of Parkinson's disease in Yonago City, Japan: comparison with a studied carried out 12 years ago. Neuroepidemiology 1996; 15(4):201–207.
18. Chen RC, Chang SF, Su CL, et al. Prevalence, incidence, and mortality of PD: a door-to-door survey in Ilan County, Taiwan. Neurology 1996; 57(9):1679–1686.
19. Vines JJ, Larumbe R, Gaminde I, Artazcoz MT. Incidencia de la enfermedad de Parkinson idiopatica y secundaria en Navarra. Registro poblacional de casos. [Incidence of idiopathic and secondary Parkinson disease in Navarre. Population-based case registry.] (Spanish). Neurologia 1999; 14:16–22.
20. Melcon MO, Anderson DW, Vergara RH, Rocca WA. Prevalence of Parkinson's disease in Junin, Buenos Aires Province, Argentina. Mov Disord 1997; 12(2):197–205.
21. Zhang Z, Roman G. Worldwide occurrence of Parkinson's disease: an updated review. Neuroepidemiology 1993; 12(4):195–208.
22. Korell M, Tanner CM. Epidemiology of Parkinson's Disease: An Overview. In Ebadi M and Pfeiffer RF, eds. Parkinson's Disease. New York: CRC Press, 2005:39–50.
23. Mutch WJ, Smith WC, Scott RF. A screening and alerting questionnaire for parkinsonism. Neuroepidemiology 1991; 10(3):150–156.
24. Tanner CM, Gilley DW, Goetz CG. A brief screening questionnaire for parkinsonism. Ann Neurol 1990; 28:267–268.
25. Duarte J, Claveria LE, de Pedro Cuesta J, et al. Screening Parkinson's disease: a validated questionnaire of high specificity and sensitivity. Mov Disord 1995; 10(5):643–649.

26. Van Den Eeden S, Tanner CM, Bernstein AL, et al. Incidence of Parkinson's disease: variation by age, gender, and race/ethnicity. Am J Epidemiol 2003; 157(11):1015–1022.
27. Aquilonius S, Hartvig P. A Swedish county with unexpectedly high utilization of antiparkinsonian drugs. Acta Neurol Scand 1986; 74(5):379–382.
28. Strickland D, Bertini JM, Pfeiffer RF. Descriptive epidemiology of Parkinson's disease through proxy measures. Can J Neurol Sci 1996; 23(4):279–284.
29. de Pedro-Cuesta J, Petersen IJ, Vassilopoulos D, et al. Epidemiological assessment of levodopa use by populations. Acta Neurol Scand 1991; 83(5):328–335.
30. Louis ED, Marder K, Cote L, et al. Mortality from Parkinson's disease. Arch Neurol 1997; 54(3):260–264.
31. Morgante L, Salemi G, Meneghini F, et al. Parkinson's disease survival: a population-based study. Arch Neurol 2000; 57(4):507–512.
32. Di Rocco A, Molinari SP, Kollmeier B, Yahr MD. Parkinson's disease: Progression and mortality in the L-DOPA era. Adv Neurol 1996; 69:3–11.
33. Lilienfeld DE, Sekkor D, Simpson S, et al. Parkinsonism death rates by race, sex and geography: an 1980s update. Neuroepidemiology 1990; 9(5):243–247.
34. Pressley J, Tang M, Marder K, Cote L, Mayeux R. Disparities in the recording of Parkinson's disease on death certificates. Mov Disord 2005; 20(3):315–321.
35. Ashok PP, Radhakrishan K, Sridharan R, et al. Parkinsonism in Benghazi, East Libya. Clin Neurol Neurosurg 1986; 88(2):109–113.
36. Bharucha NE, Bharucha EP, Bharucha AE, et al. Prevalence of Parkinson's disease in the Parsi community of Bombay, India. Arch Neurol 1988; 45(12):1321–1323.
37. Twelves D, Persins K, Counsell. Systematic review of incidence studies of Parkinson's disease. Mov Disord 2003; 18(1):19–31.
38. Betemps EJ, Buncher CR. Birthplace as a risk factor in motor neuron disease and Parkinson's disease. Int J Epidemiol 1993; 22(5):898–904.
39. Kurtzke JV, Goldberg ID. Parkinsonism death rates by race, sex, and geography. Neurology 1988; 38(10):1558–1561.
40. Svenson LW, Platt GH, Woodhead SE. Geographic variations in the prevalence rates of Parkinson's disease in Alberta. Can J Neurol Sci 1993; 20(4):307–311.
41. Tanner CM, Goldman SM, Webster Ross G. Etiology of Parkinson's Disease. In: Jankovic J, Tolosa E, eds. Parkinson's Disease and Movement Disorders. Philadelphia: Lippincott Williams & Wilkins, 2002:90–103.
42. Marras C, Tanner CM. Epidemiology of Parkinson's Disease. In: Watts RL, Koller WC, eds. Movement Disorders, Neurologic Principles and Practice. New York: McGraw-Hill 1997:177–195.
43. Rocca WA, Bower JH, McConnell SK, et al. Time trends in the incidence of parkinsonism in Olmsted County, Minnesota. Neurology 2001; 57(3):462–467.
44. Tanner CM, Thelen JA, Offord KP, et al. Parkinson's disease incidence in Olmsted County, MN: 1935–1988. Neurology 1992; 42(suppl 3):194.
45. Kuopio A, Marttila RJ, Helenius H, Rinne UK. Changing epidemiology of Parkinson's disease in southwestern Finland. Neurology 1999; 52(2):302–308.
46. Chan DK, Dunne M, Wong A, et al. Pilot study of prevalence of Parkinson's disease in Australia. Neuroepidemiology 2001; 20(2):112–117.
47. Zhang ZX, Anderson DW, Huang JB, et al. Prevalence of Parkinson's disease and related disorders in the elderly population of greater Beijing, China. Movement Disord 2003; 18(7):764–72.
48. Rosati G, Granieri E, Pinna L, et al. The risk of Parkinson disease in Mediterranean people. Neurology 1980; 30(3):250–255.
49. Baldereschi M, Di Carlo A, Rocca W, et al. Parkinson's disease and parkinsonism in a longitudinal study: two-fold higher incidence in men. ILDS Working Group, Italian Longitudinal Study on Aging. Neurology 2000; 55(9):1358–1363.
50. Kusumi M, Nakashima K, Haranda M, et al. Epidemiology of Parkinson's disease in Yonago City, Japan: comparison with a studied carried out 12 years ago. Neuroepidemiology 1996; 15(4):201–207.
51. Kimura H, Kurimura M, Wada M, et al. Female preponderance of Parkinson's disease in Japan. Neuroepidemiology 2002; 21(6):292.
52. de Rijk MC, Breteler MM, Graveland GA, et al. Prevalence of Parkinson's disease in the elderly: the Rotterdam study. Neurology 1995; 45(12):2143–2146.

53. Morens D, Davis J, Grandinetti A, et al. Epidemiology observations on Parkinson's disease: Incidence and mortality in a prospective study of middle-aged men. Neurology 1996; 46(4):1044–1050.
54. Marttila RJ, Rinne UK. Epidemiology of Parkinson's disease—an overview. J Neural Transm 1981; 51(1–2):135–148.
55. Richards M, Chaudhuri KR. Parkinson's disease in populations of African origin: a review. Neuroepidemiology 1996; 15(4):214–21.
56. Schoenberg BS, Anderson DW, Haerer AF. Prevalence of Parkinson's disease in the biracial population of Copiah County, Mississippi. Neurology 1985; 35(6):841–845.
57. Langston JW, Ballard P, Tetrud JW, et al. Chronic parkinsonism in humans due to a product of meperidine-analog synthesis. Science 1983; 219(4587):979–980.
58. Burns RS, Chuieh CC, Markey SP, et al. A primate model of parkinsonism: selective destruction of dopaminergic neurons in the pars compacta of the substantia nigra by N-methyl-4-phenyl-1,2,3,6-tetrahydropine. Proc Nat Acad Sci 1983; 80(14):4546–4550.
59. Langston JW, Forno LS, Rebert CS, Irwin I. Selective nigral toxicity after systemic administration of 1-methyl-4-phenyl-1,2,3,6-tetrahydropine (MPTP) in the squirrel monkey. Brain Research 1984; 292(2):390–394.
60. Forno LS, Langston JW, DeLanney LE, et al. Locus cereleus lesions and eosinophilic inclusions in MPTP-treated monkeys. Ann Neurol 1986; 20(4):449–455.
61. Ricaurte GA, Delanney LE, Irwin I, Langston JW. Older dopaminergic neurons do not recover from the effects of MPTP. Neuropharmacology 1987; 26(1):97–99.
62. Davis GC, Williams AC, Markey SP, et al. Chronic parkinsonism secondary to intravenous injection of meperidine analogues. Psychiatr Res 1979; 1(3):249–254.
63. Brooks, AL, Chadwick, CA, Gelbhard, HA, et al. Paraquat elicited neurobehavioral syndrome caused by dopaminergic neuron loss. Brain Res 1999; 823(1–2):1–10.
64. Rajput, AH, Uitti RJ, Stern W, et al. Geography, drinking water chemistry, pesticides and herbicides and the etiology of PD. Can J Neurol Sci 1987; 14(3 suppl):414–418.
65. Liou HH, Tsai MC, Chen CJ, et al. Environmental risk factors and PD: a case—control study in Taiwan, Neurology 1997; 48(6):1583–1588.
66. Barbeau A, Roy M, Bernier G, et al. Ecogenetics of PD; prevalence and environmental aspects in rural areas. Can J Neurol Sci 1987; 14(1):36–41.
67. Gonzalez-Polo RA, Rodriguez-Martin A, Moran JM, et al. Paraquat-induced apoptotic cell death in cerebellar granule cells. Brain Res 2004; 1011(2):170–176.
68. Thiruchelvam M, McCormack A, Richfield EK, et al. Age-related irreversible progressive nigrostriatal dopaminergic neurotoxicity in the paraquat and maneb model of the PD phenotype. Eur J Neurosci 2003; 18(3):589–600.
69. Barlow BK, Lee DW, Cory-Slechta DA, et al. Modulation of antioxidant defense systems by the environmental pesticide maneb in dopaminergic cells. Neurotoxicology 2005; 26(1):63–75.
70. Priyardarshi A, Khuder SA, Schaub EA, Shrivastava S. A meta-analysis of Parkinson's disease and exposure to pesticides. Neurotoxicology 2000; 21(4):435–440.
71. Seidler A, Hellenbrand W, Robra BP, et al. Possible environmental, occupational, and other etiologic factors for Parkinson's disease: a case control study in Germany. Neurology 1996; 46(5):1275–1284.
72. Semchuk KM, Love EJ, Lee RG. Parkinson's disease and exposure to agricultural work and pesticide chemicals. Neurology 1992; 42:1328–1335.
73. Fleming L, Mann JB, Bean J, et al. Parkinson's disease and brain levels of organochlorine pesticides. Ann Neurol 1994; 36(1):100–103.
74. Koller W, Vetere-Overfield B, Cray C, et al. Environmental risk factors and Parkinson's disease. Neurology 1990; 40(8):1218–1221.
75. De Michele G, Filla A, Volpe G, et al. Environmental and genetic risk factors in Parkinson's disease: a case-control study in southern Italy. Mov Disord 1996; 11(1):17–23.
76. Wong GF, Gray CS, Hassanein RS, Koller WC. Environmental risk factors in siblings with Parkinson's disease. Arch Neurol 1991; 48(3):287–289.
77. Werneck AL, Alvarenga H. Genetics, drugs and environmental factors in Parkinson's disease. A case-control study. Arq Neuropsiquiatr 1999; 57(2B):347–55.
78. Smargiassi A, Mutti A, De Rosa A, et al. A case-control study of occupational and environmental risk factors for Parkinson's disease in the Emilia-Romagna region of Italy. Neurotoxicology 1998; 19(4–5):709–712.

79. Tanner CM. The role of environmental toxins in the etiology of Parkinson's disease. Trend Neurosci 1989; 12(2):49–54.
80. Rybicki BA, Johnson CC, Uman J, Gorell JM. Parkinson's disease mortality and the industrial use of heavy metals in Michigan. Mov Disord 1993; 8(1):87–92.
81. Elbaz A, Levecque C, Clavel J, et al. CYP2D6 polymorphism, pesticide exposure, and Parkinson's disease. Ann Neurol 2004; 55(3):430–434.
82. Bharat S, Hsu M, Kaur D, et al. Glutathione, iron and PD. Biochem Pharmacol 2002; 64(5–6):1037–1048.
83. Kaur D, Yantiri F, Rajagopalan S, et al. Genetic or pharmacological iron chelation prevents MPTP-induced neurotoxicity in vivo: a novel therapy for PD. Neuron 2003; 37(6):899–909.
84. Normandin L, Hazell AS. Manganese neurotoxicity: an update of pathophysiologic mechanisms. Metab Brain Dis 2002; 17(4):375–387.
85. Powers KM, Smith-Weller T, Franklin GM, et al. PD risks associated with dietary iron, manganese and other nutrients intakes. Neurology 2003; 60(11):1761–1766.
86. Hauser RA, Zesiewicz TA, Rosemurgy AS, et al. Manganese intoxication and chronic liver failure. Ann Neurol 1994; 36(6):871–875.
87. Stern M, Dulaney E, Gruber SB, et al. The epidemiology of Parkinson's disease. A case-control study of young-onset and old-onset patients. Arch Neurol 1991; 48(9): 903–907.
88. Tsai CH, Lo SK, See LC, et al. Environmental risk factors of young-onset Parkinson's disease: a case-control study. Clin Neurol Neurosurg 2002; 104(4):328–333.
89. Tanner CM, Chen B, Wang WZ, et al. Environmental factors in the etiology of Parkinson's disease. Can J Neurol Sci 1987; 14(supp l3):419–423.
90. Morano A, Jimenez-Jimenez FJ, Molina JA, Antolin MA. Risk-factors for Parkinson's disease: case-control study in the province of Caceres, Spain. Acta Neurol Scand 1994; 89(3):164–170.
91. McGeer PL, McGeer EG. Inflammation and the degenerative diseases of aging." Ann NY Acad Sci 2004; 1035:104–116.
92. Schulte PA, Burnett CA, Boeniger MF, Johnson J. Neurodegenerative diseases: occupational occurrence and potential risk factors, 1982–1991. Am J Public Health 1996; 86(9):1281–1288.
93. Tanner CM. Occupation and risk of Parkinson's disease (PD): A preliminary investigation of Standard Occupational Codes (SOC) in twins discordant for disease. Neurology 2003; 60:A415.
94. Tsui JK, Calne DB, Wang Y, et al. Occupational risk factors in Parkinson's disease. Can J Public Health 1999; 90(5):334–337.
95. Kobbata S, Beaman BL. L-dopa-responsive movement disorder caused by Nocardia asteroides localized in the brains of mice. Infect Immune 1991; 59(1):181–191.
96. Hubble JP, Cao T, Kjelstrom JA, et al. Nocardia species as an etiologic agent in Parkinson's disease: serological testing in a case-control study. J Clin Microbiol 1995; 33(10): 2768–2769.
97. Logroscino G, Marder K, Cote L, et al. Dietary lipids and antioxidants in Parkinson's disease: a population-based case-control study. Ann Neurol 1996; 39(1):89–84.
98. Johnson CC, Gorell JM, Rybicki BA, et al. Adult nutrient intake as a risk factor for Parkinson's disease. Int J Epidemiol 1999; 28(6):1102–1109.
99. Anderson KC, Checkoway L, Franklin G, et al. Dietary factors in Parkinson's disease: The role of food groups and specific foods. Mov Disord 1999; 14(1):21–27.
100. Chen H, Zhang SM, Hernan MA, Willett WC, Ascherio A. Diet and Parkinson's disease: a potential role of dairy products in men. Ann Neurol 2002; 52(6):793–801.
101. Park M, Ross GW, Petrovitch H, et al. Consumption of milk and calcium in midlife and the future risk of Parkinson disease. Neurology 2005; 64(6):1047–1051.
102. Martinez MP, Angulo R, Pozo R, Jodral M. Organochlorine pesticides in pasteurized milk and associated health risks. Food Chem Toxicol 1997; 35:621–624.
103. Snyder A, Stricker E, Zigmond M. Stress-induced neurological impairments in an animal model of parkinsonism. Ann Neurol 1985; 18(5):544–551.
104. Spina M, Cohen G. Dopamine turnover and glutathione oxidation: Implications for Parkinson's disease. Proc Natl Acad Sci USA 1989; 86(4):1398–1400.

105. Gibberd FB, Simmonds JP. Neurological disease in ex-far-east prisoners of war. Lancet 1980; 2(8186):135–137.
106. Treves T, Rabey J, Korczyn A. Case-control study: use of temporal approach for evaluation of risk factors in Parkinson's disease. Mov Disord 1990; 5:11.
107. Page WF, Tanner CM. Parkinson's disease and motor-neuron disease in former prisoners of war. Lancet 2000; 355(9206):843.
108. Menza M. The personality associated with Parkinson's disease. Curr Psychiatry Rep 2000; 2(5):421–426.
109. Abbott RD, Ross GW, White LR, et al. Environmental, life-style, and physical precursors of clinical Parkinson's disease: recent findings from the Honolulu-Asia Aging Study. J Neurol 2003; 250(suppl 3):III30– III39.
110. Chen H, Zhang SM, Schwarzschild MA, et al. Obesity and the risk of Parkinson's disease. Am J Epidemiol 2004; 159(6):547–555.
111. Stern MB. The preclinical detection of Parkinson's disease: ready for prime time? Ann Neurol 2004; 56(2):169–171.
112. Amino T, Orimo S, Itoh Y, et al. Profound cardiac sympathetic denervation occurs in Parkinson disease. Brain Pathol 2005; 15(1):29–34.
113. Bonifati V, Fabrizio E, Vanacore N, et al. Familial Parkinson's disease: A clinical genetic analysis. Can J Neurol Sci 1995; 22(4):272–279.
114. Payami H, Larsen K, Bernard S, Nutt JG. Increased risk of Parkinson's disease in parents and siblings of patients. Am Neurol 1994; 36(4):659–661.
115. Vieregge P, Heberlein I. Increased risk of Parkinson's disease in relatives of patients. Ann Neurol 1995; 37(5):685.
116. Autere JM, Moilanen JS, Myllyla VV, Majamaa K. Familial aggregation of Parkinson's disease in Finnish population. J Neurol Neurosurg Psychiatry 2000; 69(1):107–109.
117. Taylor CA, Saint-Hilaire MH, Cupples LA, et al. Environmental, medical, and family history risk factors for Parkinson's disease: A New England-based case control study. Am J Med Genet 1999; 88(6):742–749.
118. Preux PM, Condet A, Anglade C, et al. Parkinson's disease and environmental factors. Matched case-control study in the Limousin region, France. Neuroepidemiology 2000; 19(6):333–337.
119. Rocca WA, McDonnell, SK, Strain KJ, et al. Familial aggregation of Parkinson's disease: The Mayo Clinic family study. Ann Neurol 2004; 56(4):495–502.
120. Marder K, Tang M, Mejia H, et al. Risk of Parkinson's disease among first-degree relatives: a community-based study. Neurology 1996; 47(1):155–160.
121. Elbaz A, McDonnell SK, Maraganore DM, et al.Validity of family history data on PD: evidence for a family information bias. Neurology 2003; 61(1):11–17.
122. de Rijk MC, Breteler MM, van der Meche FG, Hofman A. The risk of Parkinson's disease among persons with a family history of Parkinson's disease or dementia: The Rotterdam study. Neurology 1997; 48:A333.
123. Marsden CD. Parkinson's disease in twins. J Neurol Neurosurg Psychiatry 1987; 50(1):105–106.
124. Marttila RJ, Kaprio J, Koskenvuo M, Rinne UK. Parkinson's disease in a nationwide twin cohort. Neurology 1999; 38(8):1217–1219.
125. Vieregge P, Schiffke KA, Friedrich HJ, et al. Parkinson's disease in twins. Neurology 1992; 42:1453–1461.
126. Ward C, Duvoisin R, Ince S, et al. Parkinson's disease in 65 pairs of twins and in a set of quadruplets. Neurology 1983; 33(7):815–824.
127. Zimmerman TR Jr, Bhatt M, Calne DB, Duvoisin RC. Parkinson's disease in monzygotic twins: a follow-up study. Neurology 1991; 41(suppl 1):255.
128. Tanner CM, Ottman R, Goldman SM, et al. Parkinson disease in twins: an etiologic study. JAMA 1999; 281(4):341–346.
129. Wirdefeldt K, Gatz M, Schalling M, Pedersen NL. No evidence for heritability of Parkinson disease in Swedish twins. Neurology 2004; 63(2):305–311.
130. Sveinbjornsdottir S, Hicks AA, Jonsson T, et al. Familial aggregation of Parkinson's disease in Iceland. New Engl J Med 2000; 343(24):1765–1770.
131. Zayed J, Ducic S, Campanella G, et al. [Environmental factors in the etiology of Parkinson's disease] [Article in French], Can J Neurol Sci 1990; 17(3):286–291.

132. Tanner CM, Goldman SM, Aston DA, et al. Smoking and Parkinson's disease in twins. Neurology 2002; 26:58(4):581–588.

133. Ross GW, Petrovitch H. Current evidence for neuroprotective effects of nicotine and caffeine against Parkinson's disease. Drugs Aging 2001, 18(11):797–806.

134. Checkoway H, Powers K, Smith-Weller T, et al. Parkinson's disease risks associated with cigarette smoking, alcohol consumption, and caffeine intake. Am J Epidemiol 2002; 15:155(8):732–738.

135. Hernan MA, Takkouche B, Caamano-Isorna F, Gestal-Otero JJ. A meta-analysis of coffee drinking, cigarette smoking, and the risk of Parkinson's disease. Ann Neurol 2002; 52(3):276–284.

136. Gorell JM, Rybicki BA, Johnson CC, Peterson EL. Smoking and Parkinson's disease: a dose-response relationship. Neurology 1999; 52(1):115–119.

137. Mayeux R, Tang MX, Marder K, et al. Smoking and Parkinson's disease. Mov Disord 1994; 9(2):207–212.

138. Rajput AH, Offord KP, Beard CM, Kurland LT. A case-control study of smoking habits, dementia, and other illnesses in idiopathic Parkinson's disease. Neurology 1987; 37(2):226–232.

139. Menza MA , Golbe LI, Cody RA, Forman NE. Dopamine-related personality traits in PD. Neurology 1993, 43(3):505–508.

140. Heberlein I, Ludin H, Scholz J, Vieregge P. Personality, depression, and premorbid lifestyle in twin pairs discordant for PD. JNNP 1998; 64(2):262–266.

141. Kaasinen V, Nurmi E, Bergman J, et al. Personality traits and brain dopaminergic function in PD. PNAS 2001; 98(6):3272–3277.

142. Fowler JS, Volkow ND, Wang GJ, et al. Inhibition of monoamine oxidase B in the brains of smokers. Nature 1996; 379(6567):733–736.

143. Mendez-Alvarez E, Soto-Otero R, Sanchez-Sellero I, Lopez-Rivadulla Lamas M. Inhibition of brain monoamine oxidase by adducts of 1,2,3,4 tetrahydroisoquinoline with components of cigarette smoke. Life Sci 1997; 60(19):1719–1727.

144. Salach JI, Singer TP, Castagnoli N Jr, Trevor A. Oxidation of the neurotoxic amine 1-methyl-4-phenyl-1,2,3,6-tetrahydropyridine (MPTP) by monoamine oxidases A and B and suicide inactivation of the enzymes by MPTP. Biochem Biophys Res Commun 1984; 125(2):831–835.

145. Ferger B, Spratt C, Earl CD, et al. Effects of nicotine on hydroxyl free radical formation in vitro and on MPTP-induced neurotoxicity in vivo. Naunyn Schmiedebergs. Arch Pharmacol 1998; 358(3):351–359.

146. Pauly JR, Charriez CM, Guseva MC, et al. Nicotinic receptor modulation for neuroprotection and enhancement of functional recovery following brain injury or disease. Ann NY Acad Sci 2004; 1035:316–334.

147. Quik M, Kulak JM. Nicotine and nicotinic receptors; relevance to Parkinson's disease. Neurotoxicology 2002; 23(4–5):581–594.

148. Ascherio A, Zhang SM, Hernan MA, et al. Prospective study of caffeine consumption and risk of Parkinson's disease in men and women. Ann Neurol 2001; 50(1):56–63.

149. Paganini-Hill A. Risk factors for parkinson's disease: the leisure world cohort study. Neuroepidemiology 2001; 20(2):118–124.

150. Ascherio A, Chen H. Caffeinated clues from epidemiology of Parkinson's disease. Neurology 2003; 61(11 suppl 6):S51–4

151. Popoli P, Caporali MG, Scotti de Carolis A. Akinesia due to catecholamine depletion in mice is prevented by caffeine. Further evidence for an involvement of adenosinergic system in the control of motility. J Pharm Pharmacol 1991; 43(4):280–281.

152. Nehlig A, Daval JL, Debry G. Caffeine and the central nervous system: mechanisms of action, biochemical,metabolic and psychostimulant effects. Brain Res Brain Res Rev 1992; 17(2):139–170.

153. Kanda T, Tashiro T, Kuwana Y, Jenner P. Adenosine A2A receptors modify motor function in MPTP-treated common marmosets. Neuroreport 1998; 9(12):2857–2860.

154. Richardson PJ, Kase H, Jenner PG. Adenosine A2A receptor antagonists as new agents for the treatment of Parkinson's disease. Trends Pharmacol Sci 1997; 18(9):338–344.

155. Chen JF. The adenosine A(2A) receptor as an attractive target for Parkinson's disease treatment. Drug News Perspect 2003; 16(9):597–604.

156. Ragonese PG, Salemi G, Morgante L, et al. A case-control study on cigarette, alcohol, and coffee consumption preceding Parkinson's disease. Neuroepidemiology 2003; 22(5):297–304.

157. Willems-Giesenbergen P. Smoking, alcohol, and coffee consumption and the risk of PD: results from the Rotterdam study. Neurology 2000; 54:A347.

158. in t' Veld BA, Ruitenberg A, Hofman A, et al. Nonsteroidal antiinflammatory drugs and the risk of Alzheimer's disease. N Engl J Med 2001; 345(21):1515–1521.

159. McGeer PL, McGeer EG. The inflammatory response system of brain: implications for therapy of Alzheimer and other neurodegenerative diseases. Brain Res Brain Res Rev 1995; 21(2):195–218.

160. McGeer PL. Cyclo-oxygenase-2 inhibitors: rationale and therapeutic potential for Alzheimer's disease. Drugs Aging 2000; 17(1):1–11.

161. Stewart WF, Kawas C, Corrada M, Metter EJ. Risk of Alzheimer's disease and duration of NSAID use. Neurology 1997; 48(3):626–632.

162. Aubin N, Curet O, Deffois A, Carter C. Aspirin and salicylate protect against MPTP-induced dopamine depletion in mice. J Neurochem 1998; 71(4):1635–1642.

163. Ferger B, Teisman P, Earl CD, et al. Salicylate protects against MPTP-induced motor impairments in the dopaminergic neurotransmission at the striatal and nigral level in mice. Naunyn Schmiedebergs Arch Pharmacol 1999; 360(3):256–261.

164. Mohanakumar KP, Muralikrishnan D, Thomas B. Neuroprotection by sodium salicylate against 1-methyl-4-phenyl-1,2,3,6-tetrahydropyridine-induced neurotoxicity. Brain Res 2000; 864(2):281–290.

165. Teismann P, Ferger B. Inhibition of the cyclooxygenase isoenzymes COX-1 and COX-2 provide neuroprotection in the MPTP-mouse model of PD. Synapse 2001; 39(2): 167–174.

166. Chen H, Zhang SM, Hernan MA, et al. Nonsteroidal anti-inflammatory drugs and the risk of Parkinson disease. Arch Neurol 2003; 60(8):1059–1064.

4 Treatment of Parkinson's Disease

Stanley Fahn
Neurological Institute, Columbia University, New York, New York, U.S.A.

PRINCIPLES OF THERAPY OF PARKINSON'S DISEASE
Keep the Patient Functioning Independently as Long as Possible

A number of drugs have a favorable impact on the clinical features of Parkinson's disease (PD), by reducing its symptoms, but, to date, none have been proven to stop the progression of the disease. Since PD is a progressive disease, and since no medication prevents ultimate worsening, the long-term goal in treating PD is to keep the patient functioning independently for as long as possible. Clearly, if medications that provide symptomatic relief can continue to be effective without producing adverse effects, this would be excellent. For example, if levodopa therapy could persistently reverse parkinsonian signs and symptoms, no additional therapy would be needed. The difficulty is that 75% of patients have serious complications after six years of levodopa therapy (1), and younger patients (less than 60 years of age) are particularly prone to develop the motor complications of fluctuations and dyskinesias (2,3). When beginning therapy, some physicians therefore recommend using dopamine agonists rather than levodopa in younger patients, in an attempt to delay the onset of these problems (4,5). Controlled, clinical trials comparing dopamine agonists and levodopa as the initial therapeutic agent have proven that motor complications are less likely to occur with dopamine agonists (6,7,8). But each of these studies also showed that levodopa was more effective in improving parkinsonian symptoms and signs, as measured quantitatively by the Unified Parkinson's Disease Rating Scale (UPDRS).

Encourage Patients to Remain Active and Mobile

PD leads to decreased motivation and increased passivity. An active exercise program, even early in the disease, can often avoid this. Furthermore, such a program involves patients in their own care, allows muscle stretching and full range joint mobility, and enhances a better mental attitude toward fighting the disease. By encouraging the patient to take responsibility in fighting the devastations of the disease, the patient becomes an active participant. Physical therapy, which can be implemented in the form of a well-constructed exercise program, is useful in all stages of disease. Physical therapy forces the patient to become an activist in regards to his illness and helps him develop a positive commitment to battling the disease. For physical benefit, exercise aids the patient by stretching joints that tend to be utilized in PD with a reduced range of motion; it tones up muscles and builds up strength. In advanced stages of PD, physical therapy may be even more valuable by keeping joints from becoming frozen, and providing guidance how best to remain independent in mobility. It has been shown that PD patients who exercise regularly and intensively have better motor performance (9,10). If exercise is not maintained, the benefit is lost (11).

A number of basic science studies have discovered that exercise, particularly enriched exercise, can reduce the loss of dopaminergic neurons after 1-methyl-4-phenyl-1,2,3,6-tetrahydropyridine (MPTP) exposure. When such exercise was

53

initiated shortly after rodents were given experimental lesions of the nigrostriatal dopamine pathway, the result was significantly less damage to the dopamine pathway (12–18). The mechanism appears to be to the induction of increased trophic factors, such as glial-derived neurotrophic factor (GDNF) (19) and brain-derived neurotrophic factor (BDNF) (16).

Individualize Therapy

The treatment of PD needs to be individualized; each patient presents with a unique set of symptoms, signs, response to medications, and a host of social, occupational, and emotional problems that need to be addressed. As mentioned above, a major goal is to keep the patient functioning independently as long as possible. The practical guidelines for how to direct treatment are to consider the patient's symptoms, the degree of functional impairment, and the expected benefits and risks of available therapeutic agents. Ask the patient what specific symptoms trouble him the most. Also, keep in mind that younger patients are more likely to develop motor fluctuations and dyskinesias; older patients are more likely to develop confusion, sleep-wake alterations, and psychosis from medications.

NEUROPROTECTIVE THERAPY

If any drug could slow the progression of the disease process, it would make sense to use it as soon as the disease is diagnosed. No proven protective or restorative effect of a drug has been demonstrated with certainty. But, based on controlled, clinical trials, four drugs give some support in that they may offer neuroprotection, namely selegiline, coenzyme Q_{10}, rasagiline, and levodopa. Other studies in progress are looking at various agents to determine if they have such an effect.

The first controlled, clinical trial for the purpose of evaluating medications as neuroprotective agents was the DATATOP (deprenyl and tocopherol antioxidative therapy of parkinsonism) study (20). Deprenyl (now called selegiline) is an irreversible monoamine oxidase B (MAO-B) inhibitor and thus an antioxidant. Selegiline was tested along with the antioxidant, alpha-tocopherol (vitamin E), in a 2×2 design. Patients were enrolled in the study early in the course of the illness and did not require symptomatic therapy. The primary endpoint was the need for dopaminergic therapy. The study showed that tocopherol had no effect in delaying parkinsonian disability, but selegiline delayed symptomatic treatment by nine months (Fig. 1). It also reduced the rate of worsening of the UPDRS by half (Table 1).

Because the DATATOP study found that selegiline had a mild symptomatic effect that was long lasting, one could explain its ability to delay progression of disability entirely on this symptomatic effect. After the DATATOP study was concluded, many of the subjects now on levodopa therapy volunteered to be studied in a subsequent double-blind study (BLIND-DATE study) for 21 months and evaluated for the progression of clinical PD. The subjects were assigned to selegiline or matching placebo. The former group required a lower dosage of levodopa, had a slower rate of worsening of symptoms and signs of PD (Table 2), and had less freezing of gait than those assigned to placebo (Fig. 2) (21). These results support the view that selegiline does provide some neuroprotective effect. There is a likely possibility that this benefit is derived from an antiapoptotic effect rather than its antioxidative effect.

Rasagiline

Like selegiline, rasagiline is also a noncompetitive inhibitor of MAO-B. It was tested in a controlled clinical trial in patients with early PD not requiring symptomatic

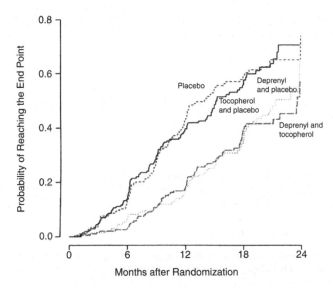

FIGURE 1 Kaplan-Meier curves of the cumulative probability of reaching the endpoint (need for dopaminergic therapy) in the DATATOP study. Subjects receiving selegiline (deprenyl) averaged about nine months longer before requiring dopaminergic therapy compared to placebo and alpha-tocopherol (which had the same outcome as placebo). *Abbreviation*: DATATOP, deprenyl and tocopherol antioxidative therapy of parkinsonism. *Source*: From Ref. 20.

TABLE 1 Average Annual Rate of Worsening of Unified Parkinson's Disease Rating Scale Scores in the Deprenyl and Tocopherol Antioxidative Therapy of Parkinsonism Study

Treatment	Total UPDRS
Placebo	14.02 ± 12.32
Tocopherol	15.16 ± 16.12
Selegiline	7.00 ± 10.76
Tocopherol and selegiline	7.28 ± 11.11
p Value between the selegiline groups and the placebo/tocopherol groups	<0.001

Note: Results are expressed as mean ± S.D.
Abbreviation: UPDRS, Unified Parkinson's Disease Rating Scale.
Source: From Ref. 20.

TABLE 2 Change in Total Unified Parkinson's Disease Rating Scale in the Blind-Date Study

Duration	Placebo	Selegiline	Difference
1 month	0.50 ± 7.73	-1.52 ± 7.54	2.02
3 months	1.57 ± 9.41	-0.85 ± 9.42	2.42
9 months	4.18 ± 10.12	1.63 ± 10.61	2.55
15 months	5.63 ± 10.73	0.46 ± 10.88	5.17
21 months	7.06 ± 12.70	1.51 ± 10.36	5.55

Note: The difference in progression of UPDRS was statistically significant ($p = 0.0002$). The placebo group required a larger increase in dosage of levodopa (181 ± 246, mean mg/day ± S.D.) than did the selegiline group (106 ± 205, mean mg/day ± S.D.) which was statistically significane ($p = 0.003$).
Source: From Ref. 21.

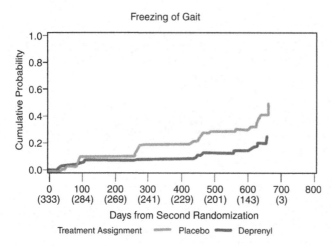

FIGURE 2 Kaplan-Meier curve showing development of freezing of gait in the treatment arms of selegiline or placebo in the presence of levodopa therapy. *Source*: From Ref. 21.

therapy for the purpose of determining an anti-PD effect. After six months of treatment, the placebo group was switched to 2 mg/day rasagiline for the next six months. Both groups were on active treatment with selegiline at the 12-month time point. Therefore each group was receiving identical symptomatic therapy at that time. The comparison between the two groups at that time showed that the group with the more prolonged treatment resulted in less progression of UPDRS scores (Fig. 3) (22). This result suggests that neuroprotection might be occurring with rasagiline treatment.

Coenzyme Q$_{10}$

Coenzyme Q$_{10}$ is the electron acceptor for mitochondrial complexes I and II and also a potent antioxidant. Complex I activity was found to be impaired by MPTP, and subsequently found to be selectively decreased in postmortem substantia nigral in patients with PD (23). Coenzyme Q$_{10}$ is reduced in the mitochondria (24) and in sera of patients with PD (25). Oral supplementation of coenzyme Q$_{10}$ in rats results in

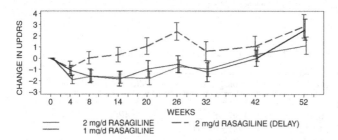

FIGURE 3 Rasagiline versus placebo therapy in untreated PD subject. Two dosages of rasagiline (1 mg/day and 2 mg/day) were evaluated. After six months, the placebo-treated group was given 2 mg/day of rasagiline. The results are expressed in the mean±SE change in total UPDRS for each treatment group, as indicated. *Abbreviation*: UPDRS, Unified Parkinson's Disease Rating Scale. *Source*: From Ref. 22.

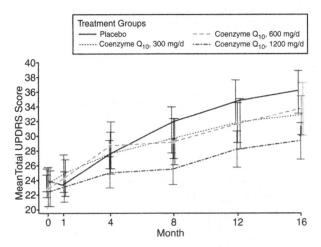

FIGURE 4 Change in total UPDRS with different dosages of coenzyme Q_{10}. *Abbreviation*: UPDRS, Unified Parkinson's Disease Rating Scale. *Source*: From Ref. 26.

increase of coenzyme Q_{10} in cerebral cortex mitochondria. A pilot trial of coenzyme Q_{10} has been carried out. Eighty patients with early PD were randomized into four equal arms and assigned 300, 600, 1200 mg/day, or placebo and followed up to 16 months (26). There was a positive trend ($p = 0.09$) for a linear trend between the dosage and the mean change in the total UPDRS score. The highest dose group (UPDRS change of +6.69) was statistically less than the UPDRS change of +11.99 for the placebo group (Fig. 4). The change in UPDRS for the lower doses showed no significant difference from the placebo group. There was slower decline in the change of all three components of the UPDRS scores in the 1200 mg/day group, with the greatest effect in Part II [the subjective Activities of Daily Living (ADL) component] (Fig. 5). This raises the question of whether patients on 1200 mg/day of coenzyme Q_{10} might simply feel better rather than have an objective improvement of their motoric features of PD. After one month of treatment, there was improvement of the Part II UPDRS (ADL) score in the 1200 mg/day group of –0.66, compared to worsening in the placebo group of +0.52. This wash-in effect supports the concern that there might be a "feel good" effect from coenzyme Q_{10} rather than a neuroprotective effect. Another secondary outcome was the need for dopaminergic therapy; there was no significant difference between active drug and placebo. The study investigators urged caution in interpretation of the results until a larger study could be conducted and evaluated.

Levodopa as a Neuroprotective Agent
The levodopa may also have neuroprotective properties in addition to its well-known symptomatic effects came to light in the ELLDOPA study (27). This topic and the results of that study are discussed below when levodopa therapy is reviewed.

TREATMENT OF PARKINSON'S DISEASE BY SEVERITY OF SYMPTOMS

Before discussing levodopa therapy, it should be mentioned that the type of treatment depends in large part upon the severity of the disease facing the patient. The earliest

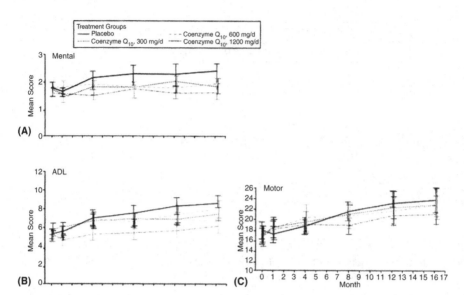

FIGURE 5   Change in the different components (**A**) mental, (**B**) ADL, and (**C**) motor of the Unified Parkinson's Disease Rating Scale with coenzyme Q_{10}. *Abbreviation*: ADL, activities of daily living. *Source*: From Ref. 26.

stage of PD begins when the symptoms are first noticed and the diagnosis is made. The designation of "early stage" lasts until the symptoms begin to become troublesome to the patient, and intervention with symptomatic medications is needed. All symptomatic drugs can induce side effects, and if a patient is not troubled by mild symptoms socially or occupationally, the introduction of these drugs can be delayed until symptoms become more pronounced. The clinician needs to discuss this choice with the patient and his/her family. Most neurologists do not use levodopa or other potent antiparkinson agents when the diagnosis is first established and the disease presents with no threat to physical, social, or occupational activities (28). Because symptomatically beneficial medications are not needed, patients in the early, recently diagnosed stage of PD are excellent candidates for participating in a clinical trial in which a placebo is one of the treatment arms. Another elective option is to use one of the drugs described in the previous section, which have demonstrated hints of neuroprotection in controlled clinical trials.

The mild stage of PD is when the signs and symptoms of the illness are beginning to interfere with daily activities or with quality of life. The judgment to initiate symptomatic drug therapy is made in discussions between the patient and the treating physician. According to a survey (29), the most common problems that clinicians consider important in the decision to initiate symptomatic agents are (*i*) threat to employability, (*ii*) threat to ability to handle domestic, financial, or social affairs, (*iii*) threat to handle activities of daily living, and (*iv*) appreciable worsening of gait or balance. The choice of drugs is wide, but the degree of disability and the age (or mental acuity) of the patient are two critical factors. If the delay in initiating symptomatic treatment was so prolonged that the symptoms now threaten employment or endanger falling, one needs to begin levodopa in order to get a quick response. The advantages of using levodopa when the symptoms are this pronounced, in preference to a dopamine agonist or other medications, are that a therapeutic response is both rapid and virtually guaranteed, because nearly all patients with PD will respond to levodopa relatively quickly. In contrast, only a minority of patients with severe symptoms will benefit sufficiently from a dopamine agonist given alone, and it takes more time (often months) to build up the dose to adequate levels to discover this. If levodopa is to be utilized, inhibitors of MAO-A must be discontinued. If selegiline (or another selective MAO-B inhibitor) were the MAO-I utilized, this drug can be continued.

If the symptoms are not severe enough to require levodopa and the patient is younger than 60 years (younger than 70 if the patient is mentally young), employing a dopa-sparing strategy is a common approach in order to avoid for as long as possible the development of levodopa-induced dyskinesias and motor fluctuations (mainly the "wearing-off" effect). These complications are more likely to occur in younger patients (2,3). The choices are dopamine agonists, amantadine, and anticholinergics. Dopamine agonists are the most potent antiparkinsonian agent among this group of drugs. Controlled trials comparing levodopa with dopamine agonists (pramipexole, ropinirole, and pergolide) consistently revealed that levodopa is more potent in reducing UPDRS scores (Fig. 6), but it is also the drug most likely to induce dyskinesias and motor fluctuations (Fig. 7) (30).

For patients older than 70 years or those with any cognitive decline, employ levodopa therapy. Not only is there less need for a dopa-sparing strategy in these elderly patients, they are more susceptible to confusion, psychosis, or drowsiness from other antiparkinson drugs, including dopamine agonists. Levodopa provides the greatest benefit at the lowest risk of these adverse effects, compared to the others.

Adverse effects that are more common with dopamine agonists than levodopa are orthostatic hypotension, nausea (because nausea from levodopa is blocked by carbidopa), drowsiness, hallucinations, and leg edema. All agonists have a propensity to produce ankle and leg edema (31), which is not an early problem, but tends to occur after a few years of treatment. The edematous skin is often red, and some clinicians, unaware of this adverse effect, assume that there is a deep vein thrombosis. The edema and redness persist unless the drug is stopped. Diuretics are usually not effective in relieving the edema. Pramipexole and ropinirole appear more readily to produce drowsiness and sleep attacks where patients fall asleep without warning, including while driving, although there have now been rare incidences of sleep

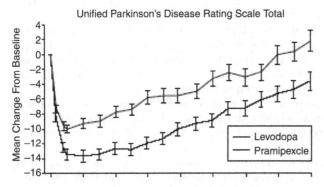

FIGURE 6 Mean and standard error of change in total Unified Parkinson's Disease Rating Scale with pramipexole (*upper curve*) and levodopa (*lower curve*) treatment arms. *Source*: From Ref. 30.

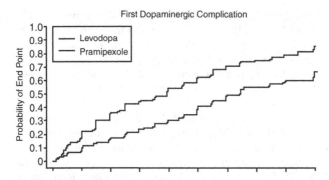

FIGURE 7 Cumulative probability of reaching the first dopaminergic complication of dyskinesia or wearing off with pramipexole (lower curve) and levodopa (upper curve) treatment arms. *Source*: From Ref. 30.

attacks with all dopamine agonists and levodopa (32–34). The Epworth Sleepiness Scale is not predictive as to which patient may develop a sleep attack (35).

LEVODOPA THERAPY FOR PARKINSON'S DISEASE
Historical Introduction
Following the discovery of striatal dopamine deficiency in PD (36,37), Birkmayer and Hornykiewicz (38) injected small doses of levodopa (up to 150 mg) intravenously and reported a transient reversal of akinesia. Levodopa was previously shown by Carlsson et al. (39) to reverse reserpine-induced parkinsonism in rabbits. Barbeau et al. (40) also reported benefit with small oral doses of levodopa (200 mg). Subsequently, many other investigators using small oral or intravenous doses reported similar results in very brief communications (41–45). However, not every investigator reported benefit from such small doses of levodopa. Greer and Williams (46) failed to find benefit in two patients after 1 gm of D, L-dopa orally. Aebert (47) saw no benefit after 70 to 100 mg L-dopa intravenously, nor did Rinaldi et al. (48) even with inhibition of MAO. Double-blind trials with low-dosage levodopa also failed to provide benefit (49,50) using up to 1.5 mg/kg of intravenous levodopa. McGeer and Zeldowicz (51) were the first to use high doses of D, L-dopa that were later found to be successful by Cotzias et al. (52). They used up to 5 gm/day in 10 patients for several days, and in one patient, 3 gm daily for two years, but only two patients showed any objective improvement.

The breakthrough in establishing levodopa as a therapeutically useful drug was the report of Cotzias et al. (52). They treated 16 patients with doses of D, L-dopa of 3–16 gm/day, building the dosage up slowly to avoid anorexia, nausea, and vomiting, which had been dose-limiting complications with previous investigators. They reported marked improvement in eight patients and less improvement in two others. Of the eight who received 12 gm or more per day, seven showed marked benefit. Granulocytopenia was seen in four patients, and bone marrow examination revealed vacuoles in the myeloid cells in four of the 12 patients with bone marrow examinations.

Because of the hematologic problems and because D-dopa is not metabolized to form dopamine, Cotzias et al. subsequently used L-dopa, and these problems were no longer encountered. The first double-blind study with high dosage levodopa was carried out by Yahr et al. (54). Many subsequent reports showed significant improvement in approximately 75% of patients with parkinsonism. Although a complete remission is rarely obtained, akinesia and rigidity were generally most benefited, and many who had been unable to turn in bed or arise from a chair became able to do so. Tremor has a more variable response; sometimes it is eliminated by levodopa, and in other patients, the tremor is resistant. A number of other symptoms, including postural instability and speech disturbance, are typically unaffected by levodopa therapy, suggesting that these symptoms are not solely due to dopamine deficiency. The introduction of levodopa therapy by Cotzias was a revolutionary treatment for PD, not just an evolutionary one.

The development of inhibitors of L-aromatic amino acid decarboxylase that do not cross the blood-brain barrier was the next major step. Carbidopa and benserazide are such peripheral decarboxylase inhibitors. When given with levodopa, they allow for a four-fold increase in the effectiveness of a given dose because peripheral metabolism to dopamine was blocked. More importantly, these agents block the gastrointestinal side effects, which were due to peripheral dopamine acting upon the vomiting center of the area postrema, which is not protected by the blood-brain barrier. The combination of levodopa with carbidopa was commercially marketed under the trade name of Sinemet®, to indicate without ("sine") emesis. Sinemet (carbidopa/levodopa) is sold in 10/100, 25/100, and 25/250 mg strengths. Many patients require at least 50–75 mg of carbidopa a day to have adequate inhibition of peripheral dopa decarboxylase. If the dose of levodopa is less than 300 mg/day, one should use the 25/100 mg strength tablets and not the 10/100 mg tablets. In some patients even 75 mg/day of carbidopa is inadequate, and nausea, anorexia, or vomiting still occur. In such patients, one needs to use higher doses of carbidopa, which are available under the trade name of Lodosyn®. The combination of benserazide and levodopa is marketed under the brand name of Madopar®.

The other enzyme that metabolizes levodopa is catechol-O-methyltransferase (COMT), and two inhibitors of this enzyme have also become available, namely tolcapone and entacapone. These COMT inhibitors delay the peripheral decay of levodopa plasma levels, allowing a slightly longer half-life. An enzyme that metabolizes dopamine centrally and peripherally is MAO, which comes in two genetically distinct forms, known as MAO-A and MAO-B. Inhibition of the A type makes patients susceptible to dietary tyramine, and can trigger hyper- and hypotensive episodes if levodopa is taken with MAO-A inhibitors. But inhibition of MAO-B alone does not create this hazard, commonly known as the cheese-effect because of the presence of high levels of tyramine in some fermenting cheeses. Inhibitors of MAO-B can be taken safely with levodopa, which potentiate the symptomatic benefit of levodopa by about one-third. Two such MAO-B inhibitors are now commercially available, selegiline (formerly called deprenyl) and rasagiline.

Drugs that act directly on the dopamine receptor have also been developed. None are as powerful as levodopa, except possibly apomorphine, which is administered parenterally and easily induces nausea and vomiting, and which has a very short half-life. However, a number of orally active dopamine agonists have received considerable use in the treatment of PD, because their side effect profile is different from that of levodopa's.

To provide a longer plasma half-life of levodopa, delayed-release formulations have been developed. One product is Sinement CR (for continuous release); another is Madopar hydrodynamically balanced system (HBS). As seen in the early days of levodopa therapy, this drug is now known not to have an immediate antiparkinsonian effect. It takes several days to weeks of high dosage therapy to achieve the desired degree of benefit. Once a patient has been primed, though, then restarting levodopa after a withdrawal period brings on the benefit almost immediately.

Clinical Benefit from Levodopa Therapy

Levodopa remains today the most powerful drug available to treat PD. In fact, the absence of a robust response to high-dose levodopa essentially excludes the diagnosis of PD and suggests that there must be another explanation for the parkinsonian symptoms. In contrast, a marked and sustained response strongly supports the diagnosis of PD (55). Although numerous other treatment options are available in early PD when the disease is mild, virtually all patients will eventually require levodopa therapy as the disease worsens.

However, as mentioned above, not all symptoms of PD are equally responsive to levodopa. Bradykinesia and rigidity generally show the most dramatic improvement with dopaminergic therapy. In fact, the presence of residual rigidity is a good means by which to determine if a patient would further improve by increasing the dose. Tremor has a more variable (and often incomplete) response to levodopa. A number of other symptoms, including postural instability, micrographia, and speech disturbance, are typically poorly responsive to dopaminergic therapy; suggesting they are likely due to deficits in other neurotransmitter systems. Recognition of the differential responsiveness of these symptoms to levodopa is critical for setting realistic treatment goals.

Early in the course of disease, levodopa provides a long-duration response that can last several days even if levodopa is discontinued. This continuous response occurs in the presence of a short plasma half-life of a little more than 30 minutes (56,57).

Problems with Levodopa Therapy

As PD worsens or with long-term usage of levodopa, more serious and persistent complications, such as "wearing off" fluctuations and dyskinesias (abnormal involuntary movements) emerge; these motor complications affect 75% of patients after six years of levodopa therapy (1). These problems markedly impair the quality of life and functional status of affected patients and prove challenging not only for the patient but also for the treating physician. Today, these motor complications, especially clinical fluctuations and dyskinesias, have limited the usefulness of levodopa.

The initial paper by Cotzias et al. (52) describing the successful use of high dosage D, L-dopa in patients with PD did not mention motor complications. The adverse effects mentioned were predominantly anorexia, nausea, vomiting, faintness, and hematologic changes. Cotzias et al. (53) then substituted levodopa for D, L-dopa, which eliminated the hematologic adverse effects. This paper also presents the first report of levodopa-induced dyskinesias, as well as mental symptoms of irritability, anger, hostility, paranoia, insomnia, and an awakening effect. The dyskinesias described were chorea, myoclonus, hemiballism (ipsilateral to the side of a prior thalamotomy), and dystonia. These investigators noted that the adverse effects would subside with a lowering of the dosage of levodopa. They also reported that the appearance of dyskinesias is not an early occurrence after initiating levodopa therapy. Dyskinesias were not seen during the first three weeks of treatment, but occurred later on.

The next paper reporting on the use of levodopa was by Yahr et al. (54). In their 60 patients, gastrointestinal adverse effects were encountered in 51, dyskinesias in

37, hypotension in 14, cardiac abnormalities in 13, and psychiatric symptoms in 10. By 1970, McDowell et al. and Schwarz and Fahn (58,59) reported that dyskinesias were as common as gastrointestinal side effects. They noted that the gastrointestinal effects could often be avoided by building up the dose of levodopa very slowly and that patients would often build up tolerance, with the result that few patients would have persistent gastrointestinal difficulties. On the other hand, dyskinesias, although occurring later, would persist and increase, becoming more prominent with continuing treatment. By 1971, dyskinesias were noted to be the most common dose-limiting adverse effect (60). The abnormal movements were seen in all parts of the body and most often were choreic in nature.

The first review article on levodopa-induced dyskinesias was presented by Duvoisin (61), based on an analysis of levodopa therapy in 116 patients with PD. He found that by six months of treatment, 53% of patients had developed dyskinesias; by 12 months, 81% had. Although described earlier by Cotzias, myoclonic jerking in patients with PD, especially as a toxic reaction to levodopa, was further elaborated by Klawans et al. (62).

Besides dyskinesias, the treating physician began to become more aware of motor fluctuations, especially as the return of parkinsonian symptoms during these episodes was more prominent due to the underlying worsening of the disease. Various terms were coined to label these fluctuations. "On-off" was coined in 1974 to describe a sudden loss of levodopa's benefit and replacement with the parkinsonian state (the "off" state) (63–66). The speed of this change was likened to that of a light switch turning on and off. The "on" state was equated with the time when the patient was having a good response from levodopa; the re-emergence of the "on" state was sometimes sudden, even without the benefit of another dose of levodopa. But the "on" state would often not appear until another dose of levodopa was ingested. The more common gradual development of the "off" state, taking many minutes to develop and appearing as the plasma levels of levodopa had fallen, was labeled in 1976 as the "wearing-off" phenomenon (67) and also the "end-of-dose" deterioration (68). Both of these terms refer to the identical clinical situation and have been used interchangeably since.

A new dyskinetic state related to the timing of levodopa dosing was described in 1977. Up to this point, all dyskinesias were considered to occur at the peak effect of the levodopa dose. Muenter et al. (69) described dyskinesias appearing at the beginning and at the end of the dose, which they called "D-I-D" for dystonia (dyskinesia)-improvement-dystonia (dyskinesia). These workers contrasted this to the much more common peak-dose dyskinesia, labeled by Muenter as "I-D-I." Subsequently, the D-I-D phenomena have been labeled diphasic dyskinesias (70,71).

Not all dyskinesias appear at the peak, the beginning, or the end of the dose. Melamed (72) described painful dystonia occurring in the foot early in the morning, when the effect of the previous night's dose of levodopa has completely worn off. This is a dyskinesia, appearing as a dystonia, that occurs during the "off" state, a time when bradykinesia and other signs of the parkinsonian state would be manifested. Instead, the "off" state dystonia is seen in place of parkinsonism. Early morning dystonia is the most common type of "off" dystonia, but these tight, cramped muscles can appear at other times of the day when the medication wears off.

In addition to the motor offs, a phenomenon known as "sensory offs" or equivalently "behavioral offs" is now recognized. These sensory and behavioral phenomena may accompany a motor (parkinsonian) "off" or be present as an "off"

TABLE 3   Major Fluctuations and Dyskinesias as Complications of Levodopa

Fluctuations ("offs")	Dyskinesias	Sensory and behavioral "offs"
Slow "wearing off"	Peak-dose chorea,	Pain
Sudden "off"	ballism, and dystonia	Akathisia
	Diphasic chorea and dystonia	Depression
Random "off"		Anxiety
Yo-yo-ing	*"Off" dystonia*	Dysphoria
Episodic failure to respond	Myoclonus	Panic
Delayed "on"	Simultaneous dyskinesia	
Weak response at end of day	and parkinsonism	
Response varies in		
relationship to meals		
Sudden transient freezing		

in the absence of much parkinsonian signs. Sensory "offs" can consist of pain, akathisia, depression, anxiety, dysphoria, or panic, and usually a mixture of more than one of these. Sensory "offs," like dystonic "offs," are extremely poorly tolerated. It is often the presence of one of these sensory and behavioral phenomena—more so than parkinsonian or dystonic "offs"—which drives the patient to take more and more levodopa, turning them into "levodopa junkies."

Levodopa-related motor and sensory complications can be subdivided according to the clinical phenomena that occur (Table 3). They can also be classified according to their temporal relationship with levodopa dosing. The latter approach is useful when discussing the treatment of motor complications (see below).

There is usually a pattern of progressively worsening response fluctuations in patients who are on chronic levodopa therapy (Table 4). Response fluctuations usually begin as mild wearing-off (end-of-dose failure). Wearing-off can be defined

TABLE 4   Temporal Development of Response Fluctuations and Dyskinesias

Dyskinesias	Myoclonus
Peak-dose dyskinesias	Myoclonic jerks during sleep
Diphasic dyskinesias	Myoclonic jerks while awake
Chorea → dystonia	Behavioral and cognitive
Yo-yo-ing	Vivid dreams
Fluctuations	Benign hallucinations
Mild wearing-off	Malignant hallucinations
Deeper wearing-off; shorter time "on"	Delusions
Delayed "ons"	Paranoia
Dose failures	Confusion
Sudden, unpredictable "offs" (on-offs)	Dementia
Early morning dystonia	Sensory offs
Off dystonia during day	Pain
Somatotopic response (e.g., dyskinetic in	Akathisia
neck, off in legs)	Depression
Freezing phenomenon	Anxiety
Freezing when "off"	Dysphoria
Freezing when "on"	Panic
Alertness	
Drowsy from a dose of levodopa	
Reverse sleep-wake cycle	

to be present when an adequate dosage of levodopa does not last at least four hours. Typically, in the first couple of years of treatment, there is a long-duration response (56). As the disease progresses or as levodopa treatment continues, the long-duration response fades, and the short-duration response becomes predominant, leading to the wearing-off effect.

The "offs" tend to be mild at first, but over time often become deeper with more severe parkinsonism; simultaneously, the duration of the "on" response becomes shorter. Eventually, many patients develop sudden "offs" in which the deep state of parkinsonism develops over minutes rather than tens of minutes, and they are less predictable in terms of timing with the dosings of levodopa. Many patients who develop response fluctuations also develop abnormal involuntary movements, that is, dyskinesias.

A number of investigators have found that the major risk factors for motor complications are the duration (73,74) or dosage (27,75) of levodopa therapy. Several studies have also shown that using dopamine agonists is much less likely to induce these motor complications, therefore using them initially to treat PD symptoms rather than levodopa can delay the start of the "wearing off" and dyskinesias effects (76–78). In a double-blind, direct comparison of starting with levodopa or the dopamine agonists pramipexole and ropinirolr, the CALM-PD and 056 trials, respectively, also showed that levodopa was statistically more likely than these agonists to induce both motor fluctuations and dyskinesias (6,7,30).

The mechanism by which levodopa induces these motor complications is not understood. A current hypothesis is that these may be a function of the higher potency and shorter half-life of levodopa as compared to dopamine agonists. Since the development of motor complications relates, in part, to the dose (27), it is probably best to use the lowest dose of levodopa possible to achieve adequate clinical benefit. In light of concerns that pulsatile administration of levodopa may contribute to the development of motor complications (79–81), there is some rationale for the initial use of extended-release levodopa preparations or COMT inhibitors to extend the half-life of levodopa. Unfortunately, clinical trials of early use of regular (Sinemet) versus long-acting (Sinemet CR) carbidopa/levodopa failed to show differences in the rate of development of motor fluctuations in the two treatment groups (82–85). There are as yet no clinical trials to determine whether the early use of COMT inhibitors will delay motor complications.

Is Levodopa Neurotoxic or Neuroprotective?

One of the most controversial questions regarding the treatment of PD is whether levodopa is neurotoxic. The results of many in vitro studies have suggested that levodopa may be injurious to dopaminergic neurons (86,87). These findings have raised concerns that chronic levodopa exposure might hasten disease progression in PD patients. Accordingly, some physicians and patients have opted to defer the use of levodopa for as long as possible (28). Other physicians have continued to use levodopa as first-line therapy, arguing that in the absence of clinical evidence of toxicity (88–90), it is inappropriate to withhold the most potent symptomatic treatment for PDO.

Until very recently, there was little clinical data to support or refute the possibility of levodopa toxicity. In 2002, however, two studies were published in which functional neuroimaging techniques had been used to compare patients initially treated with pramipexole versus levodopa comparison of the agonist pramipexole with levopoda on motor complications of Parkinson's disease study

(CALM-PD study) or ropinirole versus levodopa ropinirole evaluated against levopoda with positron emission tomography (REAL-PET study) respectively. The CALM-PD trial used single-photon emission computerized tomography (SPECT) to look at striatal dopamine transporter (DAT) activity [123]iodine 2-β-carboxymethoxy-3-β-(4-iodophenyl) tropane (β-CIT uptake) as a marker for intact axons of nigrostriatal dopaminergic neurons. This four-year trial showed a more rapid rate of decline of β-CIT uptake in the group assigned to early levodopa compared with early pramipexole treatment (91). A similar result was found in the REAL-PET trial, which used positron emission tomography (PET) to look at putaminal ^{18}F accumulation (due to ^{18}F-DOPA uptake and decarboxylation) as a marker for functional dopaminergic terminals. This two-year study showed a more rapid rate of reduction of ^{18}F accumulation in patients who were initially treated with levodopa versus ropinirole (92). Since there was no placebo group in either study, the findings of the two studies could be interpreted to show that dopamine agonists slow the progression of PD or levodopa hastens the progression of PD, or both. They also raise the question of whether levodopa or dopamine agonists have direct pharmacologic effects on DAT or L-aromatic amino acid (dopa) decarboxylase that might confound the interpretation of these results. Thus, caution must be taken in interpreting these and other studies that use imaging markers to document "neuroprotection" (93–95).

Because of ongoing controversy about whether levodopa is toxic, a large, multicenter, randomized, controlled clinical trial comparing three different doses of levodopa with placebo treatment in patients with early PD (the ELLDOPA study) was designed to answer this question (27). This was a double-blind, placebo-controlled, parallel group, multicenter trial of patients with early PD who had not been previously treated with symptomatic therapy. A total of 361 patients were enrolled, and were randomized to receive treatment with either low- (150 mg/day), middle- (300 mg/day), or high-dosage (600 mg/day) levodopa, or placebo. After 40 weeks of treatment, the patients underwent a three-day taper of their medications, followed by a two-week washout period during which they received no treatment for their PD. The primary outcome measure was the change in the total UPDRS score between baseline and after the washout period at week 42. The goal of this study was to determine whether levodopa treatment affects the rate of progression of PD.

At the end of the two-week washout period, the UPDRS scores of patients treated with all three doses of levodopa were lower (better) than those of the placebo-treated group, in a dose–response pattern (Fig. 8). These findings suggest that levodopa is not neurotoxic, and may even be neuroprotective, though the possibility that patients were experiencing a longer duration of symptomatic response to levodopa that had extended beyond the two-week washout period could not be excluded. The highest dosage of levodopa was, however, associated with a higher incidence of motor complications, including dyskinesias and a trend to develop the "wearing-off" phenomenon. The ELLDOPA study publication provides a listing of the different adverse events from different dosages of levodopa as well as placebo.

In addition to the clinical data, a subset of patients in the ELLDOPA trial was also evaluated with β-CIT SPECT imaging, which (as in the CALM-PD trial) was used as a marker for intact nigrostriatal dopaminergic neurons by labeling the DAT. These neuroimaging studies showed that there was a larger decrease in striatal DAT binding in patients treated with levodopa, in a dose-response pattern (Fig. 9). Thus, in contrast with the clinical data, the imaging findings suggested that levodopa might hasten the progression of PD. As with other neuroimaging studies, however,

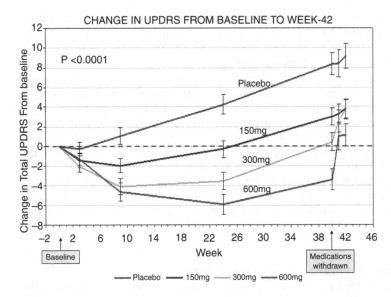

FIGURE 8   Change in total UPDRS with different dosages of levodopa treatment until week 40, followed by a two-week washout until week 42. *Abbreviation*: UPDRS, Unified Parkinson's Disease Rating Scale. *Source*: From Ref. 27.

it is possible that the observed changes in the levels of uptake of this marker reflected a pharmacologic effect of levodopa on DAT activity, rather than evidence of injury to dopaminergic neurons.

Thus, intriguing as the results of the ELLDOPA study are, it remains unclear whether levodopa may, either positively or negatively, affect the natural history of PD. Given the evidence from the ELLDOPA study that the dosage of levodopa is

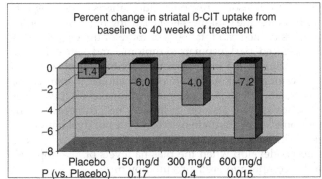

P (dose-response) = 0.036

FIGURE 9   Change in striatal beta-CIT binding from baseline to week-40 while receiving levodopa. *Abbreviations*: SPECT, single photon emission computerized tomography; CIT, carboxymethoxy-3-β-(4-iodophenyl) tropane. *Source*: From Ref. 27.

important in the development of motor complications, it is reasonable to customize the dose of levodopa to fit the specific needs of each patient.

Levodopa in Patients with a History of Melanoma
Levodopa is an intermediary metabolite in the synthesis of melanin. For this reason, there has been long-standing concern that this medication might potentially promote the growth of melanoma. While melanoma obviously occurs in patients on levodopa therapy, there is no evidence that the incidence differs from that in the general population (96–99), other than that there seems to be a higher risk for melanoma in patients with PD, even without levodopa treatment (100). In studies of patients with melanoma, levodopa exposure is rare (101). Thus, although the package insert warns that levodopa should not be used in patients with melanoma or suspicious skin lesions (102–105), there is no clinical evidence to support this admonition (106–109). Nonetheless, in patients with PD and a history of melanoma, it would seem prudent to both defer levodopa therapy until other medications prove inadequate and to monitor closely for recurrent melanoma.

Summary of Clinical Phases of Levodopa Therapy
One can usually discern four clinical phases of PD in relation to treatment with levodopa.

Phase 1—Honeymoon Period
When levodopa is first introduced, there is a "long-duration response" from each dose, with few motoric complications. This is the initial period of maximum benefit without adverse motor effects. The duration of this phase varies, but usually lasts two to three years.

Phase 2—Motoric Complication Period
With continuing treatment, the duration of beneficial response gradually shortens in almost all patients (56), who then need to take levodopa more frequently during the day to minimize the duration of the "off" (relatively immobile) periods; in addition, patients often develop dyskinesias at peak plasma levels of levodopa parallel to the timing of their doses. After approximately five years of levodopa therapy, 75% of patients have either developed troublesome response fluctuations ("wearing-off" and "on-off" phenomena) or troublesome dyskinesias (1). During the "wearing-off," dose-failures, and "on-off" states (which can total 50% or more of the waking day), there is disability with pronounced parkinsonian symptoms and signs, leaving patients immobile or akinetic for hours at a time, sometimes with painful sustained contractions, known as "off" dystonia. Dyskinesias are usually choreic in nature, and classically show a temporal correlation with peak plasma levodopa levels (peak-dose dyskinesias). Peak-dose dyskinesias may also be dystonic ("on" dystonia). Some patients, particularly younger ones, may alternate between states of dyskinesia and "off," with little normal periods in between, a state referred to as "yo-yo-ing" (70,71). Sometimes, diphasic dyskinesias develop when the plasma levels of levodopa are low (69); the mechanism of this complication remains unknown.

Whether the motor complications seen with chronic levodopa therapy in PD patients are actually caused by long-term levodopa therapy or simply reflect the progression of the disease is unknown and widely debated (2,74,110–113). The ELLDOPA study showed that dyskinesias are more common with higher doses of levodopa (27).

Phase 3—Period of Progression and Drug-Resistant Parkinsonism

Also, after two to three years of levodopa therapy, the degree of benefit begins to fade, and the signs and symptoms of parkinsonism increasingly recur. By five years of levodopa treatment, the clinical severity of PD, even while on levodopa, has been shown to reach the level it was prior to initiating levodopa, and the severity steadily continues to increase with time (7,114,115). Thus, levodopa therapy can be considered to set back the signs and symptoms by about five years. Beyond this time period, there is development of new symptoms that are resistant to treatment: loss of postural reflexes, falling, freezing, dysphonia, dysarthria, and flexed posture.

Phase 4—Dementia Period

The development of dementia in patients with PD is a most ominous sign, for there is no satisfactory reversal of this feature. Besides causing great physical and emotional stress for the caregivers, the presence of dementia often leads to nursing home placement. The leading cause patients with PD are admitted to nursing homes is the presence of hallucinations (116), which occur commonly in demented PD patients receiving anti-PD medications. The presence of dementia greatly limits the amount of levodopa the patient can tolerate because confusion and hallucinations are easily induced as the dosage of levodopa is increased. Atypical antipsychotics, such as clozapine and quetiapine, can ease the hallucinations.

REFERENCES

1. Fahn S. Adverse effects of levodopa. In: Olanow CW, Lieberman AN, eds. The Scientific Basis for the Treatment of Parkinson's Disease. Carnforth, England: Parthenon Publishing Group, 1992:89–112.
2. Quinn N, Critchley P, Marsden CD. Young onset Parkinson's disease. Mov Disord 1987; 2:73–91.
3. Kostic V, Przedborski S, Flaster E, Sternic N. Early development of levodopa-induced dyskinesias and response fluctuations in young-onset Parkinson's disease. Neurology 1991; 41:202–205.
4. Quinn NP. A case against early levodopa treatment of Parkinson's disease. Clin Neuropharmacol 1994; 17:S43–S49.
5. Fahn S. Medical treatment of Parkinson's disease. J Neurol 1998; 245:P15–P24.
6. Rascol O, Brooks DJ, Korczyn AD, et al. A five-year study of the incidence of dyskinesia in patients with early Parkinson's disease who were treated with ropinirole or levodopa. 056 Study Group. N Engl J Med 2000; 342(20):1484–1491.
7. Parkinson Study Group. Pramipexole versus levodopa as the initial treatment for Parkinson's disease: a randomized controlled trial. JAMA 2000; 284:1931–1938.
8. Oertel WH, Wolters E, Sampaio C, et al. Pergolide versus levodopa monotherapy in early Parkinson's disease patients: The PELMOPET study. Mov Disord 2005 [Epub ahead of print].
9. Reuter I, Engelhardt M, Stecker K, Baas H. Therapeutic value of exercise training in Parkinson's disease. Med Sci Sport Exercise 1999; 31:1544–1549.
10. Behrman AL, Cauraugh JH, Light KE. Practice as an intervention to improve speeded motor performance and motor learning in Parkinson's disease. J Neurol Sci 2000; 174:127–136.
11. Lokk J. The effects of mountain exercise in Parkinsonian persons—a preliminary study. Arch Gerontol Geriatr 2000; 31:19–25.
12. Tillerson JL, Cohen AD, Philhower J, Miller GW, Zigmond MJ, Schallert T. Forced limb-use effects on the behavioral and neurochemical effects of 6-hydroxydopamine. J Neurosci 2001; 21(12):4427–4435.
13. Tillerson JL, Cohen AD, Caudle WM, Zigmond MJ, Schallert T, Miller GW. Forced nonuse in unilateral parkinsonian rats exacerbates injury. J Neurosci 2002 ; 22(15):6790–6799.

14. Tillerson JL, Caudle WM, Reveron ME, Miller GW. Exercise induces behavioral recovery and attenuates neurochemical deficits in rodent models of Parkinson's disease. Neuroscience 2003; 119(3):899–911.
15. Cohen AD, Tillerson JL, Smith AD, Schallert T, Zigmond MJ. Neuroprotective effects of prior limb use in 6-hydroxydopamine-treated rats: possible role of GDNF. J Neurochem 2003; 85(2):299–305.
16. Bezard E, Dovero S, Belin D, et al. Enriched environment confers resistance to 1-methyl-4-phenyl-1,2,3,6-tetrahydropyridine and cocaine: involvement of dopamine transporter and trophic factors. J Neurosci 2003; 23(35):10999–11007.
17. Mabandla M, Kellaway L, Gibson AS, Russell VA. Voluntary running provides neuroprotection in rats after 6-hydroxydopamine injection into the medial forebrain bundle. Metab Brain Dis 2004; 19(1–2):43–50.
18. Fisher BE, Petzinger GM, Nixon K, et al. Exercise-induced behavioral recovery and neuroplasticity in the 1-methyl-4-phenyl-1,2,3,6-tetrahydropyridine-lesioned mouse basal ganglia. J Neurosci Res 2004; 77(3):378–390.
19. Smith AD, Zigmond MJ. Can the brain be protected through exercise? Lessons from an animal model of parkinsonism. Exp Neurol 2003; 184(1):31–39.
20. Parkinson Study Group. Effects of tocopherol and deprenyl on the progression of disability in early parkinson's disease. N Engl J Med 1993; 328:176–183.
21. Shoulson I, Oakes D, Fahn S, et al. Impact of sustained deprenyl (selegiline) in levodopa-treated Parkinson's disease: a randomized placebo-controlled extension of the deprenyl and tocopherol antioxidative therapy of parkinsonism trial. Ann Neurol 2002; 51:604–612.
22. Parkinson Study Group. A controlled, randomized, delayed-start study of rasagiline in early Parkinson disease. Arch Neurol 2004; 61(4):561–566.
23. Schapira AH, Mann VM, Cooper JM, et al. Anatomic and disease specificity of NADH CoQ1 reductase (complex I) deficiency in Parkinson's disease. J Neurochem 1990; 55:2142–2145.
24. Shults CW, Haas RH, Passov D, Beal MF. Coenzyme Q(10) levels correlate with the activities of complexes I and II/III in mitochondria from parkinsonian and nonparkinsonian subjects. Ann Neurol 1997; 42:261–264.
25. Matsubara T, Azuma T, Yoshida S, Yamagami T. Serum coenzyme Q_{10} level in Parkinson syndrome. In: Folkers K, Littarru GP, Yamagami T, eds. Biomedical and Clinical Aspects of Coenzyme Q_{10}. New York: Elsevier Science Publishers, 1991:159–166.
26. Shults CW, Oakes D, Kieburtz K, et al. Effects of coenzyme Q(10) in early Parkinson disease—evidence of slowing of the functional decline. Arch Neurol 2002; 59:1541–1550.
27. Parkinson Study Group. Levodopa and the progression of Parkinson's disease. N Engl J Med 2004; 351(24):2498–2508.
28. Fahn S. Parkinson disease, the effect of levodopa, and the ELLDOPA trial. Arch Neurol 1999; 56:529–535.
29. Parkinson Study Group. DATATOP: a multicenter controlled clinical trial in early Parkinson's disease. Arch Neurol 1989; 46:1052–1060.
30. Parkinson Study Group. Pramipexole vs levodopa as initial treatment for Parkinson disease—a 4-year randomized controlled trial. Arch Neurol 2004; 61(7):1044–1053.
31. Tan EK, Ondo W. Clinical characteristics of pramipexole-induced peripheral edema. Arch Neurol 2000; 57:729–732.
32. Frucht S, Rogers JD, Greene PE, Gordon MF, Fahn S. Falling asleep at the wheel: motor vehicle mishaps in persons taking pramipexole and ropinirole. Neurology 1999; 52:1908–1910.
33. Hoehn MM. Falling asleep at the wheel: motor vehicle mishaps in people taking pramipexole and ropinirole. Neurology 2000; 54:275.
34. Ferreira JJ, Galitzky M, Montastruc JL, Rascol O. Sleep attacks and Parkinson's disease treatment. Lancet 2000; 355:1333–1334.
35. Hobson DE, Lang AE, Martin WR, Razmy A, Rivest J, Fleming J. Excessive daytime sleepiness and sudden-onset sleep in Parkinson disease: a survey by the Canadian Movement Disorders Group. JAMA 2002; 287(4):455–463.
36. Ehringer H, Hornykiewicz O. Verteilung von noradrenalin und dopamin (3-hydroxytyramin) im gehirn des menschen und ihr Verhalten bei erkrankungen der extrapyramidalen systems. Klin Wochenschr 1960; 38:1236–1239.

37. Bernheimer H, Birkmayer W, Hornykiewicz O, Jellinger K, Seitelberger F. Brain dopamine and the syndromes of Parkinson and Huntington. J Neurol Sci 1973; 20:415–455.
38. Birkmayer W, Hornykiewicz O. Der L-3,4-dioxyphenylalanin (DOPA)-effekt bei der Parkinson-akinese. Wien Klin Wochenschr 1961; 73:787–788.
39. Carlsson A, Lindqvist M, Magnusson T. 3,4-Dihydroxyphenylalanine and 5-hydroxy-tryptophan as reserpine antagonists. Nature 1957; 180:1200.
40. Barbeau A, Sourkes TL, Murphy GF. Les catecholamines dans la maladie de Parkinson. In: de Ajuriaguerra J, ed. Symposium Sur les Monoamines et Systeme Nerveux Central. Geneve: Georg & Cie, 1962:247–262.
41. Friedhoff AJ, Hekiman L, Alpert M, Tobach E. Dihydroxyphenylalanine in extrapyramidal disease. JAMA 1964; 184:285.
42. Umbach W, Bauman D. Die Wirksamkeit von L-Dopa bei Parkinson-Patienten mit und ohne sterotaktischen Herneingriff. Arch Psychiat Nervenkr 1964; 205:281.
43. Hirschmann J, Mayer K. Zur beeinflussung von L-dopa (L-dihydroxyphenylananin) deutsch med wschr 1964; 89:1877.
44. Fazzagli A, Amaducci L. La Sperimentazione clinica del Dopa nelle sindromi parkinso-niane. Riv Neurobiol 1966; 12:138.
45. Bruno A, Bruno SC. Effetti dell L-2,4-dihydossifenilalanina (l-Dopa) nei pazienti parkin-soniani. Riv Sper Freniat 1966; 90:39.
46. Greer M, Williams CM. Dopamine metabolism in Parkinson's disease. Neurology 1963; 13:73.
47. Aebert K. Was leistet L-DOPA bei der Behandlung der Parkinson-Akinese? Deutsch Med Wschr 1967; 92:483.
48. Rinaldi F, Marghertia G, De Divitus E. Effetti della somministrazione de DOPA a pazienti parkinsoniani pretrattati con inhibitore delle monoaminossidasi. Ann Fren Scienze Affini 1965; 78:105–113.
49. Fehling C. Treatment of Parkinson's syndrome with L-DOPA, a double-blind study. Acta Neurol Scand 1966; 42:367–372.
50. Rinne UK, Sonninen V. A double-blind study of L-dopa treatment in Parkinson's disease. Eur Neurol 1968; 1:180–191.
51. McGeer PL, Zeldowicz LR. Administration of dihydroxyphenylalanine to parkinsonian patients. Can Med Assoc J 1964; 90:463–466.
52. Cotzias GC, Van Woert MH, Schiffer LM. Aromatic amino acids and modification of parkinsonism. N Engl J Med 1967; 276:374–379.
53. Cotzias GC, Papavasiliou PS, Gellene R. Modification of parkinsonism-chronic treatment with L-dopa. N Engl J Med 1969; 280:337–345.
54. Yahr MD, Duvoisin RC, Schear MJ, Barrett RE, Hoehn MM. Treatment of parkinsonism with levodopa. Arch Neurol 1969; 21:343–354.
55. Marsden CD, Fahn S. Problems in Parkinson's disease. In: Marsden CD, Fahn S, eds. Movement Disorders. London: Butterworth Scientific, 1982:1–7.
56. Muenter MD, Tyce GM. L-dopa therapy of Parkinson's disease: Plasma L-dopa concen-tration, therapeutic response, and side effects. Mayo Clin Proc 1971; 46:231–239.
57. Tolosa ES, Martin WE, Cohen HP, Jacobson RL. Patterns of clinical response and plasma dopa levels in Parkinson's disease. Neurology 1975; 25:177–183.
58. McDowell F, Lee JE, Swift T, Sweet RD, Ogsbury JS, Kessler JT. Treatment of Parkinson's syndrome with dihydroxyphenylalanine (levodopa). Ann Int Med 1970; 72:29–35.
59. Schwarz GA, Fahn S. Newer medical treatments in parkinsonism. Med Clin North Am 1970; 54:773–785.
60. Calne DB, Reid JL, Vakil SD, Pallis C. Problems with L-dopa therapy. Clin Med 1971; 78:21–23.
61. Duvoisin RC. Hyperkinetic reactions with L-DOPA. In: Yahr MD, ed. Current Concepts in the Treatment of Parkinsonism. New York: Raven Press, 1974:203–210.
62. Klawans HL, Goetz C, Bergen D. Levodopa-induced myoclonus. Arch Neurol 1975; 32:331–334.
63. Sweet RD, McDowell FH. The "on-off" response to chronic L-DOPA treatment of parkinsonism. Adv Neurol 1974; 5:331–338.
64. Duvoisin RC. Variations in the "on-off" phenomenon. Adv Neurol 1974; 5:339–340.
65. Yahr MD. Variations in the "on-off" effect. Adv Neurol 1974; 5:397–399.

66. Fahn S. "On-off" phenomenon with levodopa therapy in parkinsonism: clinical and pharmacologic correlations and the effect of intramuscular pyridoxine. Neurology 1974; 24:431–441.
67. Fahn S. Medical treatment of movement disorders. In: Davis FA, ed. Neurological Reviews 1976. Minneapolis: American Academy of Neurology, 1976:72–106.
68. Marsden CD, Parkes JD. 'On-off' effects in patients with Parkinson's disease on chronic levodopa therapy. Lancet 1976; 1:292–295.
69. Muenter MD, Sharpless NS, Tyce GM, Darley FL. Patterns of dystonia ('I-D-I' and 'D-I-D') in response to L-dopa therapy of Parkinson's disease. Mayo Clin Proc 1977; 52:163–174.
70. Marsden CD, Parkes JD, Quinn N. Fluctuations of disability in Parkinson's disease-clinical aspects. In: Marsden CD, Fahn S, eds. Movement Disorders. London: Butterworth Scientific, 1982:96–122.
71. Fahn S. Fluctuations of disability in Parkinson's disease: pathophysiological aspects. In: Marsden CD, Fahn S, eds. Movement Disorders. London: Butterworth Scientific, 1982:123–145.
72. Melamed E. Early-morning dystonia: a late side effect of long-term levodopa therapy in Parkinson's disease. Arch Neurol 1979; 36:308–310.
73. Horstink MW, Zijlmans JC, Pasman JW, et al. Which risk factors predict the levodopa response in fluctuating Parkinson's disease? Ann Neurol 1990; 27(5):537–543.
74. Roos RAC, Vredevoogd CB, van der Velde EA. Response fluctuations in Parkinson's disease. Neurology 1990; 40:1344–1346.
75. Poewe WH, Lees AJ, Stern GM. Low-dose L-dopa therapy in Parkinson's disease: a 6-year follow-up study. Neurology 1986; 36(11):1528–1530.
76. Montastruc JL, Rascol O, Senard JM, et al. A randomised controlled study comparing bromocriptine to which levodopa was later added, with levodopa alone in previously untreated patients with Parkinson's disease: a five year follow up. J Neurol Neurosurg Psychiatry 1994; 57(9):1034–1038.
77. Przuntek H, Welzel D, Gerlach M, et al. Early institution of bromocriptine in Parkinson's disease inhibits the emergence of levodopa-associated motor side effects. Long-term results of the PRADO study. J Neural Transm Gen Sect 1996; 103(6):699–715.
78. Rinne UK, Bracco F, Chouza C, et al. Early treatment of Parkinson's disease with caber-goline delays the onset of motor complications. Results of a double-blind levodopa controlled trial. The PKDS009 Study Group. Drugs 1998; 55(suppl 1):23–30.
79. Mouradian MM, Heuser IJE, Baronti F, Chase TN. Modification of central dopaminergic mechanisms by continuous levodopa therapy for advanced Parkinson's disease. Ann Neurol 1990; 27:18–23.
80. Chase TN. The significance of continuous dopaminergic stimulation in the treatment of Parkinson's disease. Drugs 1998; 55(suppl 1):1–9.
81. Zappia M, Oliveri RL, Bosco D, et al. The long-duration response to L-dopa in the treatment of early PD. Neurology 2000; 54(10):1910–1915.
82. Block G, Liss C, Reines S, et al. Comparison of immediate-release and controlled release carbidopa/levodopa in Parkinson's disease. A multicenter 5-year study. The CR First Study Group. Eur Neurol 1997; 37(1):23–27.
83. Capildeo R. Implications of the 5-year CR FIRST trial. Sinemet CR Five-Year International Response Fluctuation Study. Neurology 1998; 50(6 suppl 6):S15–S17; discussion S44–S18.
84. Wasielewski PG, Koller WC. Quality of life and Parkinson's disease: the CR FIRST Study. J Neurol 1998; 245(suppl 1):S28–S30.
85. Koller WC, Hutton JT, Tolosa E, et al. Immediate-release and controlled-release carbidopa/levodopa in PD: a 5-year randomized multicenter study. Carbidopa/Levodopa Study Group. Neurology 1999; 53(5):1012–1019.
86. Fahn S. Is levodopa toxic? Neurology 1996; 47:S184–S195.
87. Fahn S. Levodopa-induced neurotoxicity: Does it represent a problem for the treatment of Parkinson's disease? CNS Drugs 1997; 8:376–393.
88. Agid Y. Levodopa: is toxicity a myth? Neurology 1998; 50(4):858–863.
89. Weiner WJ. The initial treatment of Parkinson's disease should begin with levodopa. Mov Disord 1999; 14(5):716–724.

90. Factor SA. The initial treatment of Parkinson's disease. Mov Disord 2000; 15(2):360–361.
91. Parkinson Study Group. Dopamine transporter brain imaging to assess the effects of pramipexole vs levodopa on Parkinson disease progression. JAMA 2002; 287(13): 1653–1661.
92. Whone AL, Watts RL, Stoessl AJ, et al. Slower progression of Parkinson's disease with ropinirole versus levodopa: the REAL-PET study. Ann Neurol 2003; 54(1):93–101.
93. Morrish PK. Brain imaging to assess the effects of dopamine agonists on progression of Parkinson disease. JAMA 2002; 288(3):312; author reply 312–313.
94. Marek K, Jennings D, Seibyl J. Do dopamine agonists or levodopa modify Parkinson's disease progression? Eur J Neurol 2002; 9(suppl 3):15–22.
95. Albin RL, Frey KA. Initial agonist treatment of Parkinson disease: a critique. Neurology 2003; 60(3):390–394.
96. Skibba JL, Pinckley J, Gilbert EF, et al. Multiple primary melanoma following administration of levodopa. Arch Pathol 1972; 93(6):556–561.
97. Przybilla B, Schwab U, Landthaler M, et al. Development of two malignant melanomas during administration of levodopa. Acta Derm Venereol 1985; 65(6):556–557.
98. Rampen FH. Levodopa and melanoma: three cases and review of literature. J Neurol Neurosurg Psychiatry 1985; 48(6):585–588.
99. Fiala KH, Whetteckey J, Manyam BV. Malignant melanoma and levodopa in Parkinson's disease: causality or coincidence? Parkinsonism Relat Disord 2003; 9(6):321–327.
100. Olsen JH, Frils S, Frederiksen K, McLaughlin JK, Mellemkjaer l, Moller H. Atypical cancer pattern in patients with Parkinson's disease. Br J Cancer 2004; 92:1–5.
101. Sober AJ, Wick MM. Levodopa therapy and malignant melanoma. JAMA 1978; 240(6):554–555.
102. Sinemet CR [package insert]. Princeton, NJ: Bristol-Myers Squibb Co., 2002.
103. Madopar [summary of product characteristics]. Welwyn Garden City, Hertfordshire: Roche Products, Ltd., 2002.
104. Madopar HBS [summary of product characteristics]. Wellwyn Garden City, Hertfordshire: Roche Products, Limited, 2002.
105. Stalevo [package insert]. East Hanover, NJ: Novartis Pharmaceuticals Corp., 2003.
106. Weiner WJ, Singer C, Sanchez-Ramos JR, et al. Levodopa, melanoma, and Parkinson's disease. Neurology 1993; 43(4):674–677.
107. Woofter MJ, Manyam BV. Safety of long-term levodopa therapy in malignant melanoma. Clin Neuropharmacol 1994; 17(4):315–319.
108. Pfutzner W, Przybilla B. Malignant melanoma and levodopa: is there a relationship? Two new cases and a review of the literature. J Am Acad Dermatol 1997; 37(2 Pt 2):332–336.
109. Siple JF, Schneider DC, Wanlass WA, et al. Levodopa therapy and the risk of malignant melanoma. Ann Pharmacother 2000; 34(3):382–385.
110. de Jong GJ, Meerwaldt JD, Schmitz PIM. Factors that influence the occurrence of response variations in Parkinson's disease. Ann Neurol 1987;22:4–7.
111. Blin J, Bonnet A-M, Agid Y. Does levodopa aggravate Parkinson's disease? Neurology 1988; 38:1410–1416.
112. Caraceni T, Scigliano G, Musicco M. The occurrence of motor fluctuations in parkinsonian patients treated long term with levodopa: role of early treatment and disease progression. Neurology 1991; 41:380–384.
113. Cedarbaum JM, Gandy SE, McDowell FH. Early initiation of levodopa treatment does not promote the development of motor response fluctuations, dyskinesias, or dementia in Parkinson's disease. Neurology 1991; 41:622–629.
114. Yahr MD. Evaluation of long-term therapy in Parkinson's disease: mortality and therapeutic efficacy. In: Birkmayer W, Hornykiewicz O, eds. Advances in Parkinsonism. Basle: Editiones Roche, 1976;444–455.
115. Markham CH, Diamond SG. Long-term follow up of early dopa treatment in Parkinson's disease. Ann Neurol 1986; 19:365–372.
116. Goetz CG, Stebbins GT. Risk factors for nursing home placement in advanced Parkinson's disease. Neurology 1993; 43:2227–2229.

5   Genetics of α-Synuclein

Andrew Whittle and Matt Farrer
Neurogenetics, Department of Neuroscience, Mayo Clinic Jacksonville,
Jacksonville, Florida, U.S.A.

INTRODUCTION
Disorders Characterized by α-Synuclein Pathology

α-Synucleinopathy is a generic term used to describe a heterogeneous group of neurodegenerative disorders including Parkinson's disease (PD), PD and dementia (PDD), dementia with Lewy bodies (DLB) (1), and multiple system atrophy (MSA) (2,3). Postmortem, these diseases have abundant α-synuclein inclusions within the brain, but the cellular and anatomical distribution of pathology is quite different (4). PD, PDD, and DLB are often considered an overlapping spectrum of disorders; however, there is little practical benefit (5,6). Each has a distinct clinical presentation, disease course, and response to therapeutic medication. Pathologically, PD is characterized neuronal loss and depigmentation of the substantia nigra, with Lewy body inclusions within surviving neurons in the brain stem (7,8). These are generally spherical in the perikarya, ~15 mm in diameter, with a dense, granular core surrounded by a radiating rim of 8–10 nm α-synuclein filaments (9). Intraneuritic Lewy bodies are also commonly found within cell processes of the dorsal motor nucleus of the vagus and in the basal nucleus of Meynert. Neocortical Lewy bodies and Lewy neurites are infrequent. Staging criteria have recently been proposed but have yet to be validated (7,8).

PD represents a clinical syndrome of resting tremor, rigidity, bradykinesia, and postural instability, two or more of which, with a positive response to dopamine replacement/levodopa therapy, are sufficient for a diagnosis (10,11). Abnormalities of affect and cognition frequently occur, including depression, bradyphrenia, and dementia, especially in older patients (11,12). Indeed, incidence studies suggest that PD patients have an approximately six-fold increased risk of developing dementia, compared to age-matched controls (13).

In DLB the amount of α-synuclein Lewy body and Lewy neuritic pathology is far more widespread. Other than the brainstem, the temporal and limbic cortex and the corticomedial region of the amygdala are affected, and Lewy neuritic pathology is often observed in the CA2/3 region of the hippocampus (4). DLB represents a spectrum of disorders that have been classified according to the distribution of Lewy pathology, brainstem predominant, limbic (14) or neocortical depending on regional involvement (15). Alternate pathologic classifications are based on whether there are just Lewy body inclusions (pure) or whether there is an overlap with Alzheimer pathology (15–17). DLB presents with visual hallucinations and/or fluctuating cognition, with variability in attention and alertness (18). The consensus criteria require progressive cognitive decline of sufficient magnitude to interfere with normal social and occupational function (19). Parkinsonism occurs in more than 75% of cases at some point during the illness (20).

A related disorder with considerable clinical and pathologic overlap is PDD (1). The differential diagnosis is based on the duration of extrapyramidal signs prior to the onset of dementia; somewhat arbitrarily, "motor only" symptoms must be apparent for at least a year before the onset of DLB syndrome. There is no prospective data on whether the extrapyramidal features of PDD differ from those of DLB (21). The clinical spectrum of PD might be distinguished from PDD and DLB by motor subtype and affective disturbance. Cross-sectional studies highlight that the frequency/severity of depression in PD is more often reported in patients with postural instability/gait difficulty than in tremor-predominant types; postural instability motor subtype is more commonly observed in PDD and DLB patients (1,21).

In MSA, α-synuclein–positive inclusions are primarily found in white matter oligodendrocytes, rather than neurons (2). These lesions are morphologically quite distinctive from Lewy bodies and are termed glia cytoplasmic inclusions (22,23). MSA encompasses at least three clinical disorders: Shy-Drager syndrome, olivopontocerebellar atrophy, and striatonigral degeneration (24), for which parkinsonism, gait ataxia, and autonomic dysfunction, including orthostatic hypotension, and bowel and bladder incontinence are symptomatic (25).

PD affects approximately 1% to 2% of persons over 65 years and presently afflicts 0.75 million US citizens (26). DLB may constitute a further 15% to 20% of dementia cases referred to memory disorders clinics, but data on postmortem confirmation is lacking (27). MSA is rare and accounts for approximately 1% of patients with parkinsonism; however, its symptoms are perhaps more disabling and its course more rapid (25).

GENETICS OF α-SYNUCLEIN

Genetic studies in familial parkinsonism rekindled with the discovery of pathogenic missense mutations in the α-synuclein gene (*SNCA*) (28,29). The *SNCA* 209 g > a (A53T) mutation was identified through genome-wide linkage analysis in an Italian family, the Contursi kindred, with autosomal-dominant PD that manifests within the fifth and sixth decades (30). A number of families of Greek descent were shown to harbor the same mutation and a common founder haplotype (31,32). A German family with *SNCA* 88 g > c (A30P) and a Spanish/Basque family with *SNCA* 188 g > a (E46K) and familial PD provide confirmation (28,33). Our group recently discovered that genomic triplication of the *SNCA* locus was linked to familial PD in the Spellman-Muenter kindred (34). Segregation with disease is unequivocal (mLOD = 3.50, θ = 0.0 at D4S2460). Independent confirmation of this mutational mechanism was provided by a Swedish-American family with early-onset parkinsonism and de novo α-synuclein triplication (35). Brain tissue available from affected individuals in both families has provided an opportunity to compare their clinical, pathologic, and biochemical phenotypes. Studies of brain mRNA and soluble protein levels demonstrate a doubling of α-synuclein expression, consistent with molecular genetic data. Besides profuse Lewy body and Lewy neurite pathology, CA2/3 hippocampal neuronal loss appears to be a consistent feature of *SNCA* multiplication and missense mutations (30,35–39).

There has long been contention as to whether PD, PDD, and DLB represent a continuum of one disorder or are distinct disorders (15,40). Paradoxically, data from *SNCA*-triplication families provide a unifying hypothesis, as simple, overexpression of *SNCA* may lead to parkinsonism, dementia, and autonomic phenotypes. Indeed, the patients' ages of onset and disease severity suggest that excess wild type α-synuclein has more devastating consequences than mutant α-synuclein. More recently three French families with de novo *SNCA* duplications have been characterized. In affected carriers, the ages of onset, progression, and severity of disease more closely resembles idiopathic, late-onset PD. In contrast to patients with an *SNCA*-triplication mutation, cognitive decline was not a prominent or early feature of disease in *SNCA* duplication. In total, these results suggest *SNCA* dosage and wild type–α-synuclein expression is a critical determinant of disease susceptibility and severity (35).

Molecular genetic results in familial α-synucleinopathy are in good agreement with previous *SNCA* haplotype analysis showing variability within the α-synuclein promoter, including Rep1, a mixed polypurine-pyrimidine repeat around 10 Kb upstream of the start of transcription, is associated idiopathic PD (41–43). Rep1 is a negative modulator of the transcriptional activity of α-synuclein, but within the *SNCA* gene there are many regulatory enhancers that contribute to expression (44). The relationship between risk and protective promoter haplotypes is gradually becoming better defined with additional population genetic and functional studies.

Molecular Biology of α-Synuclein

SNCA maps to chromosome 4q21.3–22 (45). The gene is composed of six exons encoding a ~19 kDa, 140 amino acid protein. Alternative splicing leads to two minor transcripts, 128 amino acids, and 112 amino acids (46) that are poorly expressed relative to the full-length gene (47) (unpublished data). The amino terminus (1–67 amino acids) is composed of a consensus motif of 11 amino acids (XKTKEGVXXXX) conserved within synuclein homologues (48). Combined immunocytochemical and subcellular fractionation studies in human brain have shown α-, β-, and γ-synuclein are abundant in the neuronal cytosol and present in enriched amounts at presynaptic terminals (49). Early studies on the zebra finch suggest that α-synuclein has a role in development and in the regulation or support of synaptic plasticity (50). In vitro, both α- and β-synucleins have been shown to selectively inhibit phosphatidylcholine specific phospholipase D2 (51) whose product, phosphatidic acid, mediates processes controlling vesicular transport and changes in cell morphology (51,52). Ex vivo, the association of α-synuclein to synaptic vesicles is abolished by mutation (53) and studies in yeast have proven insightful as regards the detrimental consequence of overexpression. In vivo, α-synuclein knockout mice show impairment in the ability to replenish the presynaptic vesicular pool after paired-stimulus depression (54,55). α-synuclein has also been shown to directly bind to and inhibit tyrosine hydroxylase, the rate limiting step in dopamine production, via a competitive interaction with 14-3-3 protein (56). Theoretically, this is an attractive means to regulate dopamine synthesis and packaging.

Structurally, synucleins are natively unfolded and are prone to aggregate into β-amyloid when concentrated in aqueous solution (57–59). α-synuclein has an affinity for synaptosomes (55), and in lipid the N-terminus adopts an amphipathic α-helical conformation (48,60–62), which is partially buried in the bilayer (63) much like that found in other proteins that bind reversibly to the membrane (64). Disruption of the equilibrium between cytoplasmic and lipid-associated protein has been suggested as a mechanism underlying α-synucleinopathy (50). α-synuclein's propensity to aggregate is mediated by a central motif (NAC75-91aa), for which the negatively charged carboxy terminus is inhibitory (65,66). Overexpression of β-synuclein in vitro and in vivo may also prevent α-synuclein aggregation (67), whereas β-amyloid peptide may enhance it and seed α-synuclein fibrillization (68). Toxicity may be mediated by oligomeric species that stabilize in the presence of catecholamines perhaps, in part, explaining the selective vulnerability of dopaminergic neurons, although the relationship between aggregate formation and neurodegeneration is not straightforward (67). Both C-terminal-truncated and serine129-phosphorylated α-synuclein may precede the formation of higher molecular weight species.

α-synuclein protein degradation appears to be mediated by at least two pathways, the proteosome and chaperone-mediated autophagy (CMA) (69,70). The latter is a preferred mechanism to sequester and degrade proteins with a long half; for α-synuclein this is approximately 30 hours (unpublished data). The protein also has the CMA consensus motif (95VKKDQ99). Mutant α-synuclein is not degraded by the lysosomal pathway CMA as efficiently as wild type protein (70). Overexpression of an unfolded protein such as α-synuclein, with its propensity to aggregate when not associated with lipid, with concomitant defects in protein degradation, either through proteosomal or lysosomal pathways, may underpin Lewy body formation.

Models of α-Synucleinopathy

Many overexpression models of wild type and mutant α-synuclein have been created in cells, worms, flies, mice, and rats (71–76). In general these studies show that transgenic overproduction of α-synuclein causes neurotoxicity, whereas its ablation is not associated with neuropathology (54,77). Human genetic studies in dominant families highlight a toxic "gain-of-function" (28,29,35). Mice demonstrate a variety of neuropathologic changes, including neuronal atrophy, dystrophic neurites, and astrocytosis, accompanied by α-synuclein positive Lewy body–like inclusions, with no abnormal accumulation of α-synuclein in spinal cord or glial cells (71,74,78). In contrast to other species, murine dopaminergic neurons in vivo appear resistant to α-synuclein-induced neurotoxicity (71,79). Paradoxically, tyrosine hydroxylase-positive neurons in primary cultures do show selective vulnerability to α-synuclein overexpression. Viral delivery methods within the substantia nigra of adult rats also results in marked dopaminergic neuronal loss, dystrophic changes, and aggregated α-synuclein pathology (72,80). Differences in mice in vivo may result from developmental adaptation to constitutive transgene overexpression or may be due to congenic background. Drosophila models have been most successful in that mutant or wild type α-synuclein overexpression leads to Lewy body–like inclusions and selective loss of dopaminergic neurons, as well as a movement disorder ameliorated by levodopa or dopamine agonists (81–83). These models may be particularly useful for genetic screens to identify novel genes involved in α-synuclein mediated neurodegeneration by classical complementation, linkage analysis within congenic strains, or through microarray gene profiling. Microarray analysis of wild type α-synuclein overexpression in clonal BE2-M17 cells has previously highlighted the coordinated downregulation of mRNA/protein involved in the regulation of dopamine synthesis (84). Complementary transcriptional changes have been observed in transgenic Drosophila and mouse models, with stage-dependent disregulation of lipid processing, membrane transport, and energy metabolism (76).

CONCLUDING REMARKS

Although α-synucleinopathies are a heterogeneous group of complex, multifactorial disorders, α-synuclein expression is a central and downstream event in disease pathogenesis. There is now compelling genetic and biochemical evidence that overexpression of wild type α-synuclein is the major risk factor for rare, familial Lewy body disorders. In addition, a subset of sporadic α-synucleinopathies is likely to be explained by disregulation of temporal, regional, and/or quantitative levels of wild type α-synuclein expression. Further studies are required to understand the relationship between common genetic variability within regulatory elements of the *SNCA* locus, gene expression and protein metabolism, and the parkinsonism, cognitive decline and dementia associated with Lewy body disease. The functional consequence of wild type α-synuclein overexpression, in humans and model systems, in disease pathogenesis also requires a consensus.

Genetic studies in α-synucleinopathies may provide fundamental insights into the biology of these disorders and the molecular tools with which to study them. Genetic findings can provide direct translational benefit for patient diagnosis and for future treatments, as reduction of α-synuclein expression now represents a novel target for therapeutic intervention. Such an approach promises to provide more than just symptomatic benefit with the opportunity to halt disease progression.

REFERENCES

1. Aarsland D, Ballard C, Larsen JP, et al. A comparative study of psychiatric symptoms in dementia with Lewy bodies and Parkinson's disease with and without dementia. Int J Geriatr Psychiatry 2001; 16(5):528–536.
2. Dickson DW, Lin W, Liu WK, et al. Multiple system atrophy: a sporadic synucleinopathy. Brain Pathol 1999; 9(4):721–732.
3. Spillantini MG, Goedert M. The alpha-synucleinopathies: Parkinson's disease, dementia with Lewy bodies, and multiple system atrophy. Ann NY Acad Sci 2000; 920:16–27.
4. Dickson DW. Dementia with Lewy bodies: neuropathology. J Geriatr Psychiatry Neurol 2002; 15(4):210–216.
5. Poewe W, Wenning G. The differential diagnosis of Parkinson's disease. Eur J Neurol 2002; 9(suppl 3):23–30.
6. Jellinger KA. Neuropathological spectrum of synucleinopathies. Mov Disord 2003; 18(suppl 6):S2–S12.
7. Braak H, Del Tredici K, Bratzke H, et al. Staging of the intracerebral inclusion body pathology associated with idiopathic Parkinson's disease (preclinical and clinical stages). J Neurol 2002; 249(suppl 3):III/1–5.
8. Braak H, Del Tredici K, Rub U, et al. Staging of brain pathology related to sporadic Parkinson's disease. Neurobiol Aging 2003; 24(2):197–211.
9. Spillantini MG, Schmidt ML, Lee VM, et al. Alpha-synuclein in Lewy bodies. Nature 1997; 388(6645):839–840.
10. Gelb DJ, Oliver E, Gilman S. Diagnostic criteria for Parkinson disease. Arch Neurol 1999; 56(1):33–39.
11. Fahn S. Description of Parkinson's disease as a clinical syndrome. Ann NY Acad Sci 2003; 991:1–14.
12. Troster AI, Stalp LD, Paolo AM, et al. Neuropsychological impairment in Parkinson's disease with and without depression. Arch Neurol 1995; 52(12):1164–1169.
13. Emre M. Dementia associated with Parkinson's disease. Lancet Neurol 2003; 2(4): 229–237.
14. Colosimo C, Hughes AJ, Kilford L, et al. Lewy body cortical involvement may not always predict dementia in Parkinson's disease. J Neurol Neurosurg Psychiatry 2003; 74(7):852–856.
15. McKeith IG, Burn DJ, Ballard CG, et al. Dementia with Lewy bodies. Semin Clin Neuropsychiatry 2003; 8(1):46–57.
16. Biere AL, Wood SJ, Wypych J, et al. Parkinson's disease-associated alpha-synuclein is more fibrillogenic than beta- and gamma-synuclein and cannot cross-seed its homologs. J Biol Chem 2000; 275(44):34574–34579.

17. Mega MS, Masterman DL, Benson DF, et al. Dementia with Lewy bodies: reliability and validity of clinical and pathologic criteria. Neurology 1996; 47(6):1403–1409.
18. Harding AJ, Broe GA, Halliday GM. Visual hallucinations in Lewy body disease relate to Lewy bodies in the temporal lobe. Brain 2002; 125(Pt 2):391–403.
19. McKeith IG, Galasko D, Kosaka K, et al. Consensus guidelines for the clinical and pathologic diagnosis of dementia with Lewy bodies (DLB): report of the consortium on DLB international workshop. Neurology 1996; 47(5):1113–1124.
20. Sulkava R. Differential diagnosis between early Parkinson's disease and dementia with Lewy bodies. Adv Neurol 2003; 91:411–413.
21. Burn DJ, Rowan EN, Minett T, et al. Extrapyramidal features in Parkinson's disease with and without dementia and dementia with Lewy bodies: a cross-sectional comparative study. Mov Disord 2003; 18(8):884–889.
22. Burn DJ, Jaros E. Multiple system atrophy: cellular and molecular pathology. Mol Pathol 2001; 54(6):419–426.
23. Duda JE, Giasson BI, Gur TL, et al. Immunohistochemical and biochemical studies demonstrate a distinct profile of alpha-synuclein permutations in multiple system atrophy. J Neuropathol Exp Neurol 2000; 59(9):830–841.
24. Dickson DW, Liu W, Hardy J, et al. Widespread alterations of alpha-synuclein in multiple system atrophy. Am J Pathol 1999; 155(4):1241–1251.
25. Gilman S, Low PA, Quinn N, et al. Consensus statement on the diagnosis of multiple system atrophy. J Neurol Sci 1999; 163(1):94–98.
26. Twelves D, Perkins KS, Counsell C. Systematic review of incidence studies of Parkinson's disease. Mov Disord 2003; 18(1):19–31.
27. Heidebrink JL. Is dementia with Lewy bodies the second most common cause of dementia? J Geriatr Psychiatry Neurol 2002; 15(4):182–187.
28. Kruger R, Kuhn W, Muller T, et al. Ala30Pro mutation in the gene encoding alpha-synuclein in Parkinson's disease. Nat Genet 1998; 18(2):106–108.
29. Polymeropoulos MH, Lavedan C, Leroy E, et al. Mutation in the alpha-synuclein gene identified in families with Parkinson's disease. Science 1997; 276(5321):2045–2047.
30. Golbe LI, Di Iorio G, Lazzarini A, et al. The Contursi kindred, a large family with autosomal dominant Parkinson's disease: implications of clinical and molecular studies. Adv Neurol 1999; 80:165–170.
31. Markopoulou K, Wszolek ZK, Pfeiffer RF. A Greek-American kindred with autosomal dominant, levodopa-responsive parkinsonism and anticipation. Ann Neurol 1995; 38(3):373–378.
32. Bostantjopoulou S, Katsarou Z, Papadimitriou A, et al. Clinical features of parkinsonian patients with the alpha-synuclein (G209A) mutation. Mov Disord 2001; 16(6):1007–1013.
33. Zarranz JJ, Alegre J, Gomez-Esteban JC, et al. The new mutation, E46K, of alpha-synuclein causes Parkinson and Lewy body dementia. Ann Neurol 2004; 55(2):164–173.
34. Singleton AB, Farrer M, Johnson J, et al. Alpha-Synuclein locus triplication causes Parkinson's disease. Science 2003; 302(5646):841.
35. Farrer M, Kachergus J, Forno L, et al. Comparison of kindreds with parkinsonism and alpha-synuclein genomic multiplications. Ann Neurol 2004; 55(2):174–179.
36. Langston JW, Sastry S, Chan P, et al. Novel alpha-synuclein-immunoreactive proteins in brain samples from the Contursi kindred, Parkinson's, and Alzheimer's disease. Exp Neurol 1998; 154(2):684–690.
37. Muenter MD, Forno LS, Hornykiewicz O, et al. Hereditary form of parkinsonism—dementia. Ann Neurol 1998; 43(6):768–781.
38. Gwinn-Hardy K, Mehta ND, Farrer M, et al. Distinctive neuropathology revealed by alpha-synuclein antibodies in hereditary parkinsonism and dementia linked to chromosome 4p. Acta Neuropathol (Berl) 2000; 99(6):663–672.
39. Duda JE, Giasson BI, Mabon ME, et al. Concurrence of alpha-synuclein and tau brain pathology in the Contursi kindred. Acta Neuropathol (Berl) 2002; 104(1):7–11.
40. Farrer M, Gwinn-Hardy K, Hutton M, et al. The genetics of disorders with synuclein pathology and parkinsonism. Hum Mol Genet 1999; 8(10):1901–1905.
41. Chiba-Falek O, Nussbaum RL. Effect of allelic variation at the NACP-Rep1 repeat upstream of the {alpha}-synuclein gene (SNCA) on transcription in a cell culture luciferase reporter system. Hum Mol Genet 2001; 10(26):3101–3109.

42. Chiba-Falek O, Touchman JW, Nussbaum RL. Functional analysis of intra-allelic variation at NACP-Rep1 in the alpha-synuclein gene. Hum Genet 2003; 113(5):426–431.
43. Pals P, Lincoln S, Manning J, et al. Alpha-synuclein promoter confers susceptibility to Parkinson's disease. Ann Neurol 2004; 56(4):591–595.
44. Touchman JW, Dehejia A, Chiba-Falek O, et al. Human and mouse alpha-synuclein genes: comparative genomic sequence analysis and identification of a novel gene regulatory element. Genome Res 2001; 11(1):78–86.
45. Xia Y, Saitoh T, Ueda K, et al. Characterization of the human alpha-synuclein gene: Genomic structure, transcription start site, promoter region and polymorphisms. J Alzheimer's Dis 2001; 3(5):485–494.
46. Ueda K, Saitoh T, Mori H. Tissue-dependent alternative splicing of mRNA for NACP, the precursor of non-A beta component of Alzheimer's disease amyloid. Biochem Biophys Res Commun 1994; 205(2):1366–1372.
47. Clayton DF, George JM. The synucleins: a family of proteins involved in synaptic function, plasticity, neurodegeneration and disease. Trends Neurosci 1998; 21(6):249–254.
48. Davidson WS, Jonas A, Clayton DF, et al. Stabilization of alpha-synuclein secondary structure upon binding to synthetic membranes. J Biol Chem 1998; 273(16):9443–9449.
49. Galvin JE, Schuck TM, Lee VM, et al. Differential expression and distribution of alpha-, beta-, and gamma-synuclein in the developing human substantia nigra. Exp Neurol 2001; 168(2):347–355.
50. Clayton DF, George JM. Synucleins in synaptic plasticity and neurodegenerative disorders. J Neurosci Res 1999; 58(1):120–129.
51. Jenco JM, Rawlingson A, Daniels B, et al. Regulation of phospholipase D2: selective inhibition of mammalian phospholipase D isoenzymes by alpha- and beta-synucleins. Biochemistry 1998; 37(14):4901–4909.
52. Chen YG, Siddhanta A, Austin CD, et al. Phospholipase D stimulates release of nascent secretory vesicles from the trans-Golgi network. J Cell Biol 1997; 138(3):495–504.
53. Jensen PH, Nielsen MS, Jakes R, et al. Binding of alpha-synuclein to brain vesicles is abolished by familial Parkinson's disease mutation. J Biol Chem 1998; 273(41):26292–26294.
54. Abeliovich A, Schmitz Y, Farinas I, et al. Mice lacking alpha-synuclein display functional deficits in the nigrostriatal dopamine system. Neuron 2000; 25(1):239–252.
55. Murphy DD, Rueter SM, Trojanowski JQ, et al. Synucleins are developmentally expressed, and alpha-synuclein regulates the size of the presynaptic vesicular pool in primary hippocampal neurons. J Neurosci 2000; 20(9):3214–3220.
56. Perez RG, Waymire JC, Lin E, et al. A role for alpha-synuclein in the regulation of dopamine biosynthesis. J Neurosci 2002; 22(8):3090–3099.
57. Han H, Weinreb PH, Lansbury PT Jr. The core Alzheimer's peptide NAC forms amyloid fibrils which seed and are seeded by beta-amyloid: is NAC a common trigger or target in neurodegenerative disease? Chem Biol 1995; 2(3):163–169.
58. Weinreb PH, Zhen W, Poon AW, et al. NACP, a protein implicated in Alzheimer's disease and learning, is natively unfolded. Biochemistry 1996; 35(43):13709–13715.
59. el-Agnaf OM, Irvine GB. Aggregation and neurotoxicity of alpha-synuclein and related peptides. Biochem Soc Trans 2002; 30(4):559–565.
60. Sharon R, Goldberg MS, Bar-Josef I, et al. Alpha-synuclein occurs in lipid-rich high molecular weight complexes, binds fatty acids, and shows homology to the fatty acid-binding proteins. Proc Natl Acad Sci USA 2001; 98(16):9110–9115.
61. Hatters DM, Howlett GJ. The structural basis for amyloid formation by plasma apolipoproteins: a review. Eur Biophys J 2002; 31(1):2–8.
62. Bussell R Jr, Eliezer D. A structural and functional role for 11-mer repeats in alpha-synuclein and other exchangeable lipid binding proteins. J Mol Biol 2003; 329(4):763–778.
63. Bussell R Jr, Ramlall TF, Eliezer D. Helix periodicity, topology, and dynamics of membrane-associated alpha-synuclein. Protein Sci 2005; 14(4):862–872.
64. Davidson WS, Arnvig-McGuire K, Kennedy A, et al. Structural organization of the N-terminal domain of apolipoprotein A-I: studies of tryptophan mutants. Biochemistry 1999; 38(43):14387–14395.
65. Giasson BI, Murray IV, Trojanowski JQ, et al. A hydrophobic stretch of 12 amino acid residues in the middle of alpha-synuclein is essential for filament assembly. J Biol Chem 2001; 276(4):2380–2386.

66. Murray IV, Giasson BI, Quinn SM, et al. Role of alpha-synuclein carboxy-terminus on fibril formation in vitro. Biochemistry 2003; 42(28):8530–8540.
67. Caughey B, Lansbury PT. Protofibrils, pores, fibrils, and neurodegeneration: separating the responsible protein aggregates from the innocent bystanders. Annu Rev Neurosci 2003; 26:267–298.
68. Masliah E, Rockenstein E, Veinbergs I, et al. Beta-amyloid peptides enhance alpha-synuclein accumulation and neuronal deficits in a transgenic mouse model linking Alzheimer's disease and Parkinson's disease. Proc Natl Acad Sci USA 2001; 98(21): 12245–12250.
69. Meredith GE, Totterdell S, Petroske E, et al. Lysosomal malfunction accompanies alpha-synuclein aggregation in a progressive mouse model of Parkinson's disease. Brain Res 2002; 956(1):156–165.
70. Webb JL, Ravikumar B, Atkins J, et al. Alpha-synuclein is degraded by both autophagy and the proteasome. J Biol Chem 2003; 278(27):25009–25013.
71. Barbieri S, Hofele K, Wiederhold KH, et al. Mouse models of alpha-synucleinopathy and Lewy pathology. Alpha-synuclein expression in transgenic mice. Adv Exp Med Biol 2001; 487:147–167.
72. Lo Bianco C, Ridet JL, Schneider BL, et al. alpha -Synucleinopathy and selective dopaminergic neuron loss in a rat lentiviral-based model of Parkinson's disease. Proc Natl Acad Sci USA 2002; 99(16):10813–10818.
73. Lotharius J, Barg S, Wiekop P, et al. Effect of mutant alpha-synuclein on dopamine homeostasis in a new human mesencephalic cell line. J Biol Chem 2002; 277(41):38884–38894.
74. Hashimoto M, Rockenstein E, Masliah E. Transgenic models of alpha-synuclein pathology: past, present, and future. Ann NY Acad Sci 2003; 991:171–188.
75. Lakso M, Vartiainen S, Moilanen AM, et al. Dopaminergic neuronal loss and motor deficits in Caenorhabditis elegans overexpressing human alpha-synuclein. J Neurochem 2003; 86(1):165–172.
76. Scherzer CR, Jensen RV, Gullans SR, et al. Gene expression changes presage neurodegeneration in a Drosophila model of Parkinson's disease. Hum Mol Genet 2003; 12(19):2457–2466.
77. Specht CG, Schoepfer R. Deletion of the alpha-synuclein locus in a subpopulation of C57BL/6J inbred mice. BMC Neurosci 2001; 2(1):11.
78. Masliah E, Rockenstein E, Veinbergs I, et al. Dopaminergic loss and inclusion body formation in alpha-synuclein mice: implications for neurodegenerative disorders. Science 2000; 287(5456):1265–1269.
79. Matsuoka Y, Vila M, Lincoln S, et al. Lack of nigral pathology in transgenic mice expressing human alpha-synuclein driven by the tyrosine hydroxylase promoter. Neurobiol Dis 2001; 8(3):535–539.
80. Lauwers E, Debyser Z, Van Dorpe J, et al. Neuropathology and neurodegeneration in rodent brain induced by lentiviral vector-mediated overexpression of alpha-synuclein. Brain Pathol 2003; 13(3):364–372.
81. Feany MB, Bender WW. A Drosophila model of Parkinson's disease. Nature 2000; 404(6776):394–398.
82. Auluck PK, Bonini NM. Pharmacological prevention of Parkinson disease in Drosophila. Nat Med 2002; 8(11):1185–1186.
83. Auluck PK, Chan HY, Trojanowski JQ, et al. Chaperone suppression of alpha-synuclein toxicity in a Drosophila model for Parkinson's disease. Science 2002; 295(5556):865–868.
84. Baptista MJ, O'Farrell C, Daya S, et al. Co-ordinate transcriptional regulation of dopamine synthesis genes by alpha-synuclein in human neuroblastoma cell lines. J Neurochem 2003; 85(4):957–968.

6 Clinical and Genetic Features of *PARKIN*-Related Parkinson's Disease

Ebba Lohmann and Alexis Brice
Neurology and Experimental Therapeutics, INSERM U679, Université Pierre and Marie Curie and Fédération des Maladies du Système Nerveux and Department de Génétique, Cytogénétique, Groupe Hospitalier Pitié-Salpetriere, Paris, France

Alexandra Durr
Neurology and Experimental Therapeutics, INSERM U679, Université Pierre and Marie Curie and Department de Génétique, Cytogénétique, Groupe Hospitalier, Pitié-Salpetriere, Paris, France

Merle Ruberg
Neurology and Experimental Therapeutics, INSERM U679, Université Pierre and Marie Curie, Paris, France

INTRODUCTION

Mutations in the *PARKIN* gene cause the most common monogenic form of autosomal recessive early-onset parkinsonism. Autosomal recessive juvenile parkinsonism was recognized as a clinical entity decades ago in Japanese families (1). It is characterized by early onset (before the age of 40, sometimes before 20), dystonia (mainly in the feet), resting tremor that is less frequent than in idiopathic Parkinson's disease, brisk reflexes, sleep benefit, and a good response to levodopa. Dementia and autonomic failure were not part of the phenotype. In addition to this unique clinical phenotype, these patients also had a selective loss of pigmented neurons in the substantia nigra and locus ceruleus, but no Lewy bodies (2).

The individualization of this clinical entity led to mapping of the corresponding locus *PARK2* (3) and the responsible gene *PARKIN* (4) to the long arm of chromosome 6, first in Japanese families, then in families from other geographic regions (5,6). Initially associated with autosomal recessive juvenile parkinsonism in Japanese families (4), *PARKIN* was subsequently found to be implicated in both early- and late-onset, sporadic and familial Parkinson's disease in patients from different ethnic backgrounds. However, monogenic forms of Parkinson's disease represent only a small percentage of familial cases, and the number of patients with *PARKIN* mutations is small, in spite of its being the most frequent autosomal recessive form of the disease. The clinical spectrum of the disease is, however, large and includes atypical cases, some of which resemble dopa-responsive dystonia or are associated with peripheral neuropathies. The kinds of mutations found in patients are extremely varied, complicating genetic testing.

PARKIN GENE AND PROTEIN

PARKIN is one of the largest genes in the genome. It spans 1.35 Mb of genomic DNA, and contains 12 exons that encode a 465 amino acids protein (4,7). The PARK2 locus, adjacent to the 6q telomere, is highly subject to recombination and lies within FRA6E, the third most common fragile site in tumors (8,9), although there is as yet no evidence that *PARKIN* may be implicated in cancer.

The *PARKIN* promoter is very small. Surprisingly, it is also bidirectional. In addition to *PARKIN*, it drives the expression of the *PARKIN* coregulated gene or PACRG, which lies just upstream of *PARKIN* and is transcribed in the opposite direction (10). Neither the function of the coregulated gene nor its role, if any, in Parkinson's disease are known. Interestingly, the *PARKIN* gene is highly conserved across species, including invertebrates such as Caenorhabditis elegans and Drosophila melanogaster (11), suggesting that it might play an important role in many organisms.

The *PARKIN* protein is widely expressed in the processes and cell bodies of neurons, but not in glial cells, in the midbrain, basal ganglia, cerebral cortex, and cerebellum (12). It is characterized by the presence of an ubiquitin-like domain (UBL) at its NH_2 terminus and two ring finger motifs flanking an IBR (in between ring finger) motif at its COOH-terminus, and has been shown to be an E3 ubiquitin ligase, a critical component of the ubiquitine-proteasome pathway for protein processing and degradation (13–15). In conjunction with E2 ubiquitin conjugating enzymes, *PARKIN* ubiquitinates specific substrates. Several of the substrates, with highly diverse cell functions, have been identified: PaelR (16), cyclin E (17), alpha and beta tubulin (18), p38 (19), CDCRel-1 (15), synaptotagmin IX (20), septin (21), synphilin (22), O-glycosylated alpha synuclein (23) and element-binding protein 1 (24). It is believed that *PARKIN* mutations cause disease through a loss of function mechanism, in which reduced E3 ubiquitin ligase activity leads to accumulation of potentially neurotoxic substrates (14,25). However, some mutations seem to cause more severe disease than others, even in the heterozygous state, suggesting possible dominant negative effects (see below). *PARKIN* has also been shown to protect against a variety of stresses in different experimental paradigms, and has been proposed to act as a multipurpose protective protein in several cell compartments including mitochondria (26).

PARKIN MUTATIONS
Frequency
PARKIN gene mutations are very frequent cause of early onset Parkinson's disease. Large series of patients with either familial or apparently sporadic early-onset parkinsonism were analyzed in several studies (27–41). In one study, *PARKIN* mutations were found to be responsible for over 50% of patients autosomal recessive Parkinson's disease, with onset up to age 35 (33). Other causative genes for autosomal recessive early-onset parkinsonism such as *DJ-1* and Pink1 are less prevalent.

Most surprising was the frequency with which *PARKIN* mutations were found in early-onset cases without family histories (sporadic cases). In a study of 246 such cases with onset before the age of 45 (33), *PARKIN* mutations accounted for at least 15% of the patients. However, the relative frequency of apparently sporadic cases with *PARKIN* mutations varies greatly with age at onset. It is approximately 60% before the age of 20, 25% between 20 and 29 and less than 10% after 30. Fewer studies have dealt with late-onset cases (42–46), but all have shown that *PARKIN* mutations are rare (2%) in this population.

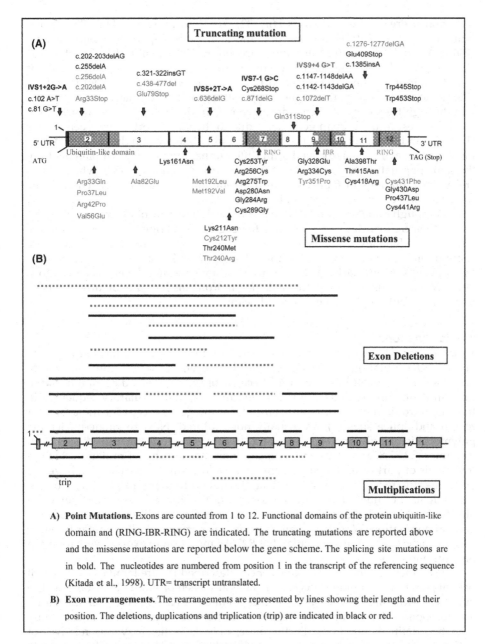

FIGURE 1 Mutations identified in the *PARKIN* gene.

Range of Mutations

In the 53 articles reporting *PARKIN* mutations (4,27–29,31–41,43,47–85) (Fig. 1), 473 apparently unrelated mutation carriers have been identified, and a total of 109 different mutations were found: 49 exon rearrangements (31 deletions and 18 multiplications of one or more exons), 48 single-base pair substitutions and 12 small deletions or insertions of one- or several-base pairs. The most common mutations were deletions of exons 4 (n = 32), 3 (n = 30), and 3 and 4 (n = 23), a point mutation in exon 7 (924C > T; n = 38), and a single-base-pair deletion in exon 2 (256delA, n = 17). These five alterations account for 35% of all *PARKIN* mutations.

In general, deletions tend to occur in exons 2 to 5, whereas point mutations have been found mainly in exons 6 to 12 where the two ring finger motifs and the IBRs are located, consistent with the functional role of these domains. It is suspected that the high frequency of exon rearrangements in the *PARKIN* gene, which is the second largest in the human genome, is due to the disproportion between its size (1350 Kb) and the small number of coding exons (12). Interestingly, most exon rearrangements have been associated with different haplotypes even in patients from the same population, suggesting that they occur independently (30), whereas several point mutations in families from different countries are associated with the same haplotype, suggesting a founder effect (30,76).

Although mutations in *PARKIN* are not limited to a particular region or ethnic group, their frequencies vary according to geographical origin. Point mutations are infrequent in Japanese patients compared with Caucasians, but exonic deletions are common in both populations. The mutations may be homozygous or compound heterozygous, particularly in families that are not consanguineous. Heterozygous *PARKIN* mutations and nonpathogenic polymorphisms have apparently also been found in patients, and will be discussed below.

Single Mutations

Variable proportions of patients have been found in several studies to carry only one *PARKIN* mutation (35–37,43,45,82,86). However, the second mutation might have been overlooked in some cases. Because of their variety, detection of mutations in the coding regions is intrinsically difficult, and regulatory sequences in the vast intronic regions or at a distance from the gene, except for the promotor region and splice sites (7), are usually not explored. Next to single-nucleotide polymorphisms only one exon rearrangement has been detected in the *PARKIN* promoter (32,87,87a). Furthermore, uncommon mechanisms of mutation, such as inversions of part or of the entire gene that could result in inactivation, have not been investigated. The presence of a single mutation might also be fortuitous in the patients and unrelated to their disease, but this hypothesis cannot be evaluated without knowledge of the frequency of carriers of the different variants in the general population. Where such an analysis was performed (76), similar frequencies for some variants, in particular, the R275W mutation in exon 7, were found in patients and controls.

Pseudodominant inheritance has been described in rare families in which all patients carry two mutations (56,88,89). It has also been proposed that some heterozygous *PARKIN* mutations may act in true dominance (29,58). However, the nature and location of the mutations were similar in heterozygous patients and in those with two defined mutations. Furthermore, only 1/34 heterozygous relatives of patients with two *PARKIN* mutations was found to have Parkinson's disease, a rate similar to the prevalence of Parkinson's disease in the general population (90). These observations do not argue in favor of dominance, but the hypothesis that single *PARKIN* mutations may be risk factors for Parkinson's disease and decrease the onset age of PD (91) has received some support from clinical and functional studies (see below).

Polymorphisms

Many different polymorphisms, including some which involve amino acid substitutions, have been detected in the *PARKIN* gene (29,43,92–97). The frequency of several of the polymorphisms varies greatly with geographical origin (93,98). Several studies have found an association between polymorphisms in the coding sequences of the gene and susceptibility to Parkinson's Disease (29,43,92,93). However, the associated polymorphisms differed in the studies, and the magnitude of the associated risk was always small.

PHENOTYPE OF *PARKIN*-RELATED PARKINSON'S DISEASE
Clinical Features

The most typical features of Parkinson's disease caused by *PARKIN* mutations are early-onset typical parkinsonism with a slow clinical course, good or excellent response to low doses of levodopa, frequent treatment-induced dyskinesias and the absence of dementia (47,99). Other frequent signs, that occur in less than 50% of the cases, however, are foot dystonia, brisk reflexes, sleep benefit, and psychiatric or behavioral disorders (Table 1).

Two studies (47,90) have compared the frequency of clinical signs in Parkinson's disease patients with and without *PARKIN* mutations, recruited according to the same clinical criteria. Although the range of ages at onset was similar in both groups of patients, the mean age at onset was significantly earlier in patients with mutations (31.4 ± 11.9 vs. 38.1 ± 11.2; p < 0.001), and dystonia, symmetry at onset and

TABLE 1 Phenotype of *PARKIN*-Related Parkinson's disease

Major features of *PARKIN* carriers
  Early- or juvenile-onset
  Excellent and sustained response to low doses of L-Dopa
  Slow progression
  Absence of dementia
  Typical parkinsonism
  Foot dystonia
  Levodopa induced dyskinesias
  No reduced olfaction
Atypical or rare additional features
  Late-onset (IPD-like) (29,43,47,67)
  DRD-like (99)
  Leg tremor in orthostatism (34)
  Focal dystonia (105)
  Mild cerebellar signs (33,59,103)
  Pyramidal tract dysfunction (59)
  Peripheral neuropathy (6,84,90)
  White matter abnormalities on brain MRI (90)
Psychiatric or behavioral manifestations
  Psychosis (99,106)
  Panic attacks (90)
  Depression (6,90,99)
  Disturbed sexual behavioral (90,99)
  Obsessive-compulsive behaviors (90,105)

Abbreviations: DRD, dopa-responsive dystonia; IPD, idiopathic Parkinson's disease; MRI, magnetic resonance imaging.

brisk reflexes were significantly more frequent. In addition, despite longer treatment, the daily dose of levodopa was significantly lower in the group with mutations. However, there was no individual sign or symptom that distinguished *PARKIN* mutation carriers from noncarriers with early-onset parkinsonism, and there was no effect of gender on the phenotype.

Interestingly, dystonia at onset was not specific to *PARKIN* carriers, but was associated with young-onset parkinsonism regardless of the cause. Freezing, festination, retropulsion, instability, and falls, which are usually considered to be late features in patients with idiopathic Parkinson's disease and often assumed to be extranigral or nondopaminergic in origin, can be early or presenting features in some patients with *PARKIN* mutations who have in principle no nondopaminergic lesions (99). Reduced olfaction, which is a frequent early frequent finding in idiopathic Parkinson's disease, is not associated with *PARKIN* mutations (100), but rapid eye movement sleep behavior disorder is frequent in both (101).

Atypical presentations or additional signs are observed as well, including onset as late as age 72 (29,43,47,67), pyramidal tract dysfunction (59) peripheral neuropathy (6,84,90,102), cerebellar ataxia (33,59,103), tremor mainly during orthostatism (34), and white matter abnormalities on brain MRI (90). One study found corticospinal dysfunction in *PARKIN* carriers suggesting extended involvment of the central nervous system in Parkinson's disease (104). Some phenotypes resemble dopa-responsive dystonia (99,105) or hemiparkinsonism-hemiatrophy (69).

Cognitive function remains normal in the majority of patients with *PARKIN* mutations (47,90,99), even after 45 years of evolution (99), but behavioral disorders have been reported, included anxiety, psychosis, panic attacks, depression, disturbed sexual behavioral, and obsessive-compulsive behaviors (6,90,99,106,107). However, since psychiatric manifestations are frequent in the general population and delirium and hypersexuality can be triggered by antiparkinsonism drugs, it cannot yet be concluded whether they are part of the phenotype or if they occurred by chance in some of the patients.

Neuronal Loss or Dysfunction

Neuropathologic studies have been performed in at least eight cases with autosomal recessive juvenile parkinsonism (4) or proven *PARKIN* mutations (54,58,72,103,108–110). Loss of dopaminergic neurones in the substantia nigra pars compacta was severe and generalized in all patients. Other abnormalities were variable. These included additional involvement of the substantia nigra pars reticulate (54), neurofibrillary tangles and argyrophilic astrocytes in the cerebral cortex and brainstem nuclei (109), neuronal loss in parts of the spinocerebellar systems (103), reactive gliosis (110) and mild histopathological changes in muscles (111).

All but one of the patients with Parkinson's disease associated with *PARKIN* mutations that have been analysed did not have Lewy bodies, suggesting that the pathogenetic mechanisms underlying this disease differ from idiopathic Parkinson's disease. The exception was a compound heterozygote whose symptoms were those of typical Parkinson's disease (58). Since he also had a family history of autosomal dominant transmission, it may be asked whether this clinically and pathologically typical case of Parkinson's disease can be explained by one or both of the *PARKIN* mutations in this patient, or whether an unidentified factor contributed to his disease. Another case had basophilic inclusions in the pedunculopontine nucleus and the mesencephalic reticular formation, which were α-synuclein-positive and ubiquitin-positive. Another exceptional case had tau aggregates as in progressive supranuclear palsy (112), but he had only one detected *PARKIN* mutation which might also be responsible for an autosomal dominant form of parkinsonism or simply be fortuitous.

Several studies aimed at determining the integrity of the dopaminergic system in patients with *PARKIN* mutations have been performed by positon emission tomagraphy, most often with [18F]fluorodopa (69,82,113–118). The reduction in [18F]fluorodopa uptake in these patients was similar in magnitude to the decrease in patients with idiopathic Parkinson's disease (113–115). When only early-onset cases with and without *PARKIN* mutations were compared, there was either no difference in [18F]fluorodopa uptake in the two groups (117) or a more severe and widespread deficit in patients with mutations that was notably bilateral and affected the caudate nucleus as much as the putamen (114,116,118,119). The difference in the pattern of the deficit has been confirmed by others with [18F]fluorodopa and with dopamine transporter (DAT) ligand [123I]FP-CIT (120) (Fig. 2), as well as by [11C] Raclopride binding (115,118) and MR segmented inversion recovery ratio imaging (SIRRIM) (121). The decline in [18F]fluorodopa uptake in patients with *PARKIN* mutations (1.47% per year), however, appears to be slower than in patients with idiopathic Parkinson's disease (5.71% per year) (116), suggesting that nigrostriatal cell loss progresses more slowly in these patients.

PHENOTYPE-GENOTYPE CORRELATIONS

There have been several attempts to establish correlations between patient phenotypes and the nature or number of their mutations (43,45,90). The nature of the mutation does not account for much of the phenotypical variability (123), since the same two mutations have been reported in patients with as much as a 27-year difference in age at onset, and can thus cause both early to late onset disease (90). However, carriers of missense mutations had more severe disease [higher United Parkinson's

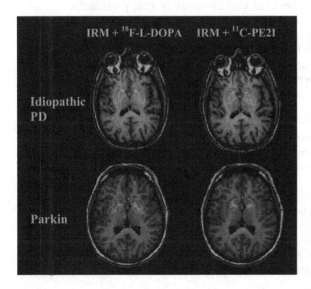

FIGURE 2 Striatal dopaminergic metabolism and dopamine transporter density in young-onset Parkinson. *Abbreviation*: PD, Parkinson's disease. *Source*: From Ref. 126.

Disease Rating Scale (UPDRS) motor score] than those carrying truncating mutations, suggesting that missense mutations result in more than a loss of function (90). The localization of the mutations also seems important, since missense mutation located within known functional domains of the protein (UBL and RING-IBR-RING) result in a significantly earlier onset than other missense mutations (90).

Intriguingly, patients with only one detected mutation, despite thorough molecular analyses of the *PARKIN* gene including the promotor region (90), were characterized by a later and more asymmetrical onset and more frequent motor fluctuations and dystonia than patients with two mutations. Furthermore, the age at onset in these patients extended up to 68 years, 10 years later than in patients with two *PARKIN* mutations. These features are those of typical Parkinson's disease, suggesting that a single *PARKIN* mutation might predispose to later onset idiopathic disease. Similar results have been reported in a number of other clinical (58,91,125) and functional studies. Significant reductions in [^{18}F]fluorodopa uptake have been observed in carriers of only one *PARKIN* mutation (82,115,116), with a pattern similar to what is observed in patients with two mutations (82), and a study of the substantia nigra by brain parenchyma sonography has confirmed the alteration of the dopaminergic system in patients with one *PARKIN* mutation, although they are affected to a lesser degree than those with two mutated alleles (122). Some of the heterozygous patients with reduced [^{18}F]fluorodopa uptake were reported to have subtle extrapyramidal signs, such as resting tremor, reduced arm swing or a mask-like face (82,99,115,116). Haploinsufficiency or a dominant effect caused by single *PARKIN* mutations may therefore be sufficient to cause dopaminergic cell loss and subclinical disease, and might therefore represent a risk factor for developing late-onset Parkinson's disease (31,32,64).

GENETIC TESTING FOR *PARKIN* MUTATIONS

Because of the extreme variety of mutations in the *PARKIN* gene, screening is complex and requires a combination of sequencing to detect point mutations as well as dosage experiments for exon rearrangements (48,124). Before undertaking a genetic test for *PARKIN* mutations, however, it is important to ask the following questions: Is the indication appropriate? Will the result be interpretable?

There are two reasons to look for *PARKIN* mutations. The first is to confirm a diagnosis. Given the frequency of dystonia in patients with *PARKIN* mutations, they may be difficult to distinguish from those with dopa-responsive dystonia. Correct diagnosis is also important for patients with juvenile onset, because it can affect prognosis and treatment; patients with *PARKIN* mutations are, for example, good candidates for deep brain stimulation. *PARKIN* should also be tested in view of genetic counselling. The identification of *PARKIN* as the cause of their disease is reassuring for patients and their sibs, since it excludes the high risk recurrence in subsequent generations by autosomal dominant transmission. In situations where the spouses are related, testing should also be performed. If both are carriers, prenatal diagnosis can be envisaged.

Before testing for *PARKIN* mutations, however, the probability of obtaining a positive test result should be evaluated. At present, patients with early-onset parkinsonism and a good response to treatment appear to be the most appropriate candidates for *PARKIN* analysis. In isolated cases, the yield is over 25% when onset is before the age of 30, although it drops sharply with age, particularly at 40 or above. When two or more sibs are affected, the yield exceeds 50%, even in patients who are 45- or 50-years. With later onset, the proportion will again decline.

The results of genetic testing for *PARKIN* mutations, as for other autosomal recessive disorders, are not easy to interpret. It is crucial that all coding exons be analysed for point mutations by sequencing and for exon rearrangements by gene dosage. In this case, the absence of mutations strongly excludes the possibility of *PARKIN*-related disease. The presence of one or more sequence variants is more difficult to interpret. When two different mutations are found, they must be in trans (affecting both copies of the gene) before it can be concluded that they are responsible for the phenotype. This is often difficult when two consecutive exons (e.g., exons 3 and 4) are deleted, since both can be deleted on the same allele or each on a different allele. However, this ambiguity can be resolved by RT-PCR analysis or when other family members can be tested. Further complicating analysis, the *PARKIN* gene carries many rare polymorphisms that vary among populations and are difficult to distinguish from pathogenic mutations. The fact that a sequence variant, even in the coding region, is not found on hundreds of control chromosomes is not sufficient proof that it is a disease-causing mutation.

These problems underline the importance of good communication between the practitioner requesting a genetic test and the biologist performing the analysis. Patients must be sure to receive reliable information, including a clear understanding of its limits.

CONCLUSION

Stimulated by the identification of causative mutations in *PARKIN*, α-synuclein, and several other genes, research on the monogenic forms of Parkinson's disease has been fruitful. Studies on *PARKIN* have been particularly important, firstly because mutations in this gene were found to be relatively frequent in early-onset cases, but also because the consequences of *PARKIN* mutations suggest that a defective ubiquitin-proteasome pathway may play a role in Parkinson's disease. Furthermore, although the clinical features of patients with *PARKIN* mutations are often indistinguishable from idiopathic Parkinson's disease, the absence of Lewy bodies despite severe loss of nigral dopaminergic neurons challenges the traditional definition of Parkinson's disease based on neuropathlogical criteria. The observations suggest that dysfunction of more than one pathway may lead to degeneration of the nigrostriatal pathway and parkinsonism, thus multiplying the number of potential targets for future therapies.

ACKNOWLEDGMENTS

The authors thank the patients and the members of the French Parkinson's Disease Genetic Study Group for their participation. This work was supported by grants from the National Institutes for Health (grant NS41723-01A1), INSERM and the French Ministry of Research and Technology "Cohortes et collections 2001" (contract 4CH03G).

REFERENCES

1. Yamamura Y, Sobue I, Ando K, et al. Paralysis agitans of early onset with marked diurnal fluctuation of symptoms. Neurology 1973; 23:239–244.
2. Matsumine H, Yamamura Y, Hattori N, et al. A microdeletion of D6S305 in a family of autosomal recessive juvenile parkinsonism (PARK2). Genomics. 1998; 49(1):143–146.
3. Kitada T, Asakawa S, Hattori N, et al. Mutations in the parkin gene cause autosomal recessive juvenile parkinsonism. Nature 1998; 392:605–608.

4. Takahashi H, Ohama E, Suzuki S, et al. Familial juvenile parkinsonism: clinical and pathologic study in a family. Neurology 1994; 44(3 Pt 1):437–441.
5. Jones AC, Yamamura Y, Almasy L, et al. Autosomal recessive juvenile parkinsonism maps to 6q25.2–q27 in four ethnic groups:detailed genetic mapping of the linked region. Am J Hum Genet 1998; 63(1):80–87.
6. Tassin J, Durr A, de Broucker T, et al. Chromosome 6-linked autosomal recessive early-onset Parkinsonism: linkage in European and Algerian families, extension of the clinical spectrum, and evidence of a small homozygous deletion in one family. The French Parkinson's Disease Genetics Study Group, and the European Consortium on Genetic Susceptibility in Parkinson's Disease. Am J Hum Genet 1998; 63(1):88–94.
7. West A, Farrer M, Petrucelli L, et al. Identification and characterization of the human parkin gene promoter. J Neurochem 2001; 78(5):1146–1152.
8. Denison SR, Wang F, Becker NA, et al. Alterations in the common fragile site gene Parkin in ovarian and other cancers. Oncogene 2003; 22:8370–8378.
9. Cesari R, Martin ES, Calin GA, et al. Parkin, a gene implicated in autosomal recessive juvenile parkinsonism, is a candidate tumor suppressor gene on chromosome 6q25–q27. Proc Nat Acad Sci 2003; 100:5956–5961.
10. West AB, Lockhart PJ, O'Farell C, et al. Identification of a novel gene linked to parkin via a bi-directional promoter. J Molec Biol 2003; 326:11–19.
11. Kahle PJ, Leimer U, Haass C. Does failure of parkin-mediated ubiquitination cause juvenile parkinsonism? Trends Biochem Sci 2000; 25(11):524–527.
12. Huynh DP, Scoles DR, Ho TH, et al. Parkin is associated with actin filaments in neuronal and nonneural cells Ann Neurol 2000; 48(5):737–744.
13. Shimura H, Hattori N, Kubo S, et al. Familial Parkinson disease gene product, parkin, is a ubiquitin-protein ligase. Nat Genet 2000; 25:302–305.
14. Imai Y, Soda M, Takahashi R. Parkin suppresses unfolded protein stress-induced cell death through its E3 ubiquitin-protein ligase activity. J Biol Chem 2000; 275: 35661–35664.
15. Zhang Y, Gao J, Chung KK, et al. Parkin functions as an E2-dependent ubiquitin- protein ligase and promotes the degradation of the synaptic vesicle-associated protein, CDCrel-1. Proc Natl Acad Sci USA 2000; 97:13354–13359.
16. Imai Y, Soda M, Inoue H, et al. An unfolded putative transmembrane polypeptide, which can lead to endoplasmic reticulum stress, is a substrate of Parkin. Cell 2001; 105(7): 891–902.
17. Staropoli JF, McDermott C, Martinat C, et al. Parkin is a component of an SCF-like ubiquitin ligase complex and protects postmitotic neurons from kainate excitotoxicity. Neuron 2003; 37(5):735–749.
18. Ren Y, Zhao J, Feng J. Parkin binds to alpha/beta tubulin and increases their ubiquitination and degradation. J Neurosci 2003; 23(8):3316–3324.
19. Corti O, Hampe C, Koutnikova H, et al. The p38 subunit of the aminoacyl-tRNA synthetase complex is a Parkin substrate: linking protein biosynthesis and neurodegeneration. Hum Mol Genet 2003; 12(12):1427–37.
20. Huynh DP, Scoles DR, Nguyen D, et al. The autosomal recessive juvenile Parkinson disease gene product, parkin, interacts with and ubiquitinates synaptotagmin XI. Hum Mol Genet 2003; 12(20):2587–2597. Epub 2003 Aug 12.
21. Choi P, Snyder H, Petrucelli L, et al. SEPT5_v2 is a parkin-binding protein. Brain Res Mol Brain Res 2003; 117(2):179–189.
22. Chung KK, Zhang Y, Lim KL, et al. Parkin ubiquitinates the alpha-synuclein-interacting protein, synphilin-1: implications for Lewy-body formation in Parkinson disease. Nat Med 2001; 7(10):1144–1150.
23. Shimura H, Schlossmacher MG, Hattori N. Ubiquitination of a new form of alpha-synuclein by parkin from human brain: implications for Parkinson's disease. Science 2001; 293(5528):263–269. Epub 2001 Jun 28.
24. Ko HS, Kim SW, Sriram SR, et al. Indentification of far upstream element-binding protein-1 as an authentic Parkin substrate. J Biol Chem 2006; 281(24):16193–16196. Epub 2006 May 3.
25. Shimura H, Hattori N, Kubo S, et al. Familial Parkinson disease gene product, parkin, is a ubiquitin-protein ligase. Nature Genet 2000; 25:302–305.

26. Corti O, Hampe C, Darios F, et al. Parkinson's disease: from causes to mechanisms. C R Biol 2005; 328(2):131–142.
27. Hattori N, Kitada T, Matsumine H, et al. Molecular genetic analysis of a novel Parkin gene in Japanese families with autosomal recessive juvenile parkinsonism: evidence for variable homozygous deletions in the Parkin gene in affected individuals. Ann Neurol 1998; 44:935–941.
28. Abbas N, Lücking CB, Ricard S, et al. A wide variety of mutations in the parkin gene are responsible for autosomal recessive parkinsonism in Europe. French Parkinson's Disease Genetics Study Group and the European Consortium on Genetic Susceptibility in Parkinson's Disease. Hum Mol Genet 1999; 8:567–574.
29. Klein C, Pramstaller PP, Kis B, et al. Parkin deletions in a family with adult-onset, tremor-dominant parkinsonism: expanding the phenotype. Ann Neurol 2000; 48:65–71.
30. Periquet M, Lücking C, Vaughan J, et al. Origin of the mutations in the parkin gene in Europe: exon rearrangements are independent recurrent events, whereas point mutations may result from Founder effects. Am J Hum Genet 2001; 68:617–626.
31. Hedrich K, Marder K, Harris J, et al. Evaluation of 50 probands with early-onset Parkinson's disease for Parkin mutations. Neurology 2002; 58:1239–1246.
32. West A, Periquet M, Lincoln S, et al. Complex relationship between Parkin mutations and Parkinson disease. Am J Med Genet 2002; 114:584–591.
33. Periquet M, Latouche M, Lohmann E, et al. Parkin mutations are frequent in patients with isolated early-onset parkinsonism. Brain 2003; 126:1271–1278.
34. Rawal N, Periquet M, Lohmann E, et al. New parkin mutations and atypical phenotypes in families with autosomal recessive parkinsonism. Neurology 2003; 60:1378–1381.
35. Bertoli-Avella AM, Giroud-Benitez JL, Akyol A, et al. Novel parkin mutations detected in patients with early-onset Parkinson's disease. Mov Disord 2005; 20(4):424–431.
36. Poorkaj P, Nutt JG, James D, et al. Parkin mutation analysis in clinic patients with early-onset Parkinson's disease. Am J Med Genet A 2004; 129(1):44–50.
37. Wu RM, Bounds R, Lincoln S, et al. Parkin mutations and early-onset parkinsonism in a Taiwanese cohort. Arch Neurol 2005; 62(1):82–87.
38. Hertz JM, Ostergaard K, Juncker I, et al. Low frequency of Parkin, Tyrosine Hydroxylase, and GTP Cyclohydrolase I gene mutations in a Danish population of early-onset Parkinson's Disease. Eur J Neurol 2006; 13(4):385–390.
39. Clark LN, Afridi S, Karlins E, et al. Case-control study of the parkin gene in early-onset Parkinson disease. Arch Neurol 2006; 63(4):548–552.
40. Madegowda RH, Kishore A, Anand A, et al. Mutational screening of the parkin gene among South Indians with early onset Parkinson's disease. J Neurol Neurosurg Psychiatry 2005; 76(11):1588–1590.
41. Sinha R, Racette B, Perlmutter JS, et al. Prevalence of parkin gene mutations and variations in idiopathic Parkinson's disease. Parkinsonism Relat Discord 2005; 11(6):341–347.
42. Oliveri RL, Zappia M, Annesi G, et al. The parkin gene is not a major susceptibility locus for typical late-onset Parkinson's disease. Neurol Sci 2001; 22(1):73–74.
43. Oliveira SA, Scott WK, Martin ER, et al. Parkin mutations and susceptibility alleles in late-onset Parkinson's disease. Ann Neurol 2003; 53:624–629.
44. Kann M, Hedrich K, Vieregge P, et al. The parkin gene is not involved in late-onset Parkinson's disease. Neurology 2002; 58(5):835.
45. Foroud T, Uniacke SK, Liu L, et al. Heterozygosity for a mutation in the parkin gene leads to later onset Parkinson disease. Neurology 2003; 60:796–801.
46. Klein C, Hedrich K, Wellenbrock C, et al. Frequency of parkin mutations in late-onset Parkinson's disease. Ann Neurol 2003; 54(3):416–417.
47. Lücking CB, Dürr A, Bonifati V, et al. Association between early-onset Parkinson's disease and mutations in the parkin gene. French Parkinson's Disease Genetics Study Group. N Engl J Med 2000; 342:1560–1567.
48. Hedrich K, Kann M, Lanthaler AJ, et al. The importance of gene dosage studies: mutational analysis of the parkin gene in early-onset parkinsonism. Hum Mol Genet 2001; 10:1649–1656.
49. Hattori N, Matsumine H, Asakawa S, et al. Point mutations (Thr240Arg and Gln311Stop) [correction of Thr240Arg and Ala311Stop] in the Parkin gene. Biochem Biophys Res Commun 1998; 249:754–758.

50. Leroy E, Anastasopoulos D, Konitsiotis S, Lavedan C, Polymeropoulos MH. Deletions in the Parkin gene and genetic heterogeneity in a Greek family with early onset Parkinson's disease. Hum Genet 1998; 103:424–427.

51. Lücking CB, Abbas N, Dürr A, et al. Homozygous deletions in parkin gene in European and North African families with autosomal recessive juvenile parkinsonism. The European Consortium on Genetic Susceptibility in Parkinson's Disease and the French Parkinson's Disease Genetics Study Group. Lancet 1998; 352:1355–1356.

52. Nisipeanu P, Inzelberg R, Blumen SC, et al. Autosomal-recessive juvenile parkinsonism in a Jewish Yemenite kindred: mutation of Parkin gene. Neurology 1999; 53:1602–1604.

53. Ujike H, Yamamoto M, Yamaguchi K, Kanzaki A, Takagi M, Kuroda S. [Two cases of sporadic juvenile Parkinson's disease caused by homozygous deletion of Parkin gene.] No To Shinkei 1999; 51:1061–1064.

54. Hayashi S, Wakabayashi K, Ishikawa A, et al. An autopsy case of autosomal-recessive juvenile parkinsonism with a homozygous exon 4 deletion in the parkin gene. Mov Disord 2000; 15:884–888.

55. Jeon BS, Kim JM, Lee DS, Hattori N, Mizuno Y. An apparently sporadic case with parkin gene mutation in a Korean woman. Arch Neurol 2001; 58:988–989.

56. Maruyama M, Ikeuchi T, Saito M, et al. Novel mutations, pseudo-dominant inheritance, and possible familial affects in patients with autosomal recessive juvenile parkinsonism. Ann Neurol 2000; 48:245–250.

57. Alvarez V, Guisasola LM, Moreira VG, Lahoz CH, Coto E. Early-onset Parkinson's disease associated with a new parkin mutation in a Spanish family. Neurosci Lett 2001; 313:108–110.

58. Farrer M, Chan P, Chen R, et al. Lewy bodies and parkinsonism in families with parkin mutations. Ann Neurol 2001; 50:293–300.

59. Kuroda Y, Mitsui T, Akaike M, Azuma H, Matsumoto T. Homozygous deletion mutation of the parkin gene in patients with atypical parkinsonism. J Neurol Neurosurg Psychiatry 2001; 71:231–234.

60. Lu CS, Wu JC, Tsai CH, et al. Clinical and genetic studies on familial parkinsonism: the first report on a parkin gene mutation in a Taiwanese family. Mov Disord 2001; 16:164–166.

61. Nisipeanu P, Inzelberg R, Abo Mouch S, et al. Parkin gene causing benign autosomal recessive juvenile parkinsonism. Neurology 2001; 56:1573–1575.

62. Terreni L, Calabrese E, Calella AM, Forloni G, Mariani C. New mutation (R42P) of the parkin gene in the ubiquitinlike domain associated with parkinsonism. Neurology 2001; 56:463–466.

63. Ujike H, Yamamoto M, Kanzaki A, Okumura K, Takaki M, Kuroda S. Prevalence of homozygous deletions of the parkin gene in a cohort of patients with sporadic and familial Parkinson's disease. Mov Disord 2001; 16:111–113.

64. Hoenicka J, Vidal L, Morales B, et al. Molecular findings in familial Parkinson disease in Spain. Arch Neurol 2002; 59:966–970.

65. Kann M, Jacobs H, Mohrmann K, et al. Role of parkin mutations in 111 community-based patients with early-onset parkinsonism. Ann Neurol 2002; 51:621–625.

66. Munoz E, Tolosa E, Pastor P, et al. Relative high frequency of the c.255delA parkin gene mutation in Spanish patients with autosomal recessive parkinsonism. J Neurol Neurosurg Psychiatry 2002; 73:582–584.

67. Nichols WC, Pankratz N, Uniacke SK, et al. Linkage stratification and mutation analysis at the Parkin locus identifies mutation positive Parkinson's disease families. J Med Genet 2002; 39:489–492.

68. Pineda-Trujillo N, Carvajal-Carmona LG, Buritica O, et al. A novel Cys212Tyr founder mutation in parkin and allelic heterogeneity of juvenile Parkinsonism in a population from North West Colombia. Neurosci Lett 2001; 298:87–90.

69. Pramstaller PP, Kunig G, Leenders K, et al. Parkin mutations in a patient with hemiparkinsonism-hemiatrophy: a clinical-genetic and PET study. Neurology 2002; 58:808–810.

70. Xu Y, Liu Z, Wang Y, Tao E, Chen G, Chen B. [A new point mutation on exon 2 of parkin gene in Parkinson's disease.] Zhonghua Yi Xue Yi Chuan Xue Za Zhi 2002; 19:409–411.

71. Chen R, Gosavi NS, Langston JW, Chan P. Parkin mutations are rare in patients with young-onset parkinsonism in a US population. Parkinsonism Relat Disord 2003; 9:309–312.

72. Gouider-Khouja N, Larnaout A, Amouri R, et al. Autosomal recessive parkinsonism linked to parkin gene in a Tunisian family. Clinical, genetic and pathological study. Parkinsonism Relat Disord 2003; 9:247–251.
73. Illarioshkin SN, Periquet M, Rawal N, et al. Mutation analysis of the parkin gene in Russian families with autosomal recessive juvenile parkinsonism. Mov Disord 2003; 18:914–919.
74. Kim JS, Lee KS, Kim YI, Lee KH, Kim HT. Homozygous exon 4 deletion in parkin gene in a Korean family with autosomal recessive early onset parkinsonism. Yonsei Med J 2003; 44:336–339.
75. Kobayashi T, Matsumine H, Zhang J, Imamichi Y, Mizuno Y, Hattori N. Pseudo-autosomal dominant inheritance of PARK2: two families with parkin gene mutations. J Neurol Sci 2003; 207:11–17.
76. Lincoln SJ, Maraganore DM, Lesnick TG, Bounds R, de Andrade M, Bower JH, Hardy JA, Farrer MJ. Parkin variants in North American Parkinson's disease: cases and controls. Mov Disord 2003; 18:1306–1311.
77. Slominskii PA, Miloserdova OV, Popova SN, et al. [Analysis of deletion mutations in the PARK2 gene in idiopathic Parkinson's disease.] Genetika 2003; 39:223–228.
78. Wang T, Liang Z, Sun S, Cao X, Peng H, Cao F, Liu H, Tong E. A novel point mutation in parkin gene was identified in an early-onset case of Parkinson's disease. Zhonghua Yi Xue Yi Chuan Xue Za Zhi 2003; 20:111–113.
79. Munhoz RP, Sa DS, Rogaeva E, Salehi-Rad S, et al. Clinical findings in a large family with a parkin ex3delta40 mutation. Arch Neurol 2004; 61(5):701–704.
80. Inzelberg R, Schecthman E, Paleacu D, et al. Onset and progression of disease in familial and sporadic Parkinson's Am J Med Genet A 2004; 124(3):255–258.
81. Dogu O, Johnson J, Hernandez D, et al. A consanguineous Turkish family with early-onset Parkinson's disease and an exon 4 parkin deletion. Mov Disord 2004; 19(7): 812–816.
82. Khan NL, Horta W, Eunson L, et al. Parkin disease in a Brazilian kindred: Manifesting heterozygotes and clinical follow-up over 10 years. Mov Disord 2005; 20(4):479–484.
83. Wiley J, Lynch T, Lincoln S, et al. Parkinson's disease in Ireland: clinical presentation and genetic heterogeneity in patients with parkin mutations. Mov Disord 2004; 19(6): 677–681.
84. Abbruzzese G, Pigullo S, Schenone A, et al. Does parkin play a role in the peripheral nervous system? A family report. Mov Disord 2004; 19(8):978–981.
85. Poorkaj P, Moses L, Montimurro JS, et al. Parkin mutation dosage and the phenomenon of anticipation: a molecular genetic study of familial parkinsonism. BMC Neurol 2005; 5(1):4.
86. Tan LC, Tanner CM, Chen R, et al. Marked variation in clinical presentation and age of onset in a family with a heterozygous parkin mutation. Mov Disord 2003; 18(7):758–763.
87. Mata IF, Alvarez V, Garcia-Moreira V, et al. Single-nucleotide polymorphisms in the promoter region of the PARKIN gene and Parkinson's disease. Neurosci Lett 2002; 329(2):149–152.
87a. Lesage S, Periquet M, Lohmann E, et al. Deletion of the Parkin and PACRG gene promotes in early-onset parkinsonism. Hum Mut 2007; 28(1):27–30.
88. Bonifati V, Lücking CB, Fabrizio E, et al. Three parkin gene mutations in a sibship with autosomal recessive early onset parkinsonism. J Neurol Neurosurg Psychiatry 2001; 71:531–534.
89. Lücking CB, Bonifati V, Periquet M, et al. Pseudo-dominant inheritance and exon 2 triplication in a family with parkin gene mutations. Neurology 2001; 57:924–927.
90. Lohmann E, Periquet M, Bonifati V, et al. How much phenotypic variation can be attributed to parkin genotype? Ann Neurol 2003; 54(2):176–185.
91. Sun M, Latourelle CL, Wooten GF, et al. Influence of heterozygosity for Parkin mutation on onset age in familial Parkinson diease. Arch Neurol 2006; 63:826–832.
92. Zou HQ, Chen B, Ma QL, et al. [New polymorphism (IVS3-20 T—>C) of the parkin gene associated with the early-onset Parkinson's disease in Chinese] Zhonghua Yi Xue Yi Chuan Xue Za Zhi 2004; 21(3):219–223.
93. Lucking CB, Chesneau V, Lohmann E, et al. Coding polymorphisms in the parkin gene and susceptibility to Parkinson disease. Arch Neurol 2003; 60(9):1253–1256.

94. Mellick GD, Buchanan DD, Hattori N, et al. The parkin gene S/N167 polymorphism in Australian Parkinson's disease patients and controls. Parkinsonism Relat Disord 2001; 7(2):89–91.

95. Hu CJ, Sung SM, Liu HC, et al. Polymorphisms of the parkin gene in sporadic Parkinson's disease among Chinese in Taiwan. Eur Neurol 2000; 44(2):90–93.

96. Satoh J, Kuroda Y. Association of codon 167 Ser/Asn heterozygosity in the parkin gene with sporadic Parkinson's disease. Neuroreport 1999; 10(13):2735–2739.

97. Wang M, Hattori N, Matsumine H, et al. Polymorphism in the parkin gene in sporadic Parkinson's disease. Ann Neurol 1999; 45(5):655–658.

98. Li X, Kitami T, Wang M. Geograohic and ethnic differences in frequencies of two polymorphisms (D/N394 and L/I272) of the parkin gene in sporadic Parkinson's disease. Parkinsonism Relat Discord 2005; 11(8):485-491. Epub 2005 Nov.

99. Khan NL, Graham E, Critchley P, et al. Parkin disease: a phenotypic study of a large case series. Brain 2003; 126(Pt 6):1279–1292.

100. Khan NL, Katzenschlager R, Watt H, et al. Olfaction differentiates parkin disease from early-onset parkinsonism and Parkinson disease. Neurology 2004; 62(7):1224–1226.

101. Kumru H, Santamaria J, Tolosa E, et al. Rapid eye movement sleep behavior disorder in parkinsonism with parkin mutations. Ann Neurol 2004; 56(4):599–603.

102. Ohsawa Y, Kurokawa K, Sonoo M. Reduced amplitude of the sural nerve sensory action potential in PARK2 patients. Neurology 2005; 65(3):459–462.

103. van de Warrenburg BP, Lammens M, Lucking CB, et al. Clinical and pathologic abnormalities in a family with parkinsonism and parkin gene mutations. Neurology 2001; 56:555–557.

104. De Rosa A, Volpe G, Marcantonio L. Neurophysiological evidence of corticospinal tract abnormality in patients with Parkin mutations. J Neurol 2006; 253(3):275–279. Epub 2006 Mar 6.

105. Tassin J, Durr A, Bonnet AM, et al. Levodopa-responsive dystonia. GTP cyclohydrolase I or parkin mutations? Brain 2000; 123:1112–1121.

106. Yamamura Y, Hattori N, Matsumine H, et al. Autosomal recessive early-onset parkinsonism with diurnal fluctuation: clinicopathologic characteristics and molecular genetic identification. Brain Dev 2000; 22(suppl 1):S87–S91.

107. Wu RM, Shan DE, Sun CM, et al. Clinical, 18F-dopa PET, and genetic analysis of an ethnic chinese kindred with early-onset parkinsonism and parkin gene mutations. Mov Disorders 2002; 17:670–67558.

108. Sasaki S, Shirata A, Yamane K, et al. Parkin-positive autosomal recessive juvenile Parkinsonism with alpha-synuclein-positive inclusions. Neurology 2004; 63(4):678–682.

109. Mori H, Kondo T, Yokochi M, et al. Pathologic and biochemical studies of juvenile parkinsonism linked to chromosome 6q. Neurology 1998; 51:890–892.

110. Pramstaller PP, Schlossmacher MG, Jacques TS. Lewy body Parkinson's disease in a large pedigree with 77 Parkin mutation carriers. Ann Neurol 2005; 58(3):411–422.

111. Serdaroglu P, Hanagasi H, Tasli H. Parkin expression in muscle from three patients with autosomal recessive Parkinson's disease carrying Parkin mutation. Acta Myol 2005; 24(1):2–5.

112. Morales B, Martinez A, Gonzalo I, et al. Steele-Richardson-Olszewski Syndrome in a patient with single C212Y mutation in the Parkin protein. Mov Disorders 2002; 17(6):1374–1380.

113. Broussolle E, Lucking CB, Ginovart N, et al. [18 F]-dopa PET study in patients with juvenile-onset PD and parkin gene mutations. Neurology 2000; 55(6):877–879.

114. Portman AT, Giladi N, Leenders KL, Maguire P, Veenma-van der Duin L, Swart J, et al. The nigrostriatal dopaminergic system in familial early onset parkinsonism with parkin mutations. Neurology 2001; 56:1759–1762.

115. Hilker R, Klein C, Ghaemi M, Kis B, et al. Positron emission tomographic analysis of the nigrostriatal dopaminergic system in familial parkinsonism associated with mutations in the parkin gene. Ann Neurol 2001; 49(3):367–376.

116. Khan NL, Brooks DJ, Pavese N, et al. Progression of nigrostriatal dysfunction in a parkin kindred: an [18F]dopa PET and clinical study. Brain 2002; 125(Pt 10):2248–2256.

117. Thobois S, Ribeiro MJ, Lohmann E, et al. Young-onset Parkinson disease with and without parkin gene mutations: a fluorodopa F 18 positron emission tomography study. Arch Neurol 2003; 60(5):713–718.
118. Scherfler C, Khan NL, Pavese N, et al. Striatal and cortical pre- and postsynaptic dopaminergic dysfunction in sporadic parkin-linked parkinsonism. Brain 2004; 127(Pt 6):1332–1342. Epub 2004 Apr 16.
119. Sawle GV, Leenders KL, Brooks DJ, et al. Dopa-responsive dystonia: [18F]dopa positron emission tomography. Ann Neurol 1991; 30(1):24–30.
120. Varrone A, Pellecchia MT, Amboni M, et al. Imaging of dopaminergic dysfunction with [123I]FP-CIT SPECT in early-onset parkin disease. Neurology 2004; 63(11):2097–2103.
121. Hu MT, Scherfler C, Khan NL. Nigral degeneration and striatal dopaminergic dysfunction in idiopathic and Parkin-linked Parkinson's disease. Mov Discord 2006; 21(3): 299–305.
122. Walter U, Klein C, Hilker R, et al. Brain parenchyma sonography detects preclinical parkinsonism. Mov Disord 2004; 19(12):1445–1449.
123. Deng H, Le WD, Hunter CB. Heterogeneous phenotype in a family with compound heterozygous parkin gene mutations. Arch Neurol 2006; 63(2):273–277.
124. Lücking CB, Brice A. Semiquantitative PCR for the detection of exon rearrangements in the parkin gene, in: "Methods in Molecular Medicine—Neurogenetics: Methods and Protocols, edt: Nicholas Potter, Humana Press Inc. Totowa, NJ, USA. 217:13–26, 2003.
125. Schlitter AM, Kurz M, Larsen JP. Parkin gene variations in late-onset Parkinson's disease: comparison between Norwegian and German cohorts. Acta Neurol Scand 2006; 113(1):9–13.
126. Santiago-Ribeiro MJ, Lohmann E, Brice A, et al. Striatal dopaminergic metabolism and DAT density in young onset Parkinson's disease patients: a PET stuy with [18F] Fluoro-L-Dopa and [11C]PE2I (Poster, 2005).

7   Genetics: *DJ-1* in Parkinson's Disease

Peter Heutink
Section of Medical Genomics, Department of Human Genetics, VU University Medical Center, Amsterdam, The Netherlands

INTRODUCTION

Our genetic knowledge of Parkinson's disease (PD) is moving forward at an impressive speed. In less than 10 years, family-based linkage analysis and positional cloning have led to the identification of several genes for autosomal recessive PD [*PARKIN* (1), *DJ-1* (2), and *PINK-1* (3)], autosomal dominant PD, [α-synuclein (4), *UCHL1* (5), *NR4A2* (6), and *LRRK2* (7,8)] and a number of potential genetic risk factors for idiopathic PD (9).

PD is characterized by resting tremor, bradykinesia, postural instability, rigidity, and a clinically significant response to treatment with levodopa (10). The disabling symptoms of PD are predominantly caused by selective loss of dopaminergic neurons in the substantia nigra pars compacta, which determines a profound reduction in striatal dopamine content. In addition, insoluble protein aggregates—known as Lewy bodies and Lewy neurites—containing many proteins, including α-synuclein and ubiquitin, are seen in the cytoplasm and neuronal processes of dopaminergic neurons and other subcortical and cortical structures in postmortem brain material of most patients.

Even though PD is generally a sporadic disorder, a significant proportion of cases (10–15%) have a positive family history (11), and the study of Mendelian forms of the disease has been of critical importance to the scientific advance of PD research, as the causal genes have offered new tools to model and understand pathways leading to neurodegeneration in PD, even though only a small proportion of cases have mutations in these genes. In the light of our current genetic knowledge, PD is etiologically heterogeneous, and the disease can result from disturbances in several molecular pathways, which can be initiated both by environmental and genetics risk factors, including rare Mendelian mutations (12–14).

Combining evidence observed through pathology and laboratory studies on the biological function of genes such as *PARKIN*, *UCHL1*, and α-synuclein, suggests that PD is a disorder of the cellular protein quality-control system, which is associated with neuronal accumulation of misfolded proteins and presence of protein aggregates. Although there is indeed strong evidence of the involvement of the protein quality-control system in PD, there is also biochemical evidence that suggests that oxidative stress and mitochondrial dysfunction can lead to the disease, as oxidation-modified proteins have been shown to accumulate in the context of normal aging and PD and may participate in the generation of protein aggregates in neurodegenerative disorders (12,13,15,16).

The recent identification of additional genes for Mendelian forms of PD provides evidence for pathways other than the disturbance of the protein quality-control system that can lead to the disease. This chapter will focus on the recent finding that mutations in *DJ-1* can lead to early-onset PD.

IDENTIFICATION OF *PARK7/DJ-1*

The PARK7 locus was identified as part of a research program Genetic Research in Isolated Populations (GRIP) (17). This study population from the southwest of the Netherlands has been genetically isolated for several centuries. Since ~1750, this population has grown with minimal immigration from ~150 individuals to an estimated 20,000 descendants, now scattered over eight adjacent villages, suggesting that the genetic background of this population could be more homogeneous than that of the general Dutch population, making it useful for genetic mapping studies. The genealogic history up to the 15th century has been computerized to a large extent, holding information on more then 60,000 individuals. Within this GRIP population, patients with PD were traced through local general practitioners, neurologists, and nursing home physicians. Parkinsonism was diagnosed when at least two out of three cardinal symptoms (bradykinesia, rigidity, resting tremor), as well as clinical improvement on dopaminergic therapy, were present. The diagnosis of idiopathic PD was established after exclusion of other possible causes of parkinsonism and was verified by two independent neurologists according to the EURPARKINSON criteria. Data on the presence of PD, essential tremor, and dementia in first-, second-, and third-degree relatives were collected by means of a family history questionnaire. In order to detect any subclinical or untreated parkinsonism, first-degree relatives of patients also underwent neurologic examination. Genealogic information was extended up to 16 generations. A total of 109 patients with parkinsonism were ascertained. Three patients with onset of disease before age 40 could be connected to a common ancestor six generations ago, and the pedigree showed several consanguineous loops (18). Parents of the identified patients were unaffected, strongly suggesting an autosomal recessive mode of inheritance. Given the genetic isolation of the population, homozygosity for a single pathogenic mutation was likely, and therefore three affected individuals, three unaffected sibs, and two parents were used for a genome-wide scan for linkage by homozygosity mapping. Significant evidence for linkage (LOD_{max}=4.3) was obtained to a locus on chromosome 1p36, distinct from the PARK6 locus and was therefore designated PARK7. Genetic analysis of a newly diagnosed patient from within the family was consistent with linkage (18). This linkage finding was confirmed in a different dataset of several small families (19) of which a single Italian family (three affected individuals) showed a lodscore >2.10, which is the suggested threshold for significance for a replication study (20). The critical region spanned approximately 20 cM. At the time, the human genome reference sequence was far from complete, and therefore a detailed recombination map was constructed on all available contigs using the Dutch and Italian families. This reduced the critical region to 5.6 cM containing approximately 90 genes. Several functional candidates did not show pathogenic mutations, but, since the region had been implicated in gross chromosomal abnormalities (21–23) and a loss-of-function mutation can be expected for a recessive disorder, a systematic screening was performed for expression of all the transcripts in the region, on mRNA derived from lymphoblast cell lines of patients and controls. One of the transcripts analyzed (*DJ-1*) could not be amplified from the mRNA of the Dutch patient but was normally amplified from healthy individuals and the Italian patient, suggesting a deletion; it was therefore a candidate for further analysis (2).

The human *DJ-1* gene contains eight exons spanning ~24 kb at genomic level (Fig. 1) (24,25). Exons 1A and 1B are noncoding and subject to alternative splicing of which the biologic significance is unknown. The protein encoded by the human

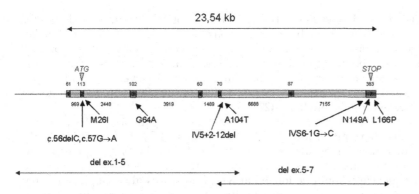

FIGURE 1 Genomic structure of the *DJ-1* gene on chromosome 1p36 and mutations identified in PD *arrows*). Purple boxes indicate exons, *Gray boxes* are intronic sequence. Intron/exon sizes are indicated in basepairs. Positions of start (ATG) and stop codons are indicated by triangles. *Abbreviation*: PD, Parkinson's disease.

DJ-1 gene consists of 189 amino acids, and its function has remained largely unknown. All patients in the Dutch kindred in whom PARK7 was originally identified carry a homozygous deletion which removes 1482 bp of genomic sequence, including ~4 kb upstream of the *DJ-1* start codon, and a large part of the coding region (Fig. 1). Sequence analysis of the deletion breakpoints revealed the presence of two flanking ALU elements. The most likely explanation for the presence of the deletion is that an unequal crossing-over event between the two ALU repeats must have occurred resulting in the intervening sequence to be lost. The crossing-over can be specifically located within a short stretch of 16 bases that is identical in both flanking ALU repeats (2).

In the patients of an Italian PARK7-linked family a homozygous missense mutation replaces a leucine at position 166 with proline (L166P) in the *DJ-1* protein (2). Several additional mutations in *DJ-1* have now been reported, including missense, truncating, splice site mutations, and large deletions (Fig. 1, Table 1). In particular, an additional patient with early-onset PD carrying compound heterozygous *DJ-1* mutations, one truncating (c.56delC c.57G → A) and one splice site mutation (IVS6-1 G → C), provides strong support that *DJ-1* mutations are indeed pathogenic (26). The c.56delC

TABLE 1 Summary of Identified *DJ-1* Mutations

Mutation		Functional effect	Population
1482bp del (Δex.1-5)	Homozygous	Loss of expression	Dutch
L166P	Homozygous	Protein stability	Italian
M26I	Homozygous		Ashkenazi Jewish
E64D	Homozygous		Turkish
IVS6-1 G → C	Compound heterozygous	Aberrant transcript	Hispanic (U.S.)
c.56delC c.57G → A	Compound heterozygous	Protein truncation	Hispanic (U.S.)
D149A	Heterozygous	Afro-Caribean	
A104T	Heterozygous	Latino	
IVS5+2-12del	Heterozygous	Aberrant transcript	Russian
(Δexon 5-7)	Heterozygous	Aberrant transcript	South Tyrol

c.57G → A is predicted to result in a truncated protein of only 18 amino acids and the IVS6-1 G → C results in a single-base substitution of the conserved invariant AG splice acceptor site of intron 6 and is predicted to result in aberrant transcription. For most other mutations, especially the heterozygous ones where no second mutation was identified, a pathogenic role remains to be demonstrated. However, for mutations like the Ex5-7del and the 11 bp deletion (IVS5+2-12del), severe effects on transcription or on the protein level can be predicted (27).

On the basis of the first screening in larger series of patients, the frequency of *DJ-1* mutations seems rather low (~1–2% in early-onset PD) (26–31). However, the occurrence of genomic rearrangements such as deletions in *DJ-1* emphasizes the importance of gene dose assays for a sensitive screening. Therefore, the observed mutation frequencies should be looked at with care since only a single study has included dosage analysis so far (27). In addition, there might be geographical differences in mutation frequencies as suggested by the absence of mutations in two cohorts from Southeast Asia (29,30). Further work, including population specific screens, is therefore needed to determine accurately the frequency of this form among early-onset PD forms in different populations and to characterize the associated phenotype.

Evidence for linkage to the PARK7 region was not found in genome scans for late-onset familial PD, suggesting that *DJ-1*, as with the other known genes for Mendelian PD, is not a major locus in common familial forms. However, whether genetic variation in *DJ-1* modifies the susceptibility to or modulates the expression of sporadic late-onset PD or other neurodegenerative diseases remains to be systematically explored.

MOLECULAR PROPERTIES OF *DJ-1*

The promoter region of *DJ-1* and the regulation of expression has not been studied in detail but a Specificity Protein 1 (SP1)–binding site at position-100 from the transcription initiation site appears to contribute most of the promoter activity (25). SP1 is a general transcription factor that directs expression of genes in many tissues, and, indeed, expression of the *DJ-1* transcripts can be detected in most body tissues, brain areas, and extracerebral tissues. Expression seems more abundant in subcortical than in cortical brain areas (2). A more detailed study on mouse brain largely confirmed these results but provided more details (32). Most structures involved in the regulation of motor activities (neurons in the motor cortex, caudate putamen, substantia nigra, red nucleus) were strongly labeled. Furthermore, cerebellum (granule cell layers and deep cerebellar nuclei, Purkinje cells) lateral globus pallidus and other nuclei such as hippocampus, piriform cortex, olfactory cortex, reticular cortex of the thalamus also showed high expression. In contrast, the molecular cell layer in the cerebellum was only weakly labeled. Expression was observed in cells with neuronal morphology, and no signal was observed in surrounding white matter. Although expression on the protein level has not yet been systematically investigated, several studies report widespread protein expression of *DJ-1* in human brain in both neurons and glial cells (33–35).

DJ-1 is strongly conserved throughout evolution and belongs to the ThiJ/PfpI superfamily of proteins (Pfam01965), which contain a highly conserved domain (ThiJ) and include members in all kingdoms of life (2,36). Prokaryotic members of this family with known function include: ThiJ, involved in the thiamine synthetic pathway, PfpI and other proteases, araC and other transcription factors, the glutamine amidotransferase family, which includes some bacterial catalases, and a recently recognized family of bacterial chaperones (EcHsp31) (2,36). In several organisms two paralogs of *DJ-1* are present [for example in *Caenorhabditis elegans* and *Drosophila Melanogaster*, each with 40% identity with the human protein (36)]. The functional divergence within this protein family makes it difficult to predict the function of human *DJ-1* on the basis of sequence homology alone. A computer-assisted model of the *DJ-1* protein based on the known crystal structure of protease PH1704 *Pyrococcus horikoshii* has been described (2), and in addition several independent groups have resolved the crystal structure of human *DJ-1* at resolutions of 1.1–1.95 Å (37–42). All the structures are very similar to each other, with the *DJ-1* monomer assuming an $\alpha\beta$ sandwich fold similar to the so-called flavodoxin-like, or Rossmann fold that is conserved in the *DJ-1*-ThiJ-PfpI superfamily. Interestingly, the structure is similar to another protein with a lower-sequence homology, the Hsp31 chaperone of *Escherichia coli* (37). Although a putative catalytic cysteine (C106) is present, which might suggest that *DJ-1* is a protease, the structural evidence does not support this since the catalytic triad (C106, H126, and perhaps G18) is present in an unfavorable confirmation for the proton transfer, which is typical of the cysteine protease catalysis (2,37,41). Biochemical approaches have failed to detect convincing protease or kinase activity of *DJ-1* so far (41).

An important finding in all these crystal studies is that *DJ-1* probably exists as a dimer, a finding that was confirmed by a series of gel filtration and circular dichroism experiments (37,38,41,43–45).

The Effect of *DJ-1* Mutations

The homozygous deletion found in the patients of the Dutch PARK7 family represents a natural knockout of *DJ-1*, indicating that the loss of function of *DJ-1* is pathogenic. The L166P mutation probably also induces a loss of *DJ-1* function because the mutant *DJ-1*[L166P] protein is unstable and rapidly degraded by the 20S/26S proteasome system, resulting in much lower steady-state levels in both transfected cells and patient lymphoblasts. The crystal structures confirmed that the residue mutated in the Italian PARK7 patients (L166) is located in a C-terminal α-helix and show that this helix is part of a hydrophobic core formed by three helices (two contributed by the C-terminal and one by the N-terminal part of the monomer), which is involved in the dimerization (37,38,41,43–47). The L166P mutation appears to disrupt the C-terminal domain and the dimerization capability, suggesting that the dimerization is functionally important. Gel filtration studies suggest that the L166P mutant does not form dimers but either adopts a different higher order structure or complexes with other proteins or is severely misfolded. Interestingly, a deletion mutant lacking residues 173–189 is also reported to form higher aggregates. Taken as a whole, these findings suggest that the dimeric structure is important for the function of *DJ-1*.

Two other homozygous disease-linked missense mutations, M26I (48) and E64D (49), seem to have distinct molecular and biochemical properties. The highly conserved residue M26 is located in the N-terminal helix, which contributes to the same hydrophobic core and is spatially close to L166; furthermore, this N-terminal helix contributes to the putative active site of *DJ-1* (34). The E64D protein is predicted to require a higher thermal energy for unfolding which might explain why available antibodies did not recognize the protein, however, whether this is relevant in vivo in unknown (45). In contrast to the L166P mutant, expression of M26I and E64D mutant proteins is stable and they can form homodimers, although less efficient than WT *DJ-1*, and are not susceptible to proteasomal degradation (45,50). At this point the functional consequences of these mutations are therefore not understood.

In addition to having a low steady-state level, the subcellular localization of the mutant *DJ-1*^{L166P} protein in transfection experiments is changed in comparison with the pattern seen with the wild type *DJ-1*. While the wild type *DJ-1* shows uniform localization in the cytosol and nucleus, the *DJ-1*^{L166P} mutant retains the nuclear localization but has lost the uniform cytosolic distribution in a fraction of the cells (between 10% and 50% of the cells depending on the study) and colocalizes with mitochondria (2,43,44,46). However, due to the high levels of expression in cell systems analyzed, it cannot be excluded that a fraction of wild type *DJ-1* also localizes to mitochondria, and in fact there is evidence to indicate this (44). However, the mitochondrial localization has not yet been confirmed for endogenous protein in human brain tissue or primary mouse neurons. The observation that the mutant (or perhaps also the wild type) *DJ-1* can colocalize with mitochondria suggests links to the function of these organelles, such as energy production, oxidative stress, and apoptosis.

DJ-1 Function

Early evidence suggested the involvement of *DJ-1* in cell-cycle regulation and oncogenesis, sperm maturation and fertilization, control of gene transcription, regulation of mRNA stability, and response to cell stress. Initially, a human cDNA termed *DJ-1* was identified as a novel oncogene that transformed NIH3T3 cells in cooperation with H-Ras (24). More recent proteomic-based studies found increased expression of the *DJ-1* protein in various human tumors, confirming the involvement of *DJ-1* in cell proliferation (51–53). Subsequently, a human protein named RS (identical to *DJ-1*) was identified as the regulatory subunit of a RNA-binding protein complex (54). It was suggested that *DJ-1* is a multifunctional protein involved in cytoskeleton-coupled RNA sorting, RNA degradation, and functions in the nucleus. Interestingly, in this study *DJ-1* was copurified with glyceraldehyde 3-phosphate dehydrogenase (GAPDH). GAPDH is increasingly recognized as a multifunctional protein involved, not only in glycolysis, but also in the induction of a neuronal apoptotic pathway (55–57). Evidence also links GAPDH to the pathogenesis of classical PD, as nuclear translocation of GAPDH has been detected in nigral neurons in postmortem PD brains, and GAPDH colocalizes with α-synuclein in Lewy bodies (58). Interestingly, the yeast genes encoding *DJ-1* and GAPDH homologs are both induced during cell stress, together with chaperones, antioxidants, and other stress-response genes (59).

Finally, two groups cloned the rat homologs of *DJ-1*, SP22, or CAP1 (60), as a protein found at reduced levels in sperm following the exposure of rats to infertility-inducing toxicants (61,62). Whether *DJ-1* is involved in these processes in humans remains unclear. *DJ-1* is present in human sperm, mainly as a flagellum protein, whereas in rats the homolog CAP1 or SP22 is also abundant in sperm heads (63). In the tail *DJ-1* colocalizes with β-tubulin, a major axoneme component. The issue of fertility has not been studied in humans with *DJ-1* related parkinsonism but knock-out mice for *DJ-1* have no fertility problems (64).

In a yeast two-hybrid screen the protein inhibitor of activated STAT (PIAS)xα/ARIP3 has been identified as a *DJ-1* binding protein (60). PIASxα/ARIP3 is expressed predominantly in the testis and is a modulator of the androgen receptor (AR) transcriptional activity (65). In cell cultures the effects of PIASxα/ARIP3 on AR activity depend from the cell lines and the reporter genes used (66). However, in most cell lines, including Sertoli cells, PIASxα/ARIP3 is a negative modulator of the AR transcriptional activity (60). *DJ-1* might therefore positively regulate the AR-mediated transcriptional activity by recruiting PIASxα and thereby removing its inhibitory activity. PIASxα/ARIP3 belongs to a family of proteins that modulate the activity of transcription factors by functioning as small ubiquitin-like modifier (SUMO) 1 ligases (67). Interestingly, a *DJ-1* mutant K130R was unable to regulate the AR activity (60). The lysine 130 of *DJ-1* is reported to be sumoylated (although experimental data have not been published) and it is possible that this modification is necessary for the full activity of *DJ-1*. More recently another *DJ-1* binding protein (DJBP) was identified (68). DJBP is also an AR-binding protein, which is highly expressed in the testis and appears to inhibit AR activity by recruiting a histone deacetylase (HDAC) complex. The binding of *DJ-1* to the DJBP-AR complex abrogates the HDAC–DJBP interaction, resulting in the enhancement of the AR activity. *DJ-1* appears therefore to positively regulate AR by antagonizing the inhibitory effects of PIASxα and DJBP (60,68). The fact that DJBP is expressed exclusively and PIASxα/ARIP3 predominantly in the testis suggests that these proteins are not relevant for the neuronal function of *DJ-1* (65,68). However, other members of the PIAS family, PIAS3 and PIASy, have also been shown to bind *DJ-1* (60). These interactions remain to be characterized and could be more relevant for the effects of *DJ-1* on gene expression in neurons.

Another group of interactors that have recently been identified are SUMO-1, the SUMO activating enzyme Uba2, and the SUMO conjugating enzyme Ubc9, all components of the sumoylation system, suggesting that *DJ-1* is sumoylated or regulates the function of sumo (69) (and unpublished data). Recent observations suggest that sumoylation plays an important role in brain function and neurodegeneration (70). There is evidence that sumoylated proteins are increased in the brain of patients with polyglutamine diseases, and altered sumoylation increases neurodegeneration in Drosophila models of polyglutamine disease (71,72).

Most of the known substrates for sumoylation are nuclear proteins, and sumoylation might influence protein function by changing the substrate localization, by competing with ubiquitylation, thereby inhibiting substrate degradation, and by directly modulating the functional properties of the substrate (70). Intriguingly, sumoylation regulates the activity not only of the steroid receptor superfamily but also of transcription factors mediating the heat-shock response, such as HSF1 and HSF2 (70). It will be interesting to see whether these transcription factors are also targeted by *DJ-1*.

A recent study has reported the interaction of *PARKIN* with mutant (L166P, M26I) *DJ-1* protein (50). *PARKIN* exists in a macromolecular protein complex with CHIP and Hsp70 that participates in the ubiquitilation and degradation of parkins substrates (73). *PARKIN* however does not ubiquitinilate or enhance the degradation of mutant *DJ-1* proteins but instead promotes their stability. Oxidative stress promotes the interaction of *PARKIN* and wild type *DJ-1*. However, this also does not lead to ubiquitilation and degradation of *DJ-1*. *DJ-1* appears not to be a target for *PARKIN* suggesting that *PARKIN* does not interact directly with *DJ-1* but is part of a protein complex of *PARKIN*, CHIP and Hsp70 that interacts with mutant *DJ-1*.

Oxidative Stress and Chaperone Activity

Important clues for the role of *DJ-1* in neurodegeneration have come from the evidence that human *DJ-1* is converted into a variant having more acidic isoelectric point in response to sublethal doses of paraquat (74,75), a toxin that generates reactive oxygen species (ROS) within cells and has been associated with dopamine neuron toxicity (76). Replacement of the C53 residue of *DJ-1*, located in the dimer interface of *DJ-1*, abolishes the pI shift of *DJ-1* in response to oxidative stimuli, suggesting that this shift is mediated by the oxidative conversion of the sulfydrylic group of cysteine to cysteine sulfinic acid (40). This modification might therefore lead to the functional activation of the protein in response to oxidative stress. However, the observation that another conserved cysteine (C106) displays extreme sensitivity to radiation damage suggests that C106 also mediates the oxidative conversion of *DJ-1* (41). The analysis of the crystal structure of oxidized *DJ-1* confirmed that C106 undergoes modification to sulfinic acid (37,77). Detailed analysis of C46, C53, and C106 revealed that mutation of C106 but not C46 or C53 prevents formation of an oxidized isoform in intact cells (77). Furthermore, the C106 also blocks oxidation-induced mitochondrial localization and protection against 1-methyl-4-phenylpyridinium (MPP+) toxicity in neuronal cells suggesting that C106 controls the previously reported neuroprotective function of *DJ-1* (77).

Gene expression of a yeast homolog of *DJ-1*, YDR533C (*Saccharomyces cerevisiae*), is upregulated in response to sorbic acid (59) an inducer of cellular oxidative stress, raising the question of whether *DJ-1* also plays a role as a molecular chaperone similar to another, recently identified member of the *DJ-1*-ThiJ-PfpI superfamily, the *Escherichia coli* Hsp31 (78). The possible function of *DJ-1* as molecular chaperone is intriguing in the light of the role of the molecular chaperones in the pathogenesis of PD and other neurodegenerative diseases since ROS and proteasomal inhibition have been correlated with PD pathology (79). These proteins function in assisting the proper folding of nascent polypeptides and the refolding of damaged proteins; they are also involved in targeting and/or delivering of protein to the proteasomal system for degradation. The *E. coli* stress-inducible chaperone Hsp31 possesses protease activity as well (37,78). It has been suggested that it switches from chaperone to protease function on the basis of the temperature shift as observed with another bacterial protein. Similarly, one could speculate that *DJ-1* has also dual function of chaperone and enzyme, depending on the cell stress level.

DJ-1-deficient embryonic stem (ES) cell derived dopamine neurons (DNs) and primary DNs with *DJ-1* levels reduced by RNAi "knockdown," display increased sensitivity to oxidative stress in the form of H_2O_2 (80). The initial accumulation of H_2O_2 induced ROS in these appears normal in *DJ-1*-deficient dopamine neurons (DNs), but over time the cellular defenses to ROS seem impaired, leading to increased apoptosis. Additionally, *DJ-1* deficiency sensitizes cells to the proteasomal inhibitor lactacystin but not other toxic stimuli such as tunicamycin. Proteasomal inhibition induces the accumulation of short-lived and misfolded cytoplasmic proteins, leading to oxidative stress and apoptosis (81) and one might hypothesize that *DJ-1* mutations lead to PD because of an increased sensitivity of *DJ-1*-deficient DNs to such stressors. There is evidence that *DJ-1* can function as an adenosine triphosphate (ATP)-independent cytoplasmic redox-sensitive molecular chaperone for multiple targets (82). However, others also have investigated the chaperone activity of *DJ-1* in vitro as well and in these studies redox regulation appeared not to be a significant factor (37,83). L166P mutant *DJ-1* fails to function as a molecular chaperone in vivo or in vitro and consistent with this, this mutant fails to complement *DJ-1* knockout cells in vivo, even when overexpressed at artificially high levels (80). The L166P loss of function seems not due simply to reduced levels of *DJ-1* protein, but might also be a consequence of altered structure and resultant loss of function (82).

Candidate substrates for *DJ-1* chaperone activity in the context of PD include α-synuclein and neurofilament proteins (NFL), based on their presence in PD protein inclusions. Indeed *DJ-1* inhibits the aggregation of α-synuclein in differentiated cells in vivo, and loss of *DJ-1* leads to increased accumulation of insoluble α-synuclein (82). The *DJ-1* chaperone activity is inhibited by reducing conditions, and can be stimulated by oxidation. Thus, in the normal reducing environment of the cell, *DJ-1* may be inactive. Production of ROS and alteration of the redox state of the cytoplasm may activate *DJ-1* chaperone activity as a mechanism of coping with protein aggregation and misfolding. This might explain some of the differences described in the literature since studies used different environmental conditions for their experiments (37,83).

PATHOLOGY

Pathologic analysis of brains from patients with *DJ-1* related forms is of great importance, but brain material is not currently available. However, investigating the presence of the *DJ-1* protein in brain from patients with Lewy body disease and other neurodegenerative diseases might provide clues on the involvement of *DJ-1* in common forms of neurodegeneration. While no convincing evidence of *DJ-1* immunoreactivity in Lewy bodies has been reported (33,35,84), in transfection studies *DJ-1* appears to associate with α-synuclein in the Triton X-100-soluble fraction of FeCl2-treated lysates. However, *DJ-1* does not colocalize with the punctate protein aggregates visible by immunostaining in the case of either α-synuclein or NFL, supporting the notion that *DJ-1* functions at an early step in the aggregation process, when the substrate protein may be misfolded, but has not yet formed a mature aggregate. It can be hypothesized that *DJ-1* may promote the degradation of such misfolded proteins, either through the proteasome or through other cellular pathways such as chaperone-mediated autophagy.

In human postmortem material, *DJ-1* immunoreactivity colocalizes within a subset of pathologic tau inclusions in various neurodegenerative disorders, including Pick's disease, Alzheimer's disease, Lewy body dementia, progressive supranuclear palsy, cortical basal degeneration, multiple system athrophy, and frontotemporal dementia with parkinsonism linked to chromosome 17 (33,35,84). At, first this might seem contradictory, however, these last findings could represent an end stage of protein aggregates in the situation when *DJ-1* is not able to cope with the amount of misfolded proteins (33,35). These data suggest that *DJ-1* could function to suppress protein aggregates in the cytoplasm, possibly in an early step in the formation of protein aggregates. It has been suggested that such protofibrils, rather than the large fibrillar aggregates, may underlie toxicity in vivo in several neurodegenerative diseases.

The colocalization of *DJ-1* and tau raises the question of whether tau pathology is also present in the brain of patients with *DJ-1* mutations. Interestingly, tau pathology has been found in patients with *PARKIN* disease (85,86). Therefore, if this would also be the case in *DJ-1* related disease, it would suggest the existence of a common pathological signature in *DJ-1-* and *PARKIN*-related forms. A strong signal for *DJ-1* was also observed in activated astrocytes both in neurodegenerative disorders and in material from other brain diseases such as Schizophrenia, in agreement with a more general role for *DJ-1* as a chaperone (33,84).

On the basis of all the available evidence, one can propose that *DJ-1* is involved in the cellular response to stress at multiple levels (2) (Fig. 2). First, it might directly

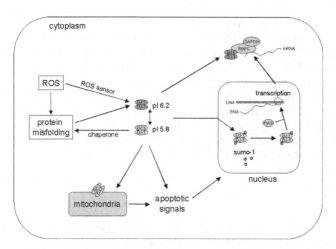

FIGURE 2 Model of *DJ-1* as a stress responsive protein. *DJ-1* is a sensor to ROS by changing its isoelectric point (from pI 6.2 to pI 5.8 under stress conditions. *DJ-1* has chaperone activity induced by such (oxidative) stress conditions. Possibly to protect the cell from damage, *DJ-1* has been colocalized with α-synuclein, neurofilament proteins, and the microtubule associated protein tau, and these proteins might be targets of the chaperone activity. In addition *DJ-1* is part of a RBPC that includes GAPDH and might be involved in post-transcriptional regulation of mRNA. In addition *DJ-1* is involved in the regulation of expression of a number of proteins some of which might play a role in response to stress. *Abbreviations*: GAPDH, glyceraldehyde 3-phosphate dehydrogenase; RBPC, RNA-binding protein complex; ROS, reactive oxygen species.

react to stress signals (e.g., redox changes, misfolded proteins) being a molecular chaperone. Second, *DJ-1* might modulate the gene expression of the stress response at the post-transcriptional level by the known interaction with RNA-binding protein complexes. Interestingly, the post-transcriptional regulation of gene expression is important for both neuronal function and spermatogenesis. Third, *DJ-1* might translocate to the nucleus in response to stress signals. In the nucleus it might interact with PIAS or other cofactors and modulate the gene expression at the transcriptional level. Although the exact involvement of human *DJ-1* in the oxidative stress response or in the response to misfolded protein stress remains to be shown, the proposed model is intriguing in the light of the evidence of oxidative stress and protein misfolding documented in the brains of patients with PD. Especially since recent studies have shown that mutations in α-synuclein and *PARKIN*, two other PD-related genes, might also be linked to oxidative stress (87,88) supporting the view that different forms of PD may have similar pathogenetic mechanisms, which likely includes a role for *DJ-1*.

CLINICAL ASPECTS

Early onset of parkinsonism, slow disease progression, and good response to levodopa are uniform clinical features in the different autosomal recessive forms of early-onset. This makes their differentiation difficult on clinical grounds, indicating the importance of genetic testing. The average age at onset is in the early 30s in the *PARKIN*- and *DJ-1* related families, whereas onset in PARK6-linked families might be slightly later (late 30s–early 40s). Interestingly, psychiatric disturbances (including severe anxiety in three cases, and psychotic episodes in one), early behavioral disturbances (one case), and dystonic features (including blepharospasm in two cases) are reported in both the original *DJ-1* related families, and they might be clinically useful for suspecting *DJ-1* involvement. The presence of severe anxiety and panic attacks has indeed been noted in two further *DJ-1* related patients identified in a recent screen. However, a note of caution is warranted, as these psychiatric disturbances are nonspecific; they occur in PD in general and have also been reported in patients with mutations in the *PARKIN* gene. Analyzing larger case series is therefore needed to investigate whether psychiatric disturbances are more frequent in the *DJ-1* related form than in other PD forms. Recent positron emission tomography studies in *DJ-1* related patients showed more uniform patterns of caudate/putamen dopaminergic terminal dysfunction than that observed in classical PD, and a greater dopaminergic dysfunction than the one expected on the basis of clinical severity. These features also resemble the pattern observed in *PARKIN*-related and PARK6-linked disease, suggesting that these three autosomal recessive forms of early-onset are similar to each other on pathophysiologic grounds.

Very recently, a mouse model was reported bearing a germline disruption of *DJ-1* by the genetic deletion of *DJ-1* exon 2, which contains the ATG (64). These *DJ-1* null mice are healthy and reproduce normally. No reduction of dopaminergic neurons in the substantia nigra was observed in the brains of *DJ-1* mutants up to 12 months of age. The mice are also did not show an increased sensitivity to paraquat. However, they did show a dopaminergic deficit. Real-time electrochemical measurements of acute striatal slices revealed reduced evoked dopamine overflow in the knockout mice. This reduction was primarily due to an increased reuptake of dopamine by the dopamine transporter in the absence of an upregulation of this gene at the mRNA or protein level (64).

No effects were detected on induction of corticostriatal long-term potentiation (LTP) but the induction of long-term depression (LTD) was impaired. Since induction of LTP requires activation of Dopamine 1 receptors (D1R) and LTD the activation of both D1 and D2 receptors this suggests that *DJ-1* is required for normal dopamine D2 receptor (D2R) regulation of dopamine reuptake in the presynaptic terminal of nigral neurons. In agreement with this, behavioral and electrophysiologic studies showed a blunted response of the D2R to pharmacologic challenges and the mice showed impaired perfromance in behavioral and locomotor tests. This study demonstrates a link between *DJ-1* and dopaminergic physiology in the nigrostriatal system in which *DJ-1* plays a role in mediating the downstream effects of the Dopamine D2 receptor activation in nigral neurons.

CONCLUSIONS

The effect of the loss of *DJ-1* function, either alone or in combination with mutations in other PD-related genes, can now be investigated in cell culture and animal models, including models of PD induced by dopaminergic neurotoxins, including 1-methyl-4-phenyl-1,2,3,6-tetrahydropyridine and rotenone. In lower organisms such as transgenic flies, *C. elegans*, or yeast, it will be possible to rapidly screen for genetic modifiers, either enhancers or suppressors of any resulting *DJ-1* related phenotype.

Apart from the knockout mice, transgenic mice overexpressing the human *DJ-1* gene have been generated and these mice might also be useful to investigate putative brain functions of *DJ-1*, including resistance to dopaminergic toxins, oxidative stress, and protein misfolding. Expression profiling in cell cultures or animal models where the *DJ-1* gene is manipulated or in patient-derived cells might facilitate the characterization of *DJ-1*-related pathways. Biochemical and cell biology studies have also been initiated to understand further the function of *DJ-1*, identify its interacting partners, and explore possible relationships between *DJ-1* and the proteins encoded by genes which are firmly implicated in PD and other common neurodegenerative disease.

The *DJ-1* gene has been highly conserved in evolution and is abundantly and ubiquitously expressed in the brain and other body tissues. However, its function has remained elusive, and no one has previously linked the *DJ-1* protein to brain function or brain disorders. The discovery that mutations in *DJ-1* cause autosomal recessive early-onset forms of PD establishes that the loss of the *DJ-1* function leads to human neurodegeneration. Clarifying the mechanisms of *DJ-1*-related disease might also potentially shed light on novel mechanisms of brain neuronal maintenance and promote the understanding of pathogenesis of common forms of PD. Although much work remains to be done to clarify the biology of this protein, the chaperone activity of *DJ-1* and/or its possible role as oxidative sensor are intriguing in the light of the current pathogenetic scenarios for PD. However, the importance of identifying a novel gene causing PD is even greater if it leads to innovative ideas about pathogenesis. In the case of *DJ-1*, potentially novel insights are the focus on the nuclear and cytoplasmic control of gene expression in PD pathogenesis.

ACKNOWLEDGMENTS

This work was supported in part by the Michael J. Fox Foundation, the Parkinson Disease Foundation/National Parkinson Foundation (USA), and the "Prinses Beatrixs Fonds."

REFERENCES

1. Kitada T, Asakawa S, Hattori N, et al. Mutations in the parkin gene cause autosomal recessive juvenile parkinsonism. Nature 1998; 392(6676):605–608.
2. Bonifati V, Rizzu P, van Baren MJ, et al. Mutations in the DJ-1 gene associated with autosomal recessive early-onset parkinsonism. Science 2003; 299(5604):256–259.
3. Valente EM, Salvi S, Ialongo T, et al. PINK1 mutations are associated with sporadic early-onset parkinsonism. Ann Neurol 2004; 56(3):336–341.
4. Polymeropoulos MH, Lavedan C, Leroy E, et al. Mutation in the alpha-synuclein gene identified in families with Parkinson's disease. Science 1997; 276(5321):2045–2047.
5. Leroy E, Boyer R, Polymeropoulos MH. Intron-exon structure of ubiquitin c-terminal hydrolase-L1. DNA. Res 1998; 5(6):397–400.
6. Le WD, Xu P, Jankovic J, et al. Mutations in NR4A2 associated with familial Parkinson's disease. Nat Genet 2003; 33(1):85–89.
7. Zimprich A, Biskup S, Leitner P, et al. Mutations in LRRK2 cause autosomal-dominant parkinsonism with pleomorphic pathology. Neuron 2004; 44(4):601–607.
8. Paisan-Ruiz C, Jain S, Evans EW, et al. Cloning of the gene containing mutations that cause PARK8-linked Parkinson's disease. Neuron 2004; 44(4):595–600.
9. Bertoli-Avella AM, Oostra BA, Heutink P. Chasing genes in Alzheimer's and Parkinson's disease. Hum Genet 2004; 114(5):413–438.
10. Lang AE, Lozano AM. Parkinson's dsisease. First of two parts. N Engl J Med 1998; 339(15):1044–1053.
11. Golbe LI. Young-onset Parkinson's disease: a clinical review. Neurology 1991; 41 [2(Pt 1)]:168–173.
12. Dawson TM, Dawson VL. Molecular pathways of neurodegeneration in Parkinson's disease. Science 2003; 302(5646):819–822.

13. Fahn S, Sulzer D. Neurodegeneration and neuroprotection in Parkinson's disease. Neurorx 2004; 1(1):139–154.

14. Dawson TM, Dawson VL. Rare genetic mutations shed light on the pathogenesis of Parkinson's disease. J Clin Invest 2003; 111(2):145–151.

15. Orth M, Schapira AH. Mitochondria and degenerative disorders. Am J Med Genet 2001; 106(1):27–36.

16. Jenner P. Oxidative stress in Parkinson's disease. Ann Neurol 2003; 53(suppl 3):S26–S36; discussion S36–S28.

17. Dekker MC, van Swieten JC, Houwing-Duistermaat JJ, et al. A clinical-genetic study of Parkinson's disease in a genetically isolated community. J Neurol 2003; 250(9): 1056–1062.

18. van Duijn CM, Dekker MC, Bonifati V, et al. Park7, a novel locus for autosomal recessive early-onset parkinsonism, on chromosome 1p36. Am J Hum Genet 2001; 69(3):629–634.

19. Bonifati V, Breedveld GJ, Squitieri F, et al. Localization of autosomal recessive early-onset parkinsonism to chromosome 1p36 (PARK7) in an independent dataset. Ann Neurol 2002; 51(2):253–256.

20. Lander E, Kruglyak L. Genetic dissection of complex traits: guidelines for interpreting and reporting linkage results. Nat Genet 1995; 11(3):241–247.

21. Poetsch M, Woenckhaus C, Dittberner T, et al. An increased frequency of numerical chromosomal abnormalities and 1p36 deletions in isolated cells from paraffin sections of malignant melanomas by means of interphase cytogenetics. Cancer Genet Cytogenet 1998; 104(2):146–152.

22. Shapira SK, McCaskill C, Northrup H, et al. Chromosome 1p36 deletions: the clinical phenotype and molecular characterization of a common newly delineated syndrome. Am J Hum Genet 1997; 61(3):642–650.

23. Bieche I, Khodja A, Lidereau R. Deletion mapping of chromosomal region 1p32-pter in primary breast cancer. Genes Chromosomes Cancer 1999; 24(3):255–263.

24. Nagakubo D, Taira T, Kitaura H, et al. DJ-1, a novel oncogene which transforms mouse NIH3T3 cells in cooperation with ras. Biochem Biophys Res Commun 1997; 231(2): 509–513.

25. Taira T, Takahashi K, Kitagawa R, et al. Molecular cloning of human and mouse DJ-1 genes and identification of Sp1-dependent activation of the human DJ-1 promoter. Gene 2001; 263(1–2):285–292.

26. Hague S, Rogaeva E, Hernandez D, et al. Early-onset Parkinson's disease caused by a compound heterozygous DJ-1 mutation. Ann Neurol 2003; 54(2):271–274.

27. Hedrich K, Djarmati A, Schafer N, et al. DJ-1 (PARK7) mutations are less frequent than Parkin (PARK2) mutations in early-onset Parkinson's disease. Neurology 2004; 62(3):389–394.

28. Clark LN, Afridi S, Mejia-Santana H, et al. Analysis of an early-onset Parkinson's disease cohort for DJ-1 mutations. Mov Disord 2004; 19(7):796–800.

29. Tan EK, Tan C, Zhao Y, et al. Genetic analysis of DJ-1 in a cohort Parkinson's disease patients of different ethnicity. Neurosci Lett 2004; 367(1):109–112.

30. Lockhart PJ, Bounds R, Hulihan M, et al. Lack of mutations in DJ-1 in a cohort of Taiwanese ethnic Chinese with early-onset parkinsonism. Mov Disord 2004; 19(9):1065–1069.

31. Healy DG, Abou-Sleiman PM, Valente EM, et al. DJ-1 mutations in Parkinson's disease. J Neurol Neurosurg Psychiatry 2004; 75(1):144–145.

32. Shang H, Lang D, Jean-Marc B, et al. Localization of DJ-1 mRNA in the mouse brain. Neurosci Lett 2004; 367(3):273–277.

33. Rizzu P, Hinkle DA, Zhukareva V, et al. DJ-1 colocalizes with tau inclusions: a link between parkinsonism and dementia. Ann Neurol 2004; 55(1):113–118.

34. Baulac S, LaVoie MJ, Strahle J, et al. Dimerization of Parkinson's disease-causing DJ-1 and formation of high molecular weight complexes in human brain. Mol Cell Neurosci 2004; 27(3):236–246.

35. Bandopadhyay R, Kingsbury AE, Cookson MR, et al. The expression of DJ-1 (PARK7) in normal human CNS and idiopathic Parkinson's disease. Brain 2004; 127(Pt 2):420–430.

36. Bandyopadhyay S, Cookson MR. Evolutionary and functional relationships within the DJ1 superfamily. BMC Evol Biol 2004; 4(1):6.

37. Lee SJ, Kim SJ, Kim IK, et al. Crystal structures of human DJ-1 and Escherichia coli Hsp31, which share an evolutionarily conserved domain. J Biol Chem 2003; 278(45): 44552–44559.

38. Tao X, Tong L. Crystal structure of human DJ-1, a protein associated with early onset Parkinson's disease. J Biol Chem 2003; 278(33):31372–31379.

39. Honbou K, Suzuki NN, Horiuchi M, et al. The crystal structure of DJ-1, a protein related to male fertility and Parkinson's disease. J Biol Chem 2003; 278(33):31380–31384.

40. Honbou K, Suzuki NN, Horiuchi M, et al. Crystallization and preliminary crystallographic analysis of DJ-1, a protein associated with male fertility and parkinsonism. Acta Crystallogr D Biol Crystallogr 2003; 59(Pt 8):1502–1503.

41. Wilson MA, Collins JL, Hod Y, et al. The 1.1-A resolution crystal structure of DJ-1, the protein mutated in autosomal recessive early onset Parkinson's disease. Proc Natl Acad Sci USA 2003; 100(16):9256–9261.

42. Huai Q, Sun Y, Wang H, et al. Crystal structure of DJ-1/RS and implication on familial Parkinson's disease. FEBS Lett 2003; 549(1–3):171–175.

43. Macedo MG, Anar B, Bronner IF, et al. The DJ-1L166P mutant protein associated with early onset Parkinson's disease is unstable and forms higher-order protein complexes. Hum Mol Genet 2003; 12(21):2807–2816.

44. Miller DW, Ahmad R, Hague S, et al. L166P mutant DJ-1, causative for recessive Parkinson's disease, is degraded through the ubiquitin-proteasome system. J Biol Chem 2003; 278(38):36588–36595.

45. Gorner K, Holtorf E, Odoy S, et al. Differential effects of Parkinson's disease-associated mutations on stability and folding of DJ-1. J Biol Chem 2004; 279(8):6943–6951.

46. Lockhart PJ, Lincoln S, Hulihan M, et al. DJ-1 mutations are a rare cause of recessively inherited early onset parkinsonism mediated by loss of protein function. J Med Genet 2004; 41(3):e22.

47. Moore DJ, Zhang L, Dawson TM, et al. A missense mutation (L166P) in DJ-1, linked to familial Parkinson's disease, confers reduced protein stability and impairs homo-oligomerization. J Neurochem 2003; 87(6):1558–1567.

48. Abou-Sleiman PM, Healy DG, Quinn N, et al. The role of pathogenic DJ-1 mutations in Parkinson's disease. Ann Neurol 2003; 54(3):283–286.

49. Hering R, Strauss KM, Tao X, et al. Novel homozygous p.E64D mutation in DJ1 in early onset Parkinson's disease (PARK7). Hum Mutat 2004; 24(4):321–329.

50. Moore DJ, Zhang L, Troncoso J, et al. Association of DJ-1 and parkin mediated by pathogenic DJ-1 mutations and oxidative stress. Hum Mol Genet 2005; 14(1):71–84.

51. Le Naour F, Misek DE, Krause MC, et al. Proteomics-based identification of RS/DJ-1 as a novel circulating tumor antigen in breast cancer. Clin Cancer Res 2001; 7(11): 3328–3335.

52. Bergman AC, Benjamin T, Alaiya A, et al. Identification of gel-separated tumor marker proteins by mass spectrometry. Electrophoresis 2000; 21(3):679–686.

53. Srisomsap C, Subhasitanont P, Otto A, et al. Detection of cathepsin B up-regulation in neoplastic thyroid tissues by proteomic analysis. Proteomics 2002; 2(6):706–712.

54. Hod Y, Pentyala SN, Whyard TC, et al. Identification and characterization of a novel protein that regulates RNA-protein interaction. J Cell Biochem 1999; 72(3):435–444.

55. Mazzola JL, Sirover MA. Alteration of intracellular structure and function of glyceraldehyde-3-phosphate dehydrogenase: a common phenotype of neurodegenerative disorders? Neurotoxicology 2002; 23(4–5):603–609.

56. Ishitani R, Tanaka M, Sunaga K, et al. Nuclear localization of overexpressed glyceraldehyde-3-phosphate dehydrogenase in cultured cerebellar neurons undergoing apoptosis. Mol Pharmacol 1998; 53(4):701–707.

57. Fukuhara Y, Takeshima T, Kashiwaya Y, et al. GAPDH knockdown rescues mesencephalic dopaminergic neurons from MPP+ -induced apoptosis. Neuroreport 2001; 12(9):2049–2052.

58. Tatton NA. Increased caspase 3 and Bax immunoreactivity accompany nuclear GAPDH translocation and neuronal apoptosis in Parkinson's disease. Exp Neurol 2000; 166(1):29–43.

59. de Nobel H, Lawrie L, Brul S, et al. Parallel and comparative analysis of the proteome and transcriptome of sorbic acid-stressed Saccharomyces cerevisiae. Yeast 2001; 18(15):1413–1428.

60. Takahashi K, Taira T, Niki T, et al. DJ-1 positively regulates the androgen receptor by impairing the binding of PIASx alpha to the receptor. J Biol Chem 2001; 276(40): 37556–37563.

61. Wagenfeld A, Gromoll J, Cooper TG. Molecular cloning and expression of rat contraception associated protein 1 (CAP1), a protein putatively involved in fertilization. Biochem Biophys Res Commun 1998; 251(2):545–549.
62. Welch JE, Barbee RR, Roberts NL, et al. SP22: a novel fertility protein from a highly conserved gene family. J Androl 1998; 19(4):385–393.
63. Whyard TC, Cheung W, Sheynkin Y, et al. Identification of RS as a flagellar and head sperm protein. Mol Reprod Dev 2000; 55(2):189–196.
64. Goldberg MS, Pisani A, Haburcak M, et al. Nigrostriatal Dopaminergic Deficits and Hypokinesia Caused by Inactivation of the Familial Parkinsonism-Linked Gene DJ-1. Neuron 2005; 45(4):489–496.
65. Moilanen AM, Karvonen U, Poukka H, et al. A testis-specific androgen receptor coregulator that belongs to a novel family of nuclear proteins. J Biol Chem 1999; 274(6):3700–3704.
66. Kotaja N, Aittomaki S, Silvennoinen O, et al. ARIP3 (androgen receptor-interacting protein 3) and other PIAS (protein inhibitor of activated STAT) proteins differ in their ability to modulate steroid receptor-dependent transcriptional activation. Mol Endocrinol 2000; 14(12):1986–2000.
67. Kotaja N, Karvonen U, Janne OA, et al. PIAS proteins modulate transcription factors by functioning as SUMO-1 ligases. Mol Cell Biol 2002; 22(14):5222–5234.
68. Niki T, Takahashi-Niki K, Taira T, et al. DJBP: a novel DJ-1-binding protein, negatively regulates the androgen receptor by recruiting histone deacetylase complex, and DJ-1 antagonizes this inhibition by abrogation of this complex. Mol Cancer Res 2003; 1(4):247–261.
69. Junn E, Taniguchi H, Zhao X, Mouradian M. Protection of cell death by DJ-1, D.S.f.N. Program No. 558.3. 2004 Abstract Viewer/Itinerary Planner. Washington, Editor, 2004.
70. Kim KI, Baek SH, Chung CH. Versatile protein tag, SUMO: its enzymology and biological function. J Cell Physiol 2002; 191(3):257–268.
71. Chan HY, Warrick JM, Andriola I, et al. Genetic modulation of polyglutamine toxicity by protein conjugation pathways in Drosophila. Hum Mol Genet 2002; 11(23):2895–2904.
72. Ueda H, Goto J, Hashida H, et al. Enhanced SUMOylation in polyglutamine diseases. Biochem Biophys Res Commun 2002; 293(1):307–313.
73. Imai Y, Soda M, Hatakeyama S, et al. CHIP is associated with Parkin, a gene responsible for familial Parkinson's disease, and enhances its ubiquitin ligase activity. Mol Cell 2002; 10(1):55–67.
74. Mitsumoto A, Nakagawa Y. DJ-1 is an indicator for endogenous reactive oxygen species elicited by endotoxin. Free Radic Res 2001; 35(6):885–893.
75. Mitsumoto A, Nakagawa Y, Takeuchi A, et al. Oxidized forms of peroxiredoxins and DJ-1 on two-dimensional gels increased in response to sublethal levels of paraquat. Free Radic Res 2001; 35(3):301–310.
76. McCormack AL, Thiruchelvam M, Manning-Bog AB, et al. Environmental risk factors and Parkinson's disease: selective degeneration of nigral dopaminergic neurons caused by the herbicide paraquat. Neurobiol Dis 2002; 10(2):119–127.
77. Canet-Aviles RM, Wilson MA, Miller DW, et al. The Parkinson's disease protein DJ-1 is neuroprotective due to cysteine-sulfinic acid-driven mitochondrial localization. Proc Natl Acad Sci USA 2004; 101(24):9103-9108.
78. Quigley PM, Korotkov K, Baneyx F, et al. The 1.6-A crystal structure of the class of chaperones represented by Escherichia coli Hsp31 reveals a putative catalytic triad. Proc Natl Acad Sci USA 2003; 100(6):3137–3142.
79. Dauer W, Przedborski S. Parkinson's disease: mechanisms and models. Neuron 2003; 39(6):889–909.
80. Martinat C, Shendelman S, Jonason A, et al. Sensitivity to oxidative stress in DJ-1-deficient dopamine neurons: an ES- derived cell model of primary parkinsonism. PLoS Biol 2004; 2(11):e327.
81. Demasi M, Davies KJ. Proteasome inhibitors induce intracellular protein aggregation and cell death by an oxygen-dependent mechanism. FEBS Lett 2003; 542(1–3):89–94.
82. Shendelman S, Jonason A, Martinat C, et al. DJ-1 is a redox-dependent molecular chaperone that inhibits alpha-synuclein aggregate formation. PLoS Biol 2004; 2(11):e362.
83. Olzmann JA, Brown K, Wilkinson KD, et al. Familial Parkinson's disease-associated L166P mutation disrupts DJ-1 protein folding and function. J Biol Chem 2004; 279(9): 8506–8515.

84. Neumann M, Muller V, Gorner K, et al. Pathological properties of the Parkinson's disease-associated protein DJ-1 in alpha-synucleinopathies and tauopathies: relevance for multiple system atrophy and Pick's disease. Acta Neuropathol (Berl) 2004; 107(6): 489–496.
85. Mori H, Kondo T, Yokochi M, et al. Pathologic and biochemical studies of juvenile parkinsonism linked to chromosome 6q. Neurology 1998; 51(3):890–892.
86. van de Warrenburg BP, Lammens M, Lucking CB, et al. Clinical and pathologic abnormalities in a family with parkinsonism and parkin gene mutations. Neurology 2001; 56(4):555–557.
87. Hyun DH, Lee M, Hattori N, et al. Effect of wild-type or mutant Parkin on oxidative damage, nitric oxide, antioxidant defenses, and the proteasome. J Biol Chem 2002; 277(32):28572–28577.
88. Hashimoto M, Hsu LJ, Rockenstein E, et al. alpha-Synuclein protects against oxidative stress via inactivation of the c-Jun N-terminal kinase stress-signaling pathway in neuronal cells. J Biol Chem 2002; 277(13):11465–11472.

8 | *PINK1* Parkinsonism

Patrick M. Abou-Sleiman, Miratul M. K. Muqit, and Nicholas W. Wood
Department of Molecular Neuroscience, Institute of Neurology, London, U.K.

INTRODUCTION

PINK1 (PTEN-induced kinase 1) is the third gene to be associated with autosomal recessive Parkinson's disease (ARPD) following *PARKIN* and *DJ-1*. Mutations in *PINK1* were identified in three consanguineous families from Italy and Spain. Subsequent mutation screens from several groups around the world reported *PINK1* mutations in ARPD at a frequency between those in *PARKIN*, which account for approximately 50% of cases under 50 years old, and *DJ-1*, which remain quite rare at approximately 1%. Clinically, *PINK1*-positive patients present with a phenotype which is remarkably similar to idiopathic Parkinson's disease (PD), albeit with a younger age at onset and slower progression. Pathologic data from *PINK1* heterozygote cases have demonstrated the presence of Lewy bodies, eosinophilic cytoplasmic inclusions that are the pathologic hallmark of idiopathic PD. It remains to be determined if homozygote mutants also develop Lewy bodies or are more similar to *PARKIN* cases, where loss of dopaminergic neurons can occur independently of Lewy body formation.

LINKAGE AND MUTATION DISCOVERY

The ARPD locus, *PARK6*, was mapped to a 12.5-centimorgan (cM) region on chromosome 1p35–36 in a large consanguineous Sicilian family (Marsala kindred) (1). Autozygosity mapping of two additional families (one Italian and one Spanish) with ARPD provided additional evidence of linkage to *PARK6* and refinement of the critical region to a 3.7 cM interval between markers D1S2647 and D1S1539. Fine mapping of the refined region using single nucleotide polymorphisms (SNPs) further narrowed the interval to 2.8 megabases (Mb), containing approximately 40 genes. These genes were prioritized according to putative expression pattern and function prior to sequencing. Two mutations in the open reading frame (ORF) of the *PINK1* gene were identified. The mutations segregated with the disease, were predicted to adversely affect the protein product and were absent in a large cohort of control individuals (2). Taken together, this evidence indicated that the *PINK1* mutations were causal of the PD phenotype in the families.

The *PINK1* gene comprises eight exons, spanning approximately 18 kb of genomic DNA. It encodes a 581 amino acid protein that contains a mitochondrial targeting motif and a highly conserved kinase domain. The Spanish family carried a homozygous G/A substitution in exon 4, resulting in a G309D missense mutation at a highly conserved residue in the kinase domain. The Italian families carried the same homozygous G/A substitution in exon 7, which results in a nonsense mutation truncating 145 amino acids at the C-terminus. The Italian families were not knowingly

115

related, despite originating from distinct geographical regions, and were later shown to share a haplotype around the *PARK6* locus, implying common ancestry.

CLONING

The *PINK1* gene was independently cloned by two different groups analyzing differential expression profiles of cancer cell lines. Unoki and Nakamura (3), identified *PINK1* following a search for transcriptionally transactivated genes in cell lines overexpressing the phosphatase and tensin homolog (*PTEN*) gene. Using bioinformatic analysis they established that it contained a serine/threonine kinase-like domain, while *PINK1* was shown to be downregulated in ovarian tumors they could not demonstrate any growth suppressive effects of *PINK1* in an in vitro cancer cell line assay and therefore discontinued characterization of *PINK1* in the context of *PTEN* signaling. Nakajima et al. (4) cloned *PINK1* (named *BRPK*) following a differential expression screen in cell lines of varying metastatic potential. *BRPK* was consistently overexpressed in the higher metastasizes prompting the authors to characterize it further. They demonstrated that the putative serine/threonine kinase domain was functional by showing that Glutathione S-transferase (GST)-fusion proteins containing either murine or human *PINK1* kinase domains were capable of in vitro autophosphorylation. Beilina et al. (5) have subsequently confirmed human *PINK1* autophosphorylation in vitro and demonstrated that both a predicted, kinase-dead mutant and several disease-causing missense mutants of *PINK1* decreased kinase activity. However, it remains to be determined whether *PINK1* phosphorylates serine or threonine residues and what its natural cellular substrates are.

DISTRIBUTION

Unoki and Nakamura demonstrated ubiquitous *PINK1* expression by Northern blotting of mouse tissues. *PINK1* is also ubiquitously expressed in the neurons and glia of all brain regions (6). At the subcellular level, both in vitro and in vivo data indicate that *PINK1* is localized to the mitochondria. Several strands of evidence have now been accumulated to support this localization; *PINK1* is actively imported into mitochondria in vitro (7) and fractionation studies on human and rat brains suggest that *PINK1* is an integral membrane protein of the outer mitochondrial membrane (6). Additionally, imaging studies have consistently demonstrated colocalization of *PINK1* with mitochondrial markers. Determining the precise subcellular localization of the protein is an important precursor to understanding its function; it is equally important to determine if the localization or distribution of the protein is affected by mutation. In both idiopathic PD and *PINK1* heterozygous brains, the distribution of *PINK1* was unchanged compared to control tissue (6), and cell models show that the localization of the protein is unaffected by truncating or missense mutations (7). This data would therefore indicate that the action of the mutations is on the function of the protein rather than a loss of function due to misdirection in the cell. In a PD brain, *PINK1* localizes to the outer halo in a subset of Lewy bodies, indicating that while it may associate with Lewy bodies it does not form an integral component of the inclusions (6).

MITOCHONDRIAL TRAFFICKING

Most mitochondrial proteins are synthesized on cytoplasmic ribosomes as precursor proteins that are then translocated into mitochondria via a highly specialized import system (8). Two broad classes of mitochondrial proteins exist: the majority contain a cleavable N-terminal "presequence" of between 20 and 60 amino acid residues. This group interacts with a multimeric complex on the outer mitochondrial membrane, known as the translocase of the outer membrane (Tom complex), specifically Tom20. After passing through the outer membrane, they enter the matrix by passing through a pore formed by a complex known as translocase of the inner membrane (Tim complex), specifically Tim23. After entry into the matrix, the presequence is cleaved off by the mitochondrial processing peptidase (MPP), and the mature protein is usually localized to the matrix (8). The second group of mitochondrial proteins does not contain a cleavable presequence but instead has internal signal sequences often consisting of stretches of positively charged amino acids adjacent to hydrophobic domains. These proteins generally interact with the Tom70 receptor on the outer membrane, and, after entry, are localized to the inner mitochondrial membrane by interaction with the Tim22 complex (8). It is currently unclear at which residue the *PINK1* leader sequence is cleaved, mitochondrial peptidase consensus sequences are difficult to predict and multiple sites may exist. Western blot analysis suggests that cleaved *PINK1* is approximately 10 kDa shorter than the full-length protein; approximately 100 amino acids may therefore be cleaved from the preprotein (5). Currently, none of the known mutations are predicted to affect *PINK1* trafficking or processing; however, some missense mutations have been reported outside the kinase domain at the N-terminus of the protein that could affect processing or folding.

PINK1 KINASE

PINK1 was the first protein kinase to be associated with PD. Recently, another kinase, *LRRK2*, has also been shown to be mutated in PD (9,10). Kinases add phosphate groups to specific substrate proteins, altering their function, localization, and activity. The phosphorylation of proteins by kinases forms a key cellular signaling mechanism. When protein phosphorylation is combined with the action of counteracting phosphoprotein phosphatases, the result is a finely tuned system that can be used to regulate of a wide variety of cellular processes, such as cellular metabolism, gene expression, cytoskeletal architecture, cell adhesion, and cell cycle progression (11,12).

In eukaryotes, the most commonly studied kinases phosphorylate the hydroxy-amino acids serine, threonine, and tyrosine. Substrate specificity can be predicted by sequence motifs that are specific to either protein tyrosine kinases or protein serine/threonine kinases. Phosphotyrosines are commonly involved in molecular recognition and the formation of protein–protein complexes, while the phospho-serines and phosphothreonines function mainly in the modulation of enzymatic activity through the modification of conformation or substrate binding. Sequence comparisons suggest that *PINK1* is most similar to the calmodulin-dependent serine/threonine kinases (13).

The wide range of diseases resultant from mutant kinases underlines their ubiquity and importance. Neurologic diseases associated with altered kinase function include myotonic dystrophy, which is caused by decreased expression of the dystrophia myotonica (DM) serine kinase (14), Pantothenate kinase-associated neurodegeneration caused by mutations in the *PINK2* gene (15), and a variety of peripheral neuropathies. Additionally, dysregulation of protein phosphorylation has been observed in several neurodegenerative diseases most notably the hyperphosphorylation of tau that is causal of neuronal dysfunction and cell death in Alzheimer's disease (AD) and associated tauopathies (16), and the phosphorylation of α-synuclein at Ser 129 in PD and other synucleinopathies (17).

In addition to primary mutations that lead directly to loss of function, such as premature truncation and missense mutations at regulatory elements, disruption of the complex regulatory pathways of kinases can also indirectly result in disease phenotype. These include the actions of second messengers, allosteric mechanisms, inhibition through pseudosubstrate sequences, positive and negative phosphorylation events, regulatory subunit binding, inhibitor proteins and differential subcellular localization through targeting domains and anchoring proteins. The assessment and determination of changes in the mitochondrial phosphoprotein milieu arising from *PINK1* dysregulation in PD will firstly require knowledge of its upstream effectors and downstream targets. Currently very little is known about the mitochondrial phosphoprotein; however, recent studies have suggested that reversible phosphorylation of complex I subunits is required for their normal assembly, and further studies will be required to determine whether *PINK1* is involved in these processes (18,19).

PINK1 AND MITOCHONDRIAL DYSFUNCTION

Mitochondrial dysfunction has long been associated with PD. Respiratory chain enzyme deficiencies have been widely reported in the substantia nigra of sporadic PD patients (20–22). Complex I is vulnerable to modification by oxidative stress, and when deregulated is a source of free radicals or reactive oxygen species (ROS) (23,24). Mitochondria are the main providers of cellular energy, sustaining aerobic life through the flow of electrons down the electron transport system (ETS). The ETS is located on the inner mitochondrial membrane (IMM) and consists of four membrane-spanning enzyme complexes namely: complex I (NADH-ubiquinone reductase) that oxidises reduced nicotinamide adenine dinucleotide (NADH); complex II (succinate-ubiquinone oxidoreductase) that oxidises $FADH_2$; complex III (ubiquinol cytochrome c oxidoreductase); and complex IV (cytochrome c oxidase). Additionally, the ETS contains two hydrophobic electron carriers, coenzyme Q10, and cytochrome c, that are both encoded by nuclear DNA. The fundamental role of the ETS is the transfer of electrons via a series of oxidation–reduction reactions, which culminates in the reduction of oxygen to produce water [for a recent review of the ETS see (25)] (Fig. 1). The oxidation-reduction reactions are coupled to the transfer of protons across the IMM, and this proton efflux creates a proton-electrochemical gradient otherwise known as the protomotive force (26). The protomotive force consists mainly of an electrical component, called the mitochondrial membrane potential ($\Delta\Psi$m), and a transmembrane pH gradient. The $\Delta\Psi$m is usually around -150 to -180 mV and is central to mitochondrial function since it provides the force that drives the influx of protons and calcium into the mitochondria, as well as determines the generation of O_2. Protons enter through a proton channel of the F_1F_0-adenosine 5-triphosphate (ATP) synthase (or complex V). This re-entry of protons depolarises the $\Delta\Psi$m and induces a motor of the enzyme to phosphorylate matrix s-diphos adenosine 5-diphosphate (ADP) and thereby generate ATP. Thus, there is close coupling of the transfer of electrons, generation of the $\Delta\Psi$m, and ATP synthesis.

The mitochondria represent not only a major source of ROS but also a major target for their damage, thus initiating a feed-forward cycle of ROS generation and accumulation of damage that ends with cell death. Given that ROS is capable

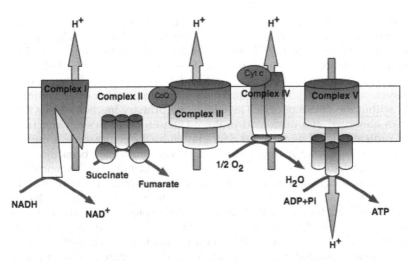

FIGURE 1 Schematic representation of the mitochondrial electron transport system. The ETS facilitates the transfer of electrons via a series of oxidation-reduction reactions. Electrons are transferred from NADH and $FADH_2$ to complex I and complex II, respectively. Both these complexes transfer electrons to coenzyme Q10 (ubiquinone), which then shuttles electrons to complex III. Complex III then transfers electrons to cytochrome c that then shuttles electrons to complex IV, which is linked to the reduction of oxygen to produce water. See the text for further details. *Abbreviations*: ADP, adenosine 5′-diphosphate; ATP, adenosine 5′-triphosphate; ETS, electron transport system; FADH, reduced flavin adenine dinucleotide; NADH, reduced nicotinamide adenine dinucleotide; NAD+, Nicotinamide adenine dinucleotide.

of inducing cell death, it still remains to be determined how ubiquitous ROS generation can precipitate the highly selective dopaminergic neuronal degeneration seen in PD. Animal models have also confirmed the highly selective aspect of cell loss; rats administered rotenone, a complex I inhibitor, develop PD-like syndromes characterized by neuronal degeneration, and the formation of α-synuclein rich inclusion bodies (27). One possible mechanism for the neuronal selectivity is the increased oxidative stres s in nigrostriatal neurons due to dopamine metabolism (28). More work is certainly required to identify the mechanism of selective neuronal degeneration.

We do not yet know if mutations of *PINK1* are sufficient to trigger mitochondrial dysfunction that has been reported in postmortem PD brains. However, preliminary results do show that homozygous missense mutations, which are predicted to disrupt kinase activity, render cells more susceptible to stress and reduce phosphorylation activity in vitro. In a cell model, overexpression of the G309D mutation resulted in decreased mitochondrial membrane potential and increased apoptopic cell death in the presence of proteasomal stress when compared to the wild type and vector constructs. Beilina et al. (5) also demonstrated that the G309D mutant has reduced kinase activity compared to wild type. Further, cells overexpressing wild type *PINK1* were protected against the stress compared to cells overexpressing the vector alone. These studies therefore suggest that *PINK1*-mediated phosphorylation of as yet unknown substrates may be critical in protecting neurons from the effects of apoptopic stress and that mutation-induced hypophosphorylation abrogates this protection.

Mitochondrial membrane potential ($\Delta\Psi$m), as discussed previously, is central to mitochondrial function. Extrapolating from this preliminary data, it would appear that at least one of the functions of *PINK1* would be to protect against mitochondrial stress-induced dysfunction. The stress used in those experiments, MG-132, is a proteasome inhibitor and suggests that stress-induced dysregulation of the ubiquitin-proteasome system (UPS) may be mitigated by protective proteins acting further downstream within the mitochondria. The UPS is the primary mechanism for the degradation of abnormal and misfolded protein. Ubiquitin moieties are attached to unwanted proteins, signaling them for degradation by the proteasome, a multi-catalytic protease complex. Impairment of the UPS has previously been directly implicated in Mendelian PD by the discovery of two genes: *PARKIN* encodes an E3-ubiquitin ligase (29,30) and the ubiquitin-carboxyl-terminal hydrolase-L1 (*UCH-L1*) gene recycles the ubiquitin moieties. While the majority of studies have characterized the effect of these gene mutations on altered protein turnover and not mitochondrial dysfunction, the interdependence of both pathways (predicted since the UPS requires ATP) has been shown in several PD models. This is well demonstrated by the finding that chronic exposure of rats to the complex I inhibitor rotenone results in the formation of Lewy body–like inclusions and parkinsonism (27). Some recent data show that the converse is also true, whereby inhibition of the UPS results in secondary mitochondrial dysfunction. In cells, low-level proteasome inhibition has been shown to result in decreased complex I and II activities accompanied by increased mitochondrial ROS and increased neuronal vulnerability to sub-toxic levels of free radicals (31,32). It was recently reported that rats exposed to proteasome inhibitors develop parkinsonism; however, it remains unknown if these animals have mitochondrial deficits and damage (33). It also remains to be seen if similar results are obtained with stresses which cause a direct increase in oxidative stress such as dopamine.

Evidence from animal models has also implicated *PINK1* mutations with substantive deleterious effects on mitochondrial function. The most striking demonstration of this linkage was obtained from *PINK1* loss-of-function mutant *Drosophila* models. Flies exhibited complete deficits in flight ability and decreased climbing speed due a reduction in the content of their indirect flight muscles. The existing muscle fibers contained massively swollen mitochondria, which had lost their outer membrane, an interesting observation in view of the localization of *PINK1* to the outer mitochondrial membrane. Functional impairment of the dysmorphic mitochondria was confirmed by the demonstration of a two-fold reduction in ATP levels compared to control flies (34,35). Significantly, all of the observed phenotypes could be reversed by the expression of either wild type *PINK1* or *PARKIN*, indicating that these two PD genes function in the same pathway.

The identification of *PINK1*'s mitochondrial substrates will be instrumental in delineating the *PINK1/PARKIN* protective pathway and may begin to address the wider role of mitochondrial dysfunction in PD. If, as *PINK1* mutations and the rotenone models suggest, primary mitochondrial lesions are causal of PD, then the relationship between mitochondrial dysfunction and the other known pathways needs to be reassessed.

PATHWAYS TO PARKINSONISM

Functional analysis of the protein products of the five genes (α-synuclein, *PARKIN*, *DJ-1*, *PINK1*, and *LRRK2*) associated with Mendelian forms of PD, has begun to uncover the underlying disease pathways that result in the nigral degeneration, which ultimately leads to the clinical phenotype. In recent years the prevailing model has become synuclein-centric, associated with protein misfolding. Its two central tenets are the protein accumulation associated with α-synuclein mutations and the dysfunction of the UPS, which is associated with *PARKIN* mutants. However, preliminary data obtained from two of the recently identified genes, *DJ-1* and *PINK1*, indicates that these genes are involved in protection against oxidative damage and mitochondrial dysfunction. *DJ-1* and *PINK1* may therefore promote neuronal, survival, and loss of their activity may also be a major molecular route in the development of PD in both familial and sporadic forms of disease.

Furthemore, these apparently disparate pathways may yet be shown to be related as it is increasingly evident that inhibition of the mitochondrial respiratory chain enzymes and ROS production are linked to protein accumulation and proteasome dysfunction.

MUTATION ANALYSIS

Several studies have now been carried out to evaluate the *PINK1* mutation burden in PD patients around the world. These data demonstrate that *PINK1* mutations account for 5% to 10% of ARPD cases. The emerging phenotype is of early-onset PD (range 18–39 years) lacking major atypical features. This suggests that *PINK1* is distinct from parkinsonism associated with *PARKIN* or *DJ-1*. While *PINK1* is unequivocally associated with young-onset ARPD, it remains difficult to quantify the overall proportion of *PINK1* positive cases in ARPD due to the preselection of cases. Familial parkinsonism remains extremely rare, estimated to account for 1% to 5% of PD patients; therefore, studies have also sought to estimate the frequency of *PINK1* mutations in the more common, sporadic manifestation. Approximately 1% of PD patients, with varying ages of onset, carry heterozygous missense mutations. Clinically, a similar absence of atypical features was observed in the single mutation carriers albeit with a later age of onset. This suggests that while heterozygous and homozygous *PINK1* carriers share the same "idiopathic PD" phenotype, the number of mutations may determine the age and severity of symptom onset, providing pathogenecity of the heterozygotes is proven.

None of the studies identified two mutations in a patient with a negative family history. The pathogenecity of these heterozygous *PINK1* mutations, like that of the *PARKIN* and *DJ-1* heterozygotes preceding them, is likely to cause controversy as they may either simply represent the *PINK1* carrier frequency in the population, bearing no relation to the disease phenotype, or they may contribute to the risk of developing PD; currently there is insufficient data to rule out either hypothesis. Under a purely Mendelian model, single-mutation carriers would not be expected to display a phenotype; however, data from an 18F-dopa positron emission tomography (PET)–study that is capable of measuring presynaptic dopamine-terminal function, has revealed a 20% to 30% reduction in caudate and putamen 18F-dopa uptake in *PINK1* heterozygotes compared to controls (36). Heterozygous *PINK1* mutations do therefore appear to confer a subclinical phenotype, which may or may not develop into the full clinical syndrome. The penetrance of the mutations must, however, be quite low, as they have been identified in patients with no significant family history. Furthermore, the subclinical manifestations may not necessarily progress to the clinical syndrome within each carrier's lifetime; this risk may therefore be modulated by environmental exposure or genetic background. This can clearly be demonstrated by the presence of hetero-zygous mutations in control samples. In some instances, identical mutations, such as the D525N and E476K, have been identified in PD patients and controls.

The attribution of pathogenecity to mutations by genetics alone is inherently limited by their penetrance. Fully penetrant mutations that always manifest with a phenotype can easily be differentiated by comparing cases to controls. Statistical comparison of mutations with reduced penetrance can give an indication of patho-genecity in situations where the case-control partition is significantly skewed. Therefore, in addition to the genetic approaches clinical and functional data will also be required to accurately classify heterozygous *PINK1* mutations.

Determining the functional effects of *PINK1* mutations is difficult at present due to the lack of a reliable kinase assay. To date, two indirect assays have been used to characterize the mutants experimentally. Valente et al. (2) demonstrated that the G309D mutation reduces mitochondrial membrane potential ($\Delta\Psi$m) which, as described in the mitochondrial physiology section, has the effect of rendering cells more susceptible to cellular stress. Autophosphorylation assays have also been used, the G309D mutation was shown to reduce kinase activity by 40% compared to the wild type (5). Beilina et al. also tested a second mutation using an autophos-phorylation assay, the L347P, which appears to be quite common in the Philippines having been identified in two, separate Filipino PD cohorts and in approximately 3% of controls (37,38). The L347P had drastically decreased kinase activity (10% of wild type), most likely due to a destabilizing effect of the mutation on the protein.

Qualitatively, the majority of mutations reported to date map within the kinase domain; however, there are a few exceptions such as the R147H mutation reported by Healy et al. (39) and the R68P, C92F, and A168P reported by Valente et al. (40). The effects of these mutations remain to be determined as the N-terminal segment of the protein between the mitochondrial targeting motif and the kinase domain is of undefined significance. Of the mutations that map within the kinase domain, there is no evidence of subclustering to any functionally significant regions (Fig. 2). However, as demonstrated by the autophosphorylation assays with the G309D and L347P mutants, even changes in nonregulatory regions of the kinase can have a dramatic effect on its activity.

ASSOCIATION STUDIES

Mutations in the Mendelian PD genes identified to date contribute only modestly to the overall incidence of the late onset sporadic form of the disease. The *LRRK2* G2019S mutation is perhaps the most numerically significant having been identified in approximately 1.5% of sporadic cases (41). The aetiology of the remainder of cases may be either environmental or genetic. To determine whether common genetic variation in the *PINK1* gene influences non-Mendelian forms of the disease, two groups have performed *PINK1* case-control association studies. Groen et al. (42) selected three coding polymorphisms in a small study of 91 cases preselected for young age of onset and/or positive family history. No association was detected between the coding polymorphisms and PD; however, having enriched their cases for Mendelian mutation carriers by preselection for early age of onset and positive family history, this study may be underpowered to accurately estimate the risk of developing sporadic PD due to common variation in *PINK1*. A more rigorous, haplotype-tagging approach was adopted by Healy et al. (43). The haplotype-struc-ture and linkage-disequilibrium patterns in and around *PINK1* were determined

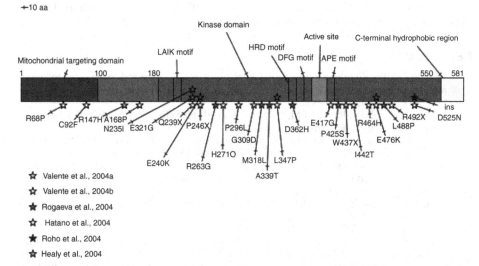

FIGURE 2 Graphical representation of the *PINK1* protein (to scale). Annotated with some of the published mutations and predicted domains. Sequence alignments indicate the kinase domain is likely to be encoded between amino acids 180 and 550. Bioinformatic and cell-transfection studies suggest that the first 100 amino acids may contain several mitochondrial-targeting domains and mitochondrial-cleavage sites and that *PINK1* undergoes sequential cleavage. The 80 amino acids between 100 and 180 are currently of unknown significance; however, it is likely that when the domain boundaries are better defined these will form part of either the kinase domain or the protease cleavage site. Also included on the annotation are selected regions of functional importance, which are essential for kinase function and therefore highly conserved. The LAIK motif forms the ATP orientation site, the HRD motif an active catalytic base and the DFG and APE motifs flank the active site. *Abbreviations*: ATP, adenosine 5´-triphosphate.

using a set of 18 SNPs spanning the *PINK1* gene and neighboring *DDOST* gene. Tagging SNPs, which are selected through a process of statistical distillation, will capture the maximum amount of information from the total genetic variation present. Healy et al. (43) selected a set of four tagging SNPs from the original set of 18 genotyped SNPs, estimating 90% power to detect association. The tagging SNPs were genotyped in a panel of 576 PD samples and 514 controls. However, no significant difference in frequency was detected in the case control partition, indicating that common genetic variants in *PINK1* are not a risk factor in the development of sporadic PD.

CONCLUSION

These are still early days for *PINK1* research; as a mitochondrial kinase, it is likely to increase our understanding of the effects of oxidative stress and complex I inhibition in PD. It may also begin to shed some light on the relationship between oxidative stress and proteasome-related protein accumulation. Numerically, mutations in *PINK1* do not appear to be as common as *PARKIN* mutations in autosomal recessive early-onset PD. However, the frequency of heterozygous mutations in sporadic PD is significant. Therefore, if *PINK1* hemizygosity is shown to be significantly deleterious, then these mutations will represent a considerable risk factor for the development of PD. Finally, as an enzyme with a protective function, *PINK1* may also represent a promising, druggable target for the treatment of PD.

REFERENCES

1. Valente EM, Bentivoglio AR, Dixon PH, et al. Localization of a novel locus for autosomal recessive early-onset parkinsonism, PARK6, on human chromosome 1p35–p36. Am J Hum Genet 2001; 68:895–900.
2. Valente EM, Abou-Sleiman PM, Caputo V, et al. Hereditary early-onset Parkinson's disease caused by mutations in *PINK1*. Science 2004; 304:1158–1160.
3. Unoki M, Nakamura Y. Growth-suppressive effects of BPOZ and EGR2, two genes involved in the PTEN signaling pathway. Oncogene 2001; 20:4457–4465.
4. Nakajima A, Kataoka K, Hong M, Sakaguchi M, Huh NH. BRPK, a novel protein kinase showing increased expression in mouse cancer cell lines with higher metastatic potential. Cancer Lett 2003; 201:195–201.
5. Beilina A, Van Der Brug M, Ahmad R, et al. Mutations in PTEN-induced putative kinase 1 associated with recessive parkinsonism have differential effects on protein stability. Proc Natl Acad Sci USA 2005; 102:5703–5708.
6. Gandhi S, Muqit MM, Stanyer L, et al. *PINK1* protein in normal human brain and Parkinson's disease. Brain 2006; 129:1720–1731.
7. Silvestri L, Caputo V, Bellacchio E, et al. Mitochondrial import and enzymatic activity of *PINK1* mutants associated to recessive parkinsonism. Hum Mol Genet 14:3477–3492.
8. Chacinska A, Pfanner N, Meisinger C. How mitochondria import hydrophilic and hydrophobic proteins. Trends Cell Biol 2002; 12:299–303.
9. Paisan-Ruiz C, Jain S, Evans EW, et al. Cloning of the gene containing mutations that cause PARK8-linked Parkinson's disease. Neuron 2004; 44:595–600.
10. Zimprich A, Biskup S, Leitner P, et al. Mutations in LRRK2 cause autosomal-dominant parkinsonism with pleomorphic pathology. Neuron 2004; 44:601–607.
11. Hunter T. Signaling—2000 and beyond. Cell 2000; 100:113–127.
12. Nolen B, Taylor S, Ghosh G. Regulation of protein kinases; controlling activity through activation segment conformation. Mol Cell 2004; 15:661–675.
13. Krupa A, Srinivasan N. The repertoire of protein kinases encoded in the draft version of the human genome: atypical variations and uncommon domain combinations. Genome Biol 2002; 3:RESEARCH0066.
14. Brook JD, McCurrach ME, Harley HG, et al. Molecular basis of myotonic dystrophy: expansion of a trinucleotide (CTG) repeat at the 3′ end of a transcript encoding a protein kinase family member. Cell 1992; 69:385.
15. Zhou B, Westaway SK, Levinson B, Johnson MA, Gitschier J, Hayflick SJ. A novel pantothenate kinase gene (PANK2) is defective in Hallervorden-Spatz syndrome. Nat Genet 2001; 28:345–349.
16. Goedert M, Jakes R, Spillantini MG, Hasegawa M, Smith MJ, Crowther RA. Assembly of microtubule-associated protein tau into Alzheimer-like filaments induced by sulphated glycosaminoglycans. Nature 1996; 383:550–553.
17. Spillantini MG, Crowther RA, Jakes R, Hasegawa M, Goedert M. Alpha-synuclein in filamentous inclusions of Lewy bodies from Parkinson's disease and dementia with lewy bodies. Proc Natl Acad Sci USA 1998; 95:6469–6473.
18. Schulenberg B, Aggeler R, Beechem JM, Capaldi RA, Patton WF. Analysis of steady-state protein phosphorylation in mitochondria using a novel fluorescent phosphosensor dye. J Biol Chem 2003; 278:27251–27255.
19. Chen R, Fearnley IM, Peak-Chew SY, Walker JE. The phosphorylation of subunits of complex I from bovine heart mitochondria. J Biol Chem 2004; 279:26036–26045.
20. Hattori N, Tanaka M, Ozawa T, Mizuno Y. Immunohistochemical studies on complexes I, II, III, and IV of mitochondria in Parkinson's disease. Ann Neurol 1991; 30:563–571.
21. Jenner P, Olanow CW. Understanding cell death in Parkinson's disease. Ann Neurol 1998; 44:S72–S84.
22. Schapira AH, Cooper JM, Dexter D, Jenner P, Clark JB, Marsden CD. Mitochondrial complex I deficiency in Parkinson's disease. Lancet 1989; 1:1269.

23. St-Pierre J, Buckingham JA, Roebuck SJ, Brand MD. Topology of superoxide production from different sites in the mitochondrial electron transport chain. J Biol Chem 2002; 277:44784–44790.
24. Nicklas WJ, Vyas I, Heikkila RE. Inhibition of NADH-linked oxidation in brain mitochondria by 1-methyl-4-phenyl-pyridine, a metabolite of the neurotoxin, 1-methyl-4-phenyl-1,2,5,6-tetrahydropyridine. Life Sci 1985; 36:2503–2508.
25. Duchen MR. Mitochondria in health and disease: perspectives on a new mitochondrial biology. Mol Aspects Med 2004; 25:365–451.
26. Nicholls DG. Mitochondrial function and dysfunction in the cell: its relevance to aging and aging-related disease. Int J Biochem Cell Biol; 34:1372–1381.
27. Betarbet R, Sherer TB, MacKenzie G, Garcia-Osuna M, Panov AV, Greenamyre JT. Chronic systemic pesticide exposure reproduces features of Parkinson's disease. Nat Neurosci 2000; 3:1301–1306.
28. Schulz JB, Lindenau J, Seyfried J, Dichgans J. Glutathione, oxidative stress and neurodegeneration. Eur J Biochem 2000; 267:4904–4911.
29. Kitada T, Asakawa S, Hattori N, et al. Mutations in the parkin gene cause autosomal recessive juvenile parkinsonism. Nature 1998; 392:605–608.
30. Shimura H, Hattori N, Kubo S, et al. Familial Parkinson disease gene product, parkin, is a ubiquitin-protein ligase. Nat Genet 2000; 25:302–305.
31. Hoglinger GU, Carrard G, Michel PP, et al. Dysfunction of mitochondrial complex I and the proteasome: interactions between two biochemical deficits in a cellular model of Parkinson's disease. J Neurochem 2003; 86:1297–1307.
32. Sullivan PG, Dragicevic NB, Deng JH, et al. Proteasome inhibition alters neural mitochondrial homeostasis and mitochondria turnover. J Biol Chem 2004, 279:20699–20707.
33. McNaught KS, Perl DP, Brownell AL. Systemic exposure to proteasome inhibitors causes a progressive model of Parkinson's disease. Ann Neurol 2004; 56:149–162.
34. Clark IE, Dodson MW, Jiang C, et al. Drosophila *PINK1* is required for mitochondrial function and interacts genetically with parkin. Nature 2006; 441:1162–1166.
35. Park J, Lee SB, Lee S, et al. Mitochondrial dysfunction in Drosophila *PINK1* mutants is complemented by parkin. Nature 2006; 441:1157–1161.
36. Khan NL, Valente EM, Bentivoglio AR, et al. Clinical and subclinical dopaminergic dysfunction in PARK6-linked parkinsonism: an 18F-dopa PET study. Ann Neurol 2002; 52:849–853.
37. Hatano Y, Li Y, Sato K, Asakawa S, et al. Novel *PINK1* mutations in early-onset parkinsonism. Ann Neurol 2004; 56:424–427.
38. Rogaeva E, Johnson J, Lang AE, et al. Analysis of the *PINK1* gene in a large cohort of cases with Parkinson disease. Arch Neurol 2004; 61:1898–1904.
39. Healy DG, Abou-Sleiman PM, Gibson JM, et al. *PINK1* (PARK6) associated Parkinson disease in Ireland. Neurology 2004; 63:1486–1488.
40. Valente EM, Salvi S, Ialongo T, et al. PINK1 mutations are associated with sporadic early-onset parkinsonism. Ann Neurol 2004, 56:336–341.
41. Gilks WP, Abou-Sleiman PM, Gandhi S, et al. A common LRRK2 mutation in idiopathic Parkinson's disease. Lancet 2005; 365:415–416.
42. Groen JL, Kawarai T, Toulina A, et al. Genetic association study of *PINK1* coding polymorphisms in Parkinson's disease. Neurosci Lett 2004; 372:226–229.
43. Healy DG, Abou-Sleiman PM, Ahmadi KR, et al. The gene responsible for PARK6 Parkinson's disease, *PINK1*, does not influence common forms of parkinsonism. Ann Neurol 2004; 56:329–335.

9 | *LRRK2*: Genetics and the Pathogenic Mechanisms of Parkinsonism

Mark R. Cookson
*Cell Biology and Gene Expression Unit, Laboratory of Neurogenetics,
National Institute on Aging, Bethesda, Maryland, U.S.A.*

In 1997, Hasegawa and Kowa reported a family from the Sagamihara area of Japan with autosomal dominant inheritance of Parkinson's disease (PD)–like symptoms (1). In 2002, after excluding known loci (2), the same group reported linkage to the long arm of chromosome 12 and named the locus *PARK8* (3). By 2004, two groups simultaneously published the identification of the gene responsible, *LRRK2* (for leucine-rich repeat kinase 2), for the *PARK8* locus in four additional families from different parts of the world (4,5). Within a year of that discovery, the *LRRK2* gene was shown to be the most common genetic cause of PD to date (6). This short chronology says a great deal about the accelerating pace of discovery in the genetics of PD, which, as others have pointed out (7), was once considered the archetype of a nongenetic disease. But, as is discussed in this chapter, these discoveries have blurred the boundaries between PD and atypical parkinsonian disorders and raise interesting questions about the etiopathogenesis of these diseases.

LRRK2 GENETICS: FROM RARE CAUSE TO COMMON ASSOCIATION

The large family from Sagamihara suggested that the *PARK8* locus was probably a rare cause of atypical parkinsonism, without the typical Lewy pathology found in sporadic PD (see below). However, groups in other parts of the world were able to find evidence of linkage to the same chromosomal region (8,9), indicating that one gene was likely to be responsible for autosomal dominant disease in several families.

The cloning of *LRRK2* revealed that there are indeed multiple variants associated with disease in different families. *LRRK2* is a large gene, with an ~7.5 kb coding sequence. The 2458 amino acid protein was named dardarin by Paisan-Ruiz et al. from the Basque word for tremor, as that group reported four families from the Basque region of northern Spain carrying a common *LRRK2* mutation. The protein has a characteristic domain structure with guanosine triphospate (GTP)–binding (Roc, for Ras in complex proteins) and kinase domains separated by a region called a COR (C-terminal of Ras) domain. Outside of this central catalytic region are at least three protein-protein interaction domains, ankyrin-like and leucine-rich repeats in the N-terminal region, and a WD40 domain at the extreme C-terminus [for a diagram of this domain structure see (10)]. There are about 20 mutations identified to date, spread throughout the more C-terminal regions of the protein coding sequence, of which at least eight are clearly pathogenic. Most are missense-point mutations, with the exception of one variant that may affect splicing. There are some "hotspots" for mutations: residue R1441 near the Roc domain is mutated to C, G, or H in different families, and there are two adjacent mutations, G2019S and I2020T, in the kinase domain.

These last two mutations are of particular interest. I2020T was identified by Zimprich et al. (5) but was subsequently shown to be the cause of disease in the Sagamihara family (11), thus confirming that all families known to be linked to the *PARK8* locus have a deficit in the same gene. Shortly after the initial cloning of *LRRK2* deficits, several groups published a large number of cases with G2019S mutations (12–14). Subsequent studies have shown that G2019S is the single most common gene variant associated with PD. Estimates vary depending in part on the study sample. Perhaps unsurprisingly, the proportion of cases carrying G2019S is higher in sample sets containing patients with some family history compared to studies that include only "sporadic" cases. However, in several studies even apparently sporadic cases do occasionally turn out to have a G2019S mutation. The frequency also varies with population. In most Caucasian populations, the frequency is between 1% and 5% of all cases. However, G2019S is vanishingly rare in Taiwanese PD patients (15) but accounts for approximately 20% and 40% of PD cases in Ashkenazi Jewish (16) and North African Arab (17) patients, respectively. Haplotype analyses showed that there are strong founder effects for G2019S within populations but that the European founder haplotype (18,19) differs from the rare Japanese G2019S haplotype (20). This suggests that the same mutation arose at least twice but became widely dispersed within populations. Other common mutations may also have founder effects such as the R1441G mutation in Spain (21) or the I2020T mutation in Japan (22).

It is worth noting that, within the original families, there are unaffected persons carrying mutations who are older than the fifth decade of life, when symptoms normally begin. Furthermore, several elderly people have been reported to be carriers of the G2019S mutation but are clinically free of disease (23,24), and in populations with high prevalence of specific mutations, there are neurologically normal controls with mutations (16,17). These cases do not imply that G2019S is not pathogenic as there is still a robust association with disease, but that penetrance is incomplete and age dependent. Presumably this explains why mutations occur in people without a clear family history of PD. The robust association is not seen with Alzheimer's disease (25–27) or other dementia (28) or with pathologically confirmed PSP (29,30), suggesting a true and strong association only with PD. One case is reported of a G2019S patient with Alzheimer's but this frequency would be compatible with the frequency seen in controls, so presumably is coincidental. Also of interest is that homozygous cases do not have earlier age at onset compared to heterozygotes (14,17). These genetic data show that G2019S and other common LRRK2 mutations are inherited in a true dominant fashion, with incomplete, age-dependent penetrance, and cause PD, not generalized, neurodegeneration.

Although there is such a robust association with point mutations of *LRRK2* and PD, there is no evidence for association of common variants across the gene with disease, either as single nucleotide polymorphism (SNPs) or as haplotypes (31–33). This contrasts with the genetics of α-synuclein, where common promoter variants (and gene multiplications) are associated with PD [reviewed in (6)]. If we interpret the genetics of α-synuclein to mean that there is a quantitative association with the disease process, presumably, the lack of association with common variants of *LRRK2* means mutations in that gene are qualitative in nature. However, it is also possible that there is little common variation in *LRRK2* that affects gene function.

Overall, *LRRK2* demonstrates a great deal of the complex contributions of gene mutations to a "nongenetic" disease. Within any population there are multiple genes that can cause PD-like symptoms, of which *LRRK2* is the most common but only one. The association is age-dependent but not fully penetrant and varies across different populations. Therefore, at a population level, it might be quite easy to miss any genetic contribution to "sporadic" PD, and one might conclude that there are no major gene effects. These considerations are complicated further by the fact that the pathology and clinical presentation of cases with *LRRK2* mutations are quite variable.

PATHOLOGY OF *LRRK2* CASES

One of the most difficult, and therefore most interesting, questions about PD is what pathology tells us about etiology. One might assume that it is axiomatic that pathology will tell us which molecules are involved in the neurodegenerative disease process. For example, amyloid and tau are the major components of the pathologic hallmarks of Alzheimer's disease, and mutations in either or in the processing enzyme for the amyloid precursor lead to inherited dementias. A similar argument can be constructed for α-synuclein, which is a building block of Lewy bodies and a single gene associated with Lewy body diseases, including PD. However, the pathology of cases with *LRRK2* mutations is more variable than might be expected from a simple cause-effect correlation between disease mechanism and pathologic outcome. In fact, using a strict definitional approach, we would be forced to conclude that *LRRK2* does not always cause PD.

At this time, only a small number of cases with *LRRK2* mutations have been autopsied. The majority are associated with Lewy body pathology and neuronal loss in the brainstem, similar to sporadic PD (34). Most of these case reports come from the most frequent mutation, G2019S. It is interesting that most cases with this mutation do not show widespread α-synuclein pathology, although patients with Lewy bodies in cortical areas and attendant signs of demetia have been reported (13,35).

The next most common type of pathology is exemplified by the I2020T mutations originally reported in Japan. These cases had nigral depigmentation (i.e., loss of dopaminergic neurons) without evidence of Lewy bodies (1). However, this pathology is not unique to this mutation, as one recently reported autopsy case with G2019S also lacked Lewy bodies or neurites (36). This type of pathology has also been reported in one case each carrying R1441C or Y1699C mutations (5).

The remaining cases are a mixed set invariably, with nigral cell loss but also pathologic deposits other than Lewy bodies or Lewy neurites. For example, in the R1441C family, there is one patient with glial tau deposits reminiscent of the atypical parkinsonian syndrome progressive supranuclear palsy (PSP) but not frequent enough to reach that diagnosis (5). Some cases have Alzheimer's like tau lesions, but whether these are part of the *LRRK2* disease process or coincidental in elderly subjects is not clear (13,35). Overall, although the tau pathology has been emphasized in some reports, it is perhaps not a major part of the pathology, although more cases are needed to answer this question. Similarly rare are reports of "ubiquitin-only" inclusions, some of which are nuclear (one Y1699C case), and *LRRK2*-positive neurites (one G2019S case). Two cases have been reported with loss of large motor neurons in the ventral horn of the spinal cord and the attendant symptoms of a motor neuron disease (5).

What do these reports add up to? First, the invariant feature of *LRRK2* disease is parkinsonism with attendant nigral cell loss, even in cases that also have other clinical features. Second, the deposition of other proteins commonly associated with neurodegenerative disease, α-synuclein and tau, is not an invariant component of the disease. The balance of evidence to date is that α-synuclein–positive Lewy bodies are the more common corollary of *LRRK2* disease and that the involvement of tau is rarer and might even be coincidental given the age range of the cases. The fact that several cases have parkinsonian symptoms in the absence of inclusion bodies suggests that the formation of Lewy bodies cannot be the underlying mechanism producing the disease. Whether this also means that synuclein and tau are not involved in disease mechanisms is a more difficult question, as the relationship between a toxic protein's involvement in disease and its deposition into pathologic structures is complex (6).

Overall, these observations support the conclusion that a single genetic cause can lead to either the typical Lewy body pathology of PD or parkinsonism in the absence of inclusion body pathology. There is no clean separation between different mutations, as originally emphasized by Zimprich et al. in their studies of several family members with Y1699C mutation, but also as illustrated by the presence of both types of pathology with the G2019S mutation. Although the argument seems obscure, the fact that synuclein deposition is variable has important implications for how we interpret the relationships between "true" PD and disorders such as the recessive genes, *PINK1*, *PARKIN*, and *DJ-1*, which sometimes also present as cell loss only, without Lewy bodies.

MOLECULAR BIOLOGY OF DARDARIN

As stated above, the *LRRK2* gene encodes a large multidomain protein, including a kinase domain named dardarin. There are two kinases with similar domain structure, *LRRK1* and *LRRK2*/dardarin, that form a small unique branch of the human kinome. Given that kinases are critical in many cellular processes, and that kinase activity is the target of many drugs, much attention has focused on the kinase activity of dardarin. Two mutations, G2019S and I2020T, are at the N-terminal end of the activation loop in the kinase domain. G2019 is actually the third residue in the DFG motif that chelates the magnesium ion in the active site of the kinase. That both mutations introduce potential phosphorylation sites around the activation loop might argue that mutations work by increasing activity. However, one might also argue that substituting the absolutely conserved glycine might disrupt the metal binding site and lead to decreased activity. In fact, arguments for either gain (37) or loss (38) of function have been made. Experimental measurements of G2019S (39,40) and I2020T (41) have suggested that there is a small but significant increase in net kinase activity compared to wild type protein, supporting a gain of function mechanism. In contrast, two studies examining mutations outside of the kinase domain/activation loop did not find significant increases in kinase activity. West et al. found that while R1441C increased activity, the increase was not statistically significant (40). In our hands, R1441C or Y1699C does not increase activity using similar assays (39).

These results would suggest that, by currently undefined mechanisms, mutations in the active site loop increase activity, but mutations in other domains do not have the same effect and thus might cause disease in a different way. However, at the time of writing, this is a premature conclusion because the assays we have for kinase activity are quite crude. All of the above studies immunoprecipitated dardarin from mammalian cells in autophosphorylation assays. As we do not yet know if dardarin is capable of autophosphorylation under physiologic circumstances, it remains possible that the observed activity is an artifact of high concentrations of the enzyme in, in vitro assays. We also do not yet know any of the physiologic substrates of dardarin. Therefore, it is possible that mutations outside of the kinase domain do in fact increase activity toward authentic substrates. It is interesting that dardarin has multiple protein-protein interaction domains (see below), reminiscent of other kinases that act as scaffolds as well as enzymes. Therefore, further studies are required to see if mutations outside of the kinase domain do increase activity toward authentic substrates.

Although these results leave the question of whether mutations are gain-of-function for kinase activity, there are other ways to ask if the same activity makes a contribution to the toxic effects of mutant dardarin. Overexpression of mutant dardarin in susceptible cell types in vitro, namely primary cultured neurons or SH-SY5Y cells, causes a loss of viability over several days (39,42). We have recently shown that, if the kinase activity of dardarin is inactivated using artificial mutations, the molecule is no longer toxic, even if pathogenic mutations are present in the same construct (39). This result implies that the kinase activity of mutant dardarin makes a significant, perhaps essential, contribution to the toxic effects of the protein, at least in cell culture models. The interpretation of these results is currently unclear. On the one hand, they could mean that the kinase phosphorylates one or more substrates, triggering cell death. Increased activity or altered substrate specificity, would increase cell death and be prevented in the kinase-dead versions. On the other hand, it is possible that dardarin is, like other proteins associated with neurodegenerative disease, somewhat prone to misfolding in its active conformation. Under this hypothesis, whether kinase activity is increased or not is less relevant—the key to the mutations is understanding how they affect folding. It is important to note that the data available to date, both on kinase activity and the contribution of the kinase domain to toxicity, are compatible with either hypothesis. Although the details of the mechanism(s) involved in the toxic effects of mutant dardarin need to be elucidated, the data available suggest that developing kinase inhibitors for this protein is a novel avenue for therapeutics in PD.

What about the other parts of the molecule? This question is especially relevant as mutations are present in other domains of dardarin. One region that might be worth studying is the GTP-binding region in the center of dardarin. It has been shown in the homologous kinase *LRRK1* that GTP binding stimulates kinase activity (43). Therefore, mutations that affected GTP binding, or the turnover of GTP to GDP, might be expected to indirectly contribute to increased activity under some conditions. The protein-protein interaction domains are also of interest, especially if the protein acts as a scaffold. Mutations in these regions may, therefore, alter the strength of association with interacting proteins, potentially adding to toxic effects.

CONCLUSION

Genetic studies showed that mutations in *LRRK2* are the single most common cause of parkinsonism found to date. Because of the complexities of inheritance of pathogenic mutations, with mixed pathologic outcomes and incomplete penetrance, the presence of an inherited cause of PD in 1% to 30% of patients may not have been obvious. Although studies on the biology of the protein are only beginning, and in vivo models are required, early results show that the kinase activity of dardarin is important in its damaging effects and may suggest a novel therapeutic approach.

The role(s) of the protein in the development of sporadic PD has not yet been identified, but if there are common mechanisms for neurologic damage between patients with *LRRK2* mutations and sporadic disease, then we may have a place to try and develop neuroprotective strategies for PD.

ACKNOWLEDGMENTS

This research was supported by the Intramural Research Program of the NIH, National Institute on Aging.

REFERENCES

1. Hasegawa K, Kowa H. Autosomal dominant familial Parkinson disease: older onset of age, and good response to levodopa therapy. Eur Neurol 1997; 38(suppl 1):39–43.
2. Hasegawa K, Funayama M, Matsuura N, et al. Analysis of alpha-synuclein, parkin, tan, and UCH-L1 in a Japanese family with autosomal dominant parkinsonism. Eur Neurol 2001; 46(1):20–24.
3. Funayama M, Hasegawa K, Kowa H, et al. A new locus for Parkinson's disease (PARK8) maps to chromosome 12p11.2-q13.1. Ann Neurol 2002; 51(3):296–301.
4. Paisan-Ruiz C, Jain S, Evans EW, et al. Cloning of the gene containing mutations that cause PARK8-linked Parkinson's disease. Neuron 2004; 44(4):595–600.
5. Zimprich A, Biskup S, Leitner P, et al. Mutations in LRRK2 cause autosomal-dominant parkinsonism with pleomorphic pathology. Neuron 2004; 44(4):601–607.
6. Cookson MR. The biochemistry of Parkinson's disease. Annu Rev Biochem 2005; 74:29–52.
7. Farrer M, Gwinn-Hardy K, Hutton M, et al. The genetics of disorders with synuclein pathology and parkinsonism. Hum Mol Genet 1999; 8(10):1901–1905.
8. Zimprich A, Muller-Myhsok B, Farrer M, et al. The PARK8 locus in autosomal dominant parkinsonism: confirmation of linkage and further delineation of the disease-containing interval. Am J Hum Genet 2004; 74(1):11–19.
9. Paisan-Ruiz C, Saenz A, Lopez de Munain A, et al. Familial Parkinson's disease; clinical and genetic analysis of four Basque families. Ann Neurol 2005; 57(3):365–372.
10. Guo L, Wang W, Chen SG. Leucine-rlch repeat kinase 2: Relevance to Parkinson's disease. Int J Biochem Cell Biol 2006; 38(9):1469–1475.
11. Funayama M, Hasegawa K, Ohta E, et al. An LRRK2 mutation as a cause for the parkinsonism in the original PARK8 family. Ann Neurol 2005; 57(6):918–921.
12. Di Fonzo A, Rohe CF, Ferrcira J, et al. A frequent LRRK2 gene mutation associated with autosomal dominant Parkinson's disease. Lancet 2005; 365(9457):412–415.
13. Gilks WP, Abou-Sleiman PM, Gandhi S, et al. A common LRRK2 mutation in idiopathic Parkinson's disease. Lancet 2005; 365(9457):415–416.
14. Nichols WC, Pankratz N, Hernandez D, et al. Genetic screening for a single common LRRK2 mutation in familial Parkinson 's disease. Lancet 2005; 365(9457): 410–412.
15. Fung HC, Chen CM, Hardy J, et al. Lack of G2019S LRRK2 mutation in a cohort of Taiwanese with sporadic Parkinson's disease. Mov Disord 2006; 21(6):880–881.
16. Ozelius LJ, Senthil G, Saunders-Pullman R, et al. LRRK2 G2019S as a cause of Parkinson's disease in Ashkenazi Jews. N Engl J Med 2006; 354(4):424–425.
17. Lesage S, Durr A, Tazir M, et al. LRRK2 G2019S as a cause of Parkinson's disease in North African Arabs. N Engl J Med 2006; 354(4):422–423.
18. Gosal D, Ross OA, Wiley J, et al. Clinical traits ofLRRK2-associated Parkinson's disease in Ireland: a link between familial and idiopathic PD. Parkinsonisin Relat Disord 2005;11(6):349–352.
19. Kachergus J, Mata IF, Hulihan M, et al. Identification of a novel LRRK2 mutation linked to autosomal dominant parkinsonism: evidence of a common founder across European populations. Am J Hum Genet 2005; 76(4):672–680.
20. Zabetian CP, Morino H, Ujike H, et al. Identification and haplotype analysis of LRRK2 G2019S in Japanese patients with Parkinson disease. Neurology 2006; 79(4): 697–699.

21. Mata IF, Taylor IP, Kachergus J, et al. LRRK2 R144JG in Spanish patients with Parkinson's disease. Neurosci Lett 2005;382(3):309–11.
22. Tomiyama H, Li Y, Funayama M, et al.Clinicogenetic study of mutations in LRRK2 exon 41 in Parkinson's disease patients from 18 countries. Mov Disord 2006; 21(8):1102–1108.
23. Kay DM, Kramer P, Higgins D, et al. Escaping Parkinson's disease; a neurologically healthy octogenarian with the LRRK2 G2019S mutation. Mov Disord 2005; 20(2):1077–1078.
24. Carmine Belin A, Westerlund M, Sydow O, et al. Leucine-rich repeat kinase 2 (LRRK2) mutations in a Swedish Parkinson cohort and a healthy nonagenarian. Mov Disord 2006; 21(10):1731–1734.
25. Hemandez D, Paisan Ruiz C, Crawley A, et al. The dardarin G 2019 S mutation is a common cause of Parkinson's disease but not other neurodegenerative diseases. Neurosci Lett 2005; 389(3):137–139.
26. Lee E, Hui S, Ho G, et al. LRRK2 G2Q19S and 12020T mutations are not common in Alzheimer's disease and vascular dementia. Am J Med Genet B Neuropsychiatr Genet 2006; 141(5):549–550.
27. Zabetian CP, Lauricella CJ, Tsuang DW, et al. Analysis of the LRRK2 G2019S mutation in Alzheimer Disease. Arch Neurol 2006; 63(1):156–157.
28. Saunders-Pullman R, Lipton RB, Senthil G, et al. Increased frequency of the LKRK2 G20I9S mutation in an elderly Ashkenazi Jewish population is not associated with dementia. Neurosci Lett 2006; 402(1–2):92–96.
29. Ross OA, Whittle AJ, Cobb SA, et al. Lrrk2 R1441 substitution and progressive supranu-clear palsy. Neuropathol Appl Neurobiol 2006; 32(1):23–25.
30- Tan EK, Skipper L, Chua R, et al. Analysis of 14 LRRK2 mutations in Parkinson's plus syndromes and late-onset Parkinson's disease. Mov Disord 2006; 21(7):997–1001.
31. Biskcup S, Mueller JC, Sharma M, et al. Common variants of LRRK2 are not associated with sporadic Parkinson's disease. Ann Neurol 2005; 58(6):905–908.
32. Paisan-Ruiz C, Evans EW, Jain S, et al. Testing association between LRRK2 and Parkinson's disease and investigating linkage disequilibrium. J Med Genet 2006; 43(2):e9.
33. Skipper L, Li Y, Bonnard C, et al. Comprehensive evaluation of common genetic varia-tion within LRRK2 reveals evidence for association with sporadic Parkinson's disease. Hum Mol Genet 2005; 14(23):3549–3556.
34. Taylor JP, Mata IF, Fairer MJ. LRRK2: a common pathway for parkinsonism, pathogene-sis and prevention? Trends Mol Med 2006; 12(2):76–82.
35. Ross OA, Toft M, Whittle AJ, et al. Lrrk2 and Lewy body disease. Ann Neurol 2006; 59(2):388–393.
36. Giasson BI, Covy JP, Bonini NM, et al. Biochemical and pathological characterization of Lrrk2. Ann Neurol 2006; 59(2):315–322.
37. Toft M, Mata IF, Kachergus JM, et al. LRRK2 mutations and Parkinsonism. Lancet 2005; 365(9466):1229–1230.
38. Albrecht M. LRRK2 mutations and Parkinsonism. Lancet 2005; 365(9466):1230.
39. Greggio E, Jain S, Kingsbuiy A, et al. Kinase activity is required for the toxic effects of mutant LRRK2/dardarin. Neurobioi Dis 2006; 23(2):329–341.
40. West AB, Moore DJ, Biskup S, et at. Parkinson's disease-associated mutations in leucine-rich repeat kinase 2 augment kinase activity. Proc Natl Acad Sci USA 2005; 102:16842–16847.
41. Gloeckner CJ, Kinkl N, Schumacher A, et al. The Parkinson disease causing LRRK2 mutation 12020T is associated with increased kinase activity. Hum Mol Genet 2006; 15(2):223–232.
42. Smith WW, Pel Z, Jiang H, et al. Leucine-rich repeat kinase 2 (LRRK2) interacts with parkin, and mutant LRRK2 induces neuronal degeneration. Proc Natl Acad Sci USA 2005; 102(51):18676–18681.
43. Korr D, Toschi L, Donner P, et al. LRRK1 protein kinase activity is stimulated upon bind-ing of GTP to its Roc domain.Cell Signal 2005; 18(6):910–920.

10 Genetics of Tau in Parkinsonism

Rosa Rademakers, Marc Cruts, and
Christine van Broeckhoven
*Department of Molecular Genetics, Neurodegenerative Brain Diseases Group,
Laboratory of Neurogenetics, Institute Born-Bunge, University of Antwerp,
Antwerpen, Belgium*

INTRODUCTION

Tau belongs to the family of microtubule-associated proteins (MAP) with a central role in the assembly of tubulin monomers into microtubules to constitute the microtubule network (1–3). Tau is highly expressed in the axons of mature and growing neurons, although low levels are also present in oligodendrocytes and astrocytes (4,5). In non-neuronal cells, tau can be detected in several peripheral tissues such as heart, kidney, lung, muscle, pancreas, and testis (6–8). In addition to the polymerization and stabilization of microtubules, neuronal tau is important for morphogenesis, axonal extension, and the regulation of motor protein–mediated transport of vesicles and organelles along the microtubules (9–11). In human brain, six different tau isoforms are generated by alternative splicing from a single unique gene, *MAPT*, located over a 140 kb region on the long arm of chromosome 17 (12). Alternative splicing is an important mechanism, generating different protein isoforms from a single gene, which occurs in about 60% of all human genes (13,14). It is expected that the diverse tau isoforms produced in human brain each have specific physiological roles since they are differentially expressed during development and may be differentially distributed in neuronal subpopulations (15–17).

A wide variety of neurodegenerative diseases are characterized by neuronal loss and the accumulation of intracellular and/or extracellular protein aggregates. The deposition of hyperphosphorylated tau in insoluble filaments in brain is the pathological hallmark of the group of disorders collectively known as tauopathies (18,19). These include frontotemporal dementia (FTD), Pick's disease (PiD), Alzheimer's disease (AD), as well as rare parkinsonian disorders, such as progressive supranuclear palsy (PSP) and corticobasal degeneration (CBD). In Parkinson's disease (PD) the affected neurons contain intracytoplasmic protein aggregates called Lewy bodies, which are mainly composed of α-synuclein (20). Although PD is therefore referred to as a synucleinopathy, rather than a tauopathy, it can be expected that parallel disease mechanisms are involved in the polymerization of either tau or α-synuclein into fibrils that accumulate to form pathological inclusions.

Recently, biochemical and pathological evidence suggested a direct role for tau in the pathogenesis of PD. Postmortem brain examination of two PD patients from the Contursi kindred with the rare A53T missense mutation in the gene encoding α-synuclein (*SNCA*) revealed widespread α-synuclein and tau inclusions (21,22). Concomitant tau and α-synuclein pathology was also described in two patients from the Western Nebraska kindred in whom the R1441C missense mutation in the gene dardarin, encoding the leucine-rich repeat kinase 2 (*LRRK2*), was identified (23,24). Aggregation of tau proteins in the absence of Lewy bodies was reported in

PD patients with mutations in the *PARKIN* gene (*PARK2*) (25,26). Furthermore, in vitro studies supported the interaction between the negatively charged C-terminus of α-synuclein and the positively charged microtubule-binding region of tau and demonstrated that tau and α-synuclein synergistically promote and propagate each other's polymerization into fibrils (27,28). Finally, it was shown that α-synuclein could modulate the phosphorylation of tau by protein kinase A (28), and mice over-expressing A30P α-synuclein developed abnormally phosphorylated tau in parallel with the accumulation of aggregated α-synuclein (29).

In this chapter, we highlight the genetic findings that support the involvement of tau in the pathogenesis of PD and related parkinsonian syndromes. To understand the effect of genetic variation in *MAPT* on the development of neurodegenerative diseases we will first describe the genomic organization and regulation of *MAPT* and its location within the complex genomic region at 17q21. Next, we will review the current knowledge on the rare *MAPT* mutations as well as the common genetic variants in *MAPT*, emphasizing the role of *MAPT* in PD where appropriate.

GENOMIC ORGANIZATION OF THE TAU GENE
Gene Structure and Splicing
MAPT is located in chromosome 17q21 and consists of a noncoding exon 0 followed by 14 coding or partially coding exons (Fig. 1A) (30). Intron 13 is always retained in human *MAPT* transcripts, resulting in a single last exon comprising exon 13, intron 13, exon 14, and containing the 3' untranslated region (3'UTR). Restriction analyses showed that *MAPT* contains two CpG islands, one associated with the promoter region upstream of exon 0, the other with exon 9 (31). *MAPT* produces three

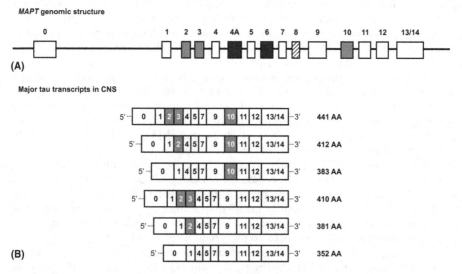

FIGURE 1 (A) Schematic presentation of the *MAPT* genomic structure with 15 exons shown as boxes. White boxes represent constitutively spliced exons. Human brain–specific, alternatively spliced exons are in dark gray. The black exons 4A and 6 are predominantly expressed in the peripheral nervous system. Exon 8 (hatched box) is not expressed in human *MAPT* transcripts. Introns and exons are not drawn to scale. (B) The six major tau transcripts resulting from the alternative splicing of exons 2, 3, and 10 observed in human brain. For each transcript the number of amino acids is indicated. *Abbreviation*: CNS, central nervous system.

transcripts of 2, 6, and 9 kb that are differentially expressed and localized in the nervous system, depending upon the stage of neuronal maturation and neuron type (12,16,32,33). The 2 kb and 6 kb transcripts are generated by the alternative use of two distinct polyadenylation signals (34). In humans, *MAPT* exons 2, 3, 4A, 6, 8, and 10 undergo tissue-specific and developmentally regulated alternative splicing.

In brain, *MAPT* exons 4A, 6, and 8 are not usually transcribed, however, alternative splicing of *MAPT* exons 2, 3, and 10 produces six major tau isoforms composed of 352 to 441 amino acids (Fig. 1B). The interaction of tau with the microtubules occurs at the C-terminus of the protein (35), by four imperfect repeat domains encoded by exons 9–12, and alternative splicing of exon 10 results in two classes of tau isoforms with either three (3R) or four (4R) microtubule binding repeat domains. This alternative splicing is under developmental regulation with only 3R tau expression in fetal brain, but near equal amounts of 3R and 4R tau in adult human brain (15). Since 4R tau binds to microtubules three-fold more strongly (36) and assembles microtubules more efficiently than 3R tau (16), this differential regulation clearly has an important biological relevance and correlates with increased stability of the cytoskeleton in adult as compared to developing neurons. Alternative splicing of exon 2, or exons 2 and 3 together, further results in the inclusion of zero, one, or two 29 amino acid inserts in the amino-terminal half of the protein. These N-terminal inserts are part of the projection domain that mediates the interaction of tau with the neural plasma membrane, establishing the interaction of the microtubules with the plasma membrane (37). Only the shortest isoform lacking exons 2 and 3 is expressed during fetal brain stages (15).

Exon 4A is an unusually long exon and is only included in the 9 kb tau transcript detected in the retina and peripheral nervous system, where it encodes a higher molecular weight tau protein nicknamed big tau (38,39) (Fig. 1B). Exon 6, included in both 6 and 9 kb tau mRNAs, is most prominent in the peripheral nervous system where the corresponding tau proteins are involved in increased microtubule spacing (40,41). Unexpectedly, it was shown that apart from the originally described acceptor splice site, exon 6 utilizes two cryptic splice sites that would generate cryptic splice variants lacking the C-terminal microtubule binding domains (42,43). Thus far, exon 8 has never been observed in human *MAPT* transcripts (44).

ARCHITECTURE OF THE *MAPT* GENOMIC REGION

MAPT is located in a complex region characterized by the presence of an unusual long stretch of complete linkage disequilibrium (LD) that extends into the genes encoding the corticotrophin releasing hormone receptor 1 (*CRHR1*) and LOC284058, flanking *MAPT* (45). In fact, a recent assessment of LD across the genome in different populations suggested that the *MAPT* locus was the longest region of LD in Europeans (46). The atypical LD structure of *MAPT* was first described in 1999, when Baker et al. performed mutation analyses of *MAPT* exons and flanking intronic sequences and identified a series of eight common single nucleotide polymorphisms (SNPs) that were transmitted in complete LD and defined two extended *MAPT* haplotypes, H1 and H2 (47). They recognized the complete lack of recombination between H1 and H2, and suggested that the establishment of the *MAPT* haplotypes was an ancient event and that either recombination was suppressed in this chromosomal region due to a genomic mutation, or that recombinants were selected against. By use of additional SNPs and single tandem repeat (STR) polymorphisms subsequent studies further expanded the extent of the nonrecombining

H1 and H2 haplotypes, first by an additional 68 kb to the promoter region 5′ of *MAPT* exon 0 (48,49), and then to a 363 kb interval between rs937 and rs1816 (50). In 2004, Pittman et al. delineated the outer edges of the extended LD region, defining a maximum LD block of ~2 Mb at 17q21.31 (45).

The recent construction of a refined physical map of the *MAPT* genomic region finally provided an explanation for the suppressed recombination and extended LD at 17q21 (51). By genotyping 60 STR markers in genomic clones derived from a single H1/H2 individual and assembling the clones in two chromosome-specific contigs, Stefansson et al. uncovered a 900 kb genetically balanced inversion that is present in the Caucasian population as a common inversion polymorphism (51). This inverted region included *MAPT* as well as the known genes *CRHR1*, presenilin homologue 2 (*PSH2*), and Saitohin (*STH*), and three putative genes FLJ25268, BC018135, and LOC284058. A consequence of this paracentric inversion is that meiotic recombinations within the inverted region in H1/H2 individuals, lead to genetically unstable acentric and dicentric chromosomes, and recombination products are not observed in the population (52). However, meiotic recombinations in H1/H1 and H2/H2 individuals are not hampered by this inversion, and define H1 and H2 specific LD maps of *MAPT*, presenting as two distinct haplotype clades. A comparison of the H1 and H2 frequencies in different racial groups from the CEPH diversity panel indicated that H2 is almost exclusively Caucasian in origin with middle eastern and European populations having frequencies of ~25%, central Asian populations of ~5% and other populations (African, East Asian and native American) having essentially zero (53).

Simultaneously with the identification of the H1-H2 inversion polymorphism, we constructed a genomic sequence contig of the *MAPT* region at 17q21 (54). We showed that *MAPT* was flanked by duplicated sequences and subsequent annotation of ~2 Mb genomic sequence surrounding *MAPT* identified three low copy repeats (LCR A-C) with >97% sequence similarity. LCR A was located 250 kb centromeric of *MAPT*, whereas LCR B and LCR C were inverted relative to LCR A and located at 180 and 950 kb telomeric of *MAPT*, respectively. The location of LCR A and LCR B coincided with the boundaries of the 900 kb inverted region, suggesting that the historical H1-H2 inversion polymorphism resulted from non-allelic homologous recombination between LCR A and LCR B. Synteny mapping of human, mouse and chimpanzee further supported this hypothesis, and demonstrated that at least two inversions in the chromosomal segments located between LCR A-C must have occurred during evolution, most likely before chimpanzee speciation (54).

MUTATIONS IN *MAPT*
Overview
In 1994, it was demonstrated that the Irish Mo family, presenting with a disorder then referred to as disinhibition-dementia-parkinsonism-amyotrophy complex (DDPAC), was genetically linked to a region in chromosome 17q21 including *MAPT* (55). Individual Mo family members presented with a variety of clinical phenotypes, but the combination of FTD and parkinsonism was most commonly observed. The next two years, follow-up linkage studies in families with autosomal dominantly inherited forms of FTD collected from around the world, established definite or probable linkage of 13 families to the same region on chromosome 17. In 1997, a consensus conference convened in Ann Arbor, Michigan to compare the clinical,

pathologic and genetic findings of these families, and the term frontotemporal dementia with parkinsonism linked to chromosome 17 (FTDP-17) was introduced to best categorize the predominant symptoms in these families (56). Main clinical features included a severe behavioral disorder characteristic of FTD accompanied by a parkinsonian syndrome without resting tremor. Neuropathological brain examination revealed pathological accumulations of tau proteins in nearly all patients. Therefore, *MAPT* became the obvious candidate gene for this disorder, and, shortly after, mutations in *MAPT* were identified in nine of the original 13 FTDP-17 families (57–59).

In the past nine years, 41 different pathogenic *MAPT* mutations have been reported in a total of 117 tauopathy families (FTD mutation database, www.molgen. ua.ac.be/FTDMutations) (60). These include 27 missense mutations, four silent mutations, two in-frame single codon deletions, and eight intronic mutations (Fig. 2). With the exception of two mutations in exon 1, all coding *MAPT* mutations clustered in exons 9-13 encoding the microtubule binding domains of tau and flanking regions. The intronic mutations are all located in the introns flanking the alternatively spliced exon 10 (Fig. 2B). Mutations are most frequently observed in exon 10 and intron 10, with a C to T substitution in codon 301 corresponding to P301L in exon 10 in 29 families and IVS10+16C>T in intron 10, identified in 23 different families (60). In contrast, 28 mutations were reported in one single family worldwide. In general, *MAPT* mutations are heterozygous segregating as dominant mutations within families; however, a homozygous S352L mutation was reported in two siblings of an English consanguineous family with an aggressive early-onset hereditary tauopathy (61), and a homozygous deltaN296 (Δ296N) mutation was identified in a Spanish patient diagnosed with atypical PSP (62).

Several studies have attempted to estimate the frequency of *MAPT* mutations in patient populations with a variety of clinical phenotypes including classical FTD, AD, PSP, and PD. In FTD, the frequency of *MAPT* mutations varied considerably between populations from 0% to 50% depending on the family history of dementia and the use of clinical or pathological inclusion criteria (60). Mutation analysis of all coding *MAPT* exons in 96 PSP patients identified only one mutation, R5L in exon 1, in a patient with pathological confirmed PSP (63). No *MAPT* mutations were identified in an early-onset AD population (64), in a mixed population of patients with dementia of the non-AD type (65) or in 150 PD patients from a large collection of 80 independent PD families (66).

Effect of Mutations on Tau Function

MAPT mutations can be divided in two categories depending on the primary disease mechanism that is involved (67). The first class of mutations has been referred to as *splicing regulation mutations*. These include all mutations in intron 10 and most mutations in exon 10 that disturb the normal splicing balance of exon 10, thereby producing an altered 4R/3R isoform ratio. The deregulation of alternative splicing is a frequently observed mechanism in neurodegenerative disorders, and it has been estimated that up to 15% of genetic defects caused by point mutations in humans, manifest themselves as mRNA splicing defects (68,69). In the case of *MAPT* exon 10, it was demonstrated that alternative splicing is regulated by at least two exon-splicing enhancers and one exon-splicing silencer together with an additional sequence located at the beginning of intron 10 that inhibits exon 10 splicing, most likely by the presence of a stem-loop structure that limits access of the splicing

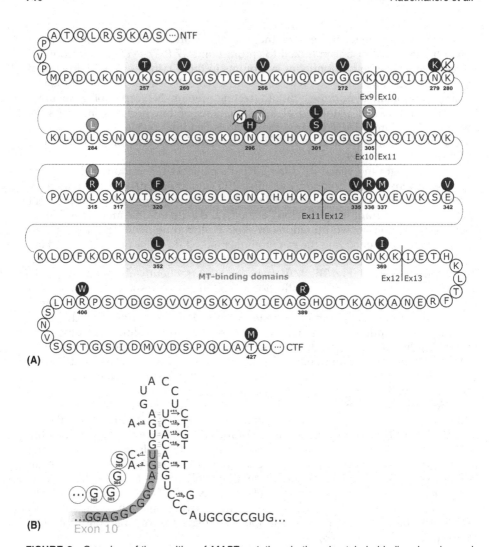

(A)

(B)

FIGURE 2 Overview of the position of *MAPT* mutations in the microtubule-binding domains and intron 10. (**A**) Schematic presentation of the four microtubule-binding domains and inter-repeat regions of tau encoded by exons 9-13. Each circle represents an amino acid. For mutations, amino acid numbering is shown relative to the longest tau isoform retaining exons 2, 3, and 10. All mutations are shown above the mutated amino acid; missense mutations are presented in black, silent mutations in gray, and single-codon deletions are shown as crossed circles. (**B**) Schematic presentation of the stem-loop structure in the pre-mRNA at the boundary between exon 10 and intron 10. The 10 mutations indicated by arrows, of which two (S305N and S305S) are located in exonic sequence, represented by a gray bar. *Abbreviations*: NTF, N-terminal fragment; CTF, C-terminal fragment; MT, microtubule.

machinery to the 5′ splice site (57,59) (Fig. 2B). The known exon 10 and all intron 10 mutations are located within these different regulatory sequences, and usually result in more inclusion of exon 10 with an increased 4R/3R tau ratio as the final outcome. At this moment, the mechanism by which a simple increase in the 4R/3R isoform ratio of normal tau causes neurodegeneration is not completely understood. It has been proposed that there are discrete microtubule binding sites for 3R and 4R tau, and that the synthesis of excess 4R tau would result in saturation of the 4R binding sites (70). The subsequent higher levels of free 4R tau might then drive tau aggregation resulting in abnormal tau filaments that cause cellular dysfunction. The frequent exon 10 mutations at codon 301, P301L and P301S, are exceptional since they are not located in regulatory sequence elements and therefore do not affect the splicing of *MAPT* exon 10.

The second class of *MAPT* mutations, referred to as *protein function mutations*, have their primary effect at the protein level of tau. Based on their location within the microtubule binding domains and flanking regions, it was predicted that most coding mutations would interfere with the correct binding of tau to tubulin, thereby decreasing the ability of tau to promote microtubule assembly (Fig. 2A). Therefore, much research focused on the ability of mutant tau to maintain the integrity of the cytoskeleton, and for almost all missense mutations, including the two single-codon deletions, in vitro microtubule assembly and/or binding assays showed a reduced ability of mutant tau to assemble microtubules (71–78). The degree of reduction has been controversial and varies not only between different *MAPT* mutations, but also between different studies of the same mutation (79). Thus far only three coding mutations, N279K and S305N in exon 10 and Q336R in exon 12, failed to show a decreased ability to promote microtubule assembly (80,81). In contrast, S305N and Q336R showed an increased ability to promote microtubule assembly. Although it can be expected that too much microtubule binding might be as detrimental to neuronal function as too little, this increased microtubule binding may also be irrelevant to the pathogenic mechanism. Interestingly, in addition to their effect on microtubule binding, a number of coding mutations were shown to accelerate the in vitro aggregation of tau to form filaments that resemble those isolated from diseased brains (82,83). The faster aggregation of free mutant tau into pathological insoluble filaments might be an additional mechanism whereby coding mutations increase the cellular dysfunction.

Finally, tau is a multipurpose protein that fullfils several functions besides the maintenance of the cytoskeleton. Only limited research has focused on the possibility that *MAPT* mutations would alter another biological relevant function of tau. One study has reported enhanced phosphorylation of tau in vitro as a result of the presence of *MAPT* mutations (84), and a number of mutations significantly decreased the binding affinity of tau for protein phosphatase 2A in vivo (85). Although it was shown that more phosphorylated tau leads to less interactions with the microtubules in vitro (86), it remains to be determined if tau hyperphosphorylation is either necessary or sufficient for filament assembly in vivo.

GENOTYPE-PHENOTYPE CORRELATIONS

The presence of a filamentous brain pathology made of hyperphosphorylated tau proteins is thus far reported in all patients with *MAPT* mutations. However, it was shown that the location of a particular mutation within the tau protein could be an important determinant of the cellular pathology and the tau isoform composition and morphology within the affected brains (86,87). Patients with mutations in exon 10 or intron 10 showed neuronal and glial tau pathology with twisted, ribbon-like filaments that were predominantly or exclusively composed of 4R tau isoforms. In contrast, patients with missense mutations outside exon 10, affecting the amino acid composition of both 3R and 4R tau isoforms, showed a selective neuronal pathology, with tau filaments composed of all six major brain isoforms deposited as neurofibrillary tangles (NFTs) or straight filaments (SF). Unexpectedly, some mutations in the constitutively spliced exon 9 resulted in the selective deposition of 3R (K257T) or 4R (I260V) tau isoforms, suggesting different biochemical properties for each mutated isoform (88,89).

Compared to the pathological manifestation, the clinical phenotypes associated with *MAPT* mutations have been more variable and resembled either FTD, PSP, CBD, AD, PiD, or PD (90). When only a few *MAPT* mutations were known, it was noticed that mutations located in exons 9 and 13 were more often associated with PiD without motor symptoms, whereas mutations altering *MAPT* splicing more frequently presented with parkinsonian features in addition to FTD (91). Also, coding mutations within the first two microtubule-binding domains usually presented with an earlier onset and shorter disease duration compared to more C-terminal located mutations, which showed a more prominent memory loss (92). However, now that an increasing number of *MAPT* mutations have been reported, several mutations do not fit this generalization. Moreover, a number of *MAPT* mutations have been reported in multiple families and occasionally more variation is observed within a single family than between families with different *MAPT* mutations (60). For example, clinical heterogeneity within a single Italian family with P301S in exon 10 resulted in the diagnosis of FTD in one patient and CBD in his son (93,94). On the contrary, N279K in exon 9, identified in one American, one French, one Italian, and four Japanese families, resulted in the presentation of highly similar clinical phenotypes (95–100). All patients uniformly showed typical parkinsonian features including bradykinesia, rigidity and postural instability with a well-defined onset age between 41 and 47 years. Personality and behavioural changes and dementia also occurred in the course of the illness, but were less prominent.

In the context of *MAPT* in PD, the Δ296N mutation identified in two families is of note. This mutation was first reported in the homozygous state in a Spanish kindred in which two brothers, born from a third-degree consanguineous marriage, were affected with atypical PSP in their late 30s (62). Interestingly, two heterozygous family members developed typical PD with onset ages of 62 and 72 years, whereas at least 10 heterozygous carriers did not show PD phenotypes even at advanced ages. Recently, heterozygous Δ296N mutation carriers were also reported in a second family (101). Again, the proband presented with an atypical PSP-like syndrome, however one paternal uncle developed atypical parkinsonism at age 51 years, while a paternal aunt was affected by classical PD with an onset age of 63 years. The identification of patients with typical PD in two independent Δ296N families, suggested that this mutation might be an important genetic factor increasing PD-risk. Systematic mutation analyses of exon 10 in 80 late-onset PD families however did not identify Δ296N (66).

The identification of *MAPT* mutations in patients that were clinically diagnosed with PD has provided new genetic evidence for a direct role of *MAPT* in the development of PD. In the near future, in-depth mutation analyses of *MAPT* in additional PD populations should be performed to further support these findings, and eventually to identify the biological mechanism underlying the *MAPT*-associated PD risk.

MAPT AS A SUSCEPTIBILITY GENE
In Primary Tauopathies

Before it became apparent that *MAPT* mutations could lead to neurodegeneration in FTDP-17 families, Conrad et al. already hypothesized that common genetic variability in *MAPT* could lead to increased risk for neurodegenerative tauopathies (102). They first studied PSP, the second most common form of parkinsonism worldwide, which is clinically distinguished from PD by the presence of ocular gaze palsy (103). Pathologically, PSP is characterized by neuronal loss and gliosis accompanied by abundant subcortical NFTs that are mainly composed of 4R tau proteins (104). The initial association study of *MAPT* in PSP was performed with a dinucleotide repeat polymorphism within intron 9, presenting with four polymorphic alleles of which two, A0 and A3, were frequently observed. Conrad et al. identified highly significant association that could be explained by an overrepresentation of the frequent A0 allele in PSP patients as compared to control individuals (102). Shortly thereafter this association was replicated in four independent PSP populations (105–108). Due to the location of *MAPT* in the 900 kb H1-H2 inversion (see "Architecture of the *MAPT* genomic region"), the A0 allele of the dinucleotide repeat was in complete LD with the H1 haplotype, while the A3 allele was always inherited with H2. Therefore it was no surprise that in all subsequent studies the positive association of PSP with A0 was replicated with the extended H1 haplotype (48,109). In most populations, genotypic (H1/H1) association was more significant than allelic (H1) association suggesting the existence of a recessive mutation or a dosage sensitive risk-allele on H1. Significant associations with H1 were also observed with two other 4R tauopathies, CBD (110,111) and argyrophilic grain disease (AGD) (112,113). In contrast, association studies in AD (114), FTD (115–119) and primary progressive aphasia (PPA) (120) populations were in general negative or inconsistent in independent populations.

In PD Populations
Association Studies with the H1–H2 Inversion Polymorphism
The potential involvement of *MAPT* in the rare parkinsonian syndromes PSP and CBD, suggested that genetic variation in *MAPT* might also confer increased susceptibility to the development of the more common PD. However, it rapidly became clear that the highly significant associations observed in PSP were not replicated in PD populations. Albeit two studies reported a moderate significant increase of the A0 frequency of the dinucleotide repeat in intron 9 (121,122), most studies only reported slightly increased A0 frequencies that were nonsignificant (107,123). Additional evidence for the involvement of *MAPT* in PD was provided when Scott et al. reported linkage with D17S1293 located on chromosome 17q, about 8 cM centromeric of *MAPT*, in a large genome screen among 174 families with idiopathic PD (124). The linkage was particularly strong in the subset of 147 families with levodopa-responsive late-onset PD. Using family-based association analyses they showed that the A0 allele was significantly overtransmitted to patients with late-onset PD.

To date, at least 15 publications reported independent association studies with the A0-A3 alleles or H1-H2 haplotypes in PD populations. A meta-analysis that pooled 10 of these studies revealed a significant 1.5 times increased PD-risk (95% CI, 1.12–2.04) for carriers of the H1 haplotype (125). In contrast to PSP the genotypic associations in PD populations were not always stronger than the allelic associations suggesting different disease mechanisms for PD and PSP. Two studies were excluded from the meta-analyses because they showed significant heterogeneity across studies. The first study was performed in a genetically isolated PD population from Trondheim in Norway, and reported association with the H1 haplotype of the same magnitude as the associations observed in PSP and CBD (126). Most likely, the low immigration rate in this geographically remote population close to the Arctic Circle, produced a genetically homogeneous population with a dramatically increased power to detect association. The second study, performed in a PD population from southern Italy, unexpectedly showed significant association with the A3 allele, which is inherited as part of the extended H2 haplotype (127). The discrepancy between these studies may be explained by genetic heterogeneity between populations with different ethnic backgrounds, and argues against the hypothesis that the H1-H2 inversion polymorphism per se underlies the *MAPT* associated PD-risk. Most likely, genetic variants that determine H1 and H2 specific subhaplotypes are responsible for the increased PD risk in the different populations.

H1 Subhaplotype Association Studies

In a first attempt to study H1 subhaplotypes, Skipper et al. performed 5 kb of resequencing in evolutionarily conserved regions of *MAPT* and *CRHR1* (128). They identified 14 H1 specific SNPs and selected a minimum set of 9 haplotype tagging (ht) SNPs that captured all haplotype diversity in the *MAPT-CRHR1* region. Systematic association analyses with these H1 specific SNPs in H1/H1 homozygous subpopulations of Norwegian PD patients and control individuals identified highly significant association with an H1 subhaplotype spanning a region of 90 kb including *MAPT* exons 1 to 4. The authors propose that this PD-associated haplotype might harbor genetic variability that influences the alternative splicing of *MAPT* exons 2 and 3. A second study was performed by Oliveira et al. with four H1 htSNPs selected from a larger genomic region spanning multiple genes in the *MAPT* genomic region (66). They also identified significant association with one specific H1 subhaplotype; however, the low H1 SNP density did not allow finemapping of the PD-associated risk to a specific *MAPT* interval. In fact, the authors could not exclude that the risk identified in their study resulted from genetic variation in *CRHR1* or LOC284058 flanking *MAPT*. A negative-association study was reported with an H1 specific insertion of a "T" nucleotide at position –568 relative to exon 0 in the *MAPT* promoter in an Australian population of late-onset PD patients (129). Interestingly, this study did identify significant association with the H1-H2 inversion polymorphism and demonstrated that the extended H1 haplotype was more efficient at driving *MAPT* expression than the H2 haplotype, suggesting that an increase in expression of *MAPT* is a susceptibility factor in PD.

Recently, additional H1 subhaplotype associations were performed in diverse ethnic PD populations. Using single marker and haplotype association analyses moderate associations were reported in Greek and Finnish populations, but not in a Taiwanese cohort (130,131). These studies further supported the hypothesis that H1 subhaplotypes confer susceptibility to PD, however, they also suggested that the nature of the association is influenced by allelic heterogeneity and ethnic variation.

Genetic Interaction of MAPT and SCNA

Recently, the genetic interaction of *SNCA* and *MAPT* genotypes was studied in a large population including >500 PD patients and control individuals (132). In this population significantly increased PD-risk was identified in carriers with either the H1/H1 genotype of *MAPT* or the *SNCA* 261/261 genotype of REP1, a polymorphic complex repeat located ~10 kb upstream of the translational start of *SNCA*. REP1 had been previously associated with PD, and luciferase reporter assays suggested that the 261 bp allele increased the expression of α-synuclein (133). Because it had been shown that α-synuclein and tau stimulated each other's assembly in vitro (27), it was hypothesized that the *MAPT* H1 and the *SNCA* 261 alleles might interact to confer PD susceptibility. However, when the *SNCA* and *MAPT* data were analyzed in an interaction model, the combined effect of the two genotypes was the same as for either of the genotypes alone (132).

CONCLUSION

Although mutations in *MAPT* have not yet been detected in extended multiplex families segregating typical PD, genetic-association studies have steadily increased the evidence that *MAPT* variants are implicated in the pathogenesis of PD. Aberrant splicing could confer increased PD risk by the production of abnormal 4R/3R tau isoform ratios. This hypothesis was supported by genotype-proteotype studies showing that FTDP-17 patients with mutations in exon 10 and intron 10, which specifically increased 4R tau isoforms, more frequently exhibited parkinsonian symptoms (91). In this context, it would be of interest to study extended populations of neuropathologically characterized PD patients to determine if certain patient subgroups specifically present with (4R) tau isoforms in addition to the α-synuclein pathology. On the other hand, the significant association with genetic variants in *MAPT* intron 0 suggested that altered tau expression levels could influence PD susceptibility. In this light it was hypothesized that an increased expression of tau might indirectly cause Lewy body formation by increasing the propensity of α-synuclein to aggregate in PD brains (27).

Finally, it is important to realize that a susceptibility gene does not have to cause gross pathological changes to be relevant, and that the effect of *MAPT* variants in PD may rather be to trigger the disease. Anyway, the actual functional *MAPT* variants underlying the PD-associated risk should now be identified to understand the precise role of tau in the pathogenesis of PD. It can be expected that a better insight into the functional relationship between tau and PD will eventually contribute to the development of novel and efficient therapeutic strategies.

ACKNOWLEDGMENTS

The research in the authors' laboratory is in part sponsored by the Special Research Fund of the University of Antwerp, the Fund for Scientific Research Flanders (FWO-F), the Interuniversity Attraction Poles program P5/19 of the Belgian Science Policy Office (BELSPO), the International Alzheimer's Research Foundation, Belgium; the EU contract LSHM-CT-2003-503330 (APOPIS), and the Alzheimer's Association USA. R.R and M.C are postdoctoral fellows of the FWO-F, Belgium.

REFERENCES

1. Cleveland DW, Hwo SY, Kirschner MW. Purification of tau, a microtubule-associated protein that induces assembly of microtubules from purified tubulin. J Mol Biol 1977; 116(2):207–225.
2. Hirokawa N. Microtubule organization and dynamics dependent on microtubule-associated proteins. Curr Opin Cell Biol 1994; 6(1):74–81.
3. Weingarten MD, Lockwood AH, Hwo SY, et al. A protein factor essential for microtubule assembly. Proc Natl Acad Sci USA 1975; 72(5):1858–1862.
4. Binder LI, Frankfurter A, Rebhun LI. The distribution of tau in the mammalian central nervous system. J Cell Biol 1985; 101(4):1371–1378.

5. LoPresti P, Szuchet S, Papasozomenos SC, et al. Functional implications for the microtubule-associated protein tau: localization in oligodendrocytes. Proc Natl Acad Sci USA 1995; 92(22):10369–10373.

6. Gu Y, Oyama F, Ihara Y. Tau is widely expressed in rat tissues. J Neurochem 1996; 67(3):1235–1244.

7. Ingelson M, Vanmechelen E, Lannfelt L. Microtubule-associated protein tau in human fibroblasts with the Swedish Alzheimer mutation. Neurosci Lett 1996; 220(1):9–12.

8. Vanier MT, Neuville P, Michalik L, et al. Expression of specific tau exons in normal and tumoral pancreatic acinar cells. J Cell Sci 1998; 111(Pt 10):1419–1432.

9. Couchie D, Faivre-Bauman A, Puymirat J, et al. Expression of microtubule-associated proteins during the early stages of neurite extension by brain neurons cultured in a defined medium. J Neurochem 1986; 47(4):1255–1261.

10. Ebneth A, Godemann R, Stamer K, et al. Overexpression of tau protein inhibits kinesin-dependent trafficking of vesicles, mitochondria, and endoplasmic reticulum: implications for Alzheimer's disease. J Cell Biol 1998; 143(3):777–794.

11. Sato-Harada R, Okabe S, Umeyama T, et al. Microtubule-associated proteins regulate microtubule function as the track for intracellular membrane organelle transports. Cell Struct Funct 1996; 21(5):283–295.

12. Goedert M, Spillantini MG, Jakes R, et al. Multiple isoforms of human microtubule-associated protein tau: sequences and localization in neurofibrillary tangles of Alzheimer's disease. Neuron 1989; 3(4):519–526.

13. Lee CJ, Irizarry K. Alternative splicing in the nervous system: an emerging source of diversity and regulation. Biol Psychiatry 2003; 54(8):771–776.

14. Mironov AA, Fickett JW, Gelfand MS. Frequent alternative splicing of human genes. Genome Res 1999; 9(12):1288–1293.

15. Goedert M, Spillantini MG, Potier MC, et al. Cloning and sequencing of the cDNA encoding an isoform of microtubule-associated protein tau containing four tandem repeats: differential expression of tau protein mRNAs in human brain. EMBO J 1989; 8(2): 393–399.

16. Goedert M, Jakes R. Expression of separate isoforms of human tau protein: correlation with the tau pattern in brain and effects on tubulin polymerization. EMBO J 1990; 9(13): 4225–4230.

17. Kosik KS, Orecchio LD, Bakalis S, et al. Developmentally regulated expression of specific tau sequences. Neuron 1989; 2(4):1389–1397.

18. Spillantini MG, Goedert M, Crowther RA, et al. Familial multiple system tauopathy with presenile dementia: a disease with abundant neuronal and glial tau filaments. Proc Natl Acad Sci USA 1997; 94(8):4113–4118.

19. Tolnay M, Probst A. REVIEW: tau protein pathology in Alzheimer's disease and related disorders. Neuropathol Appl Neurobiol 1999; 25(3):171–187.

20. Spillantini MG, Schmidt ML, Lee VM, et al. Alpha-synuclein in Lewy bodies. Nature 1997; 388(6645):839–840.

21. Duda JE, Giasson BI, Mabon ME, et al. Concurrence of alpha-synuclein and tau brain pathology in the Contursi kindred. Acta Neuropathol (Berl) 2002; 104(1):7–11.

22. Kotzbauer PT, Giasson BI, Kravitz AV, et al. Fibrillization of alpha-synuclein and tau in familial Parkinson's disease caused by the A53T alpha-synuclein mutation. Exp Neurol 2004; 187(2):279–288.

23. Wszolek ZK, Pfeiffer RF, Tsuboi Y, et al. Autosomal dominant parkinsonism associated with variable synuclein and tau pathology. Neurology 2004; 62(9):1619–1622.

24. Zimprich A, Biskup S, Leitner P, et al. Mutations in LRRK2 cause autosomal-dominant parkinsonism with pleomorphic pathology. Neuron 2004; 44(4):601–607.

25. Mori H, Kondo T, Yokochi M, et al. Pathologic and biochemical studies of juvenile parkinsonism linked to chromosome 6q. Neurology 1998; 51(3):890–892.

26. van de Warrenburg BP, Lammens M, Lucking CB, et al. Clinical and pathologic abnormalities in a family with parkinsonism and parkin gene mutations. Neurology 2001; 56(4):555–557.

27. Giasson BI, Forman MS, Higuchi M, et al. Initiation and synergistic fibrillization of tau and alpha-synuclein. Science 2003; 300(5619):636–640.

28. Jensen PH, Hager H, Nielsen MS, et al. alpha-synuclein binds to Tau and stimulates the protein kinase A-catalyzed tau phosphorylation of serine residues 262 and 356. J Biol Chem 1999; 274(36):25481–25489.
29. Frasier M, Walzer M, McCarthy L, et al. Tau phosphorylation increases in symptomatic mice overexpressing A30P alpha-synuclein. Exp Neurol 2005; 192(2):274–287.
30. Andreadis A, Brown WM, Kosik KS. Structure and novel exons of the human tau gene. Biochemistry 1992; 31(43):10626–10633.
31. Andreadis A, Broderick JA, Kosik KS. Relative exon affinities and suboptimal splice site signals lead to non-equivalence of two cassette exons. Nucleic Acids Res 1995; 23(17):3585–3593.
32. Nunez J, Fischer I. Microtubule-associated proteins (MAPs) in the peripheral nervous system during development and regeneration. J Mol Neurosci 1997; 8(3):207–222.
33. Wang Y, Loomis PA, Zinkowski RP, et al. A novel tau transcript in cultured human neuroblastoma cells expressing nuclear tau. J Cell Biol 1993; 121(2):257–267.
34. Sadot E, Marx R, Barg J, et al. Complete sequence of 3′-untranslated region of Tau from rat central nervous system. Implications for mRNA heterogeneity. J Mol Biol 1994; 241(2): 325–331.
35. Gustke N, Trinczek B, Biernat J, et al. Domains of tau protein and interactions with microtubules. Biochemistry 1994; 33(32):9511–9522.
36. Goode BL, Chau M, Denis PE, et al. Structural and functional differences between 3-repeat and 4-repeat tau isoforms. Implications for normal tau function and the onset of neurodegenetative disease. J Biol Chem 2000; 275(49):38182–38189.
37. Brandt R, Leger J, Lee G. Interaction of tau with the neural plasma membrane mediated by tau's amino-terminal projection domain. J Cell Biol 1995; 131(5):1327–1340.
38. Couchie D, Mavilia C, Georgieff IS, et al. Primary structure of high molecular weight tau present in the peripheral nervous system. Proc Natl Acad Sci USA 1992; 89(10): 4378–4381.
39. Goedert M, Spillantini MG, Crowther RA. Cloning of a big tau microtubule-associated protein characteristic of the peripheral nervous system. Proc Natl Acad Sci USA 1992; 89(5):1983–1987.
40. Chen J, Kanai Y, Cowan NJ, et al. Projection domains of MAP2 and tau determine spacings between microtubules in dendrites and axons. Nature 1992; 360(6405): 674–677.
41. Frappier TF, Georgieff IS, Brown K, et al. tau Regulation of microtubule-microtubule spacing and bundling. J Neurochem 1994; 63(6):2288–2294.
42. Wei ML, Andreadis A. Splicing of a regulated exon reveals additional complexity in the axonal microtubule-associated protein tau. J Neurochem 1998; 70(4):1346–1356.
43. Wei ML, Memmott J, Screaton G, et al. The splicing determinants of a regulated exon in the axonal MAP tau reside within the exon and in its upstream intron. Brain Res Mol Brain Res 2000; 80(2):207–218.
44. Chen WT, Liu WK, Yen SH. Expression of tau exon 8 in different species. Neurosci Lett 1994; 172(1–2):167–170.
45. Pittman AM, Myers AJ, Duckworth J, et al. The structure of the tau haplotype in controls and in progressive supranuclear palsy. Hum Mol Genet 2004; 13(12):1267–1274.
46. Hinds DA, Stuve LL, Nilsen GB, et al. Whole-genome patterns of common DNA variation in three human populations. Science 2005; 307(5712):1072–1079.
47. Baker M, Litvan I, Houlden H, et al. Association of an extended haplotype in the tau gene with progressive supranuclear palsy. Hum Mol Genet 1999; 8(4):711–715.
48. de Silva R, Weiler M, Morris HR, et al. Strong association of a novel Tau promoter haplotype in progressive supranuclear palsy. Neurosci Lett 2001; 311(3):145–148.
49. Ezquerra M, Pastor P, Valldeoriola F, et al. Identification of a novel polymorphism in the promoter region of the tau gene highly associated to progressive supranuclear palsy in humans. Neurosci Lett 1999; 275(3):183–186.
50. Pastor P, Ezquerra M, Tolosa E, et al. Further extension of the H1 haplotype associated with progressive supranuclear palsy. Mov Disord 2002; 17(3):550–556.
51. Stefansson H, Helgason A, Thorleifsson G, et al. A common inversion under selection in Europeans. Nat Genet 2005; 37(2):129–137.

52. Stankiewicz P, Lupski JR. Genome architecture, rearrangements and genomic disorders. Trends Genet 2002; 18(2):74–82.
53. Evans W, Fung HC, Steele J, et al. The tau H2 haplotype is almost exclusively Caucasian in origin. Neurosci Lett 2004; 369(3):183–185.
54. Cruts M, Rademakers R, Gijselinck I, et al. Genomic architecture of human 17q21 linked to frontotemporal dementia uncovers a highly homologous family of low copy repeats in the tau region. Hum Mol Genet 2005; 14(13):1753–1762.
55. Wilhelmsen KC, Lynch T, Pavlou E, et al. Localization of disinhibition-dementia-parkinsonism-amyotrophy complex to 17q21-22. Am J Hum Genet 1994; 55(6):1159–1165.
56. Foster NL, Wilhelmsen K, Sima AA, et al. Frontotemporal dementia and parkinsonism linked to chromosome 17: a consensus conference. Ann Neurol 1997; 41(6):706–715.
57. Hutton M, Lendon CL, Rizzu P, et al. Association of missense and 5′-splice-site mutations in tau with the inherited dementia FTDP-17. Nature 1998; 393(6686):702–705.
58. Poorkaj P, Bird TD, Wijsman E, et al. Tau is a candidate gene for chromosome 17 frontotemporal dementia. Ann Neurol 1998; 43(6):815–825.
59. Spillantini MG, Murrell JR, Goedert M, et al. Mutation in the tau gene in familial multiple system tauopathy with presenile dementia. Proc Natl Acad Sci USA 1998; 95(13): 7737–7741.
60. Rademakers R, Cruts M, Van Broeckhoven C. The role of tau (MAPT) in frontotemporal dementia and related tauopathies. Hum Mutat 2004; 24(4):277–295.
61. Nicholl DJ, Greenstone MA, Clarke CE, et al. An English kindred with a novel recessive tauopathy and respiratory failure. Ann Neurol 2003; 54(5):682–686.
62. Pastor P, Pastor E, Carnero C, et al. Familial atypical progressive supranuclear palsy associated with homozygosity for the delN296 mutation in the tau gene. Ann Neurol 2001; 49(2):263–267.
63. Poorkaj P, Muma NA, Zhukareva V, et al. An R5L tau mutation in a subject with a progressive supranuclear palsy phenotype. Ann Neurol 2002; 52(4):511–516.
64. Roks G, Dermaut B, Heutink P, et al. Mutation screening of the tau gene in patients with early-onset Alzheimer's disease. Neurosci Lett 1999; 277(2):137–139.
65. Houlden H, Baker M, Adamson J, et al. Frequency of tau mutations in three series of non-Alzheimer's degenerative dementia. Ann Neurol 1999; 46(2):243–248.
66. Oliveira SA, Scott WK, Zhang F, et al. Linkage disequilibrium and haplotype tagging polymorphisms in the Tau H1 haplotype. Neurogenetics 2004; 5(3):147–155.
67. D'Souza I, Schellenberg GD. Regulation of tau isoform expression and dementia. Biochim Biophys Acta 2005; 1739(2–3):104–115.
68. Krawczak M, Reiss J, Cooper DN. The mutational spectrum of single base-pair substitutions in mRNA splice junctions of human genes: causes and consequences. Hum Genet 1992; 90(1–2):41–54.
69. Nakai K, Sakamoto H. Construction of a novel database containing aberrant splicing mutations of mammalian genes. Gene 1994; 141(2):171–177.
70. Makrides V, Massie MR, Feinstein SC, et al. Evidence for two distinct binding sites for tau on microtubules. Proc Natl Acad Sci USA 2004; 101(17):6746–6751.
71. Dayanandan R, Van Slegtenhorst M, Mack TG, et al. Mutations in tau reduce its microtubule binding properties in intact cells and affect its phosphorylation. FEBS Lett 1999; 446(2–3):228–232.
72. Grover A, DeTure M, Yen SH, et al. Effects on splicing and protein function of three mutations in codon N296 of tau in vitro. Neurosci Lett 2002; 323(1):33–36.
73. Hasegawa M, Smith MJ, Goedert M. Tau proteins with FTDP-17 mutations have a reduced ability to promote microtubule assembly. FEBS Lett 1998; 437(3):207–210.
74. Hong M, Zhukareva V, Vogelsberg-Ragaglia V, et al. Mutation-specific functional impairments in distinct tau isoforms of hereditary FTDP-17. Science 1998; 282(5395): 1914–1917.
75. Krishnamurthy PK, Johnson GV. Mutant (R406W) human tau is hyperphosphorylated and does not efficiently bind microtubules in a neuronal cortical cell model. J Biol Chem 2004; 279(9):7893–7900.
76. Rizzu P, van Swieten JC, Joosse M, et al. High prevalence of mutations in the microtubule-associated protein tau in a population study of frontotemporal dementia in the Netherlands. Am J Hum Genet 1999; 64(2):414–421.

77. Vogelsberg-Ragaglia V, Bruce J, Richter-Landsberg C, et al. Distinct FTDP-17 missense mutations in tau produce tau aggregates and other pathological phenotypes in transfected CHO cells. Mol Biol Cell 2000; 11(12):4093–4104.
78. Yoshida H, Crowther RA, Goedert M. Functional effects of tau gene mutations deltaN296 and N296H. J Neurochem 2002; 80(3):548–551.
79. DeTure M, Ko LW, Yen S, et al. Missense tau mutations identified in FTDP-17 have a small effect on tau-microtubule interactions. Brain Res 2000; 853(1):5–14.
80. Hasegawa M, Smith MJ, Iijima M, et al. FTDP-17 mutations N279K and S305N in tau produce increased splicing of exon 10. FEBS Lett 1999; 443(2):93–96.
81. Pickering-Brown SM, Baker M, Nonaka T, et al. Frontotemporal dementia with Pick-type histology associated with Q336R mutation in the tau gene. Brain 2004; 127(6): 1415–1426.
82. Goedert M, Jakes R, Crowther RA. Effects of frontotemporal dementia FTDP-17 mutations on heparin-induced assembly of tau filaments. FEBS Lett 1999; 450(3):306–311.
83. Nacharaju P, Lewis J, Easson C, et al. Accelerated filament formation from tau protein with specific FTDP-17 missense mutations. FEBS Lett 1999; 447(2–3):195–199.
84. Alonso A, Mederlyova A, Novak M, et al. Promotion of hyperphosphorylation by frontotemporal dementia tau mutations. J Biol Chem 2004; 279(33):34873–34881.
85. Goedert M, Satumtira S, Jakes R, et al. Reduced binding of protein phosphatase 2A to tau protein with frontotemporal dementia and parkinsonism linked to chromosome 17 mutations. J Neurochem 2000; 75(5):2155–2162.
86. Goedert M. Neurofibrillary pathology of Alzheimer's disease and other tauopathies. Prog Brain Res 1998; 117287–117306.
87. Hutton M. Missense and splice site mutations in tau associated with FTDP-17: multiple pathogenic mechanisms. Neurology 2001; 56(11 Suppl 4):S21–S25.
88. Grover A, England E, Baker M, et al. A novel tau mutation in exon 9 (1260V) causes a four-repeat tauopathy. Exp Neurol 2003; 184(1):131–140.
89. Rizzini C, Goedert M, Hodges JR, et al. Tau gene mutation K257T causes a tauopathy similar to Pick's disease. J Neuropathol Exp Neurol 2000; 59(11):990–1001.
90. Reed LA, Wszolek ZK, Hutton M. Phenotypic correlations in FTDP-17. Neurobiol Aging 2001; 22(1):89–107.
91. Ingram EM, Spillantini MG Tau gene mutations: dissecting the pathogenesis of FTDP-17. Trends Mol Med 2002; 8(12):555–562.
92. Heutink P. Untangling tau-related dementia. Hum Mol Genet 2000; 9(6):979–986.
93. Bugiani O, Murrell JR, Giaccone G, et al. Frontotemporal dementia and corticobasal degeneration in a family with a P301S mutation in tau. J Neuropathol Exp Neurol 1999; 58(6):667–677.
94. Bugiani O. FTDP-17: phenotypical heterogeneity within P301S. Ann Neurol 2000; 48(1):126.
95. Arima K, Kowalska A, Hasegawa M, et al. Two brothers with frontotemporal dementia and parkinsonism with an N279K mutation of the tau gene. Neurology 2000; 54(9): 1787–1795.
96. Delisle MB, Murrell JR, Richardson R, et al. A mutation at codon 279 (N279K) in exon 10 of the Tau gene causes a tauopathy with dementia and supranuclear palsy. Acta Neuropathol (Berl) 1999; 98(1):62–77.
97. Soliveri P, Rossi G, Monza D, et al. A case of dementia parkinsonism resembling progressive supranuclear palsy due to mutation in the tau protein gene. Arch Neurol 2003; 60(10):1454–1456.
98. Tsuboi Y, Uitti RJ, Delisle MB, et al. Clinical features and disease haplotypes of individuals with the N279K tau gene mutation: a comparison of the pallidopontonigral degeneration kindred and a French family. Arch Neurol 2002; 59(6):943–950.
99. Woodruff BK, Baba Y, Hutton ML, et al. Haplotype-phenotype correlations in kindreds with the N279K mutation in the tau gene. Arch Neurol 2004; 61(8):1327.
100. Yasuda M, Kawamata T, Komure O, et al. A mutation in the microtubule-associated protein tau in pallido-nigro-luysian degeneration. Neurology 1999; 53(4):864–868.
101. Rossi G, Gasparoli E, Pasquali C, et al. Progressive supranuclear palsy and Parkinson's disease in a family with a new mutation in the tau gene. Ann Neurol 2004; 55(3):448.

102. Conrad C, Andreadis A, Trojanowski JQ, et al. Genetic evidence for the involvement of tau in progressive supranuclear palsy. Ann Neurol 1997; 41(2):277–281.
103. Litvan I, Hutton M. Clinical and genetic aspects of progressive supranuclear palsy. J Geriatr Psychiatry Neurol 1998; 11(2):107–114.
104. Spillantini MG, Yoshida H, Rizzini C, et al. A novel tau mutation (N296N) in familial dementia with swollen achromatic neurons and corticobasal inclusion bodies. Ann Neurol 2000; 48(6):939–943.
105. Bennett P, Bonifati V, Bonuccelli U, et al. Direct genetic evidence for involvement of tau in progressive supranuclear palsy. European Study Group on Atypical Parkinsonism Consortium. Neurology 1998; 51(4):982–985.
106. Higgins JJ, Litvan I, Pho LT, et al. Progressive supranuclear gaze palsy is in linkage disequilibrium with the tau and not the alpha-synuclein gene. Neurology 1998; 50(1): 270–273.
107. Morris HR, Janssen JC, Bandmann O, et al. The tau gene A0 polymorphism in progressive supranuclear palsy and related neurodegenerative diseases. J Neurol Neurosurg Psychiatry 1999; 66(5):665–667.
108. Oliva R, Tolosa E, Ezquerra M, et al. Significant changes in the tau A0 and A3 alleles in progressive supranuclear palsy and improved genotyping by silver detection. Arch Neurol 1998; 55(8):1122–1124.
109. Higgins JJ, Golbe LI, De Biase A, et al. An extended 5'-tau susceptibility haplotype in progressive supranuclear palsy. Neurology 2000; 55(9):1364–1367.
110. Di Maria E, Tabaton M, Vigo T, et al. Corticobasal degeneration shares a common genetic background with progressive supranuclear palsy. Ann Neurol 2000; 47(3):374–377.
111. Houlden H, Baker M, Morris HR, et al. Corticobasal degeneration and progressive supranuclear palsy share a common tau haplotype. Neurology 2001; 56(12):1702–1706.
112. Miserez AR, Clavaguera F, Monsch AU, et al. Argyrophilic grain disease: molecular genetic difference to other four-repeat tauopathies. Acta Neuropathol (Berl) 2003; 106(4):363–366.
113. Togo T, Sahara N, Yen SH, et al. Argyrophilic grain disease is a sporadic 4-repeat tauopathy. J Neuropathol Exp Neurol 2002; 61(6):547–556.
114. Russ C, Powell JF, Zhao J, et al. The microtubule associated protein tau gene and Alzheimer's disease—an association study and meta-analysis. Neurosci Lett 2001; 314(1–2):92–96.
115. Hughes A, Mann D, Pickering-Brown S. Tau haplotype frequency in frontotemporal lobar degeneration and amyotrophic lateral sclerosis. Exp Neurol 2003; 181(1):12–16.
116. Ingelson M, Fabre SF, Lilius L, et al. Increased risk for frontotemporal dementia through interaction between tau polymorphisms and apolipoprotein E epsilon4. Neuroreport 2001; 12(5):905–909.
117. Short RA, Graff-Radford NR, Adamson J, et al. Differences in tau and apolipoprotein E polymorphism frequencies in sporadic frontotemporal lobar degeneration syndromes. Arch Neurol 2002; 59(4):611–615.
118. Sobrido MJ, Miller BL, Havlioglu N, et al. Novel tau polymorphisms, tau haplotypes, and splicing in familial and sporadic frontotemporal dementia. Arch Neurol 2003; 60(5):698–702.
119. Verpillat P, Camuzat A, Hannequin D, et al. Association between the extended tau haplotype and frontotemporal dementia. Arch Neurol 2002; 59(6):935–939.
120. Sobrido MJ, Abu-Khalil A, Weintraub S, et al. Possible association of the tau H1/H1 genotype with primary progressive aphasia. Neurology 2003; 60(5):862–864.
121. Golbe LI, Lazzarini AM, Spychala JR, et al. The tau A0 allele in Parkinson's disease. Mov Disord 2001; 16(3):442–447.
122. Pastor P, Ezquerra M, Munoz E, et al. Significant association between the tau gene A0/A0 genotype and Parkinson's disease. Ann Neurol 2000; 47(2):242–245.
123. Hoenicka J, Perez M, Perez-Tur J, et al. The tau gene A0 allele and progressive supranuclear palsy. Neurology 1999; 53(6):1219–1225.
124. Scott WK, Nance MA, Watts RL, et al. Complete genomic screen in Parkinson disease: evidence for multiple genes. JAMA 2001; 286(18):2239–2244.
125. Zhang J, Song Y, Chen H, et al. The Tau Gene Haplotype H1 Confers a Susceptibility to Parkinson's Disease. Eur Neurol 2004; 53(1):15–21.

126. Farrer M, Skipper L, Berg M, et al. The tau H1 haplotype is associated with Parkinson's disease in the Norwegian population. Neurosci Lett 2002; 322(2):83–86.
127. Zappia M, Annesi G, Nicoletti G, et al. Association of tau gene polymorphism with Parkinson's disease. Neurol Sci 2003; 24(3):223–224.
128. Skipper L, Wilkes K, Toft M, et al. Linkage disequilibrium and association of MAPT H1 in Parkinson disease. Am J Hum Genet 2004; 75(4):669–677.
129. Kwok JB, Teber ET, Loy C, et al. Tau haplotypes regulate transcription and are associated with Parkinson's disease. Ann Neurol 2004; 55(3):329–334.
130. Fidani L, Kalinderi K, Bostant Jopoulou S, et al. Association of the tau haplotype with Parkinson's disease in the Greek population. Mov Disord 2006; 21(7):1036–1039.
131. Fung HC, Xiromerisiou G, Gibbs JR, et al. Association of tau haplotype-tagging polymorphisms with Parkinson's disease in diverse ethnic Parkinson's disease cohorts. Neurodegen Dis 2006; 3(6):327–333.
132. Mamah CE, Lesnick TG, Lincoln SJ, et al. Interaction of alpha-synuclein and tau genotypes in Parkinson's disease. Ann Neurol 2005; 57(3):439–443.
133. Chiba-Falek O, Touchman JW, Nussbaum RL. Functional analysis of intra-allelic variation at NACP-Rep1 in the alpha-synuclein gene. Hum Genet 2003; 113(5):426–431.

11 Genetic Risk Factors for Parkinson's Disease

Sofia A. Oliveira
Instituto Gulbenkian de Ciência, Oeiras, Portugal

Jeffery M. Vance
Division of Human Genetics, Center for Molecular Genetics and Genomic Medicine, Miami Institute for Human Genomics, University of Miami, Miami, Florida, U.S.A.

INTRODUCTION

Theories on the etiology of Parkinson disease (PD) have changed since its first description. In the famous James Parkinson monograph (1) that gave the disease its name, Parkinson reported that "affliction to indulge in spirituous liquors, another to long lying on the damp ground" were among the suggested causes of the disease. Yet by 1888, Gowers (2) reported that 15% of his patients had a family history. Indeed, today most investigators accept that PD is due to a mixture of genetic and environmental influences interacting with each other, where the relative role of each may change from individual to individual.

There are many reasons to explore the genetic component of PD. Certainly one of the first outcomes over the past 10 years is the realization that PD is not a single disease, but rather a phenotype. We understand now that many genes can contribute to the development of PD; that is, it is genetically heterogeneous. Perhaps 10% of PD is secondary to single-gene disorders like *PARKIN* and *LRRK2*, while the remainder of cases is believed to be multifactorial. Within this majority, many different genes appear to be important, some genes are more influential than others, and more than one is likely to influence the risk of any single individual to develop PD.

The presence of this genetic heterogeneity can provide conflicting and confusing data among research studies. For environmental investigations, genetic heterogeneity can mask the identification of an agent, as half of the patients may be susceptible, while the other half is not. Without the ability to separate these groups, the observer will see the total effect, which, in this example, would appear to be none at all. Thus, as the genetic causes of PD become elucidated and more homogenous groups can be studied, a clearer picture will be obtained of how each group responds to specific environmental agents. It should also begin to provide a basis for better decisions on pharmaceutical therapy, as different genetic groups of PD may differ in their response to therapies. But the most ambitious goal in understanding the genetics of PD is prevention. If one can predict with confidence those individuals susceptible to the disorder and the environmental interactions that promote that susceptibility, physicians may be able to prevent the disease from occurring at all.

GENETIC MECHANISMS

Until recent years, investigations in medical genetics have focused on single gene, or "Mendelian" disorders. Examples of these would be sickle cell anemia, cystic fibrosis, Charcot-Marie-Tooth disease or Duchenne muscular dystrophy. Here, the disease is caused by a single genetic change (which we refer to as a *mutation*) that leads to the dysfunction of the protein that the gene produces or controls. The change caused by a mutation is so severe that, by itself, it leads to disease. These disorders are inherited in a Mendelian fashion, that is, they follow the fundamental laws first proposed by Gregor Mendel, with identifiable inheritance patterns defined by basic genetic segregation (i.e., autosomal dominant, recessive, or X-linked). In PD, these Mendelian genes explain perhaps 10% of the clinical phenotype and are discussed elsewhere in this book.

However, most genetic variability does not severely affect the gene's function, and thus variations can accumulate in the population over time. Like name brands producing the same commercial product, these variations create some differences in the proteins made, but they all perform a basic threshold level of function required for normal life. We refer to these genetic changes as *polymorphisms*, and they are numerous, with single nucleotide polymorphisms (SNP) as frequent as every 600 to 700 bases. Given that the human genome is approximately 3.3 megabases, these variations number in the millions. Thus, a polymorphism may cause the product of the gene to function a bit slower, faster, or have no effect at all, or they may have no effect unless placed in a specific situation or exposed to an environmental agent. As an analogy, in bumper-to-bumper city traffic, whether you are driving a turbocharged or production model of a car doesn't make much difference in your ability to move. But put these cars, or "automobile polymorphisms," in a new environment, such as the German Autobahn, and their differences become obvious. The interaction of the various products and functions of these polymorphisms with each other, as well as with the environment, make each of us unique and contribute to most human diseases.

As polymorphisms (not mutations), these changes are not severe enough to cause a disease themselves. Rather, the variability differs in the disease predisposition that they confer to the individual. This potential to develop disease may require the concordant presence of certain polymorphisms found in other susceptibility genes, be masked by the presence of these other genes (epistasis), or need exposure to a specific environmental agent, perhaps even at a unique time in life. Thus identifying these genes is not a trivial matter. In recent years, with the increasing power of computers, the growth of molecular genetics, and now the completion of the human genome project, human geneticists have slowly begun to unravel these "susceptibility genes," which lead to the majority of human diseases.

LINKAGE AND ASSOCIATION

The difference between association and linkage analysis is often confusing to the nongeneticist. Linkage analysis detects a chromosomal "region" or physical location that travels with a disease significantly more than expected by chance, and thus is likely to harbor the disease susceptibility gene. Linkage analysis does not focus on what genes lie within the "linked region"; only the actual physical location of the chromosome traveling with the disease is important. This is why linkage analysis can detect linkage in different families with a disease, even if they have different mutations of the same gene. On the other hand, the goal of association analysis is to identify a particular DNA-sequence variant or form of a polymorphism that is found more commonly in patients than in unaffected individuals. Here the entire population is of interest, or a representative subset is evaluated.

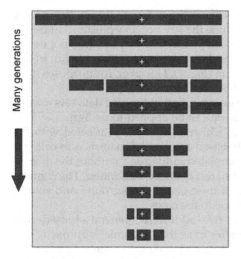

Many generations

FIGURE 1 Linkage disequilbrium. The *dark bar* represents high LD between polymorphisms across a region of DNA. The *star* represents the disease gene. As generations progress, the ends of the LD region are reduced by recombination. But the LD region is also broken up by mutation, represented by the small breaks in the dark bars of LD. Thus, after many generations LD is block-like, but is not necessarily continuous, shaped by both recombination and the rare process of mutation. *Abbreviation*: LD, linkage disequilbrium.

If human geneticists had to identify the exact susceptibility polymorphism associated with a disease at the start of the research, the task would be extremely difficult. However, we do not inherit each base separately from our parents, but we inherit patchwork quilts of small segments of each parental chromosome (Fig. 1). The size of these inherited blocks of chromosome differ among ethnicities, with Africans having the smallest blocks. That is because, as the ancestral race, they had more time to accumulate recombinations between genes, which is the main tool that breaks the chromosome into these blocks of DNA that travel together in time. In mapping human disease using allelic association, we refer to the process of the tight physical linkage of two specific forms (or alleles) of loci as *linkage disequilibrium* (LD). Why this term is used is beyond the scope of this chapter, but it reflects the lack of independent segregation of each polymorphism relative to its other LD block members. LD is generated when a susceptibility allele is first generated by a base pair change and, at that particular point in time, only exists on the single ancestral combination of alleles (haplotype) at polymorphic loci surrounding it (Fig. 1). As mentioned, this initial association due to physical linkage is gradually broken up over time, and the primary factor determining the rate of LD decay in a randomly mating population is the recombination frequency between the disease locus and the adjacent polymorphic loci. However, mutation also affects LD relationships, but is much less frequent in occurrence than recombination. LD is also strongly influenced by stochastic factors, which makes it difficult to predict the amount of LD as a function of physical distance alone. Commonly used statistical measures of LD in present-day chromosomes include D' and r^2, both of which are reviewed and comprehensively compared elsewhere (3). In a genetically homogeneous population, strong LD will only persist over many generations of chromosomes when marker and disease loci are so tightly linked that their alleles almost never recombine. Thus, any polymorphism lying in "tight" LD with the true susceptibility allele will appear as a coconspirator in association analysis. As it is traveling in time with the disease allele, it will also show association with the disease. If the most common size of LD "blocks" in Caucasians is 15 to 30 kb (4), and there is a SNP on average every 600 to 700 bp, then there are on average up to 50 SNPs lying in that same LD block that could show association with the disease. This is the conceptual idea behind the HAPMAP project (5), which seeks to determine the key polymorphisms that define each LD block in the human genome. It should be realized that LD does not necessarily always present in "blocks" of DNA, and that markers in high LD can in fact be separated by markers not in LD with them (Fig. 1). However, for purposes here, LD can be thought of as small blocks of DNA.

For LD mapping of complex disease genes, different types of data sets may be used. A family-based test of allelic association can be applied to pedigrees with at least two sampled first-degree relatives, of which at least one is affected with the disease of interest. An alternative to family-based association analysis is to collect a data set of unrelated patients (cases) and unrelated individuals without the disease of interest (controls) to perform a case-control test of allelic association. The controls need to be matched to the cases in terms of their genetic background and should represent the source population that gave rise to the cases.

To identify PD susceptibility genes, two additional, general study-design approaches have been used. The first we refer to as the "genomic" approach. This approach essentially starts with all known data and makes no assumptions on the actual biological mechanisms leading to the disease. It lets the data tell the investigator which avenues to pursue. This has been by far the most successful approach in both Mendelian and complex diseases, providing new mechanisms and genes leading to the disease. Examples of this approach are whole genome linkage analysis, whole genome association analysis and for expression analysis, serial analysis of gene expression (SAGE) (6). Their drawback is the requirement of a multidisciplinary research team, and they tend to be more expensive than the second approach, "candidate gene analysis." Here the investigator chooses the candidate genes for study, which implies some knowledge or hypothesis concerning the mechanism of disease. This approach had early successes, as obvious candidates were chosen for study of various diseases. However, given the choice of candidate genes and polymorphisms depends heavily on the presently limited understanding of the pathogenic mechanisms leading to PD, it is not surprising that candidate gene studies have had relatively few subsequent successes.

EVIDENCE FOR A GENETIC COMPONENT IN PARKINSON'S DISEASE

While familial aggregation of PD has been observed for many years (2), it has been widely debated whether it is due to genetic or environmental factors. One indication of genetic causality in a disorder is increased concordance rates in genetically identical [monozygotic (MZ)] twins compared to nonidentical [dizygotic (DZ)] twins. Early studies failed to detect differences in concordance rates and concluded that no major genetic factors for PD existed (7,8). Reappraisals of this evidence showed that these twin studies suffered from statistical imprecision due to small sample size and inadequate follow-up of the unaffected twin; thus genetic factors could neither be demonstrated nor ruled out (9,10).

In later studies, Tanner and colleagues (11) examined concordance rates in the NAS/NRC World War II Veteran Twins Registry. Screening 19,842 white male twins identified 193 twin pairs with at least one individual affected with PD. Overall there was no statistically significant difference in concordance rates in MZ twins (15.5%) compared to DZ twins (11.1%). However, when considering 16 pairs where one twin had onset of symptoms prior to age 50, concordance rates were significantly different (100% MZ vs. 16.7% DZ). The authors of the study interpreted their results as supporting a genetic etiology for early, but not late-onset PD. However, Langston (12) pointed out that an additional five to 10 years of follow-up will be necessary to ensure that the low concordance rates are not due to the inadequate follow-up, a problem also plaguing earlier twin studies of PD (9). This idea was supported by the study of Piccini et al. (13) who performed PET scans on twins in a large longitudinal study. They found that 75% of MZ twins were concordant for PET changes consistent with PD while only 25% of DZ twins both had PD changes.

The conflict of these studies with the now accepted importance of genetics in PD most likely reflects upon the initial application and design of twin studies. They have primarily been used for Mendelian diseases with high penetrance. A recent study in Swedish twins by Wirdefeldt et al. (14), again failed to find a strong genetic effect in MZ twins, and thus concluded that "genetic effects are of little importance in PD." However, as Lin and Simon (15,16) point out in a letter to the editor concerning the Wendefelt study, when it comes to susceptibility genes, twin studies are much less informative than when applied to Mendelian disorders. They demonstrate that a dominant mutation, occurring in 2.5% of the population, but with only a 10% penetrance, would fit Wirdefeldt et al. findings in the Swedish twins, and even account for half of all cases of PD. In response (15), Wirdefeldt agreed, restating their conclusions that "highly penetrant mutations do not play a substantial role in PD." The bottom line is that twin studies in PD and other complex diseases with late age-at-onset (AAO) caused primarily by susceptibility genes, are not necessarily appropriate research models and lead to conflict with other methods that have clearly defined a genetic importance in PD.

Another method to examine the importance of genetics on a trait is to identify patients with the disease and compare the recurrence rates in their relatives to the general population. This can be expressed as the risk ratio for sibs λ_s, and caculated using the recurrence rate in sibs divided by the general population prevalence (17,18). For geneticists, any value of $\lambda_s > 2$ suggests a significant genetic component exists in the disease. The higher the value of λ_s, the stronger the genetic effect, although these values are dependent on estimates of population prevalence. Estimates of λ_s for PD range from 2 to 13 (19,20). Thus relative risk studies support the presence of a genetic effect in PD.

Environmental Exposures

Conceptually, current ideas about PD would suggest potential environmental influences would be interacting with susceptibility genes, with some variations (polymorphisms) of the gene more susceptible than others to these environmental exposures. Classic examples of such gene-environment pairs are well known in pharmacogenetics, where interactions between P450 variations and drugs (21) have been well studied. However, no genes in PD have actually been described that clearly define such a gene-environment pair. There are many current reasons for this finding. As mentioned, without fully understanding the genetic heterogeneity in any randomly sampled group of PD patients, positive and negative effects of environmental influences on different members of the group will tend to cancel out. In addition, statistical methods to measure such interactions are just beginning to be worked out, and information on environmental effects is difficult to measure. For instance, while more studies than not find an influence of pesticides on the risk of PD, few individuals, other than professional agriculture workers, can remember the type or dose of their pesticide exposure. Although a few groups have been collecting both DNA and environmental data on patients, most investigators have not included it in their regular studies. However, as the different genetic causes of PD begin to be identified, the ability to place individuals in meaningful "response" groups will greatly accelerate these investigations.

That is not to say that potential environmental risk factors for PD have not been suggested. A universally accepted risk factor for PD is age, as both incidence and prevalence of the disease increase sharply after the age 60 (22). Interestingly, the other factor now accepted as inversely associated with PD is cigarette smoking. A recent meta-analysis of 48 published studies found a statistically significant "protective" effect of smoking, with a pooled estimate of 0.59 for the relative risk (23). A recent study from our group using family data, which greatly reduces many of the concerns in case-control data, also strongly supports an inverse association with risk for PD (24). Interestingly, the smoking association holds even when individuals have ceased smoking for many years. Two potential biologic mechanisms that have been discussed for this association (i) smoking decreases monoamine oxidase activity, which might be neuroprotective in PD; and (ii) nicotine might have a direct neuroprotective effect (25,26). Other environmental factors most frequently associated with PD are residential or occupational pesticide use and occupational exposure to heavy metals or chemicals. Farming occupations, living in a rural area, and drinking well water have all been associated with the risk of PD (27–29). It has been suggested that these exposures may be acting as surrogate measures for pesticide exposure (30–33).

GENOMIC LINKAGE
Screens for Risk of Parkinson's Disease
To date, four complete genomic screens of multiplex families (two or more sampled, affected family members) have been reported for PD (34–37). As with many other complex disorders, the results of these studies are not entirely consistent. However, there is substantial overlap of results in several regions, particularly those on chromosomes 5q (36–38), 6q (36,38), 9q (35,38), and 10q (35,36), suggesting that these regions may be the most promising for follow-up. The overlap on chromosome Xq is also very good in two studies (36,38). The relatively short distances between the peak markers across these independent studies provide evidence for linkage and support the existence of PD susceptibility loci on 5q, 6q, 9q, 10q, and Xq.

Follow-up studies from the Parkinson Study Group with increased sample sizes and/or more stringent definitions of PD (39) have strengthened their strongest initial findings on chromosomes 2q, 6q, and Xq (36). A meta-analysis of these linkages studies has not yet been performed mainly due to the difficulty of combining data from the different genetic markers that have been genotyped in different datasets.

Genomic Convergence
As discussed, the popular candidate-gene approach relies on selecting the right candidate gene(s) and polymorphism(s), a daunting task since the human genome harbors at least 25,000 to 30,000 genes and millions of polymorphisms. Conversely, genomic linkage studies in complex disorders like PD provide broad peaks of 25 to 30 million base pairs, again with many genes lying in the region. One approach to overcoming this numerical problem is "genomic convergence." Proposed by

Hauser et al. (40) for PD, it converges multiple geonomic sources of information to arrive at a high priority candidate.

The first convergence factor in this process is usually a whole-genome linkage screen that identifies areas of the genome that individuals affected by PD share more often than one would expect by chance. Microarray or profiling, the second convergence factor in this strategy, allows prioritizing the analysis of those genes that are significantly differentially expressed in the tissue of interest, in this case, the substantia nigra and surrounding region. Again, by itself, it produces too many changes to know which is useful. But the use of intersecting data derived from these two powerful resources present a small number of focused candidates that are high priority susceptibility genes. The third and last convergence factor is association studies on these converged genes.

As mentioned, unlike candidate gene analysis, genomic convergence has the advantage of being unbiased by preconceived models of disease. This approach has been applied to a number of genetic systems. The combination of quantitative expression analysis with genetic mapping has been used to analyze the murine NOD model of type 1 diabetes (41). Similar approaches have been used to identify complement factor 5 as a susceptibility locus for experimental allergic asthma (42). This strategy has already proven successful in the identification of the glutathione S-transferase omega-1/2 (*GSTO1/2*) as genes located in the chromosome 10q linkage region influencing the AAO in both PD and Alzheimer disease (AD) (43).

Genomic Modifiers, Age-at-Onset of Parkinson's Disease

Genes are not only involved in causing a disease; the genetic background surrounding the disease has a great influence on its phenotype as well. This is most easily seen in the well-known variations in phenotype caused by placing the same introduced mutation in different mouse backgrounds. "Modifying" genes have great potential importance. For one, it is likely that they are influential in more than one disorder, reflecting the limited number of mechanisms that the brain has available in dealing with stress. Second, they may provide excellent therapeutic targets, as slowing progression of PD or delaying its AAO for many years is clearly of great benefit to both the patient and society.

Three linkage screens for AAO genes affecting PD have thus far been performed (44–46) and reported different results. Interestingly, there are two overlaps between AAO and risk linkage peaks: The AAO linkage peak on chromosome 1p from Li et al. (44) almost exactly overlaps with the risk linkage peak (*PARK10*) in late-onset Icelandic PD families (47). Not as close but still interesting, the AAO and risk linkage peaks in chromosome 9q from the GenePD Study are only 16 cM apart (35,45). It is conceivable that a single gene is influencing both risk and AAO (Apolipoprotein E, for instance, is known to affect both risk and AAO of PD, see below) (48), but it is also possible that distinct susceptibility and AAO alleles exist at each one of these loci.

The recent study of *GSTO1/2* and AAO in PD and AD by our group demonstrated significant association for both disorders. The functions of *GSTO1* are not well understood (49). The Ala140Asp and Thr217Asn variants of *GSTO1* display reduced enzyme activity (50) and therefore might influence the susceptibility to oxidative stress. Recent data suggest that *GSTO1* may be involved in the post-translational modification of the inflammatory cytokine Interleukin-1b (51) and contribute to inflammation, which is provocative given reports of the possible role of inflammation in PD (52). Recently, our group (53) found that only 39/174 families showed both positive linkage on chromosome 10 and positive association of *GSTO1* with PD. In this set of families the average AAO difference between asparagine carriers and individuals homozygous for alanine at the *GSTO1* rs4925 polymorphism is 7.9 ± 4.78 years, much higher than 1.6 ± 7.17 observed in the overall dataset.

Since our report, four case-control studies (three small and one large) have been reported looking at *GSTO1* and AAO in AD. One found no AAO effect in Japanese (54), another no AAO effect in Caribbean hispanics (55), one no AAO effect in a large Caucasian sample (56) and another a mild effect on AAO at $p = 0.05$, but with the Asp allele with a later onset than the alanine allele (57). Interestingly, two of these studies, however, did find a significant association of *GSTO1/2* with risk for AD (55,58).

This data can be used to discuss various aspects of association studies, especially when trying to make sense of conflicting results. The first is the known genetic heterogeneity in complex diseases, which means that very large datasets are needed to be meaningful, especially in replication. If the results of Li et al. (53) are correct, and less than 25% of the families in the original report on the association of *GSTO1/2* with AAO were actually driving the association, then small sample sizes probably have very little chance of actually observing such an event. The study of Nishimura et al. (54) had only 172 affecteds, that of Kolsch et al. (57) 280 affecteds, although Ozturk et al. (56) had 990 cases. The first two studies are clearly too small in the face of genetic heterogeneity to provide much useful information in this case. Second, the difference in case-control and family based designs can complicate interpretation of analysis. As Ozturk et al. points out, the difference between the results of Li et al. and their own may be due to the difference in study design. The effect of modifying genes may be much easier to observe studying family data, with common genetic backgrounds. Indeed, we did not observe a *GSTO1/2* association in our case-control data. Third, what exactly is the relationship between risk and modifier genes, such as AAO? ApoE4 has been observed as having an effect on both risk and AAO in PD and AD. Clearly, in any given sampling of the population, if the presence of an allele moves the onset of the disease to an earlier age or more severe state, it is increasing the risk that those affected individuals will be observed in the sampled population, and thus seen as risk alleles. Perhaps the best example of this in PD is the *PARK10* locus. Hicks et al. (37) published a linkage study in Icelandic families that reported significant linkage for a risk locus for PD. Li et al. (44) reported a linkage peak for AAO with PD in the same region.

SUSCEPTIBILITY GENES
Overview
The foregoing examples highlight few of the problems inherent in association studies. Like early clinical trials, association studies will need to be held to a higher standard in the future. But they remain a powerful tool for looking at the disease genetics and will become an even major force in the future. There are many conflicting reports in the literature on many different loci. Therefore, we have tried to focus on those genes with the most consistent replicated reports.

Tau
Tau is a microtubule-associated protein that normally functions to promote assembly and stability of the microtubule. Mutations in tau are known to cause frontotemporal dementia with parkinsonism-17 (59). An intronic microsatellite

allele, A_0, was intially reported to be associated with PD by two groups (60,61). As the gene lies under the chromosome 17 peak of our genomic screen (34) we performed a family-based association study of SNP polymorphisms in the *tau* gene that detected association between the H1 haplotype (the common haplotype comprising 80% of the normal population) of tau and late-onset PD (62). Healy et al. (63) performed a meta-analysis of nine case-control studies plus their own and confirmed that the H1 haplotype was highly associated with PD ($p < 10^{-6}$).

However, Oliveira et al. (64) point out that the H1 haplotype is extremely large, encompassing 3.15 megabases and thus contains several genes including corticotropin-releasing hormone receptor 1, presenilin homolog 2, Saitohin and KIAA1267 along with Tau. They identified a subhaplotype of H1 found in 11% of the population (65) that appears to contain the association to PD ($p = 0.02$), but still spanned several loci. Thus, while Tau is known to bind to α-synuclein (66) and serves the most likely reason for this association, the genetic data at present cannot rule out other genes in the Tau haplotype as the causative factors.

α-Synuclein
Two meta-analyses in the Caucasian and Japanese populations support the association of a complex microsatellite in the α-synuclein promoter (NACP-Rep1) with susceptibility risk for PD (67,68). However, other SNPs in the α-synuclein promoter have not been associated with PD (69,70).

PARKIN
Association studies in the *PARKIN* gene have diverged widely in their conclusions. No meta-analysis has been published so far, but a large association study of the most commonly tested *PARKIN* SNPs (-258T>G, IVS2+25T>C, IVS3-20C>T, Ser167Asn, IVS7-35A>G, Val380Leu, and Asp394Asn) did not find any evidence for association with risk for PD (71).

Oliveira et al. reported a study of 16 families with *PARKIN* mutations, in which 10 *PARKIN* heterozygotes had PD and nine were unaffected (mean age at exam = 67.5 years), and suggested that heterozygotes for *PARKIN* mutations, particularly those that lie in exon 7, the first RING finger of the protein, are actually susceptibility alleles for late-onset PD. This was supported by the findings of Fouroud et al. (72) who found that in *PARKIN* families, 86% of individuals with AAO >60 years were heterozygotes. Recent functional studies also support this premise. Khan et al. (73) studied 13 unaffected first-degree relatives from eight unrelated PD *PARKIN* carriers and found a significant reduction in ^{18}F-dopa uptake in these heterozygotes relative to controls. Thus, there is mounting evidence that *PARKIN* heterozygotes are at increased risk for PD, although it still remains controversial. Interestingly, heterozygotes for *PINK1* and Gaucher carriers have also been suggested to be at risk for late-onset PD, suggesting a more general trend in these recessive forms of the disease.

Mitochondrial Genome (mtDNA)
Van der Walt et al. (74) reported that the J and K haplogroups were associated with decreased risk for PD, particularly in females (609 affected, 340 controls). While the JT haplogroup has been associated with increasing risk for PD in subsequent Irish and Finnish populations (75,76), these studies were much smaller in size (90 cases/129 controls and 238 cases/104 controls, respectively). Recently, a second large study, by Pyle et al. (77) (455 affected, 447 controls) supported van der Walt's findings with a

reduced risk for developing PD with the U, K, J, and T haplogroups. Looking at the raw data from van der Walt et al., these authors found the results of the two studies remarkably similar, and found the same p < 0.0001 for reduced risk of the U, K, J, and T haplogroups (1302 affected, 891 controls) as initially reported by van der Walt. While van der Walt suggested the causative SNP was the A10398G polymorphism, Pyle et al. suggest that other SNPs maybe causative, as this SNP has been found on other haplogroup backgrounds. Another small study looking at A10398G found it trending but not significant (78) (102 affected, 112 controls).

Inducible NOS

Under oxidative stress NOS reacts with superoxide anion to form toxic hydroxyl radicals. Inducible NOS is found in glial cells of the CNS and is induced in response to injury. Levecque et al. (79) and Hague et al. (80) both reported association of inducible NOS (iNOS) with PD in European and Finnish populations, respectively.

GENE-GENE AND GENE-ENVIRONMENT INTERACTIONS

One reason for the inconsistencies in studies of genetic and environmental factors in PD, may be that these tests are often conducted looking at a single factor at a time. Tests that consider interactions among genes or among genes and environmental factors can be critical to unraveling the complex etiology of PD. The idea that gene-gene and gene-environment interactions play an important role in human biology is not new. Wright (81) in 1932 emphasized that the relationship between genotype and phenotype is dependent on dynamic interactive networks of genes and environmental factors. This idea holds true today. Gibson (82) stresses that gene-gene and gene-environment interactions must be ubiquitous given the complexities of intermolecular interactions that are necessary to regulate gene expression and the hierarchical complexity of metabolic networks. The identification and characterization of common complex disease susceptibility genes remains one of the great challenges human geneticists face. A recent example of gene-environment interaction in PD is found in a recent study of MAO-B and smoking in PD (83). Consideration of the two factors together indicated that only in carriers of the "G" allele of a polymorphism in intron 13 was smoking protective; the opposite effect was found in the carriers of the "A" allele. Whether this holds true in other studies of MAO-B has to be seen.

The challenge in detecting and characterizing gene-gene and gene-environment interactions is partly due to the limitations of parametric statistical methods for detecting gene effects that are dependent solely or partially on interactions with other genes (84) and environmental exposures (85). To address these issues, the multifactor dimensionality reduction method has been developed (86). Studies in hypertension, coronary heart disease and breast cancer have used dimensionality reduction methods to detect interactions between candidate genes (86–88). These studies demonstrated significant interactions even though there were no significant main effects for the genes involved. These approaches should be useful in PD as well.

CONCLUSION

Understanding the role of genetics and environment in PD is crucial to future advances in research and therapy. In-depth evaluation of genetic factors will not only unravel complex inheritance patterns but will also enable a better understanding of the environmental risks, and hopefully, one day be used in preventing the disease.

REFERENCES

1. Parkinson J. An Essay on the Shaking Palsy. London: Notingham and Rowland, 1817.
2. Gowers WR. A Manual of Diseases of the Nervous System. P. Blakiston, Philadelphia, PA: Son & Co., 1888.
3. Haines JL, Pericak-Vance MA. Approaches to Gene Mapping in Complex Human Diseases, Vol. 1. New York: Wiley & Sons, Inc., 1998:1–12.
4. Costas J, Salas A, Phillips C, et al. Human genome-wide screen of haplotype-like blocks of reduced diversity. Gene 2005; 349:219–225.
5. Gibbs RA. The International HapMap Consortium. The International HapMap Project. Nature 2003; 426(6968):789–796.
6. Velculescu VE, Zhang L, Vogelstein B, et al. Serial analysis of gene expression. Science 1995; 270:484–487.
7. Duvoisin RC, Eldridge R, Williams A, et al. Twin study of Parkinson disease. Neurology 1981; 31:77–80.
8. Ward CD, Duvoisin RC, Ince SE, et al. Parkinson's disease in 65 pairs of twins and in a set of quadruplets. Neurology 1983; 33:815–824.
9. Johnson WG, Hodge SE, Duvoisin RC. Twin studies and the genetics of Parkinson's Disease—a reappraisal. Mov Disord 1990; 5(3):187–194.
10. Vieregge P, Schiffke KA, Friedrich HJ, et al. Parkinson's disease in twins. Neurology 1992; 421453–421461.
11. Tanner CM, Ottman R, Goldman SM, et al. Parkinson disease in twins: an etiologic study. JAMA 1999; 281(4):341–346.
12. Langston JW. Epidemiology versus genetics in Parkinson's disease: progress in resolving an age-old debate. Ann Neurol 1998; 44(3 suppl 1):S45–S52.
13. Piccini P, Burn DJ, Ceravolo R, et al. The role of inheritance in sporadic Parkinson's disease: evidence from a longitudinal study of dopaminergic function in twins. Ann Neurol 1999; 45(5):577–582.
14. Wirdefeldt K, Gatz M, Schalling M, et al. No evidence for heritability of Parkinson disease in Swedish twins. Neurology 2004; 63(2):305–311.
15. Lin MT, Simon DK. No evidence for heritability of Parkinson disease in Swedish twins. Neurology 2005; 64(5):932.
16. Simon DK, Lin MT, Pascual-Leone A. "Nature versus nurture" and incompletely penetrant mutations. J Neurol Neurosurg Psychiatry 2002; 72(6):686–689.
17. Risch N. Linkage strategies for genetically complex traits. I. Multilocus models. Am J Hum Genet 1990; 46(2):222–228.
18. Risch N. Linkage strategies for genetically complex traits. II. The power of affected relative pairs. Am J Hum Genet 1990; 46(2):229–241.
19. Sveinbjornsdottir S, Hicks AA, Jonsson T, et al. Familial aggregation of Parkinson's disease in Iceland. N Engl J Med 2000; 343:1765–1770.
20. Marder K, Tang MX, Mejia H, et al. Risk of Parkinson's disease among first-degree relatives: a community-based study. Neurology 1996; 47(1):155–160.
21. Wilkinson GR. Drug metabolism and variability among patients in drug response. N Engl J Med 2005; 352(21):2211–2221.
22. Tanner CM, Goldman SM. Epidemiology of Parkinson's disease. Neurol Clin 1996; 14(2):317–335.
23. Hernan MA, Takkouche B, Caamano-Isorna F, et al. A meta-analysis of coffee drinking, cigarette smoking, and the risk of Parkinson's disease. Ann Neurol 2002; 52(3):276–284.
24. Scott WK, Zhang F, Stajich JM, et al. Family-based case-control study of cigarette smoking and Parkinson disease. Neurology 2005; 64(3):442–447.
25. Tanner CM, Goldman SM, Aston DA, et al. Smoking and Parkinson's disease in twins. Neurology 2002; 58(4):581–588.

26. Castagnoli K, Murugesan T. Tobacco leaf, smoke and smoking, MAO inhibitors, Parkinson's disease and neuroprotection; are there links? Neurotoxicology 2004; 25(1–2):279–291.
27. Morano A, Jiménez-Jiménez F, Molina JA, et al. Risk-factors for Parkinson's disease: case-control study in the province of Cáceres, Spain. Acta Neurol Scand 1994; 89(164):170.
28. Marder K, Logroscino G, Alfaro B, et al. Environmental risk factors for Parkinson's disease in an urban multiethnic community. Neurology 1998; 50(1):279–281.
29. Petrovitch H, Ross GW, Abbott RD, et al. Plantation work and risk of Parkinson disease in a population-based longitudinal study. Arch Neurol 2002; 59(11):1787–1792.
30. Hubble JP, Cao T, Hassanein RE, et al. Risk factors for Parkinson's disease. Neurology 1993; 43(9):1693–1697.
31. Semchuk KM, Love EJ, Lee RG. Parkinson's disease: a test of the multifactorial etiologic hypothesis. Neurology 1993; 43(6):1173–1180.
32. Liou HH, Tsai MC, Chen CJ, et al. Environmental risk factors and Parkinson's disease: a case-control study in Taiwan. Neurology 1997; 48(6):1583–1588.
33. Gorell JM, Johnson CC, Rybicki BA, et al. The risk of Parkinson's disease with exposure to pesticides, farming, well water, and rural living. Neurology 1998; 50(5):1346–1350.
34. Scott WK, Nance MA, Watts RL, et al. Complete genomic screen in Parkinson disease: evidence for multiple genes. JAMA 2001; 286(18):2239–2244.
35. Destefano AL, Golbe LI, Mark MH, et al. Genome-wide scan for Parkinson's disease: the GenePD Study. Neurology 2001; 57(6):1124–1126.
36. Pankratz N, Nichols WC, Uniacke SK, et al. Genome screen to identify susceptibility genes for Parkinson disease in a sample without parkin mutations. Am J Hum Genet 2002; 71(1):124–135.
37. Hicks AA, Petursson H, Jonsson T, et al. A susceptibility gene for late-onset idiopathic Parkinson's disease. Ann Neurol 2002; 52(5):549–555.
38. Scott WK, Stajich JM, Scott BL, et al. Complete genomic screen in familial Parkinson disease. European Journal of Human Genetics 2001; 9:346.
39. Pankratz N, Nichols WC, Uniacke SK, et al. Genome-wide linkage analysis and evidence of gene-by-gene interactions in a sample of 362 multiplex Parkinson disease families. Hum Mol Genet 2003; 12(20):2599–2608.
40. Hauser MA, Li YJ, Takeuchi S, et al. Genomic convergence: identifying candidate genes for Parkinson's disease by combining serial analysis of gene expression and genetic linkage. Hum Mol Genet 2003; 12(6):671–677.
41. Eaves IA, Wicker LS, Ghandour G, et al. Combining mouse congenic strains and microarray gene expression analyses to study a complex trait: the NOD model of type 1 diabetes. Genome Res 2002; 12(2):232–243.
42. Karp CL, Grupe A, Schadt E, et al. Identification of complement factor 5 as a susceptibility locus for experimental allergic asthma. Nat Immunol 2000; 1(3):221–226.
43. Li YJ, Oliveira SA, Xu P, et al. Glutathione S-transferase omega-1 modifies age-at-onset of Alzheimer disease and Parkinson disease. Hum Mol Genet 2003; 12(24):3259–3267.
44. Li YJ, Scott WK, Hedges DJ, et al. Age at onset in two common neurodegenerative diseases is genetically controlled. Am J Hum Genet 2002; 70(4):985–993.
45. Destefano AL, Lew MF, Golbe LI, et al. PARK3 influences age at onset in Parkinson disease:a genome scan in the GenePD study. Am J Hum Genet 2002; 70(5):1089–1095.
46. Pankratz N, Uniacke SK, Halter CA, et al. Genes influencing Parkinson disease onset: replication of PARK3 and identification of novel loci. Neurology 2004; 62(9):1616–1618.
47. Westerman AM, Entius MM, Boor PPC, et al. Novel mutations in the LKB1/STK11 gene in Dutch Peutz-Jeghers families. Hum Mutat 1999; 13(6):476–481.
48. Li YJ, Hauser MA, Scott WK, et al. Apolipoprotein E controls the risk and age at onset of Parkinson disease. Neurology 2004; 62(11):2005–2009.
49. Board PG, Coggan M, Chelvanayagam G, et al. Identification, characterization, and crystal structure of the Omega class glutathione transferases. J Biol Chem 2000; 275(32):24798–24806.
50. Tanaka-Kagawa T, Jinno H, Hasegawa T, et al. Functional characterization of two variant human GSTO 1-1s (Ala140Asp and Thr217Asn). Biochem Biophys Res Commun 2003; 301(2):516–520.
51. Laliberte RE, Perregaux DG, Hoth LR, et al. Glutathione s-transferase omega 1-1 is a target of cytokine release inhibitory drugs and may be responsible for their effect on interleukin-1beta posttranslational processing. J Biol Chem 2003; 278(19):16567–16578.

52. McGeer PL, McGeer EG. Inflammation and the degenerative diseases of aging. Ann NY Acad Sci 2004; 1035:104–116.
53. Li Y-J, Scott WK, Zhang L, et al. Revealing the role of glutathione S-transferase Omega in age at onset of Alzheimer and Parkinson diseases. Neurobiol Aging 2006; 27(8): 1087–1093.
54. Nishimura M, Sakamoto T, Kaji R, et al. Influence of polymorphisms in the genes for cytokines and glutathione S-transferase omega on sporadic Alzheimer's disease. Neurosci Lett 2004; 368(2):140–143.
55. Lee JH, Mayeux R, Mayo D, et al. Fine mapping of 10q and 18q for familial Alzheimer's disease in Caribbean Hispanics. Mol Psychiatry 2004; 9(11):1042–1051.
56. Ozturk A, Desai PP, Minster RL, et al. Three SNPs in the GSTO1, GSTO2 and PRSS11 genes on chromosome 10 are not associated with age-at-onset of Alzheimer's disease. Neurobiol Aging 2005; 26(8):1161–1165.
57. Kolsch H, Linnebank M, Lutjohann D, et al. Polymorphisms in glutathione S-transferase omega-1 and AD, vascular dementia, and stroke. Neurology 2004; 63(12):2255–2260.
58. Michielsen PP, Francque SM, van Dongen JL. Viral hepatitis and hepatocellular carcinoma. World J Surg Oncol 2005; 3(1):27.
59. Hutton M, Lendon CL, Rizzu P, et al. Association of missense and 5'-splice-site mutations in tau with the inherited dementia FTDP-17. Nature 1998; 393(6686):702–705.
60. Pastor P, Ezquerra M, Munoz E, et al. Significant association between the tau gene A0/A0 genotype and Parkinson's disease. Neurology 2000; 47(2):242–245.
61. Golbe LI, Lazzarini AM, Spychala JR, et al. The tau A0 allele in Parkinson's disease. Mov Disord 2001; 16(3):442–447.
62. Martin ER, Scott WK, Nance MA, et al. Association of single-nucleotide polymorphisms of the tau gene with late-onset Parkinson disease. JAMA 2001; 286(18):2245–2250.
63. Healy DG, Abou-Sleiman PM, Lees AJ, et al. Tau gene and Parkinson's disease: a case-control study and meta-analysis. J Neurol Neurosurg Psychiatry 2004; 75(7):962–965.
64. Oliveira SA, Scott WK, Zhang F, et al. Linkage disequilibrium and haplotype tagging polymorphisms in the Tau H1 haplotype. Neurogenetics 2004; 5(3):147–155.
65. Koyama H, Raines EW, Bornfeldt KE, et al. Fibrillar collagen inhibits arterial smooth muscle proliferation through regulation of Cdk2 inhibitors. Cell 1996; 87(6):1069–1078.
66. Benussi L, Ghidoni R, Paterlini A, et al. Interaction between tau and alpha-synuclein proteins is impaired in the presence of P301L tau mutation. Exp Cell Res 2005; 308(1): 78–84.
67. Mizuta I, Nishimura M, Mizuta E, et al. Meta-analysis of alpha synuclein/NACP polymorphism in Parkinson's disease in Japan. J Neurol Neurosurg Psychiatry 2002; 73(3):350.
68. Mellick GD, Maraganore DM, Silburn PA. Australian data and meta-analysis lend support for alpha-synuclein (NACP-Rep1) as a risk factor for Parkinson's disease. Neurosci Lett 2005; 375(2):112–116.
69. Pastor P, Munoz E, Ezquerra M, et al. Analysis of the coding and the 5' flanking regions of the alpha-synuclein gene in patients with Parkinson's disease. Mov Disord 2001; 16(6):1115–1119.
70. Holzmann C, Kruger R, Saecker AM, et al. Polymorphisms of the alpha-synuclein promoter: expression analyses and association studies in Parkinson's disease. J Neural Transm 2003; 110(1):67–76.
71. Oliveira SA, Scott WK, Martin ER, et al. Parkin mutations and susceptibility alleles in late-onset Parkinson's disease. Ann Neurol 2003; 53(5):624–629.
72. Foroud T, Uniacke SK, Liu L, et al. Heterozygosity for a mutation in the parkin gene leads to later onset Parkinson disease. Neurology 2003; 60(5):796–801.
73. Khan NL, Scherfler C, Graham E, et al. Dopaminergic dysfunction in unrelated, asymptomatic carriers of a single parkin mutation. Neurology 2005; 64(1):134–136.
74. van der Walt JM, Nicodemus KK, Martin ER, et al. Mitochondrial polymorphisms significantly reduce the risk of Parkinson disease. Am J Hum Genet 2003; 72(4):804–811.
75. Ross OA, McCormack R, Curran MD, et al. Mitochondrial DNA polymorphism: its role in longevity of the Irish population. Exp Gerontol 2001; 36(7):1161–1178.
76. Autere JM, Hiltunen MJ, Mannermaa AJ, et al. Molecular genetic analysis of the alpha-synuclein and the parkin gene in Parkinson's disease in Finland. Eur J Neurol 2002; 9(5):479–483.

77. Pyle A, Foltynie T, Tiangyou W, et al. Mitochondrial DNA haplogroup cluster UKJT reduces the risk of PD. Ann Neurol 2005; 57(4):564–567.
78. Otaegui D, Paisan C, Saenz A, et al. Mitochondrial polymporphisms in Parkinson's Disease. Neurosci Lett 2004; 370(2–3):171–174.
79. Levecque C, Elbaz A, Clavel J, et al. Association between Parkinson's disease and poly-morphisms in the nNOS and iNOS genes in a community-based case-control study. Hum Mol Genet 2003; 12(1):79–86.
80. Hague S, Peuralinna T, Eerola J, et al. Confirmation of the protective effect of iNOS in an independent cohort of Parkinson disease. Neurology 2004; 62(4):635–636.
81. Wright S. The roles of mutation, inbreeding, crossbreeding, and selection in evolution. Proceedings of the 6th International Congress of Genetics 1932; 1:356–366.
82. Gibson G. Epistasis and pleiotropy as natural properties of transcriptional regulation. Theor Popul Biol 1996; 49(1):58–59.
83. Checkoway H, Franklin GM, Costa-Mallen P, et al. A genetic polymorphism of MAO-B modifies the association of cigarette smoking and Parkinson's disease. Neurology 1998; 50(5):1458–1461.
84. Templeton AR. Epistasis and complex traits. In: Wade M, Brodie N, Wolf J, eds. Epistasis and the Evolutionary Process. Oxford University Press, 2000:41–57.
85. Schlichting CD, Pigliucci M. Phenotypic evolution: A reaction norm perspective. Sinauer Associates, Inc., 1998.
86. Ritchie MD, Hahn LW, Roodi N, et al. Multifactor-dimensionality reduction reveals high-order interactions among estrogen-metabolism genes in sporadic breast cancer. Am J Hum Genet 2001; 69(1):138–147.
87. Williams RR, Hunt SC, Heiss G, et al. Usefulness of cardiovascular family history data for population-based preventive medicine and medical research (the Health Family Tree Study and the NHLBI Family Heart Study). Am J Cardiol 2001; 87(2):129–135.
88. Nelson MR, Kardia SLR, Ferrell RE, et al. A combinatorial partitioning method (CPM) to identify multi-locus genotypic partitions that predict quantitative trait variation. Genome Res 2001; 11:458–470.

Section III: Pathogenesis

12 α-Synuclein and Parkinson's Disease

James H. Soper, John Q. Trojanowski, and Virginia M.-Y. Lee
*Center for Neurodegenerative Disease Research, Department of Pathology and
Laboratory Medicine, Institute on Aging, University of Pennsylvania,
Philadelphia, Pennsylvania, U.S.A.*

INTRODUCTION

The synaptic protein, α-synuclein, has been associated with several neurodegenerative diseases known as α-synucleinopathies. Thus, elucidation of mechanisms leading to α-synuclein abnormalities is particularly important for understanding the
pathogenesis of Parkinson's disease (PD) and related α-synucleinopathies. Many
studies, in both cell culture models and animal models, have linked α-synuclein to
the pathogenesis of PD. In this review, we critically review data linking α-synuclein
to neurodegeneration in PD. We review several of the neurodegenerative diseases
that are linked to accumulations of α-synuclein pathologies, the structure and
proposed functions of the α-synuclein protein, and several theories concerning
α-synuclein toxicity and degradation.

α-SYNUCLEINOPATHIES

α-Synucleinopathies are a group of neurodegenerative disorders that are characterized by cytoplasmic inclusions of insoluble, filamentous α-synuclein proteins
(Fig. 1). The relationship between these different disorders is unclear; however,
the brain regions affected by α-synuclein inclusions in these neurodegenerative
diseases are directly related to their clinical manifestations.

PD is the most common neurodegenerative movement disorder, and its hallmark clinical features are bradykinesia, rigidity, tremor, and postural instability.
While it is characterized neuropathologically by the presence of cytoplasmic inclusions containing filamentous α-synuclein (1), known as Lewy bodies, in the
substantia nigra, as well as a profound loss of substantia nigral neurons and gliosis.
In addition to the substantia nigra, Lewy bodies are found in many brain regions
including the brainstem, basal forebrain, and cortex. Filamentous aggregates of
α-synuclein are also found in neuronal processes, and these inclusions are known as
Lewy neurites (2). To date, three mutations in the α-synuclein gene that are inherited in an autosomal dominant manner have been linked to familial forms of PD.
Indeed, the recognition that α-synuclein is the building block of Lewy bodies was
due to the identification in 1997 of the A53T α-synuclein gene mutation in several
Italian and Greek families with familial PD. The clinical phenotype of this autosomal disorder was similar to idiopathic PD and included the presence of Lewy
bodies. However, the individuals in these families affected with the disorder had an
earlier age of onset than individuals with idiopathic PD (3). Two other α-synuclein
missense mutations have been found that also are linked to familial PD, including
the *A30P* (4), and *E46K* mutations (5), while more recently duplications of the

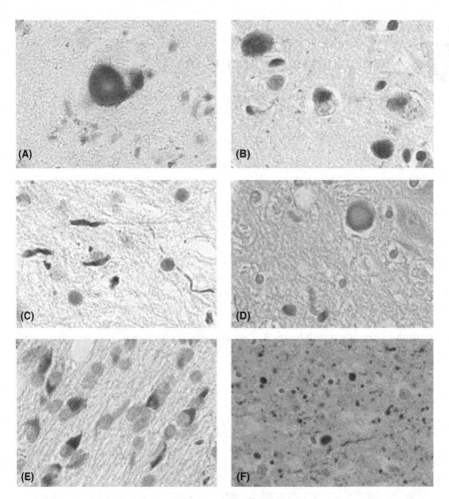

FIGURE 1 α-Synuclein inclusions in several α-synucleinopathies. (**A**) Lewy bodies from the sub-stantia nigra of a Parkinson's disease patient. (**B**) Lewy bodies from the cortex of a DLB patient. (**C**) Lewy neurite pathology from the substantia nigra of a DLB patient. (**D**) Lewy bodies from the sub-stantia nigra of a patient with early-onset Parkinson's disease due to the *A53T* α-synuclein mutation. (**E**) Glial cytoplasmic inclusions in the pons of a patient with multiple system atrophy. (**F**) α-Synuclein pathology from the putamen of a patient with neurodegeneration with brain iron accumulation, type1. *Abbreviation*: DLB, dementia with Lewy bodies. *Source*: From Ref. 140.

α-synuclein gene have also been found to be pathogenic for neurodegenerative disease (4). The discovery of these α-synuclein gene mutations led to the identifica-tion of α-synuclein as a critical component in the pathogenesis of PD and several other neurodegenerative disorders.

Dementia with Lewy bodies (DLB) is a dementia characterized pathologically by cortical Lewy bodies and Lewy neurites. DLB is clinically characterized by dementia, hallucinations, bradykinesia, and rigidity (2,6). Another type of dementia with α-synuclein inclusions is known as Lewy body variant of Alzheimer's disease (LBVAD), due to the presence of Lewy bodies in association with the signature lesions of Alzheimer's disease (AD), i.e., senile plaques formed by Aβ fibrils and neurofibrillary tangles composed of abnormal tau filaments (2). The clinical characteristics of LBVAD are similar to DLB, with progressive cognitive defects and extrapyramidal symptoms (7). These two disorders present an interesting overlap between the symptoms and neuropathological features of PD and AD, and suggest that there may be an interaction between the underlying mechanisms for the pathogenesis of these different disorders.

α-Synuclein has also been implicated in diseases affecting glial cells. α-Synuclein has been identified as a major component of glial cytoplasmic inclusions (GCIs) found in oligodendrocytes in multiple system atrophy (MSA), which is characterized clinically by parkinsonism, cognitive defects, and cerebellar symptoms. In MSA, GCIs are found in oligodendrocytes throughout the white matter and to a lesser extent gray matter of neocortex, cerebellum, brainstem, hippocampus, and spinal cord (2,8). GCIs and Lewy bodies are present in another rare disorder known as neurodegeneration with brain iron accumulation type 1 (NBIA-1), which is clinically characterized by parkinsonism, cognitive impairment, cerebellar ataxia, and bulbar symptoms (9).

The presence of α-synuclein inclusions in all of these neurodegenerative disorders strongly implicates fibrillar aggregates of α-synuclein as causative agents of the selective degeneration of the central nervous system in these diseases. Furthermore, the presence of α-synuclein inclusions in affected brain regions suggests that inclusion formation may be a pathogenic process. To understand the process of α-synuclein inclusion formation, it is important to understand the structure and function of α-synuclein.

THE SYNUCLEIN PROTEIN FAMILY
Structure

α-Synuclein is a small, synaptically localized protein that is expressed most abundantly in neurons (10,11). α-Synuclein, which has been mapped to chromosome 4q21 (12), is the major component of pathological inclusions in PD and other α-synucleinopathies (1,13), and mutations in α-synuclein (*A53T, A30P,* and *E46K*) or duplications of this gene have been linked to familial forms of PD and DLB (3–5,14). Studies of the toxicity and pathogenesis of α-synuclein have focused on the polymerization of the protein into filamentous aggregates similar to those seen in the brains of patients with PD, DLB, MSA, and related disorders (15).

α-Synuclein was originally identified when it was purified from the electric organ of *Torpedo californica* in a screen for synaptic proteins (16). α-Synuclein is 140 amino acids long and consists of an amino-terminal region containing several KTKEGV repeat sequences (16–18), a hydrophobic central region known as the non-amyloid component or NAC (18,19), and a negatively charged acidic C-terminal region (20).

At low concentrations, α-synuclein assumes a random-coil, unfolded conformation (18,21). However, the N-terminal region is similar to the lipid-binding domain of exchangeable apolipoproteins (17,22), suggesting that α-synuclein may be involved in membrane interaction. Indeed, α-synuclein can interact with small vesicles containing acidic phospholipids, and this interaction is accompanied by a shift from random coil to α-helical structure (23). Disrupting the predicted α-helices by introducing charged residues inhibits the lipid association of α-synuclein, supporting the idea that α-synuclein undergoes a conformational change in order to interact with acidic phospholipids. The disease-causing α-synuclein mutation,

A53T, appears to have no significant effect on lipid binding (24,25), while the *A30P* mutation disrupts the ability of α-synuclein to interact with lipids (24). The most recently identified mutation, *E46K*, enhances the ability of α-synuclein to bind lipids (25).

The central region of α-synuclein (residues 61–95), known as the NAC region, was originally purified from AD brains using methods to isolate Aβ amyloid plaque components (19); however, since subsequent studies showed that α-synuclein is not a prominent component of senile plaques (26), the presence of α-synuclein was most likely due to Lewy body contamination of these preparations. The NAC region of α-synuclein is hydrophobic, and a smaller portion of this region (amino acids 71–82) is necessary for the assembly of α-synuclein into fibrils (27). This central peptide region has the ability to form fibrils and β-pleated sheet structure by itself, suggesting that this region is responsible for the fibrillization of α-synuclein (27).

The C-terminus of α-synuclein is an acidic, hydrophilic series of amino acids with an abundance of glutamate residues (17). The acidic C-terminal region of α-synuclein appears to have an inhibitory effect on α-synuclein fibril formation.

Two other members of the synuclein family, β-synuclein and γ-synuclein, have been identified (28,29). β-Synuclein, which has been mapped to chromosome 5q35 (30), is highly homologous to α-synuclein, except that it lacks a large portion of the central NAC domain (10). β-Synuclein is not found in filamentous inclusions of PD or other α-synucleinopathies (31), and it does not form fibrils in vitro, as is expected due to its lack of the essential NAC domain (32), although specific nucleotide substitutions in the β-synuclein gene have been linked to familial DLB in some kindreds (33). γ-Synuclein maps to chromosome 10q23 and has less homology to α-synuclein than β-synuclein (34,35). Like β-synuclein, γ-synuclein is not found in filamentous inclusions in PD (31). γ-Synuclein can form fibrils in vitro, however, the rate of fibril formation is much slower than α-synuclein (32).

Function

α-Synuclein is expressed throughout the brain, with high levels in the olfactory bulb, cerebral cortex, striatum, hippocampus, and at lower levels in the thalamus (11). α-Synuclein is quite abundant in the brain, and has been estimated to be as much as 1% of total soluble brain protein (11). α-Synuclein is also expressed in other cell types, such as platelets (36) and neurons of the cardiac plexus (37). β-Synuclein is expressed throughout the brain at high levels, and at low levels in the peripheral nervous system and skeletal muscle (10,38). γ-Synuclein is also expressed at high levels in the brain, particularly the brainstem (39), at moderate levels in the heart and skeletal muscle, and at low levels in the peripheral nervous system, pancreas, kidneys, and lungs (38). γ-Synuclein is also highly up regulated in advanced infiltrating breast cancer tissue, indicating that it may play a role in late-stage cancer progression (40).

α-Synuclein was originally characterized as both a nuclear and synaptic protein (16); subsequent studies with more specific antibodies revealed that both α- and β-synuclein are primarily localized to synaptic terminals (10,11). α-Synuclein behaves similarly to a weak, vesicle-associated protein during biochemical fractionation experiments; however, α-synuclein is not present in purified synaptic vesicle preparations (17). Electron microscopy of rat brains, reveals that α-synuclein is associated with, or in close proximity to, synaptic vesicles. γ-Synuclein, in contrast to α- and β-synuclein, does not appear to be specifically localized to synaptic terminals. γ-Synuclein is cytosolic and present in cell bodies, processes, and growth cones of cultured dorsal root ganglia neurons, and is present in cell bodies and axons of sensory neurons (39).

Developmentally, α-synuclein is first expressed between 15 and 17 weeks gestational age, with initial localization to the cell body and processes, which shifts to an exclusively synaptic localization by week 18 of gestation (41). The absence of initial α-synuclein expression and the viability of α-synuclein knockout mice (42) indicate that α-synuclein is not essential for synaptic development or survival.

The normal function of α-synuclein is currently unknown. α-Synuclein knockout mice are healthy and fertile and have normal brain anatomy. However, these mice display an increased release of dopamine at nigro-striatal terminals in response to paired stimuli. These mice also display an attenuation of locomotor responses in response to amphetamine (42). These observations indicate that α-synuclein may be involved in regulation of dopamine neurotransmission. However, α- and β-synuclein double knockout mice do not have any detectable phenotypes, and the effects on dopamine neurotransmission were not observed in these bigenic mice (43). Studies have shown that these knockout mice have a depleted, undocked vesicle pool in hippocampal synapses, indicating that α-synuclein may be involved in maintenance of the "reserve" presynaptic vesicle pool (44), as initially suggested in studies of cultured wild-type rodent hippocampal neurons (45). α-Synuclein can also regulate the amount of dopamine transporter (DAT) in the plasma membrane. Expression of α-synuclein has the ability to both increase (46) and decrease (47) trafficking of DAT to the plasma membrane. Direct binding of the NAC region of α-synuclein to the C-terminal region of DAT has been demonstrated through coimmunoprecipitation studies (48). The A30P mutation of α-synuclein is able to bind to DAT similar to wild type; however, the A53T mutation of α-synuclein results in an inhibition of the interaction with DAT (49). Through its ability to regulate the trafficking of DAT to the membrane, α-synuclein may function as a regulator of dopamine toxicity by regulating the amount of dopamine entering the cell. α-Synuclein has also been shown to inhibit dopamine biosynthesis by reducing tyrosine hydroxylase activity (50).

Both α- and β-synuclein have been shown to be potent inhibitors of phospholipase D2 (PLD2) in vitro (51). PLD2 catalyzes the hydrolysis of phosphatidylcholine into phosphatidic acid and choline (52). Because of its ability to bind to acidic phospholipids, it is possible that α-synuclein is concentrated to areas containing high levels of phosphatidic acid and then is able to inhibit PLD2, resulting in negative feedback on phosphatidic acid production. Phosphatidic acid has been proposed to be involved in kinase activation (53), regulation of GTP binding proteins (54), actin stress fibre formation (55), and regulation of vesicle formation in the trans-golgi network (56,57). α-Synuclein also shares homology with the 14-3-3 family of cytoplasmic chaperones, and is able to bind to 14-3-3 proteins and 14-3-3 ligands (58). 14-3-3 proteins are able to bind to and stabilize an inactive form of protein kinase C (PKC), inhibiting PKC enzymatic activity (59). Some evidence indicates that α-synuclein shares a similar ability to inhibit PKC (58). Recent studies have suggested that α-synuclein may be involved in regulation of the enzyme phospholipase Cβ_2, an enzyme involved in the phosphatidylinositol signaling pathway. Regulation of phospholipase Cβ_2 by α-synuclein is disrupted by the A53T mutation (60).

Despite these observations, the normal function of α-synuclein and its relation to the pathogenesis of PD and related α-synucleinopathies remain unclear, but further study of the function of α-synuclein may lead to insights into the pathogenesis of these disorders. However, it is clear that the polymerization of α-synuclein plays an important role in neurodegeneration in PD.

α-SYNUCLEIN POLYMERIZATION

PD is characterized neuropathologically by the presence of Lewy bodies and neurites in the substantia nigra (1,61,62). α-Synuclein was first identified as a major protein component of Lewy bodies in both PD and DLB in 1997 (1). Antibodies to α-synuclein, but not β- or γ-synuclein, strongly stain Lewy bodies and neurites, as well as filamentous material isolated from these inclusions (31). The ability of α-synuclein to form fibrils in vitro that are similar to those seen in Lewy bodies (21,63), and the observation that the A53T mutation of α-synuclein accelerates in vitro fibril formation (21), suggests that the polymerization of α-synuclein may be directly related to the pathogenesis of PD.

α-Synuclein polymerization is concentration, temperature, and time dependent, and results in the conversion of soluble α-synuclein monomers into insoluble 10–19 nm-wide filaments that are readily visible by electron microscopy or atomic force microscopy (21,64). The formation of α-synuclein fibrils is depicted in Figure 2. The assembly of filamentous fibrils from monomeric α-synuclein is associated with a change from random-coil conformation to an ordered β-pleated sheet structure (27,65). These fibrils are similar in appearance, structure, and dye-binding properties to those found in Lewy bodies of PD brains (64,65). The polymerization of α-synuclein into fibrils is strikingly similar to the polymerization of other molecules involved in neurodegenerative diseases, such as tau and Aβ. Aβ can readily form fibrils of a β-pleated sheet structure when incubated in

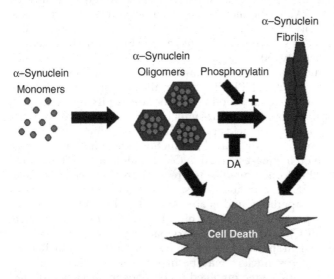

FIGURE 2 The α-synuclein fibril formation pathway. α-Synuclein monomers can aggregate into soluble oligomers. These oligomers can then form the insoluble fibrils that make up inclusion bodies. Phosphorylation of α-synuclein at serine 129 can accelerate fibril formation, while molecules such as dopomine can inhibit the conversion of oligomers to fibrils. Fibrils or oligomers may be the pathogenic species that cause cell death in Parkinson's disease. *Abbreviation:* DA, dopamine.

solution, while tau can also form fibrils in the presence of cofactors such as glycos-aminoglycans and other polyanions (66,67). Aβ and tau are implicated in the pathogenesis of AD, and tau is implicated in most forms of frontal temporal dementia (FTD) known as tauopathies (66,68).

α-Synuclein fibril formation occurs through a nucleation-dependent process, characterized by a slow lag phase followed by a faster elongation phase (69). Both the A53T and E46K mutations of α-synuclein increase the polymerization speed of the proteins, while the A30P mutation has no effect on fibril formation (21,70). Truncation of the C-terminus of α-synuclein results in faster fibril formation (20,71), and substitution of the negatively charged amino acids in this region also increases the rate of fibril formation (72). This suggests that the negatively charged amino acids in the C-terminal region of α-synuclein have an inhibitory effect on the ability of the molecule to polymerize.

The presence of other proteins in the cell may influence the speed at which α-synuclein forms fibrils. Indeed, it has been observed that incubation of α-synuclein with the cytoskeletal protein tau results in a faster rate of fibril formation for both proteins (73). Insoluble, filamentous tau is found in intracellular inclusions, called neurofibrillary tangles, in AD, FTDs, and related tauopathies (74). Not surprisingly, there is some localization of tau and α-synuclein within the same inclusions in individuals who have the A53T α-synuclein mutation, supporting the hypothesis that tau and α-synuclein can promote polymerization of each other (75).

Several observations make the fibrillization of α-synuclein a potential mechanism for the toxicity of α-synuclein and cause of neuronal death in PD. As was previously mentioned, fibrillar protein inclusions are found in many different neurodegenerative diseases, including PD, AD, DLB, MSA, and NBIA-1 (2,76,77). Two of the three α-synuclein mutations, A53T and E46K, accelerate the aggregation process in vitro, and the A53T mutation causes a form of PD with an earlier onset than idiopathic PD (3). It has been proposed that the A30P mutation may cause disease due to its decreased ability to bind lipids, resulting in an increased intracellular concentration and facilitating fibril formation (24). Triplication of the α-synuclein gene is also sufficient to cause a PD-like and DLB-like disorder, suggesting that simply increasing the amount of α-synuclein in the cell can result in neurodegeneration, possibly through increasing the rate at which α-synuclein forms fibrils (14). Expression of α-synuclein in Drosophila results in adult onset loss of dopaminergic neurons accompanied by fibrillar α-synuclein inclusions (78). Overexpression of human α-synuclein in many different mouse models results in varying degrees of neurodegeneration (61).

The mechanisms for fibril toxicity are not known; however, it is unlikely that sequestration of α-synuclein into fibrils causes neuron death due to a lack of normal α-synuclein function. Fibrillar inclusions may act in a sponge-like manner to sequester or trap many different proteins through nonspecific protein interactions, resulting in the loss of activity of proteins necessary for cell survival. Fibrils may disrupt the structural components of the cytoskeleton, resulting in axonal deterioration and eventually cell death, or they could impede cellular transport thereby preventing essential proteins and molecules from being transported down the axon and resulting in cell damage and death. α-Synuclein aggregates may have a toxic gain of function; it has been shown that the cleavage of α-synuclein by the protease Calpain I is altered when α-synuclein is in its fibrillar form. These altered cleavage products may contribute to neurodegeneration.

An alternate hypothesis for the toxicity of α-synuclein is that it is not the fibrils themselves that are toxic, but some intermediate in the fibrillization pathway, sometimes called "protofibrils" (79). Protofibrils are small, oligomeric species that contain some β-sheet structure (80). Several different types of protofibrils have been observed by electron microscopy (EM) and atomic force microscopy (AFM) in vitro, including spherical structures, ring-like structures, and tubes (79,81). The *A30P* mutation appears to form soluble oligomers at a faster rate than wild-type or A53T α-synuclein (82). Incubation of α-synuclein with dopamine under oxidizing conditions results in the formation of an α-synuclein-dopamine adduct that results in increased formation of α-synuclein oligomer while decreasing the ability of α-synuclein to form fibrils (83). The mechanisms by which α-synuclein protofibrils may cause neurotoxicity are unclear. One hypothesis is that one form of α-synuclein protofibril is a pore-like structure that is able to permeabilize membranes and disrupt ionic gradients or cellular homeostasis (79), although there is no direct evidence for this in cell culture and in vivo animal models.

Both the fibril and protofibril theories of α-synuclein toxicity are intriguing, and are not mutually exclusive. There is an abundance of evidence that supports the hypothesis that fibrillar α-synuclein causes neurotoxicity. However, it may be possible that both α-synuclein fibrils and protofibrils are toxic species and that both contribute to the pathogenesis of PD and related α-synucleinopathies. It is also a possibility that the polymerization of α-synuclein does not directly contribute to neuronal death in PD, and it may be some dysfunction of the monomeric form of α-synuclein molecule that results in neurodegeneration.

Expression of α-synuclein in human dopaminergic neurons results in increased apoptosis (84), and this proapoptotic effect requires the production of dopamine. However, in nondopaminergic cells, α-synuclein appears to have a neuroprotective effect. α-Synuclein in these human dopaminergic neurons does not form fibrils, and appears to be associated with 14-3-3 proteins. The formation of these α-synuclein-14-3-3 complexes may result in sequestration of the antiapoptotic 14-3-3 protein, resulting in increased apoptosis, and possibly an increased vulnerability to reactive oxygen species that are produced during dopamine biosynthesis (85).

It has also been demonstrated that mutant α-synuclein can increase sensitivity of cells to proteasome inhibition (86). This indicates that α-synuclein may be able to regulate proteasome function or integrity. Rat α-synuclein can interact with Tat binding protein 1, a component of the 26s proteasomal subunit, in a yeast two-hybrid screen (87). Alternatively, aggregated α-synuclein may be simply "clogging up" and inhibiting the activity of the proteasome, as has been shown with other aggregated proteins (88). Aggregated α-synuclein strongly inhibits the activity of the 26s proteasome with an IC50 of 1 nm, while monomeric α-synuclein inhibits 26s proteasome activity with a much lower potency (89). There is ample evidence to support the theory that monomeric α-synuclein is toxic to cells, although the mechanism for this toxicity is currently unknown.

α-SYNUCLEIN MODIFICATIONS
Oxidation and Nitration

Another possible mechanism for the toxicity of α-synuclein is that chemical modifications of the molecule, such as oxidation, nitration, or phosphorylation, are responsible for the neurotoxicity seen in PD and related α-synucleinopathies.

Dopaminergic neurons are thought to be more susceptible to oxidative stress due to byproducts of dopamine metabolism by monoamine oxidase, which generates hydrogen peroxide, oxygen radicals, semiquinones, and quinines (90). Because of the selective death of dopaminergic neurons in PD, oxidation of α-synuclein has been examined as a mechanism for cytotoxicity. It has been demonstrated that α-synuclein can undergo metal-catalyzed oxidative self-oligomerization when incubated with Cu^{2+} and hydrogen peroxide. This oxidation is dependent upon the C-terminus of α-synuclein (91). Oxidation of α-synuclein may cause oligomer formation, which could speed up the fibril formation process by providing oligomeric α-synuclein "seeds." Oxidation of α-synuclein by dopamine, however, stabilizes α-synuclein oligomers, and inhibits fibril formation (83). In vitro oxidation of all four methionine residues in α-synuclein by hydrogen peroxide results in complete inhibition of α-synuclein fibril formation (92). However, lower levels of oxidation do not inhibit the formation of fibrils, suggesting that inhibition of fibril formation only occurs during exposure to high concentrations of oxidizing agents (93). Susceptibility to the oxidizing agent menadione is increased in cells transfected with A30P α-synuclein, but not wild type α-synuclein (94). Expression of α-synuclein in SH-SY5Y cells results in increased levels of reactive oxygen species and increases the susceptibility of these cells to dopamine-mediated toxicity (95).

Nitration of α-synuclein is another possible mechanism for neurotoxicity. In the presence of reactive oxygen species, nitric oxide forms peroxynitrite, which is capable of converting tyrosine residues to 3-nitrotyrosine (96). Nitrotyrosine immunoreactivity has been demonstrated in Lewy bodies in PD (97), as well as in DLB, LBVAD, NBIA-1, and in the GCIs of MSA. α-Synuclein appears to be the major source of the 3-nitrotyrosine immunoreactivity in the inclusions in these diseases (98). Nitration of recombinant α-synuclein results in stabilization of α-synuclein oligomers due to *o,o'*-dityrosine cross-linking (99,100). Nitration of preformed α-synuclein filaments results in stabilization of these fibrils, making them resistant to heat and denaturing agents such as sodium dodecyl sulfate (SDS) or urea (93,99). While nitration of α-synuclein does result in the stabilization of oligomers, it also inhibits further polymerization into fibrils (93,100). Incubation of α-synuclein in the presence of small amounts of these nitrated oligomers is sufficient to inhibit fibril formation (100). In cell culture, intracellular generation of nitrating agents such as peroxynitrite result in the formation of α-synuclein aggregates in transfected cells (101). It is clear that nitration of α-synuclein occurs in PD, but its relationship to the pathogenesis of the disease is not well understood.

Phosphorylation and Glycosylation

Phosphorylation is a common mechanism for regulating the activity and function of proteins. In AD, phosphorylation of the cytoskeletal protein tau is associated with disease (102), and it is reasonable to suspect that a similar mechanism may be involved with α-synuclein in PD. In vitro, it has been shown that α-synuclein can be phosphorylated at serine 129. In transfected cells, this phosphorylation is insensitive to stimulation of PKC and protein kinase A (PKA), and at steady state the majority of α-synuclein is unphosphorylated (103). In vitro, α-synuclein can be phosphorylated by both casein kinase 1 and casein kinase 2, but not by PKA or PKC. α-Synuclein can also be phosphorylated by G-protein coupled receptor kinases (GRKs), with GRK5 preferentially phosphorylating α-synuclein, while GRK2 phosphorylates both α- and β-synuclein (104). Phosphorylation of α-synuclein by GRKs inhibits both the association of α-synuclein with lipids and its ability to inhibit PLD2. Lewy bodies in brains from DLB patients stain strongly with an antibody specific to S129 phosphorylated α-synuclein (105). Because α-synuclein is not phosphorylated at steady state conditions in cultured cells, this raises the possibility that the phosphorylation of α-synuclein at serine 129 is a pathological event that may lead to neurodegeneration. Phosphorylation of α-synuclein at serine 129 speeds up the fibril and oligomer formation process, suggesting a mechanism by which aberrant phosphorylation can cause α-synuclein to polymerize, resulting in inclusion formation and cell death (105).

A rare glycosylated form of α-synuclein, α-Sp22, has been precipitated from human brain extracts. α-Sp22, but not monomeric unglycosylated α-synuclein, was coprecipitated with the E3 ubiquitin ligase, *PARKIN* (106). It is unclear how α-Sp22 is involved in PD pathogenesis, however, it appears that α-Sp22 is a target for ubiquitination by *PARKIN*, and may accumulate in the brains of individuals with *PARKIN* mutations but this observation remains to be validated.

α-SYNUCLEIN AND TOXIC CHEMICALS

Epidemiological data suggest that risk for PD may increase with exposure to environmental toxins such as pesticides (107). Several compounds have been identified that cause PD-like symptoms in animal models, as well as in humans. Several of these compounds have interesting effects on α-synuclein in vitro and in cell culture.

1-Methyl-4-phenyl-1,2,3,6-tetrahydropyridine (MPTP) is a neurotoxin capable of producing specific degeneration of dopaminergic neurons in the substantia nigra and results in a PD-like syndrome in humans and in animals (108). MPTP is metabolized into the 1-methyl-4-phenylpyridinium (MPP+) ion by monoamine oxidase type B (109). MPP+ is required for MPTP toxicity, and is a potent mitochondrial complex 1 inhibitor. MPP+ is transported into neurons through the dopamine transporter, where it can enter mitochondria and interfere with the electron transport chain (110). Treatment of SH-SY5Y cells with MPP+ results in an increased amount of α-synuclein in the cytoplasm, release of cytochrome C, as well as DNA fragmentation and cell death (111). In addition to these effects, MPP+ treatment also results in increased phosphorylation of ERK/MAP kinases, which are involved in cellular responses to stress and other toxins. One hypothesis is that the increase in α-synuclein levels and ERK/MAP kinase phosphorylation is a protective response to the cytotoxicity of MPP+ (112). In transfected HEK-293 cells, expression of mutant α-synuclein results in increased toxicity during low levels of MPP+ treatment (113).

The pesticide rotenone is a potent inhibitor of complex I of the mitochondrial electron transport chain. Administration of rotenone to animals results in degeneration of dopaminergic neurons, motor defects, and intracellular accumulation of fibrillar α-synuclein (114). Treatment of human dopaminergic SH-SY5Y cells with rotenone increases the amount of α-synuclein found in these cells, and increases the amount of α-synuclein bound to 14-3-3 in these cells (115). In SK-N-MC human neuroblastoma cells, rotenone exposure results in increased levels of α-synuclein, and after prolonged exposure, increased levels of insoluble α-synuclein. This insoluble α-synuclein is also accompanied by increased ubiquitin immunoreactivity in the insoluble protein fraction. In addition to these effects on α-synuclein, rotenone exposure in these human neuroblastoma cells results in reduced glutathione levels, oxidative DNA damage, vulnerability to oxidative insults, and activation of caspases (116). It has also been observed that rotenone is able to accelerate α-synuclein fibril formation in vitro (117).

Another pesticide, paraquat, has also been studied as a model for PD. Paraquat is primarily used in animal models (61), however, it has been observed that paraquat is able to accelerate α-synuclein fibril formation in vitro (117).

These epidemiological and experimental observations indicate a strong possibility that pesticides or other toxins are involved in the pathogenesis of PD, and that this effect may involve α-synuclein. Many of these pesticides are inhibitors of complex I of the mitochondrial electron transport chain, and treatment of cultured cells with these chemicals results in altered expression and cellular distribution of α-synuclein.

α-SYNUCLEIN: DEGRADATION, CLEARANCE, AND CHAPERONES

Proteins can be degraded in the cell by two different pathways, the ubiquitin-proteasome pathway and the lysosomal pathway. The ubiquitin-proteasome system is responsible for degradation of many types of intracellular proteins, as well as misfolded proteins and oxidatively damaged proteins (118). Proteins are targeted for proteasomal degradation by attachment of a polyubiquitin chain to a lysine within the protein. This reaction is catalyzed by a series of enzymes. First, an ubiquitin-activating enzyme (E1) activates ubiquitin in an ATP-dependent manner, then the activated ubiquitin is conjugated to a carrier protein by an ubiquitin-conjugating enzyme (E2), and lastly the ubiquitin chain is attached to a lysine group by an ubiquitin ligase (E3). Polyubiquitin chains can then be formed by linking many ubiquitins together in tandem, and it is effete, misfolded or otherwise abnormal proteins tagged with these polyubiquitin chains that are recognized by the 26s proteasome complex and degraded, but this is preceded by the release of the polyubiquitin chains (119).

Because α-synuclein deposits are thought to be involved in neurodegeneration, many studies have focused on the mechanisms by which both soluble and filamentous α-synuclein is degraded or cleared from inclusion bodies. Lewy bodies in PD, DLB, and LBVAD are often strongly stained with antibodies to ubiquitin (120). This suggests that insoluble proteins in Lewy bodies, such as α-synuclein, are targeted for degradation by ubiquitin. Polyubiquitinated α-synuclein has been purified from insoluble brain fractions of DLB patients (121); however, mono and di-ubiquitinated α-synuclein is more abundant than polyubiquitinated forms (122). It is possible that ubiquitination of α-synuclein occurs prior to inclusion formation and is thus a pathological event, or alternatively, that it occurs after inclusion formation as a response to accumulated insoluble proteins. Ubiquitination of α-synuclein is, not required for inclusion formation, because there are abundant α-synuclein inclusions that are not labeled with ubiquitin antibodies (122). Ubiquitination of recombinant monomeric α-synuclein by mammalian cell lysates results in primarily polyubiquitinated forms of α-synuclein. Ubiquitination of recombinant α-synuclein fibrils, however, results in a predominance of mono and di-ubiquitinated α-synuclein, recapitulating the pattern seen in DLB brain (122). In vitro, recombinant α-synuclein can be degraded by the 20s proteasome (123). Proteasomal inhibition in rat cortical neurons results in formation of ubiquitinated inclusions that contain α-synuclein; however, the α-synuclein in these inclusions is not insoluble and is not ubiquitinated (124). While there is some contradicting evidence in some of these models, it appears that ubiquitination of α-synuclein could contribute to the pathology of inclusion formation, but this ubiquitination most likely occurs after inclusion formation.

It has been demonstrated that α-synuclein can be a substrate for ubiquitination, however, there is conflicting evidence about the role of the proteasome in degradation of α-synuclein. In transfected SH-SY5Y cells, α-synuclein degradation is inhibited by administration of the proteasome inhibitor β-lactone, indicating that α-synuclein is being degraded by the proteasome in this system. In this transfected cell system, A53T α-synuclein is degraded about half as fast as wild-type α-synuclein, suggesting that aggregation of mutant α-synuclein may be due to increased concentrations of the protein because of impaired degradation (125). However, α-synuclein does not appear to be ubiquitinated in transfected SH-SY5Y cells during proteasome inhibition (123,125). Proteasomal inhibition in transfected PC12 cells results in aggregation of α-synuclein, however, this effect was determined to be due to increased expression of α-synuclein, and not a decrease in degradation (126). It has also been reported that α-synuclein and A53T α-synuclein are not ubiquitinated in HEK293 cells and TSM1 neurons, and that proteasomal inhibition did not increase levels of α-synuclein in these cells (127). Proteasomal inhibition does not increase α-synuclein levels in cortical rat neurons (124). Expression of the ubiquitin ligase, *PARKIN*, can rescue toxicity caused by α-synuclein expression in primary midbrain cultures, which involves downregulation of proteasome activity (86).

The involvement of the ubiquitin-proteasome system in PD and other α-synucleinopathies is unclear. Mutations in the genes encoding the ubiquitin ligase *PARKIN* and the ubiquitin carboxy-terminal hydrolase L1 (UCH-L1) have been linked to familial forms of PD (128); however, it has not been established whether these inherited forms of PD are related to α-synuclein aggregation.

The lysosomal pathway is a protein degradation pathway that acts on extracellular or membrane-bound proteins such as immunoglobulins and lipoproteins (129), as well as intracellular proteins and organelles through a process known as autophagy (130). There are three types of lysosomal degradation, differentiated by the manner in which the target is transported into the lysosome. In macroautophagy, a target protein or organelle is surrounded by a nonlysosomal membrane, which then fuses with the lysosome, allowing the target to enter the lysosome and be degraded. In microautophagy, the lysosomal membrane itself engulfs the target protein or organelle. In chaperone-mediated autophagy, chaperone proteins can bind to the target and then interact with receptors in the lysosomal membrane that bind the target protein/chaperone complex and transport it into the lysosome (130,131). Several recent studies have suggested that α-synuclein may be degraded by the lysosome. PC12 cells stably expressing α-synuclein show an increase in α-synuclein protein levels when treated with inhibitors of autophagy, and also show a decrease in α-synuclein protein levels when treated with rapamycin, a stimulator of autophagy (132). HEK293 cells stably expressing α-synuclein also show an increase in steady-state levels of α-synuclein when treated with ammonium chloride, which disrupts lysosomal function (101). Rotenone-induced α-synuclein aggregates in stably expressing COS-7 cells show reduced clearance during lysosomal inhibition (133). In neurons from mice lacking the transmembrane protein presenilin-1, α-synuclein is localized to large degradative lysosome-like structures in the perikarya that label with antibodies to lysosomal proteins such as lamp-1 and lamp-2 (134).

Residues 95–99 (VKKDQ) of α-synuclein have been recently identified as a recognition motif for chaperone-mediated autophagy. α-Synuclein is transported into and degraded by isolated lysosomes in vitro. Saturation of the system with other established chaperone-mediated autophagy substrates results in decreased binding and uptake of α-synuclein into isolated lysosomes. Mutation of residues 95–99 results in a significant reduction in the translocation of α-synuclein into the lysosome, and this mutant is unable to compete for lysosomal binding with known chaperone-mediated autophagy substrates. One particularly interesting observation is that mutant A30P and A53T α-synuclein bind to lysosomes stronger than wild-type α-synuclein, and these mutants inhibit the lysosomal uptake of other chaperone-mediated autophagy substrates. PC12 cells expressing mutant α-synuclein show impaired degradation of proteins through chaperone-mediated autophagy (135). This study suggests that α-synuclein is normally degraded in the lysosome by chaperone-mediated autophagy. Mutant α-synuclein may impair lysosomal function by interfering with the chaperone-mediated autophagy pathway.

Chaperone proteins are thought to function by binding unfolded proteins and facilitating the transition of those proteins into different conformations. α-Synuclein fibril formation is thought to occur because of a "misfolded" β-sheet conformation, thus it is reasonable to examine whether chaperone proteins are capable of regulating the folding of α-synuclein into fibrils or oligomeric intermediates. The molecular chaperone Hsp70 is able to inhibit in vitro fibril formation of α-synuclein, and this appears to occur through binding to prefibrillar α-synuclein species (136). Coexpression of Hsp70 and α-synuclein in transfected H4 cells results in a decrease in α-synuclein expression as well as decreased insoluble α-synuclein. Hsp70 also inhibits α-synuclein-induced toxicity in transfected H4 cells (137). Expression of Hsp70 and α-synuclein in Drosophila dramatically decreases the loss of dopaminergic neurons that is normally seen in flies expressing α-synuclein; however, there is no effect on inclusion formation in the dopaminergic neurons in these flies. Mutation of the Drosophila form of Hsp70 results in increased dopaminergic cell death in the α-synuclein expressing flies. Staining of human brain tissue from PD and other α-synucleinopathy patients revealed that Lewy bodies are immunoreactive for Hsp70 and Hsp40 (138). Administration of the drug geldanomycin, which sensitizes the stress response and increases activation of chaperone proteins, results in decreased dopaminergic neuron degeneration in α-synuclein expressing Drosophila (139). These studies suggest that chaperones are able to interact with α-synuclein, and possibly prevent the folding of α-synuclein into a toxic species. Expression or activation of chaperone proteins may be a potential therapy for PD.

The data summarized here illustrate the wealth of knowledge about α-synuclein that has been obtained in the past decade. In the future it will be important to determine the exact function of α-synuclein, as well as address the question as to which form of α-synuclein is the toxic species. Inhibitors of the α-synuclein polymerization pathway, activators of α-synuclein degradation, or activators of chaperone proteins may all be viable therapies for preventing the neurotoxicity caused by α-synuclein in PD and other α-synucleinopathies.

CONCLUSION

Two recent studies have contributed new data that may be related to the function of α-synuclein. Overexpression of α-synuclein was able to rescue the toxicity caused by deletion of the CSPα gene in mice, suggesting that α-synuclein may play a protective role in the regulation of CSPα and SNARE proteins at the synapse (141).

Another study showed that toxicity caused by α-synuclein overexpression in yeast, was rescued by overexpression of the Rab-GTPase, Ypt1p. Overexpression of the Ypt1 homolog, Rab-1, was able to rescue α-synuclein-induced toxicity in *Drosophila*, *C. elegans*, and in rat midbrain neurons (142). Ypt1/Rab-1 is involved in endoplasmic reticulum-to-Golgi transport, implicating the involvement of α-synuclein in this transport pathway.

REFERENCES

1. Spillantini MG, Schmidt ML, Lee VMY, Trojanowski JQ, Jakes R, Goedert M. Alpha-synuclein in Lewy bodies. Nature 1997; 388:839–840.
2. Galvin JE, Lee VMY, Trojanowski JQ. Synucleinopathies — Clinical and pathological implications. Arch Neurol 2001; 58:186–190.
3. Polymeropoulos MH, Lavedan C, Leroy E, et al. Mutation in the alpha-synuclein gene identified in families with Parkinson's disease. Science 1997; 276:2045–2047.
4. Kruger R, Kuhn W, Muller T, et al. Ala30Pro mutation in the gene encoding alpha-synuclein in Parkinson's disease. Nat Genet 1998; 18:106–108.
5. Zarranz JJ, Alegre J, Gomez-Esteban JC, et al. The new mutation, E46K, of alpha-synuclein causes Parkinson and Lewy body dementia. Ann Neurol 2004; 55:164–173.
6. Goedert M. Filamentous nerve cell inclusions in neurodegenerative diseases:tauopathies and alpha-synucleinopathies. Philos Trans R Soc Lond B Biol Sci 1999; 354:1101–1118.
7. Forstl H. The Lewy body variant of Alzheimer's disease:clinical, pathophysiological and conceptual issues. Eur Arch Psychiatry Clin Neurosci 1999; 249(Suppl 3):64–67.
8. Tu PH, Galvin JE, Baba M, et al. Glial cytoplasmic inclusions in white matter oligodendrocytes of multiple system atrophy brains contain insoluble alpha-synuclein. Ann Neurol 1998; 44:415–422.
9. Galvin JE, Giasson B, Hurtig HI, Lee VM, Trojanowski JQ. Neurodegeneration with brain iron accumulation, type 1 is characterized by alpha-, beta-, gamma-synuclein neuropathology. Am J Pathol 2000; 157:361–368.
10. Jakes R, Spillantini MG, Goedert M. Identification of 2 distinct synucleins from human brain. FEBS Lett 1994; 345:27–32.
11. Iwai A, Masliah E, Yoshimoto M, et al. The precursor protein of non-a-beta component of Alzheimers disease amyloid is a presynaptic protein of the central nervous system. Neuron 1995; 14:467–475.
12. Spillantini MG, Divane A, Goedert M. Assignment of human alpha-synuclein (SNCA) and beta-synuclein (SNCB) genes to chromosomes 4q21 and 5q35. Genomics 1995; 27:379–381.
13. Duda JE, Giasson BI, Gur TL, et al. Immunohistochemical and biochemical studies demonstrate a distinct profile of alpha-synuclein permutations in multiple system atrophy. J Neuropathol Exp Neurol 2000; 59:830–841.
14. Singleton AB, Farrer M, Johnson J, et al. alpha-synuclein locus triplication causes Parkinson's disease. Science 2003; 302:841.
15. Crowther RA, Daniel SE, Goedert M. Characterisation of isolated alpha-synuclein filaments from substantia nigra of Parkinson's disease brain. Neurosci Lett 2000; 292:128–130.
16. Maroteaux L, Campanelli JT, Scheller RH. Synuclein — a neuron-specific protein localized to the nucleus and presynaptic nerve-terminal. J Neurosci 1988; 8:2804–2815.
17. George JM, Jin H, Woods WS, Clayton DF. Characterization of a novel protein regulated during the critical period for song learning in the Zebra Finch. Neuron 1995; 15:361–372.
18. Weinreb PH, Zhen W, Poon AW, Conway KA, Lansbury PT Jr. NACP, a protein implicated in Alzheimer's disease and learning, is natively unfolded. Biochemistry 1996; 35:13709–13715.
19. Ueda K, Fukushima H, Masliah, et al. Molecular-cloning of CDNA-encoding an unrecognized component of amyloid in Alzheimer-disease. Proc Natl Acad Sci USA 1993; 90:11282–11286.
20. Crowther RA, Jakes R, Spillantini MG, Goedert M. Synthetic filaments assembled from C-terminally truncated alpha-synuclein. FEBS Lett 1998; 436:309–312.

21. Conway KA, Harper JD, Lansbury PT. Accelerated in vitro fibril formation by a mutant alpha-synuclein linked to early-onset Parkinson disease. Nat Med 1998; 4: 1318–1320.
22. Segrest JP, Jones MK, De Loof H, Brouillette CG, Venkatachalapathi YV, Anantharamaiah GM. The amphipathic helix in the exchangeable apolipoproteins:a review of secondary structure and function. J Lipid Res 1992; 33:141–166.
23. Davidson WS, Jonas A, Clayton DF, George JM. Stabilization of alpha-synuclein secondary structure upon binding to synthetic membranes. J Biol Chem 1998; 273:9443–9449.
24. Jensen PH, Nielsen MS, Jakes R, Dotti CG, Goedert M. Binding of alpha-synuclein to brain vesicles is abolished by familial Parkinson's disease mutation. J Biol Chem 1998; 273:26292–26294.
25. Choi W, Zibaee S, Jakes R, et al. Mutation E46K increases phospholipid binding and assembly into filaments of human alpha-synuclein. FEBS Lett 2004; 576:363–368.
26. Bayer TA, Jakala P, Hartmann T, et al. Alpha-synuclein accumulates in Lewy bodies in Parkinson's disease and dementia with Lewy bodies but not in Alzheimer's disease beta-amyloid plaque cores. Neurosci Lett 1999; 266:213–216.
27. Giasson BI, Murray IV, Trojanowski JQ, Lee VM. A hydrophobic stretch of 12 amino acid residues in the middle of alpha-synuclein is essential for filament assembly. J Biol Chem 2001; 276:2380–2386.
28. Tobe T, Nakajo S, Tanaka A, et al. Cloning and characterization of the cDNA encoding a novel brain-specific 14-kDa protein. J Neurochem 1992; 59:1624–1629.
29. Ninkina NN, Alimova-Kost MV, Paterson JW, et al. Organization, expression and polymorphism of the human persyn gene. Hum Mol Genet 1998; 7:1417–1424.
30. Spillantini MG, Divane A, Goedert M. Assignment of human alpha-synuclein (SNCA) and beta-synuclein (SNCB) genes to chromosomes 4q21 and 5q35. Genomics 1995; 27:379–381.
31. Spillantini MG, Crowther RA, Jakes R, Hasegawa M, Goedert M. Alpha-synuclein in filamentous inclusions of Lewy bodies from Parkinson's disease and dementia with Lewy bodies. Proc Natl Acad Sci USA 1998; 95:6469–6473.
32. Biere AL, Wood SJ, Wypych J, et al. Parkinson's disease-associated alpha-synuclein is more fibrillogenic than beta- and gamma-synuclein and cannot cross-seed its homologs. J Biol Chem 2000; 275:34574–34579.
33. Ohtake H, Limprasert P, Fan Y, et al. Beta-synuclein gene alterations in dementia with Lewy bodies. Neurology 2004; 63:805–811.
34. Lavedan C. The synuclein family. Genome Res 1998; 8:871–880.
35. Lavedan C, Leroy E, Dehejia A, et al. Identification, localization and characterization of the human gamma-synuclein gene. Hum Genet 1998; 103:106–112.
36. Hashimoto M, Yoshimoto M, Sisk A, et al. NACP, a synaptic protein involved in Alzheimer's disease, is differentially regulated during megakaryocyte differentiation. Biochem Biophys Res Commun 1997; 237:611–616.
37. Iwanaga K, Wakabayashi K, Yoshimoto M, et al. Lewy body-type degeneration in cardiac plexus in Parkinson's and incidental Lewy body diseases. Neurology 1999; 52: 1269–1271.
38. Giasson BI, Duda JE, Forman MS, Lee VM, Trojanowski JQ. Prominent perikaryal expression of alpha- and beta-synuclein in neurons of dorsal root ganglion and in medullary neurons. Exp Neurol 2001; 172:354–362.
39. Buchman VL, Hunter HA, Pinon LGP, et al. Persyn, a member of the synuclein family, has a distinct pattern of expression in the developing nervous system. J Neurosci 1998; 18:9335–9341.
40. Ji H, Liu YE, Jia T, et al. Identification of a breast cancer-specific gene, BCSG1, by direct differential cDNA sequencing. Cancer Res 1997; 57:759–764.
41. Galvin JE, Schuck TM, Lee VMY, Trojanowski JQ. Differential expression and distribution of alpha-, beta-, gamma-synuclein in the developing human substantia nigra. Exp Neurol 2001; 168:347–355.
42. Abeliovich A, Schmitz Y, Farinas I, et al. Mice lacking alpha-synuclein display functional deficits in the nigrostriatal dopamine system. Neuron 2000; 25:239–252.
43. Chandra S, Fornai F, Kwon HB, et al. Double-knockout mice for alpha- and beta-synucleins: Effect on synaptic functions. Proc Natl Acad Sci USA 2004; 101:14966–14971.

44. Cabin DE, Shimazu K, Murphy D, et al. Synaptic vesicle depletion correlates with attenuated synaptic responses to prolonged repetitive stimulation in mice lacking alpha-synuclein. J Neurosci 2002; 22:8797–8807.
45. Murphy DD, Rueter SM, Trojanowski JQ, Lee VMY. Synucleins are developmentally expressed, alpha-synuclein regulates the size of the presynaptic vesicular pool in primary hippocampal neurons. J Neurosci 2000; 20:3214–3220.
46. Lee FJS, Liu F, Pristupa ZB, Niznik HB. Direct binding and functional coupling of alpha-synuclein to the dopamine transporters accelerate dopamine-induced apoptosis. Faseb J 2001; 15:916–926.
47. Wersinger C, Prou D, Vernier P, Sidhu A. Modulation of dopamine transporter function by alpha-synuclein is altered by impairment of cell adhesion and by induction of oxidative stress. Faseb J 2001:2151–2153.
48. Lee FJS, Liu F, Pristupa ZB, Niznik HB. Direct binding and functional coupling of alpha-synuclein to the dopamine transporters accelerate dopamine-induced apoptosis. Faseb J 2001; 15:916–926.
49. Wersinger C, Prou D, Vernier P, Niznik HB, Sidhu A. Mutations in the lipid-binding domain of alpha-synuclein confer overlapping, yet distinct, functional properties in the regulation of dopamine transporter activity. Mol Cell Neurosci 2003; 24:91–105.
50. Perez RG, Waymire JC, Lin E, Liu JJ, Guo FL, Zigmond MJ. A role for alpha-synuclein in the regulation of dopamine biosynthesis. J Neurosci 2002; 22:3090–3099.
51. Jenco JM, Rawlingson A, Daniels B, Morris AJ. Regulation of phospholipase D2: selective inhibition of mammalian phospholipase D isoenzymes by alpha- and beta-synucleins. Biochemistry 1998; 37:4901–4909.
52. Morris AJ, Hammond SM, Colley C, et al. Regulation and functions of phospholipase D. Biochem Soc Trans 1997; 25:1151–1157.
53. Khan WA, Blobe GC, Richards AL, Hannun YA. Identification, Partial-purification, characterization of a novel phospholipid-dependent and fatty acid-activated protein-kinase from human platelets. J Biol Chem 1994; 269:9729–9735.
54. Chuang TH, Bohl BP, Bokoch GM. Biologically-active lipids are regulators of rac-center-dot-gdi complexation. J Biol Chem 1993; 268:26206–26211.
55. Cross MJ, Roberts S, Ridley AJ, et al. Stimulation of actin stress fibre formation mediated by activation of phospholipase D. Curr Biol 1996; 6:588–597.
56. Ktistakis NT, Brown HA, Waters MG, Sternweis PC, Roth MG. Evidence that phospholipase D mediates ADP ribosylation factor-dependent formation golgi coated vesicles. J Cell Biol 1996; 134:295–306.
57. Chen YG, Siddhanta A, Austin CD, et al. Phospholipase D stimulates release of nascent secretory vesicles from the trans-golgi network. J Cell Biol 1997; 138:495–504.
58. Ostrerova N, Petrucelli L, Farrer M, et al. Alpha-synuclein shares physical and functional homology with 14-3-3 proteins. J Neurosci 1999; 19:5782–5791.
59. Meller N, Liu YC, Collins TL, et al. Direct interaction between protein kinase C theta (PKC theta) and 14-3-3 tau in T cells: 14-3-3 overexpression results in inhibition of PKC theta translocation and function. Mol Cell Biol 1996; 16:5782–5791.
60. Narayanan VGYSS. Fluorescence studies suggest a role for a-synuclein in the phosphatidylinositol lipid signaling pathway. Biochemistry 2005; 44:462–470.
61. Norris EH, Giasson BI, Lee VMY. Alpha-synuclein: normal function and role in neurodegenerative diseases. Stem Cell Dev Disease 2004; 60:17–54.
62. Trojanowski JQ. Role of alpha-synuclein and tau in Parkinson's disease. Mov Dis 2004; 19:S2.
63. Han HY, Weinreb PH, Lansbury PT. The core Alzheimers peptide nac forms amyloid fibrils which seed and are seeded by beta-amyloid — is nac a common trigger or target in neurodegenerative disease. Chem Biol 1995; 2:163–169.
64. Giasson BI, Uryu K, Trojanowski JQ, Lee VM. Mutant and wild type human alpha-synucleins assemble into elongated filaments with distinct morphologies in vitro. J Biol Chem 1999; 274:7619–7622.
65. Conway KA, Harper JD, Lansbury PT Jr. Fibrils formed in vitro from alpha-synuclein and two mutant forms linked to Parkinson's disease are typical amyloid. Biochemistry 2000; 39:2552–2563.

66. Goedert M, Jakes R, Spillantini MG, Hasegawa M, Smith MJ, Crowther RA. Assembly of microtubule-associated protein tau into Alzheimer-like filaments induced by sulphated glycosaminoglycans. Nature 1996; 383:550–553.

67. Serpell LC. Alzheimer's amyloid fibrils:structure and assembly. Biochimica et Biophysica Acta-Molecular Basis of Disease 2000; 1502:16–30.

68. Mirra SS, Murrell JR, Gearing M, et al. Tau pathology in a family with dementia and a P301L mutation in tau. J Neuropathol Exp Neurol 1999; 58:335–345.

69. Wood SJ, Wypych J, Steavenson S, Louis JC, Citron M, Biere AL. Alpha-synuclein fibril-logenesis is nucleation-dependent—Implications for the pathogenesis of Parkinson's disease. J Biol Chem 1999; 274:19509–19512.

70. Greenbaum EA, Graves CL, Mishizen-Eberz AJ, et al. The E46K mutation in alpha-synuclein increases amyloid fibril formation. J Biol Chem 2005;M411638200.

71. Murray IV, Giasson BI, Quinn SM, et al. Role of alpha-synuclein carboxy-terminus on fibril formation in vitro. Biochemistry 2003; 42:8530–8540.

72. Murray IV, Giasson BI, Quinn SM, et al. Role of alpha-synuclein carboxy-terminus on fibril formation in vitro. Biochemistry 2003; 42:8530–8540.

73. Giasson BI, Forman MS, Higuchi M, et al. Initiation and synergistic fibrillization of tau and alpha-synuclein. Science 2003; 300:636–640.

74. Giasson BI, Lee VM, Trojanowski JQ. Interactions of amyloidogenic proteins. Neuromolecular Med 2003; 4:49–58.

75. Kotzbauer PT, Giasson BI, Kravitz AV, et al. Fibrillization of alpha-synuclein and tau in familial Parkinson's disease caused by the A53T alpha-synuclein mutation. Exp Neurol 2004; 187:279–288.

76. Tu PH, Galvin JE, Baba M, et al. Glial cytoplasmic inclusions in white matter oligo-dendrocytes of multiple system atrophy brains contain insoluble alpha-synuclein. Ann Neurol 1998; 44:415–422.

77. Baba M, Nakajo S, Tu PH, et al. Aggregation of alpha-synuclein in Lewy bodies of sporadic Parkinson's disease and dementia with lewy bodies. Am J Pathol 1998; 152:879–884.

78. Feany MB, Bender WW. A drosophila model of Parkinson's disease. Nature 2000; 404:394–398.

79. Volles MJ, Lansbury PT. Zeroing in on the pathogenic form of alpha-synuclein and its mechanism of neurotoxicity in Parkinson's disease. Biochemistry 2003; 42: 7871–7878.

80. Volles MJ, Lee SJ, Rochet JC, et al. Vesicle permeabilization by protofibrillar alpha-synuclein: implications for the pathogenesis and treatment of Parkinson's disease. Biochemistry 2001; 40:7812–7819.

81. Ding TT, Lee SJ, Rochet JC, Lansbury PT. Annular alpha-synuclein protofibrils are pro-duced when spherical protofibrils are incubated in solution or bound to brain-derived membranes. Biochemistry 2002; 41:10209–10217.

82. Li J, Uversky VN, Fink AL. Effect of familial Parkinson's disease point mutations A30P and A53T on the structural properties, aggregation, fibrillation of human alpha-synuclein. Biochemistry 2001; 40:11604–11613.

83. Conway KA, Rochet JC, Bieganski RM, Lansbury PT Jr. Kinetic stabilization of the alpha-synuclein protofibril by a dopamine-alpha-synuclein adduct. Science 2001; 294: 1346–1349.

84. Zhou WB, Schaack J, Zawada WM, Freed CR. Overexpression of alpha-Synuclein causes human dopamine neuron death in primary mesencephalic culture. Exp Neurol 2002; 175:448–449.

85. Xu J, Kao SY, Lee FJS, Song WH, Jin LW, Yankner BA. Dopamine-dependent neurotoxic-ity of alpha-synuclein: a mechanism for selective neurodegeneration in Parkinson disease. Nat Med 2002; 8:600–606.

86. Petrucelli L, O'Farrell C, Lockhart PJ, et al. Parkin protects against the toxicity associated with mutant alpha-synuclein: proteasome dysfunction selectively affects catecholamin-ergic neurons. Neuron 2002; 36:1007–1019.

87. Ghee M, Fournier A, Mallet J. Rat alpha-synuclein interacts with Tat binding protein 1, a component of the 26S proteasomal complex. J Neurochem 2000; 75:2221–2224.

88. Bence NF, Sampat RM, Kopito RR. Impairment of the ubiquitin-proteasome system by protein aggregation. Science 2001; 292:1552–1555.

89. Snyder H, Mensah K, Theisler C, Lee J, Matouschek A, Wolozin B. Aggregated and monomeric alpha-synuclein bind to the S6 ' proteasomal protein and inhibit proteasomal function. J Biol Chem 2003; 278:11753–11759.

90. Halliwell B. Reactive oxygen species and the central-nervous-system. J Neurochem 1992; 59:1609–1623.

91. Paik SR, Shin HJ, Lee JH. Metal-catalyzed oxidation of alpha-synuclein in the presence of copper(II) and hydrogen peroxide. Arch Biochem Biophys 2000; 378:269–277.

92. Uversky VN, Yamin G, Souillac PO, Goers J, Glaser CB, Fink AL. Methionine oxidation inhibits fibrillation of human alpha-synuclein in vitro. Febs Lett 2002; 517:239–244.

93. Norris EH, Giasson BI, Ischiropoulos H, Lee VMY. Effects of oxidative and nitrative challenges on alpha-synuclein fibrillogenesis involve distinct mechanisms of protein modifications. J Biol Chem 2003; 278:27230–27240.

94. Ko LW, Mehta ND, Farrer M, et al. Sensitization of neuronal cells to oxidative stress with mutated human alpha-synuclein. J Neurochem 2000; 75:2546–2554.

95. Junn E, Mouradian MM. Human alpha-synuclein over-expression increases intracellular reactive oxygen species levels and susceptibility to dopamine. Neurosci Lett 2002; 320:146–150.

96. Ischiropoulos H. Oxidative modifications of alpha-synuclein. Parkinson's disease: the life cycle of the dopamine. Neuron 2003; 991:93–100.

97. Good PF, Hsu A, Werner P, Perl DP, Olanow CW. Protein nitration in Parkinson's disease. J Neuropathol Exp Neurol 1998; 57:338–342.

98. Duda JE, Giasson BI, Chen QP, et al. Widespread nitration of pathological inclusions in neurodegenerative synucleinopathies. Am J Pathol 2000; 157:1439–1445.

99. Souza JM, Giasson BI, Chen QP, Lee VMY, Ischiropoulos H. Dityrosine cross-linking promotes formation of stable alpha-synuclein polymers—implication of nitrative and oxidative stress in the pathogenesis of neurodegenerative synucleinopathies. J Biol Chem 2000; 275:18344–18349.

100. Yamin G, Uversky VN, Fink AL. Nitration inhibits fibrillation of human alpha-synuclein in vitro by formation of soluble oligomers. Febs Lett 2003; 542:147–152.

101. Paxinou E, Chen QP, Weisse M, et al. Induction of alpha-synuclein aggregation by intracellular nitrative insult. J Neurosci 2001; 21:8053–8061.

102. Trojanowski JQ, Lee VMY. Phosphorylation of neuronal cytoskeletal proteins in Alzheimers-disease and Lewy body dementias. Calcium Hypothesis of Aging and Dementia 1994; 747:92–109.

103. Okochi M, Walter J, Koyama A, et al. Constitutive phosphorylation of the Parkinson's disease associated alpha-synuclein. J Biol Chem 2000; 275:390–397.

104. Pronin AN, Morris AJ, Surguchov A, Benovic JL. Synucleins are a novel class of substrates for G protein-coupled receptor kinases. J Biol Chem 2000; 275:26515–26522.

105. Fujiwara H, Hasegawa M, Dohmae N, et al. Alpha-synuclein is phosphorylated in synucleinopathy lesions. Nat Cell Biol 2002; 4:160–164.

106. Shimura H, Schlossmacher MC, Hattori N, et al. Ubiquitination of a new form of alpha-synuclein by parkin from human brain: implications for Parkinson's disease. Science 2001; 293:263–269.

107. Gorell JM, Johnson CC, Rybicki BA, Peterson EL, Richardson RJ. The risk of Parkinson's disease with exposure to pesticides, farming, well water, rural living. Neurology 1998; 50:1346–1350.

108. Langston JW. Mptp — insights into the etiology of Parkinsons-disease. Eur Neurol 1987; 26:2–10.

109. Chiba K, Trevor A, Castagnoli N Jr. Metabolism of the neurotoxic tertiary amine, MPTP, by brain monoamine oxidase. Biochem Biophys Res Commun 1984; 120:574–578.

110. Kitayama S, Shimada S, Uhl GR. Parkinsonism-inducing neurotoxin MPP+: uptake and toxicity in nonneuronal COS cells expressing dopamine transporter cDNA. Ann Neurol 1992; 32:109–111.

111. Kakimura J, Kitamura Y, Takata K, Kohno Y, Nomura Y, Taniguchi T. Release and aggregation of cytochrome c and alpha-synuclein are inhibited by the antiparkinsonian drugs, talipexole and pramipexole. Eur J Pharmacol 2001; 417:59–67.

112. Gomez-Santos C, Ferrer I, Reiriz J, Vinals F, Barrachina M, Ambrosio S. MPP+ increases alpha-synuclein expression and ERK/MAP-kinase phosphorylation in human neuroblastoma SH-SY5Y cells. Brain Res 2002; 935:32–39.

113. Lehmensiek V, Tan EM, Schwarz J, Storch A. Expression of mutant alpha-synucleins enhances dopamine transporter-mediated MPP+ toxicity in vitro. Neuroreport 2002; 13:1279–1283.

114. Betarbet R, Sherer TB, MacKenzie G, Garcia-Osuna M, Panov AV, Greenamyre JT. Chronic systemic pesticide exposure reproduces features of Parkinson's disease. Nat Neuro 2000; 3:1301–1306.

115. Watabe M, Nakaki T. Rotenone induces apoptosis via activation of bad in human dopaminergic SH-SY5Y cells. J Pharmacol Exp Therap 2004; 311:948–953.

116. Sherer TB, Betarbet R, Stout AK, et al. An in vitro model of Parkinson's disease: linking mitochondrial impairment to altered alpha-synuclein metabolism and oxidative damage. J Neurosci 2002; 22:7006–7015.

117. Uversky VN, Li J, Fink AL. Pesticides directly accelerate the rate of alpha-synuclein fibril formation: a possible factor in Parkinson's disease. FEBS Lett 2001; 500:105–108.

118. Coux O, Tanaka K, Goldberg AL. Structure and functions of the 20S and 26S proteasomes. Ann Rev Biochem 1996; 65:801–847.

119. Betarbet R, Sherer TB, Greenamyre JT. Ubiquitin-proteasome system and Parkinson's diseases. Exp Neurol 2005; 191(suppl 1):S17–S27.

120. Kuzuhara S, Mori H, Izumiyama N, Yoshimura M, Ihara Y. Lewy bodies are ubiquitinated. A light and electron microscopic immunocytochemical study. Acta Neuropathol (Berl) 1988; 75:345–353.

121. Hasegawa M, Fujiwara H, Nonaka T, et al. Phosphorylated alpha-synuclein is ubiquitinated in alpha-synucleinopathy lesions. J Biol Chem 2002; 277:49071–49076.

122. Sampathu DM, Giasson BI, Pawlyk AC, Trojanowski JQ, Lee VMY. Ubiquitination of alpha-synuclein is not required for formation of pathological inclusions in alpha-synucleinopathies. Am J Pathol 2003; 163:91–100.

123. Tofaris GK, Layfield R, Spillantini MG. Alpha-synuclein metabolism and aggregation is linked to ubiquitin-independent degradation by the proteasome. Febs Lett 2001; 509: 22–26.

124. Rideout HJ, Stefanis L. Proteasomal inhibition-induced inclusion formation and death in cortical neurons require transcription and ubiquitination. Mol Cell Neurosci 2002; 21:223–238.

125. Bennett MC, Bishop JF, Leng Y, Chock PB, Chase TN, Mouradian MM. Degradation of alpha-synuclein by proteasome. J Biol Chem 1999; 274:33855–33858.

126. Biasini E, Fioriti L, Ceglia I, et al. Proteasome inhibition and aggregation in Parkinson's disease:a comparative study in untransfected and transfected cells. J Neurochem 2004; 88:545–553.

127. Ancolio K, da Costa CA, Ueda K, Checler F. Alpha-synuclein and the Parkinson's disease-related mutant Ala53Thr-alpha-synuclein do not undergo proteasomal degradation in HEK293 and neuronal cells. Neurosci Lett 2000; 285:79–82.

128. Dawson TM, Dawson VL. Rare genetic mutations shed light on the pathogenesis of Parkinson disease. J Clin Invest 2003; 111:145–151.

129. Glickman MH, Ciechanover A. The ubiquitin-proteasome proteolytic pathway: destruction for the sake of construction. Physiol Rev 2002; 82:373–428.

130. Cuervo AM. Autophagy: in sickness and in health. Trends Cell Biol 2004; 14:70–77.

131. Cuervo AM, Dice JF. Lysosomes, a meeting point of proteins, chaperones, proteases. J Mol Med-Jmm 1998; 76:6–12.

132. Webb JL, Ravikumar B, Atkins J, Skepper JN, Rubinsztein DC. Alpha-synuclein is degraded by both autophagy and the proteasome. J Biol Chem 2003; 278:25009–25013.

133. Lee HJ, Khoshaghideh F, Patel S, Lee SJ. Clearance of alpha-synuclein oligomeric intermediates via the lysosomal degradation pathway. J Neurosci 2004; 24:1888–1896.

134. Wilson CA, Murphy DD, Giasson BI, Zhang B, Trojanowski JQ, Lee VMY. Degradative organelles containing mislocalized alpha- and beta-synuclein proliferate in presenilin-1 null neurons. J Cell Biol 2004; 165:335–346.

135. Cuervo AM, Stefanis L, Fredenburg R, Lansbury PT, Sulzer D. Impaired degradation of mutant alpha-synuclein by chaperone-mediated autophagy. Science 2004; 305: 1292–1295.

136. Dedmon MM, Christodoulou J, Wilson MR, Dobson CM. Hsp70 inhibits alpha -synuclein fibril formation via preferential binding to prefibrillar species. J Biol Chem 2005; M413024200.
137. Klucken J, Shin Y, Masliah E, Hyman BT, Mclean PJ. Hsp70 reduces alpha-synuclein aggregation and toxicity. J Biol Chem 2004; 279:25497–25502.
138. Auluck PK, Chan HYE, Trojanowski JQ, Lee VMY, Bonini NM. Chaperone suppression of alpha-synuclein toxicity in a drosophila model for Parkinson's disease. Science 2002; 295:865–868.
139. Auluck PK, Meulener MC, Bonini NM. Mechanisms of Suppression of (alpha)-synuclein neurotoxicity by geldanamycin in drosophila. J Biol Chem 2005; 280:2873–2878.
140. Uryu K, Kotzbauer P. Center for Neurodegenerative Disease Research, HUP, Philadelphia, PA 19104. Unpublished data.
141. Chandra S, Gallardo G, Fernandez-Chacon R, Schluter OM, Sudhof TC. Alpha-synuclein cooperates with CSPalpha in preventing neurodegeneration. Cell 2005; 123: 383–396.
142. Cooper AA, Gitler AD, Cashikar A, et al. Alpha-Synuclein Blocks ER-Golgi Traffic and Rab1 Rescues Neuron Loss in Parkinson's Models. Science 2006; 313(5785):324–328.

13 Tau in Parkinsonian Diseases

Daniel M. Skovronsky
Avid Radiopharmaceuticals, Inc., Philadelphia, Pennsylvania, U.S.A.

Virginia M.-Y. Lee and John Q. Trojanowski
*Center for Neurodegenerative Disease Research, Department of Pathology and
Laboratory Medicine, Institute on Aging, University of Pennsylvania,
Philadelphia, Pennsylvania, U.S.A.*

AMYLOID AS A COMMON THEME IN NEURODEGENERATIVE PARKINSONIAN DISEASES

Parkinson's disease (PD) and Alzheimer's disease (AD) may be pathogenically linked by a single common mechanism: the aggregation and deposition of misfolded proteins (1–3). Indeed, as summarized in Table 1, nearly every major neurodegenerative disease is pathologically characterized by the insidious accumulation of insoluble filamentous aggregates of normally soluble proteins in the central nervous system (CNS) (3). Since these filamentous aggregates show the ultrastructural and tinctorial properties of amyloid (i.e., ~10 nm wide fibrils with crossed-β-pleated sheet structures that stain with congo red, thioflavin-S, or other related dyes), these diseases are appropriately linked together as brain amyloidoses (4). An understanding that PD and other neurodegenerative parkinsonian diseases including cortical basal degeneration (CBD), progressive supranuclear palsy (PSP), and frontal temporal dementia with parkinsonism linked to chromosome 17 (FTDP-17) are related brain amyloidoses may permit novel insights into the pathogenesis of these common movement disorders and ultimately may lead to improvements in diagnosis and therapy for these devastating diseases.

PD is one of the most common forms of brain amyloidosis, and is the archetype α-synucleinopathy (4). The discoveries that mutations and duplications in the α-synuclein gene can lead to the accumulation of insoluble filaments of α-synuclein in Lewy bodies and thus can cause PD have provided strong evidence for the role of α-synuclein in PD (5–9). However, α-synuclein is not the only type of brain amyloid seen in PD. Indeed, abnormal aggregates of tau protein are present in PD and other parkinsonian diseases, making tau pathology one of the most widespread forms of brain amyloid (10–15). A pathogenic linkage between tau abnormalities and parkinsonian neurodegeneration is suggested by three lines of evidence: (*i*) *histopathologic observations*—widespread tau pathology is seen in affected brain regions of many parkinsonian neurodegenerative patients (10–15); (*ii*) *genetic linkages*—polymorphisms and mutations in the gene for tau have been linked to PD and other parkinsonian neurodegenerative diseases, respectively (16–23); and (*iii*) *experimental data*—in vitro paradigms and transgenic mouse models link tau aggregation to parkinsonian-related abnormalities in the laboratory (24–29). This chapter reviews these lines of evidence that mechanistically link tau abnormalities to parkinsonian neurodegeneration.

TABLE 1 Amyloid in Neurodegenerative Disease

Disease	Microscopic lesion	Location	Aggregated protein
Alzheimer's disease	Amyloid plaque	Extracellular	Amyloid-β (Aβ)
	Neurofibrillary tangle	Intracytoplasmic (neurons)	Tau
	Lewy bodies (seen in Lewy body variant)	Intracytoplasmic (neurons)	α-Synuclein
Parkinson's disease	Lewy bodies	Intracytoplasmic (neurons)	α-Synuclein
Corticobasal degeneration	Tau-positive inclusions	Intracytoplasmic (neurons, oligodendroglia and astrocyes)	Tau (4R only)
Progressive supra-nuclear palsy	Tau-positive inclusions	Intracytoplasmic (neurons, oligodendroglia and astrocytes)	Tau (4R only)
Amyotrophic lateral sclerosis/parkinsonism dementia complex of Guam	Neurofibrillary tangle	Intracytoplasmic (neurons)	Tau
	α-Synuclein inclusions	Intracytoplasmic (neurons)	α-Synuclein
Dementia with Lewy bodies	Lewy bodies	Intracytoplasmic (neurons)	α-Synuclein
Multiple system atrophy	Glial cytoplasmic inclusions	Intracytoplasmic (oligodendroglia)	α-Synuclein
Huntington disease	Neuronal inclusions	Intranuclear (neurons)	Huntington (containing polyglutamine repeat expansion)
Pick's disease	Pick bodies	Intracytoplasmic (neurons)	Tau
Prion diseases	Prion plaques	Extracellular	Protease-resistant prion protein
Spinocerebellar ataxia	Neuronal inclusions	Intranuclear (neurons)	Ataxin (containing polyglutamine repeat expansion)

TAU: NORMAL BIOLOGY AND DYSFUNCTION IN DISEASE

Tau is a microtubule-binding protein that stabilizes microtubules and promotes their polymerization in neurons (15,24,30). Six isoforms of tau are present in the adult human brain. These isoforms are generated by alternative mRNA splicing of the tau gene on chromosome 17 (15). Significantly, in the carboxy-terminal half of the molecule, alternative splicing of exon 10 results in the presence of either three or four microtubule-binding motifs, yielding 3R-tau and 4R-tau isoforms, respectively (Fig. 1).

Tau protein is phosphorylated at multiple sites in a developmentally controlled manner (15); tau phosphorylation plays a role in regulating its microtubule-binding properties (31). Tau is likely involved in numerous cellular processes, including maintenance of neuronal polarity and neurite outgrowth (31). However, there is overlap of function with other microtubule-associated proteins since tau gene knockout mice show only a relatively mild phenotype (32).

Tau monomers can polymerize to form fibrils which accumulate in neurons as neurofibrillary tangles, dystrophic neurites, and neuropil threads. While tau normally is barely detected in glial cells, in disease states, tau fibrils can accumulate in oligodendroglia and astrocytes. Tau polymerization can be modeled in vitro, and shows a lag period that is heavily concentration-dependent, consistent with a nucleation-dependent process.

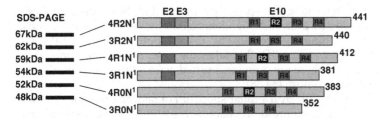

FIGURE 1 Six human brain tau isoforms are generated by alternative splicing. Alternative splicing of the *tau* gene yields six tau isoforms that are expressed in the adult brain. The isoforms differ by the inclusion of 3 or 4 microtubule-binding repeats (3R and 4R respectively) and by the inclusion of 0, 1, or 2 N-terminal repeats (0N, 1N, or 2N). The splicing diversity is generated at the mRNA level by splicing in exon 10 (E10) in the case of 4R tau and by spicing in exons 2 and 3 (E2, E3) in the case of 1N and 2N isoforms. Normal human brain contains similar amounts of 3R and 4R tau isoforms. Mobility on SDS-PAGE of each of the isoforms (in its dephosphorylated state) is shown on the left. *Abbreviation:* SDS-PAGE, sodium dodecyl sulfate–poly acrylamide gel electro phoresis.

TAU PATHOLOGY IN PARKINSONIAN DEGENERATION

Tau pathology defines several of the parkinsonian neurodegenerative diseases, including CBD, progressive supranuclear palsy (PSP), frontal temporal dementia with parkinsonism linked to chromosome 17 (FTDP-17), amylotrophic lateral sclerosis/parkinsonism–dementia complex of Guam (ALS/PDC Guam) and dementia puglistica. Together, these diseases are referred to as tauopathies—a designation that evokes the strong correlative evidence between tau pathology and neurodegeneration in these parkinsonian diseases.

Corticobasal Degeneration

CBD is a clinically heterogenous disease most commonly characterized by progressive neurodegeneration with L-dopa-resistant rigidity and focal cortical deficits accompanied by variable degrees of dementia. CBD is pathologically defined by the presence of prominent glial and neuronal intracytoplasmic filamentous immunoreactive pathology (14,33). The glial tau pathology consists of both astrocytic plaques and coiled bodies, which are immunoreactive inclusions in gray and white matter in astrocytes and oligodendrocytes (34–36). There is also very extensive accumulation of immunoreactive cell processes throughout both the gray and white matter in CBD. Unlike the neuropil threads of AD, in CBD the threads are neurofilament-negative, and likely are contained in glial processes (35,36).

The pathological filamentous inclusions in CBD are primarily composed of abnormally phosphorylated tau similar to many other sporadic and familial neurodegenerative diseases, including AD. However, in AD, the filamentous tau aggregates are composed of all six tau isoforms, while in CBD, the aggregates are composed predominantly of 4R-tau (14). The selective accumulation of specific tau isoforms in different neurodegenerative diseases adds further support to the notion that tau accumulation plays an integral role in pathogenesis.

Progressive Supranuclear Palsy

PSP is clinically characterized by a symmetrical akinetic-rigid parkinsonian syndrome with supranuclear gaze palsy and cognitive changes. Neuropathologically, PSP is defined by widespread neurofibrillary degeneration, with characteristic globose-type neurofibrillary tangles, especially prominent in the brainstem (37,38). Tau-positive argyrophilic threads and oligodendroglial inclusions similar to those seen in CBD are also commonly seen in PSP (34,38). Both CBD and PSP show astrocytic tau pathology, but in CBD, this takes the form of tau-immunoreactive astrocytic plaques; in PSP, there are numerous tufted astrocytes, most abundant in the motor cortex and neostriatum (34,38).

PSP is thus linked to CBD by a similar spectrum of neuropathologic findings. In addition, these two diseases are both characterized by selective accumulation of 4R-tau, and are both linked to the same tau gene haplotype (as described in genetics, later). It is noteworthy that the histopathologic, biochemical, and genetic symmetries between CBD and PSP all revolve around tau, further reinforcing the notion that tau pathology is mechanistically linked to neurodegeneration in both of these diseases.

Frontal Temporal Dementia with Parkinsonism Linked to Chromosome 17

FTDP-17 is a heterogenous clinical pathologic entity that can now be defined by the presence of causative mutations in the tau gene (as described subsequently). As the name implies, the clinical picture is dominated by frontal-temporal dementia and parkinsonism. Different FTDP-17 syndromes have been described, and phenotypic differences may reflect differences in regional distribution of tau pathology and degeneration in the brain (15).

While the pathology of FTDP-17 can be varied, even between different members of the same family, all cases of FTDP-17 are unified by the presence of severe filamentous hyperphosphorylated tau pathology in neurons, with accompanying regional neuronal loss (39–44). Glial involvement by tau pathology (similar to that seen in CBD and PSP) is seen in some but not all FTDP-17 cases.

Despite the fascinating phenotypic, genetic, and pathologic diversity seen in FTDP-17 cases, these cases are all defined by an insidious cascade in which pathogenic mutations in the tau gene lead to tau dysfunction and/or accumulation of brain tau pathology, which in turn lead to neurodegeneration.

Amylotrophic Lateral Sclerosis/Parkinsonism Dementia Complex of Guam

ALS/PDC Guam is a progressive neurodegenerative disorder that affects the Chamorro residents of Guam and the Mariana Islands. Clinically, these patients show a combination of motor neuron disease and progressive cognitive dysfunction with extrapyramidal signs. Neuropathologically the disease is characterized by cortical atrophy with abundant neuron loss and widely distributed tau neurofibrillary pathology similar to that observed in AD (12,45). The tau pathology of ALS/PDC Guam is similar both biochemically and immunohistochemically to that observed in AD, and is composed of all six CNS isoforms of tau (12,45). However, unlike AD, ALS/PDC Guam shows prominent astrocytic pathology and typically lacks the amyloid plaques that are characteristic of AD (46).

Interestingly, in Guamanian ALS/PDC patients, α-synuclein pathology is often present in multiple brain regions, including the substantia nigra and in the amygdala (47,48). Just as in AD and PD, the presence of multiple forms of brain amyloid in ALS/PDC Guam (i.e., α-synuclein and tau filaments) suggests an interaction between these different pathologies (48), a notion that has now been confirmed by experimental evidence (reviewed later) (24,27,49).

Dementia Pugilistica
Dementia pugilistica is a form of chronic traumatic brain injury associated with boxing and clinically characterized by motor, cognitive, and/or behavioral impairments that typically become clinically evident after the cessation of a boxing career (50). Early motor impairments may include mild dysarthria and difficulty with balance progressing to ataxia, spasticity, impaired coordination, and parkinsonism (50). Pathologically, the disease is characterized by deposition of abundant neurofibrillary tangles and amyloid plaques, similar to those seen in AD (51–53). In addition, glial tau pathology is frequently seen in dementia pugilistica. Just as in AD and ALS/PDC Guam, the hyperphosphorylated tau pathology in dementia pugilistica comprises all six brain tau isoforms, suggesting that recurrent brain injury may cause dementia pugilistica by similar mechanisms as seen in AD and other neurodegenerative diseases (51).

Parkinson's Disease
While PD is the best known of the α-synucleinopathies, tau pathology is also seen in many PD cases. Tau pathology can be seen in both sporadic PD (54) and in familial PD cases caused by mutations in α-synuclein (10,25). In sporadic PD, neurofibrillary tau pathology is typically confined to the transentorhinal and entorhinal regions, and is mild in severity, as compared to AD (54). In addition to this overt tau pathology, staining of Lewy bodies with multiple tau antibodies has been reported, suggesting cellular colocalization of these two pathologies (55). In one individual of the familial PD Contursi kindred (harboring the Ala53Thr pathogenic mutation in the α-synuclein gene), neuritic and perikaryal tau inclusions were observed (10). The finding of significant levels of insoluble, aggregated tau in this patient suggest that tau and α-synuclein may cross-seed each other in neurodegenerative disease and that α-synuclein mutations may be sufficient to induce tau pathology in the human brain (25).

GENETIC EVIDENCE LINKING TAU TO PARKINSONIAN NEURODEGENERATION
Genetic evidence now implicates tau abnormalities in at least four parkinsonian diseases: FTDP-17, PSP, CBD, and PD. Thus, mutations and polymorphisms in the tau gene are common genetic causes and risk factors for parkinsonian degeneration.

Familial Tauopathies—FTDP-17
Postmortem studies have established a strong correlation between brain tau pathology and neurodegeneration in a large number of heterogenous neurodegenerative diseases, including each of the aforementioned parkinsonian diseases. The import of this correlation has long been debated; however, the absence of other disease-specific neuropathologic hallmarks has suggested the primacy of tau pathology in neurodegeneration. Nonetheless, the possibility that pathology is merely a consequence of neurodegeneration, not its cause, could not be refuted. Controversy on this point continued until 1998, when multiple disease-causing mutations in the

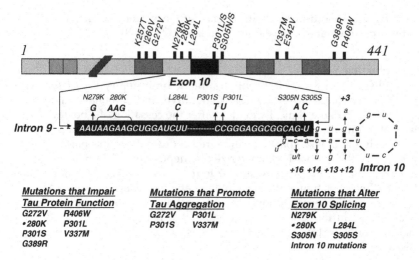

FIGURE 2 Tau mutations cause FTDP-17 by different mechanisms. Tau mutations may lead to neurodegenerative disease by impairing tau's ability to bind to and stabilize microtubules, promoting tau aggregation and altering exon 10 splicing. *Abbreviation*: FTDP-17, frontal temporal dementia with parkinsonism linked to chromosome 17.

tau gene were discovered in FTDP-17 families, thereby providing unambiguous evidence that tau gene abnormalities alone are sufficient to cause neurodegeneration (16,44,56–58). Currently, more than 30 different mutations in the tau gene have been described in over 100 families with FTDP-17 (59). Tau mutations are either missense, deletion or silent mutations in the coding region, or intronic mutations located close to the splice-donor site of the intron following the exon 10. Representative examples of these mutations are shown in Figure 2.

These mutations may lead to neurodegenerative disease by one or more distinct mechanisms, including (*i*) alterations in splicing of tau, leading to abnormal patterns of tau isoform expression (60); (*ii*) compromise of tau's ability to bind to and stabilize microtubules (61,62); and (*iii*) enhanced fibrillization of tau (63). Thus, as illustrated in Figure 3, tau mutations, and by analogy tau dysfunction in sporadic disease, may be pathogenic through mechanisms involving both loss of function (decreased microtubule stabilization) and toxic gain of function (increased fibril formation).

Polymorphisms in the Tau Gene Increase the Risk of Neurodegeneration

A polymorphic intronic dinucleotide repeat in the tau gene has been linked to PSP (64). Indeed, the tau allele *A0* is more frequently found in PSP patients than in healthy controls or AD patients (21). Two extended tau gene haplotypes that include the dinucleotide repeat polymorphism have been described. One of these haplotypes, H1, is significantly overrepresented in PSP patients (19,65–68). The functional consequences resulting from the presence of the H1 or the H2 haplotype remain controversial. Indeed, the haplotype block may also extend beyond the tau gene, so the involvement of polymorphisms in other genes cannot be ruled out.

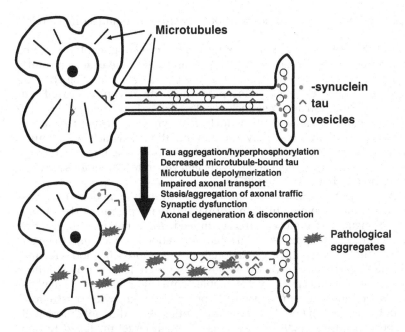

FIGURE 3 Deleterious effects of tau amyloidosis. Tau hyperphosphorylation and aggregation may lead to neuronal dysfunction through a variety of mechanisms, including microtubule depolymerization. This in turn may lead to impaired axonal transport, causing synaptic dysfunction and eventually axonal degeneration.

While the *A0* allele and H1 haplotype of tau were first associated with PSP, it quickly became apparent that they were also associated with CBD (19,65,69,70). Since PSP and CBD share biochemical, neuropathologic, and genetic overlap, these two diseases may ultimately represent different phenotypic manifestations of similar disease processes.

In addition to the association with CBD and PSP, the *A0* allele of tau shows a weak but significant overrepresentation in sporadic PD (71,72). Indeed, one of the regions giving the highest lod scores in genomic screens for PD is 17q21, the region that contains the tau gene, and multiple single-nucleotide polymorphisms in the tau gene are associated with sporadic PD (22). Furthermore, homozygosity for the tau H1 haplotype is associated with a ~57% increased risk of PD (73,74). The H1 haplotype may thus account for ~25% of the population attributable risk for PD (73). The association of tau genotype with PD must be reconciled with the apparent minor contribution of tau pathology to sporadic PD.

SUMMARY AND IMPLICATIONS FOR THERAPEUTIC INTERVENTION

The majority of sporadic and familial parkinsonian degenerative diseases are characterized by both tau protein pathology and an association with mutations or polymorphisms in the tau gene. These human data validate tau as a crucial component of both the genotype and molecular phenotype of parkinsonian neurodegeneration.

Further support for this view has come from both in vitro studies and animal models of neurodegeneration.

Various mechanisms linking tau genotypes to tau protein phenotypes can be proposed to describe pathogenesis in FTDP-17, PSP, and CBD, where tau gene mutations or polymorphisms lead to a predominantly tau-based neuropathology (Fig. 3). But how might tau polymorphisms lead to a predominantly α-synuclein based neuropathology in PD? Since tau and α-synuclein colocalize in Lewy bodies in the PD brain (55) and tau filaments can effectively nucleate α-synuclein filament formation in vitro (27), tau abnormalities may play a role in initiating α-synuclein accumulation in PD. This view is supported by experimental evidence gained from transgenic mice, since mice expressing both tau and α-synuclein generate filamentous amyloid inclusions composed of both proteins (26,27).

If this theory is correct, inhibiting tau filament formation, and/or tau phosphorylation (which may promote filament formation) may be an important therapeutic target for neurodegenerative disease. Indeed, there has been a growing emphasis on designing inhibitors of tau filament formation in an attempt to generate drugs that ameliorate tau pathology. Rationale design approaches and screening of small molecule libraries have revealed a number of different classes of inhibitors (75–78), although in vivo data are not yet available. Similarly, inhibition of tau phosphorylation has presented a tempting target for drug design, with most efforts focused on inhibiting GSK3β (79). However, difficulties generating inhibitors with appropriate specificity for GSK3β as well as issues with target-mediated toxicity complicate this approach.

Data from the subset of FTDP-17 cases caused by mutations in tau that disrupt its ability to appropriately stabilize microtubules suggest an alternative target for therapeutic intervention: stabilization of microtubules (80). Indeed, transgenic mice that overexpress tau accumulate filamentous tau inclusions and show reductions in microtubules and impaired fast axonal transport, accompanied by neurodegeneration and motor weakness (81). When these mice are treated with the microtubule-stabilizing drug paclitaxel they show improvements in microtubule numbers and fast axonal transport, accompanied by amelioration of motor impairments, thus providing in vivo evidence that microtubule-stabilizing drugs may have therapeutic benefit for human tauopathies (82).

The neurodegenerative parkinsonian diseases have long been defined by the properties of the neuropathologic lesions seen in the brain, many of which are comprised of abnormal aggregates of tau. We now know that these tau lesions are not just markers for neurodegenerative diseases, but are intrinsically tied to their pathogenesis. Genetic clues have now come into sharp focus and they have provided a strong rationale for the in vitro experiments, the mouse models, and the epidemiologic studies that have gone a long way toward verifying this hypothesis. Indeed, these experiments have laid a solid groundwork for a number of potential therapeutics that are now in preclinical development. As the efficacy of these tau-targeted drugs is further examined, valuable insights into the etiology of the neurodegenerative parkinsonian diseases will surely be gained.

ACKNOWLEDGMENTS

Studies reviewed here from the laboratory of the authors were supported by grants from the National Institute on Aging and the National Institute of Neurological Disorders and Stroke of the National Institutes of Health (AG-09215, AG-10124,

AG-14382, AG-17586, AG-17628, and NS-44233), the Marian S. Ware Alzheimer Drug Discovery Program and the Picower Foundation. VMYL is the John H. Ware 3rd Professor for Alzheimer's Disease Research and JQT is the William Maul Measey-Truman G. Schnabel Jr. M.D., Professor of Geriatric Medicine and Gerontology.

REFERENCES

1. Trojanowski JQ. Protein mis-folding emerges as a "drugable" target for discovery of novel therapies for neuropsychiatric diseases of aging. Am J Geriatr Psychiatry 2004; 12:134–135.
2. Trojanowski JQ, Goedert M, Iwatsubo T, Lee VM. Fatal attractions: abnormal protein aggregation and neuron death in Parkinson's disease and Lewy body dementia [see comments]. Cell Death & Differentiation 1998; 5:832–837.
3. Forman MS, Trojanowski JQ, Lee VM. Neurodegenerative diseases: a decade of discoveries paves the way for therapeutic breakthroughs. Nat Med 2004; 10:1055–1063.
4. Trojanowski JQ, Lee VM. Parkinson's disease and related alpha-synucleinopathies are brain amyloidoses. Ann N Y Acad Sci 2003; 991:107–110.
5. Spillantini MG, Schmidt ML, Lee VM, Trojanowski JQ, Jakes R, Goedert M. Alpha-synuclein in Lewy bodies. Nature 1997; 388:839–840.
6. Eriksen JL, Dawson TM, Dickson DW, Petrucelli L. Caught in the ac. alpha-synuclein is the culprit in Parkinson's disease. Neuron 2003; 40:453–456.
7. Singleton AB, Farrer M, Johnson J, et al. alpha-Synuclein locus triplication causes Parkinson's disease. Science 2003; 302:841.
8. Polymeropoulos MH, Lavedan C, Leroy E, et al. Mutation in the alpha-synuclein gene identified in families with Parkinson's disease. Science 1997; 276:2045–2047.
9. Goedert M. Familial Parkinson's disease. The awakening of alpha-synuclein. Nature 1997; 388:232–233.
10. Duda JE, Giasson BI, Mabon ME, et al. Concurrence of alpha-synuclein and tau brain pathology in the Contursi kindred. Acta Neuropathol (Berl) 2002; 104:7–11.
11. Lippa CF, Fujiwara H, Mann DM, et al. Lewy bodies contain altered alpha-synuclein in brains of many familial Alzheimer's disease patients with mutations in presenilin and amyloid precursor protein genes. Am J Pathol 1998; 153:1365–1370.
12. Mawal-Dewan M, Schmidt ML, Balin B, Perl DP, Lee VM, Trojanowski JQ. Identification of phosphorylation sites in PHF-Tau from patients with Guam amyotrophic lateral sclerosis/parkinsonism-dementia complex. J Neuropathol Exp Neurol 1996; 55:1051–1059.
13. Reed LA, Schmidt ML, Wszolek ZK, et al. The neuropathology of a chromosome 17-linked autosomal dominant parkinsonism and dementia ("pallido-ponto-nigral degeneration"). J Neuropathol Exp Neurol 1998; 57:588–601.
14. Forman MS, Zhukareva V, Bergeron C, et al. Signature tau neuropathology in gray and white matter of corticobasal degeneration. Am J Pathol 2002; 160:2045–2053.
15. Lee VM, Goedert M, Trojanowski JQ. Neurodegenerative tauopathies. Annu Rev Neurosci 2001; 24:1121–1159.
16. Clark LN, Poorkaj P, Wszolek Z, et al. Pathogenic implications of mutations in the tau gene in pallido-ponto-nigral degeneration and related neurodegenerative disorders linked to chromosome 17. Proc Natl Acad Sci USA 1998; 95:13103–13107.
17. Goedert M, Crowther RA, Spillantini MG. Tau mutations cause frontotemporal dementias. Neuron 1998; 21:955–958.
18. D'Souza I, Poorkaj P, Hong M, et al. Missense and silent tau gene mutations cause frontotemporal dementia with parkinsonism-chromosome 17 type, by affecting multiple alternative RNA splicing regulatory elements. Proc Natl Acad Sci USA 1999; 96:5598–5603.
19. Houlden H, Baker M, Morris HR, et al. Corticobasal degeneration and progressive supranuclear palsy share a common tau haplotype. Neurology 2001; 56:1702–1706.
20. Goedert M, Jakes R. Mutations causing neurodegenerative tauopathies. Biochim Biophys Acta 2005; 1739:240–250.
21. Morris HR, Janssen JC, Bandmann O, et al. The tau gene A0 polymorphism in progressive supranuclear palsy and related neurodegenerative diseases. J Neurol Neurosurg Psychiatry 1999; 66:665–667.

22. Martin ER, Scott WK, Nance MA, et al. Association of single-nucleotide polymorphisms of the tau gene with late-onset Parkinson's disease. JAMA 2001; 286:2245–2250.
23. Oliveira SA, Scott WK, Zhang F, et al. Linkage disequilibrium and haplotype tagging polymorphisms in the Tau H1 haplotype. Neurogenetics 2004; 5:147–155.
24. Lee VM, Giasson BI, Trojanowski JQ. More than just two peas in a pod: common amyloidogenic properties of tau and alpha-synuclein in neurodegenerative diseases. Trends Neurosci 2004; 27:129–134.
25. Kotzbauer PT, Giasson BI, Kravitz AV, et al. Fibrillization of alpha-synuclein and tau in familial Parkinson's disease caused by the A53T alpha-synuclein mutation. Exp Neurol 2004; 187:279–288.
26. Giasson BI, Lee VM, Trojanowski JQ. Interactions of amyloidogenic proteins. Neuromolecular Med 2003; 4:49–58.
27. Giasson BI, Forman MS, Higuchi M, et al. Initiation and synergistic fibrillization of tau and alpha-synuclein. Science 2003; 300:636–640.
28. Frasier M, Walzer M, McCarthy L, et al. Tau phosphorylation increases in symptomatic mice overexpressing A30P alpha-synuclein. Exp Neurol 2005; 192:274–287.
29. Lewis J, McGowan E, Rockwood J, et al. Neurofibrillary tangles, amyotrophy and progressive motor disturbance in mice expressing mutant (P301L) tau protein. Nat Genet 2000; 25:402–405.
30. Vogelsberg-Ragaglia V, Trojanowski JQ, Lee VM-Y. Cell biology of tau and cytoskeletal pathology in Alzheimer's disease. In: RD Terry, R Katzman, KL Bick, SS Sisodia, pp. eds. Alzheimer's Disease. Philadelphia: Lippincot, Williams & Wilkins, 1999:359–72
31. Mandelkow E-M, Mandelkow E. Tau in Alzheimer's disease. Trends in Cell Biology 1998; 8:425.
32. Harada A, Oguchi K, Okabe S, et al. Altered microtubule organization in small-calibre axons of mice lacking tau protein. Nature 1994; 369:488–491.
33. Dickson DW, Bergeron C, Chin SS, et al. Office of Rare Diseases neuropathologic criteria for corticobasal degeneration. J Neuropathol Exp Neurol 2002; 61:935–946.
34. Dickson DW. Neuropathologic differentiation of progressive supranuclear palsy and corticobasal degeneration. J Neurol 1999; 246(Suppl 2):II6–II15.
35. Feany MB, Dickson DW. Neurodegenerative disorders with extensive tau pathology: a comparative study and review. Ann Neurol 1996; 40:139–148.
36. Feany MB, Dickson DW. Widespread cytoskeletal pathology characterizes corticobasal degeneration. Am J Pathol 1995; 146:1388–1396.
37. Hauw JJ, Daniel SE, Dickson D, et al. Preliminary NINDS neuropathologic criteria for Steele-Richardson-Olszewski syndrome (progressive supranuclear palsy). Neurology 1994; 44:2015–2019.
38. Wakabayashi K, Takahashi H. Pathological heterogeneity in progressive supranuclear palsy and corticobasal degeneration. Neuropathology 2004; 24:79–86.
39. van Swieten JC, Stevens M, Rosso SM, et al. Phenotypic variation in hereditary fronto-temporal dementia with tau mutations. Ann Neurol 1999; 46:617–626.
40. Hulette CM, Pericak-Vance MA, Roses AD, et al. Neuropathological features of fronto-temporal dementia and parkinsonism linked to chromosome 17q21-22 (FTDP-17): Duke Family 1684. J Neuropathol Exp Neurol 1999; 58:859–866.
41. Mirra SS, Murrell JR, Gearing M, et al. Tau pathology in a family with dementia and a P301L mutation in tau. J Neuropathol Exp Neurol 1999; 58:335–345.
42. Spillantini MG, Crowther RA, Kamphorst W, Heutink P, van Swieten JC. Tau pathology in two Dutch families with mutations in the microtubule-binding region of tau. Am J Pathol 1998; 153:1359–1363.
43. Spillantini MG, Goedert M. Tau protein pathology in neurodegenerative diseases. Trends Neurosci 1998; 21:428–433.
44. Spillantini MG, Murrell JR, Goedert M, Farlow MR, Klug A, Ghetti B. Mutation in the tau gene in familial multiple system tauopathy with presenile dementia. Proc Natl Acad Sci USA 1998; 95:7737–7741.
45. Buee-Scherrer V, Buee L, Hof PR, et al. Neurofibrillary degeneration in amyotrophic lateral sclerosis/parkinsonism-dementia complex of Guam. Immunochemical characterization of tau proteins. Am J Pathol 1995; 146:924–932.

46. Schmidt ML, Lee VM, Saido T, et al. Amyloid plaques in Guam amyotrophic lateral sclerosis/parkinsonism-dementia complex contain species of A beta similar to those found in the amyloid plaques of Alzheimer's disease and pathological aging. Acta Neuropathologica 1998; 95:117–122.

47. Yamazaki M, Arai Y, Baba M, et al. Alpha-synuclein inclusions in amygdala in the brains of patients with the parkinsonism-dementia complex of Guam. J Neuropathol Exp Neurol 2000; 59:585–591.

48. Forman MS, Schmidt ML, Kasturi S, Perl DP, Lee VM, Trojanowski JQ. Tau and alpha-synuclein pathology in amygdala of Parkinsonism-dementia complex patients of Guam. Am J Pathol 2002; 160:1725–1731.

49. Trojanowski JQ, Ishihara T, Higuchi M, et al. Amyotrophic lateral sclerosis/parkinsonism dementia complex: transgenic mice provide insights into mechanisms underlying a common tauopathy in an ethnic minority on Guam. Exp Neurol 2002; 176:1–11.

50. Jordan BD. Chronic traumatic brain injury associated with boxing. Semin Neurol 2000; 20:179–185.

51. Schmidt ML, Zhukareva V, Newell KL, Lee VM, Trojanowski JQ. Tau isoform profile and phosphorylation state in dementia pugilistica recapitulate Alzheimer's disease. Acta Neuropathol (Berl) 2001; 101:518–524.

52. Hof PR, Bouras C, Buee L, Delacourte A, Perl DP, Morrison JH. Differential distribution of neurofibrillary tangles in the cerebral cortex of dementia pugilistica and Alzheimer's disease cases. Acta Neuropathol (Berl) 1992; 85:23–30.

53. Tokuda T, Ikeda S, Yanagisawa N, Ihara Y, Glenner GG. Re-examination of ex-boxers' brains using immunohistochemistry with antibodies to amyloid beta-protein and tau protein. Acta Neuropathol (Berl) 1991; 82:280–285.

54. Braak H, Rub U, Jansen Steur ENH, Del Tredici K, de Vos RAI. Cognitive status correlates with neuropathologic stage in Parkinson's disease. Neurology 2005; 64:1404–1410.

55. Ishizawa T, Mattila P, Davies P, Wang D, Dickson DW. Colocalization of tau and alpha-synuclein epitopes in Lewy bodies. J Neuropathol Exp Neurol 2003; 62:389–397.

56. Hutton M, Lendon CL, Rizzu P, et al. Association of missense and 5'-splice-site mutations in tau with the inherited dementia FTDP-17. Nature 1998; 393:702–705.

57. Poorkaj P, Bird TD, Wijsman E, et al. Tau is a candidate gene for chromosome 17 fronto-temporal dementia. Ann Neurol 1998; 43:815–825.

58. Dumanchin C, Camuzat A, Campion D, et al. Segregation of a missense mutation in the microtubule-associated protein tau gene with familial frontotemporal dementia and parkinsonism. Hum Mol Genet 1998; 7:1825–1829.

59. Goedert M, Jakes R. Mutations causing neurodegenerative tauopathies. Biochimica et Biophysica Acta (BBA)—Molecular Basis of Disease 2005; 1739:240.

60. D'Souza I, Poorkaj P, Hong M, et al. Missense and silent tau gene mutations cause fronto-temporal dementia with parkinsonism-chromosome 17 type, by affecting multiple alternative RNA splicing regulatory elements. Proc Natl Acad Sci USA 1999; 96:5598–5603.

61. Hasegawa M, Smith MJ, Goedert M. Tau proteins with FTDP-17 mutations have a reduced ability to promote microtubule assembly. FEBS Lett 1998; 437:207–210.

62. Hong M, Zhukareva V, Vogelsberg-Ragaglia V, et al. Mutation-specific functional impairments in distinct tau isoforms of hereditary FTDP-17. Science 1998; 282:1914–1917.

63. Goedert M, Jakes R, Crowther RA. Effects of frontotemporal dementia FTDP-17 mutations on heparin-induced assembly of tau filaments. FEBS Lett 1999; 450:306–311.

64. Conrad C, Andreadis A, Trojanowski JQ, et al. Genetic evidence for the involvement of tau in progressive supranuclear palsy. Ann Neurol 1997; 41:277–281.

65. Pittman AM, Myers AJ, Duckworth J, et al. The structure of the tau haplotype in controls and in progressive supranuclear palsy. Hum Mol Genet 2004; 13:1267–1274.

66. de Silva R, Weiler M, Morris HR, Martin ER, Wood NW, Lees AJ. Strong association of a novel Tau promoter haplotype in progressive supranuclear palsy. Neurosci Lett 2001; 311:145–148.

67. Higgins JJ, Golbe LI, De Biase A, Jankovic J, Factor SA, Adler RL. An extended 5'-tau susceptibility haplotype in progressive supranuclear palsy. Neurology 2000; 55:1364–1367.

68. Baker M, Litvan I, Houlden H, et al. Association of an extended haplotype in the tau gene with progressive supranuclear palsy. Hum Mol Genet 1999; 8:711–715.

69. Di Maria E, Tabaton M, Vigo T, et al. Corticobasal degeneration shares a common genetic background with progressive supranuclear palsy. Ann Neurol 2000; 47:374–377.
70. Pittman AM, Myers AJ, Abou-Sleiman P, et al. Linkage disequilibrium fine-mapping and haplotype association analysis of the tau gene in progressive supranuclear palsy and corticobasal degeneration. J Med Genet 2005; 42:837–846.
71. Pastor P, Ezquerra M, Munoz E, et al. Significant association between the tau gene A0/A0 genotype and Parkinson's disease. Ann Neurol 2000; 47:242.
72. Golbe LI, Lazzarini AM, Spychala JR, et al. The tau A0 allele in Parkinson's disease. Mov Disord 2001; 16:442–447.
73. Healy DG, Abou-Sleiman PM, Lees AJ, et al. Tau gene and Parkinson's disease: a case-control study and meta-analysis. J Neurol Neurosurg Psychiatry 2004; 75:962–965.
74. Mamah CE, Lesnick TG, Lincoln SJ, et al. Interaction of alpha-synuclein and tau genotypes in Parkinson's disease. Ann Neurol 2005; 57:439–443.
75. Wischik CM, Edwards PC, Lai RYK, Roth M, Harrington CR. Selective inhibition of Alzheimer disease-like tau aggregation by phenothiazines. PNAS 1996; 93:11213–11218.
76. Taniguchi S, Suzuki N, Masuda M, et al. Inhibition of heparin-induced tau filament formation by phenothiazines, polyphenols, and porphyrins. J Biol Chem 2005; 280:7614–7623.
77. Chirita C, Necula M, Kuret J. Ligand-dependent inhibition and reversal of tau filament formation. Biochemistry 2004; 43:2879–2887.
78. Pickhardt M, Gazova Z, von Bergen M, et al. Anthraquinones inhibit tau aggregation and dissolve Alzheimer's paired helical filaments in vitro and in cells. J Biol Chem 2005; 280:3628–3635.
79. Bhat RV, Budd Haeberlein SL, Avila J. Glycogen synthase kinase 3: a drug target for CNS therapies. J Neurochem 2004; 89:1313–1317.
80. Lee VM, Daughenbaugh R, Trojanowski JQ. Microtubule stabilizing drugs for the treatment of Alzheimer's disease. Neurobiol Aging 1994; 15 (Suppl 2):S87–S89.
81. Ishihara T, Hong M, Zhang B, et al. Age-dependent emergence and progression of a tauopathy in transgenic mice overexpressing the shortest human tau isoform. Neuron 1999; 24:751–762.
82. Zhang B, Maiti A, Shively S, et al. Microtubule-binding drugs offset tau sequestration by stabilizing microtubules and reversing fast axonal transport deficits in a tauopathy model. PNAS 2005; 102:227–231.

14   The Role of *PARKIN* in Parkinson's Disease

Andrew B. West
Institute for Cell Engineering, Department of Neurology, Johns Hopkins University School of Medicine, Baltimore, Maryland, U.S.A.

Valina L. Dawson
Institute for Cell Engineering, Department of Neurology, Neuroscience, and Physiology, Johns Hopkins University School of Medicine, Baltimore, Maryland, U.S.A.

Ted M. Dawson
Institute for Cell Engineering, Department of Neurology and Neuroscience, Johns Hopkins University School of Medicine, Baltimore, Maryland, U.S.A.

INTRODUCTION TO *PARKIN*-LINKED PARKINSON'S DISEASE

Parkinson's disease (PD) is the most common movement disorder and the second most common neurodegenerative disorder. Patients often present with heterogeneous symptoms, reflecting the underlying complex nature of pathogenesis (1). Prevalent motor-related symptoms include bradykinesia, rigidity, resting tremor, and postural instability due in large part to the loss of pigmented, dopaminergic neurons in the substantia nigra pars compacta (SNpc). However, additional brain regions that influence cognitive decline and other psychiatric conditions are affected both prior and subsequent to neurodegeneration in the midbrain, an important factor when considering pathogenic mechanisms in PD (2). In sporadic disease, lesions first occur in the dorsal motor nucleus of the glossopharyngeal and vagal nerves and anterior olfactory nucleus. Gradually, nuclear grays and cortical areas become affected as the disease process in the brain stem follows an ascending course. Lesions then appear in the anteromedial temporal mesocortex and neocortex, with end-stage dysfunction in first-order sensory association/premotor areas and primary sensory and motor fields (3).

Eosinophilic inclusions containing α-synuclein and ubiquitin are hallmarks of lesions found in PD, present in either the perikarya (Lewy bodies) and/or neuronal processes (Lewy neurites) within many of the remaining neurons in an affected area (4). It is a matter of debate whether the formation of Lewy bodies is a toxic event leading to pathology or whether Lewy bodies are protective by potentially sequestering toxic species. Nevertheless, treatment with L-dopa and dopaminergic agonists through the course of PD provides symptomatic benefit, although the therapy fails to halt disease progression and produces deleterious side effects (5). Therefore PD is a major cause of morbidity and mortality, with significant impact on the economy. While it would appear that the majority of PD patients present without a family history of disease, numerous studies have indicated the importance of underlying genetic susceptibility factors (6,7). In contrast, environmental susceptibilities that provide clear avenues for research have yet to be identified. The identification and isolation of genes that contribute to PD therefore provide a necessary foundation from which exploration of the molecular basis of disease is possible.

It is well-established that the risk for developing PD increases with age, while the disease is uncommon before the age of 30 (8). A genetic locus for juvenile-onset PD, a rare condition confined to patients with age-at-onset of less than 21 years (9) was initially mapped to chromosome 6q25.2–27 in consanguineous Japanese families (10). Examination of Japanese families with positive linkage to 6q25 revealed a proband with a homozygous deletion of a microsatellite marker, and an exon-trapping strategy revealed a nearby expressed-sequence tag belonging to a novel gene dubbed *PARKIN* (11). Homozygous exonic deletions were identified in five additional Japanese juvenile-onset PD patients from four independent families, and mutations in the *PARKIN* gene were identified as the predominant cause of recessively inherited juvenile-onset PD in the Japanese.

The identification of *PARKIN* as a major cause of a PD-like disease with juvenile onset occurred in the scientific wake of the previously discovered mutations in the α-synuclein gene (see Chapters 5 and 6). However, *PARKIN* has since established a unique role in the pathophysiology of PD with mutations now known to occur both in familial and, less commonly, in sporadic cases with both early-onset and late-onset typical PD. *PARKIN* mutations have been identified in nearly every ethnicity and PD case population yet studied, although the genetic link to sporadic PD is still speculative (12). *PARKIN* mutations are usually inherited in a recessive manner, suggesting loss of function genetic alterations (12). Some studies have challenged this notion with the identification of individuals that inherit disease in an apparent dominant manner (13). Genetic studies therefore do not provide an entirely clear mechanism that might be anticipated on a biochemical level. When considering pathogenic mechanisms related to *PARKIN*-linked disease, it is likely that loss of function of the *PARKIN* gene may be only one of several possible scenarios that can result in *PARKIN*-linked PD. The following sections discuss the relationship between *PARKIN*, PD, and neurodegeneration, with a focus on potential cellular mechanisms important in pathogenesis.

CLINICAL PRESENTATION AND PATHOLOGY OF
PARKIN-LINKED DISEASE
Clinical Characterization

The characterization of the clinical and pathological aspects of *PARKIN*-related disease is instrumental in the both design and interpretation of downstream biochemical studies involving *PARKIN* and in understanding *PARKIN*-related pathogenic pathways. If *PARKIN*-proven PD closely resembles the clinical and pathological phenotypes observed in the majority of PD cases, then a close association is more likely to exist between *PARKIN* function and the pathogenic mechanisms occurring in PD. An initial clinical evaluation of *PARKIN*-positive cases revealed that, in general, *PARKIN*-proven PD results in significantly higher frequencies of dystonia and symmetric symptoms, as well as a better and prolonged response to dopamine replacement therapy as compared to PD cases without *PARKIN* mutations (14). In a large study of 146 *PARKIN*-positive cases and 250 *PARKIN*-negative PD cases, a single clinical entity revealing the identity of either group was not identified, illustrating the close overlap between *PARKIN*-positive PD and *PARKIN*-negative PD (15). In this study, *PARKIN*-positive cases again demonstrated an earlier and more symmetrical onset, with elevated rates of dystonia and progression of disease. Differences hypothesized as potential diagnostic indicators of *PARKIN*-positive

PD include a reduced amplitude of the sural nerve sensory action potential in PD-positive cases and the lack of olfactory dysfunction in *PARKIN*-positive PD; however, these studies used relatively few patients and remained to be confirmed (16,17). In general, *PARKIN*-positive disease results in a phenotype that largely overlaps with sporadic PD, although more subtle differences hint that *PARKIN* may be related to and important in the development of sporadic PD but perhaps not the sole determinant of disease in most cases of PD.

Positron Emission Tomography Scanning

In agreement with clinical observations, imaging studies using (^{18}F)-dopa positron-emission tomography (PET) to quantitatively determine the amount of dopaminergic input from the SNpc to the striatum have suggested that *PARKIN*-positive cases resemble that of *PARKIN*-negative cases, although it was noted that a worse clinical outcome might be predicted by PET in *PARKIN* mutation cases than was actually observed (18). Likewise, no correlation between PET data and clinical presentation in *PARKIN* mutation cases was found, whereas cases without *PARKIN* mutations displayed a significant correlation (19). PET scanning performed over a number of years in a family with *PARKIN* mutations revealed a slower disease progression in *PARKIN*-positive cases *versus* cases without *PARKIN* mutations (20). Numerous studies suggest that carriers of a *PARKIN* mutation that are clinically asymptomatic have significantly reduced dopamine input to the striatum as compared with individuals with two normal *PARKIN* alleles (21–23). These observations favor the loss of function model of *PARKIN* pathogenesis and haploinsufficiency model of genetic inheritance. Taken together, PET scans in *PARKIN*-positive cases are similar to *PARKIN*-negative cases, illustrating the inability of PET to accurately predict *PARKIN* mutations. Further, PET studies demonstrate the phenotypic similarity between PD caused by *PARKIN* mutations and sporadic *PARKIN*-negative PD (24).

Neuropathologic Characterization

Ultimately, the neuropathological examination of *PARKIN*-positive cases may provide the most useful information toward understanding the pathogenic mechanisms in *PARKIN*-positive PD. The first reports of neuropathology in *PARKIN*-proven disease revealed a near-complete loss of pigmented dopaminergic neurons of the SNpc, reminiscent of advanced cases of sporadic PD (25). Autopsy of Japanese juvenile-onset *PARKIN*-positive PD showed that neuronal loss and gliosis were restricted to the SNpc and locus ceruleus, surprisingly without accompanying Lewy pathology (26). Other Japanese juvenile-onset PD cases in addition to a Dutch early-onset *PARKIN*-positive case were again described without Lewy pathology, although both cases demonstrated tau-positive neurofibrillary tangles (27,28). As Lewy pathology is a hallmark feature of PD, the lack of α-synuclein positive inclusions in *PARKIN*-positive cases suggests that the biochemical defects caused by mutations in the *PARKIN* gene are distinct on a cellular level as compared to the dysfunctional pathways occurring in *PARKIN*-negative PD. Challenging this notion is the identification of two unrelated *PARKIN*-positive PD cases that demonstrated widespread Lewy pathology in the SNpc and locus ceruleus (29,30). In addition, a Japanese juvenile-onset PD case was reported with Lewy pathology, although α-synuclein positive inclusions were restricted to the pedunculopontine nucleus (31). The *PARKIN*-positive cases with Lewy pathology were of relatively old age compared to *PARKIN*-positive cases without Lewy pathology, perhaps suggesting that the formation of Lewy bodies requires advanced age in most cases. Thus, *PARKIN*-positive cases demonstrate pleomorphic pathology with an unclear role in the formation of Lewy pathology, and, again, do not provide clear direction for biochemical analysis. Disease and pathologic lesions are clearly not restricted to the dopaminergic neurons of the substantia nigra in either *PARKIN*-linked PD or *PARKIN*-negative PD, and pathogenic mechanisms must attempt to account for widespread alterations, including degeneration in the peripheral nervous system. Thus, clinical and pathologic manifestation due to *PARKIN* mutation reveal a disease entity closely overlapping with sporadic PD, but distinct (albeit inconsistent) differences between *PARKIN*-positive and -negative disease suggest some divergence of pathogenic pathways relating to disease.

PARKIN GENE STRUCTURE AND REGULATION
Cellular Localization
Clinical, pathologic, and genetic studies suggest that *PARKIN*-linked disease is due to the loss of *PARKIN* expression and function in the majority of *PARKIN*-positive cases. Understanding the normal function of *PARKIN* would provide the initial foundation from which a biochemical pathway important to pathogenesis might be identified. Physiologically relevant gene function is usually tied to both regulation and localization of the protein product. In understanding potential pathogenic mechanisms related to mutations in the *PARKIN* gene, the normal function and distribution of *PARKIN* must be considered. Similar to the known genes associated with PD, such as α-synuclein and *UCHL-1*, *PARKIN* expression in the brain is largely restricted to neurons in both rodents and humans. In situ hybridization experiments demonstrate a broad distribution of *PARKIN* across the brain, with few non-neuronal cells expressing any appreciable amounts of *PARKIN* transcript (32,33). Importantly, the neurons susceptible to degeneration in *PARKIN*-positive disease robustly express *PARKIN*, with overlapping expression patterns of α-synuclein transcript, although *PARKIN* is also highly expressed in many brain nuclei and other organs that are presumably not affected in *PARKIN*-proven disease (34).

Antibodies raised to the *PARKIN* protein demonstrated a 50–52 kDa protein expressed in the cytosol and neuronal processes in the brain (35). Alternative splicing in *PARKIN* mRNA has been described, but likely does not constitute even a small fraction of total *PARKIN* transcript produced in the brain and no alternative protein isoforms due to splicing have been identified. Subcellular fractionation demonstrates a broad distribution of *PARKIN* protein in neurons with apparent affinity for membranes, although *PARKIN* itself is not a transmembrane protein (36). *PARKIN* is largely excluded from the nucleus, but rather associates with such components as cellular vesicles, transgolgi network, endoplasmic reticulum, and lipid rafts in postsynaptic densities (36,37). In cultured cortical neurons, *PARKIN* colocalizes to postsynaptic densities and associates with several proteins present in lipid rafts (37). The majority of Lewy bodies in PD brains were initially described as not immunoreactive with antibodies directed against *PARKIN* (38,39). Other experiments employing different antibodies suggest that *PARKIN* is present in the central core of the majority of Lewy bodies in PD (40,41).

Transcription Regulation
Transcription regulation is the primary tool with which cells tightly control downstream expression, and it often divulges the endogenous function of the associated

gene. For example, genes involved in the unfolded protein or heat-shock response may experience several orders of magnitude transcription up-regulation during critical times where such reaction is required for survival. Unfortunately, endogenous *PARKIN* expression is not tied to cell processes that immediately indicate a biochemical role for *PARKIN* in the pathogenesis of PD. Of note, *PARKIN* expression is restricted to the latest stages of embryonic development, a feature of *PARKIN* transcription regulation that is evolutionarily conserved in humans, rodents, xenopus, fugu, and drosophila (42–45). In the mouse brain, *PARKIN* expression closely tracts with neuronal maturation with the first appearance of mRNA at E10/12 followed by a marked increase in neuronal expression until adulthood (46). This feature was confirmed in humans and can also be demonstrated in vitro in neuroblastoma differentiated with retinioic acid (43).

Biochemical analysis of the *PARKIN* promoter revealed a compact CpG island that controls a second gene in the antisense orientation to *PARKIN*, although the encoded protein of the antisense gene, *PACRG*, does not appear to directly interact with *PARKIN* (47). The majority of transcription up-regulation appears to map to a region controlled in part by the myc family of transcription factors (47). In particular, the oncogene *N-myc* was identified as controlling *PARKIN* expression in neurons and may be responsible in combination with other transcription factors for the regulation of *PARKIN* during cellular maturation. Despite initial expectations that *PARKIN* may be a protective element highly responsive to various cellular stressors, numerous studies suggest *PARKIN* expression is constitutive, albeit in mature cells. Therefore, the biological regulation of *PARKIN* has not yet revealed a role for *PARKIN* protein, but implies function in the transition and maintenance of a postmitotic state.

Protein Turnover

While *PARKIN* transcription appears to be related to cellular maturation, *PARKIN* protein itself does not appear to be tightly controlled via degradation once expressed. *PARKIN* protein in the brain, while not particularly abundant, appears to exhibit a very long half life of at least five days or more ([48] and unpublished observations, ABW). The long-lived *PARKIN* protein in neurons may in fact be out of range for standard assays that estimate half life, although exogenous overexpressed *PARKIN* in cell lines displays a much shorter half life of five hours (49). Interestingly, *PARKIN* may be degraded by the ubiquitin proteasome system as exogenous ubiquitinated *PARKIN* has been detected, although no factors involved in endogenous *PARKIN* degradation have yet been described (50). Toward this end, in vitro data suggest that the ubiquitin-protein isopeptide ligase Nrdp1/FLRF may regulate *PARKIN* turnover (49). As with many proteins expressed in mammalian cells, the N-terminal amino acids of *PARKIN* (localized to the UbL domain) appear to define at least overexpressed *PARKIN* protein levels but apparently are not critical for E3 ligase–like activity (51).

In vitro ubquitination assays, as with other RING-(really interesting new gene) finger-containing proteins, show that exogenous *PARKIN* readily autoubiquitinates. However, *PARKIN* autoubiquitination is likely restricted to multiple monoubiquitination as opposed to attaching ubiquitin chains required for degradation (as is discussed in upcoming sections), thereby obscuring the physiological potential for autoregulation (52). One factor perhaps important in *PARKIN* turnover is the apparent shift in *PARKIN* solubility that occurs with age in humans. In young human brain, *PARKIN* protein is present in the high salt-extractable fraction as well as the SDS-extractable fraction, but in aged brain, *PARKIN* protein shifts to the SDS-extractable fraction, indicating a change in solubility (38). In contrast, α-synuclein undergoes an apparent age-related stabilization that may result in increased total synuclein protein (53). Thus, *PARKIN* levels may effectively decrease with age while α-synuclein protein increases, although the factors governing these alterations are unknown.

PARKIN AND THE UBIQUITIN SYSTEM
PARKIN as an E3 Ligase

Upon initial characterization of the *PARKIN* gene open-reading frame, a protein-domain homology search revealed that the most likely function of the *PARKIN* protein involves E3 ligase activity due to the presence of two conserved RING fingers near the C-terminus and homology to the ubiquitin molecule itself near the N-terminus. RING-finger domains are found in several other known E3 ligase proteins such as the MDM2 protein which targets p53 for degradation and the BRCA1 protein which functions in a number of ubiquitin-dependent pathways (11). E3 ubiquitin ligases are thought to comprise an exceptionally large family of proteins in mammals, perhaps one thousand or more encoded in the human genome, and are classified into three distinct types: N-end rule E3s; E3s containing the HECT (Homology to E6AP C-Terminus) domain; and E3's containing RING fingers (by far the most common E3-ligase protein). In an initial functional assessment of enzymatic activity, *PARKIN* interacted with the E2 ubiquitin ligase UbcH7 and UbcH8 and promoted ubiquitination in, in vitro assays while mutations associated with PD abrogated the E3-ligase-like activity (54). In understanding the function of *PARKIN* in the pathogenesis of PD, the role of *PARKIN* as an E3 ligase became the focus of research.

The RING finger motifs identified in the *PARKIN* protein are defined as a linear series of conserved cysteine and histidine residues, $Cys-X_2-Cys-X_{9-39}-Cys-X_{1-3}-Cys/His-X_2-Cys-X_{4-48}-Cys-X_2-Cys$, where X can be any amino acid (55). Although there is high conservation in the cysteine and histidine residues, there is disparate conservation between the remaining sequence structures among proteins containing RING fingers. RING fingers bind two zinc atoms in a cross-brace arrangement, and are known to be essential protein protein interaction domains (55). *PARKIN* contains two RING finger domains (otherwise known as a TRIAD motif) where the second RING finger binds only a single zinc atom with resemblance to a zinc-ribbon motif and may be principally responsible for E3 ligase activity (56). Many RING-finger-containing proteins are known to possess autoubiquitination properties in addition to binding to an often daunting number of cellular targets as evident by BRCA1-related research. The suggestion is that the RING-finger classification of E3 ligases could potentially imply a role in diverse cellular processes for the host protein thereby preventing an obvious understanding of *PARKIN* function.

While the presence of two RING-finger domains within *PARKIN* suggests functionality in ubiquitin-dependent pathways, the presence of an ubiquitin-like (UbL) domain near the N-terminus strongly suggests the ability of *PARKIN* to interact directly with the proteasome. As opposed to RING-finger domains, UbL domains are rarely encoded in the human proteasome, present in just 62 proteins, although only ~25% of these proteins contain the residues necessary to directly bind the proteasome (57). The *PARKIN* UbL encodes the rare proteasome-interacting motif and might be thought of in a conventional way to facilitate the delivery of either autoubiquitinated protein or ubiquitinated substrate protein to the proteasome for degradation.

Since the UbL domain is also present in non-E3 ligase proteins, such as ataxin-1 or zinc-finger-containing transcription factors (57), the interaction of *PARKIN*'s UbL domain and the proteasome may have altogether novel biochemical significance apart from models where *PARKIN* simply chaperones proteins to the proteasome. Indeed, the vast majority of E3 ligases accomplish efficient degradation of target substrates without a UbL domain. While the classification of *PARKIN* as an E3 ligase based on protein homology helped to focus downstream experimentation, a broad number of diverse cellular roles may still be attributed to the encoded protein domains thereby requiring the identification of physiological substrates and biochemical pathways to understand the role of *PARKIN* in neurodegeneration.

The Ubiquitin System

In understanding the role of *PARKIN* in the ubiquitin system and as an E3 ligase, a brief background concerning the ubiquitin molecule is helpful. Ubiquitin is a 76–amino acid protein produced from a number of ubiquitin precursor proteins encoded in the human genome and can be covalently attached to the lysine residue of substrate proteins in a process called ubiquitination. The process of ubiquitination occurs through the transfer of an ubiquitin molecule from an activated E1 enzyme to the conjugating E2 enzyme, where an E3 ligase catalyzes the transfer of the ubiquitin molecule from the E2 enzyme to a target substrate (58). The E3 enzyme usually confers substrate specificity and acts as a scaffold to facilitate the stoichiometric requirements of the covalent attachment of ubiquitin. The ubiquitin chain elongation factors, otherwise known as E4s, can catalyze the multiubiquitination of proteins bound to the E2 and E3 complexes.

The ubiquitination reaction may end with the attachment of a single ubiquitin molecule, a process called monoubiquitination, or the attachment of a ubiquitin molecule to several lysine residues in the target protein (multiple monoubiquitination). E3 ligase proteins can also promote the attachment of ubiquitin molecules to lysine residues in the ubiquitin molecule already attached to a target substrate (most famously on lysine residues 48 or 63 in the ubiquitin molecule) to form a chain arrangement of ubiquitin molecules. Pioneering work classically describes a role for many of the E3 ligases in the human genome as catalyzing the formation of lysine-48-linked ubiquitin chains on target proteins, a particular arrangement of ubiquitin that is efficiently recognized and degraded by the 26S proteasome. A 26S proteasome comprises a multisubunit protein complex with proteolytic activity localized on the inside of a barrel-shaped core complex dubbed the 20S complex. A 19S cap located on either end of the 20S complex can recognize lysine-48 chains composed of at least 4 ubiquitin molecules or more and unfold the ubiquitinated protein into the inner chamber of the 20S complex. Within the complex, the target protein is proteolytically cleaved in an ATP-dependent manner into small peptides that are released into the cytosol for further metabolism.

The ubiquitin system is responsible for the majority of targeted protein turnover in eukaryotic cells. As such, the proteasome is estimated to metabolize up to 30% of newly synthesized proteins via polyubiquitination that are likely improperly folded and therefore have the potential to form deleterious tertiary structures that would be difficult for a cell to metabolize (59). Besides a general housekeeping role, the ubiquitin-proteasome system degrades proteins as a means of functional control of downstream targets due to highly efficient and rapid turnover. For example, most components of the cell cycle are metabolized in a tightly controlled manner via ubiquitination and degradation. Disruption of the proteasome during cell cycle progression leads to immediate cell death through deregulating the rapid and coordinated turnover of target proteins, a feature of the ubiquitin system currently being exploited in cancer therapy (60).

As previously mentioned, at least four lysine-48-linked ubiquitin molecules are required for efficient degradation by the proteasome, implying other nondegradation roles for lysine-63-linked chains and mono/di/tri ubiquitination. In the case of the "noncanonical" attachment of ubiquitin to target substrates (e.g., anything other than lysine-48-linked chains), biological significance is still studied on a case by case basis and is largely unrecognized in most studies and perhaps underappreciated in general. In a number of proteins, monoubiquitination/diubiquitination robustly affects intracellular trafficking, perhaps implying a general mechanism albeit one that is awaiting confirmation from additional studies (61). Monoubiquitination likely provides an altered protein interaction surface thereby conferring the specificity of the trafficking to the proper cellular compartment (62). Indeed monoubiquitination of histones has been hypothesized as robustly regulating gene expression (although not necessarily trafficking) due to an altered surface confirmation acting as a scaffold for other proteins that influence the accessibility of chromatin and the factors involved in transcription (63). Ironically, the first description of the ubiquitin molecule covalently attached to a protein substrate involved monoubiquitination of a histone protein (64), a phenomenon that may be regarded today as a "noncanonical" role for ubiquitin.

Further complicating the understanding of ubiquitin chains is at least circumstantial evidence that may form as a mixture of lysine-63 and lysine-48-linked chains, the proportion defining the fate of the target protein. Lysine-63-linked polyubiquitination of proteins has been described as modifying downstream functionality of target proteins effecting such processes as postreplicative DNA repair, IkBα kinase activation, translational regulation, and some instances of endocytosis, although the mechanistic role of ubiquitin chains in these processes remains unknown (65). Polyubiquitination of Met4, a bZIP transcription factor involved in regulating methionine biosynthesis, inactivates Met4 due to both preventing recruitment of a coactivator, Cbf1, and comprising the ability of Met4 to bind to a subclass of target promoters (66,67). Lysine-63-linked polyubiquitination of Myc alters the transcriptional properties and suggests that the chains contribute to the switch between an activating and a repressive state of the protein (68). On the other hand, polyubiquitination is not always inhibitory of downstream function since ubiquitination of the HIVTat protein by Hdm2 enhances its ability to activate transcription (69).

Thus, the biological significance of the attachment of one or many ubiquitin molecules on a target protein can range from degradation to enzymatic activation of the target, an important consideration in interpreting *PARKIN*-related research. Many E3 ligase proteins are capable of conjugating ubiquitin molecules in a number of ways depending on the substrate target, the E2 ligase, and any other potential cofactors (such as E4 molecules) that regulate specificity. Ultimately, the effect of ubiquitination is defined by assessing downstream function of the target protein, be it degradation, functional activation, or inactivation.

Substrates and Interacting Proteins

RING-finger-containing E3 ubiquitin ligases are known to exist as single polypeptide or multimeric complexes and interact with an ubiquitin-conjugating enzyme

(E2) in facilitating the transfer of an ubiquitin molecule to a substrate. *PARKIN* can utilize both the ubiquitin-conjugating enzymes Ubc-H7 and Ubc-H8 and the endoplasmic-reticulum-associated E2s UBC6 and UBC7 (54,70,71). Additionally, *PARKIN* interacts with the E2 complex UbcH13/Uev1 in mediating lysine-63-linked polymerization of ubiquitin (72). The E2 enzymes interact with the RING-IBR (in between RING finger)-RING domain of *PARKIN* and have been hypothesized to mediate in part the nature of *PARKIN* ubiquitination activity, determining whether a substrate is polyubiqutinated (lysine 48 or 63) or monoubiquitinated (71,73). UbcH13 is the only described E2 ligase protein with the ability to promote lysine-63-linked chains, thus the selection of the E2 enzyme utilized by *PARKIN* may be critical toward exacting a *PARKIN*-mediated event. The cofactors that determine the choice of a particular E2 enzyme are not yet known. The UbL domain may facilitate *PARKIN* function through interactions with the Rpn10 subunit of the 26S proteasome, while the C-terminal region of *PARKIN* can interact with the α4 subunit of the 20S proteasome (74,75). Recombinant *PARKIN* purified from *E. coli* retains autoubiquitination activity in vitro suggesting that post-translational modifications or associations with other proteins apart from an E2 enzyme are not absolutely required (76).

Toward the identification of substrates of *PARKIN* E3 ligase activity, a number of groups utilized yeast two-hybrid technology with human brain libraries to attempt identify proteins that directly bind to *PARKIN*. The simplest model of *PARKIN*-linked disease might involve the accumulation of a toxic substance in human cells that *PARKIN* normally degrades. The first test is usually whether *PARKIN* ubiquitinates a target and whether this ubiquitination promotes degradation. The first *PARKIN* substrate identified, CDCrel-1, belongs to a family of GTPases called septins and is robustly expressed in the nervous system where it associates with synaptic vesicles, although mice deficient in CDCrel-1 do not display a phenotype (71,77). Overexpression of CDCrel-1 in neurons by adeno-associated viral transfer induced neurodegeneration, although there is limited evidence that CDCrel-1 accumulates in the absence of *PARKIN* and that *PARKIN* modulates CDCrel-1 levels in vivo (78,79).

A novel gene isolated in a yeast hybrid screen dubbed *PARKIN*-associated endothelin receptor-like receptor (Pael-R) is a putative G-protein-coupled transmembrane protein with homology to the endothelin receptor type B (70). As opposed to *PARKIN*, Pael-R is primarily expressed in oligodendrocytes but present in a lower level in some populations of neurons including dopaminergic neurons. Exogenous overexpressed Pael-R induces the unfolded stress response in cultured cells and loses solubility with increased expression. Coexpressed *PARKIN* abrogates the formation of insoluble Pael-R presumably through an ubiquitination-dependent mechanism. Lending some credibility to neurodegenerative specificity, pan-neuronal overexpression of human Pael-R in *Drosophila* causes age-dependent selective degeneration of dopaminergic neurons (80), but limited evidence suggests that *PARKIN* is indeed a native physiologic factor responsible for regulating levels of Pael-R.

In a candidate screening approach, *PARKIN* was found to interact with and ubiquitinate the synphilin-1 protein, which promoted the formation of protein aggregates when overexpressed with α-synuclein in cell culture (81). In follow-up reports, *PARKIN* mediated the formation of lysine-63-linked polyubiquitin chains onto synphilin and only formed lysine-48-linked chains at an unusually high *PARKIN* to synphilin-1 overexpression ratio or when primed for lysine-48-linked ubiquitination (73). In this case, *PARKIN* appears to mediate a proteasome-independent modification of synphilin, with unknown physiological consequence. Another substrate of *PARKIN* activity identified through yeast-hybrid interaction with *PARKIN*, JTV1 or p38 or AIMP2, was identified in Lewy bodies in PD (82). In vitro experiments demonstrated that overexpressed *PARKIN* can promote the degradation of overexpressed AIMP2 presumably via polyubiquitination and proteasome degradation. In a follow-up analysis, a significant up-regulation in the levels of AIMP2 was identified in both PD and *PARKIN*-null mice, suggesting *PARKIN* as a physiologic factor in the degradation of endogenous AIMP2 thereby setting this substrate apart from other proteins (83). Since AIMP2 is a ubiquitous protein implicated in protein biogenesis, the potential involvement in the development of PD remains to be understood.

Other *PARKIN* substrates have been identified via yeast-two hybrid and confirmed with coimmunoprecipitation and in vitro ubiquitination experiments. *PARKIN* interacts with α/β tubulin heterodimers and microtubules and acts to stabilize microtubule formation, potentially in an ubiquitin-dependent manner (84). In vitro steady-state levels of synaptotagmin XI expression are decreased in the presence of *PARKIN*, and protein aggregates in PD were found immunoreactive for synaptotagmin XI (85). SEPT5_v2/CDCrel-2, another member of the septin family and a close homolog to CDCrel-1, has been reported as a *PARKIN* substrate and may accumulate in disease brains (86). In another study, *PARKIN* was found to interact with cyclin E in the context of a protein complex including hSel-10 and Cullin-1, and found to prevent the accumulation of cyclin E in kainate acid-treated neurons (87). *PARKIN* also binds to the RanBP2 protein in overexpression cell culture models and apparently influences the downstream ability of exogenous RanBP2 to sumoylate the HDAC4 protein due to ubiquitination of RanBP2 via *PARKIN* (88).

In yeast hybrid and immunoprecipitation experiments, *PARKIN* interacts with a plethora of diverse proteins implicated in any number of cellular pathways. The majority of substrates are understood only by a limited number of experiments that, in general, fail to determine the effects of ubiquitination on the function of the host protein and whether the interaction has physiological relevance. Historically, an E3 ligase substrate is verified on an endogenous level by confirmation of robust up-regulation and accumulation of substrate (but not mRNA) in an E3 enzyme knockout or knock-down animal or disease model. The mouse *PARKIN* knockout model has not demonstrated a robust up-regulation of any protein as evident by several proteomic screens (78). *PARKIN* does not robustly degrade any of the identified substrates in vivo, even in the case of AIMP2 protein *PARKIN* can influence only a small proportion of total protein and then with considerable variation between matched animals (83). This is in stark opposition to dozens of described E3 ligase interactions, most famously MDM2 and p53, where the presence of the E3 ligase produces an immediate and efficient turnover of nearly all of the substrate protein when present on an equimolar level.

In the case of several of the known substrates of *PARKIN*, ubiquitination occurs in noncanonical lysine-63-linked chains or multiple monoubiquitination not linked to substrate degradation, suggesting that *PARKIN* may not robustly control the levels of any given protein substrate. When synphilin-1 and α-synuclein are cooverexpressed, a condition which forms aggregates in cells, *PARKIN* mediates ubiquitination via lysine-63 linkages and that the formation of the aggregates is enhanced by lysine-63-linked ubiquitination (73). These studies suggest *PARKIN* is involved in a number of cellular pathways independent of proteasome-mediated degradation, perhaps akin to the RING-finger-containing BRCA1 protein, another E3 ligase important in human disease that does not appear to robustly regulate the level of any particular protein. In addition, only a fraction of mutations known to cause *PARKIN*-linked disease, particularly those outside of the RING domains, appear to affect the E3 ligase activity of *PARKIN*, as will be discussed in upcoming sections. Further examination of the functional consequence of *PARKIN* enzymatic activity, particularly those functions which are independent of protein degradation, may help clarify the true downstream functions and better define the interaction of *PARKIN* with the known substrates.

FUNCTIONAL CHARACTERIZATION OF *PARKIN* PROTEIN
Neuroprotection from α-synuclein

The primary mechanisms of neurodegeneration relevant to PD are largely unknown. Oxidative stress, mitochondrial impairment, α-synucleinopathy, and proteasome dysfunction are all considered potential primary mechanisms of pathogenesis (89,90). Since the *PARKIN* gene is important in susceptibility to at least a subset of PD cases, understanding how *PARKIN* expression might protect a cell from exposures that would otherwise mediate neurodegeneration may help refine the general understanding of pathogenesis in PD. However, *PARKIN* is ubiquitously expressed throughout mammalian organisms and may have divergent and distinct roles in local environments, making a general classification of *PARKIN* function a difficult task.

Numerous groups have focused efforts on determining whether *PARKIN* expression might provide protection in various cell-death and PD-model systems, and in a handful of more refined studies, how mutations linked to *PARKIN* PD affect *PARKIN* neuroprotection. Since models of PD arguably do not recapitulate the core components of the PD, such as progressive loss of neurons with accompanying Lewy pathology, *PARKIN* function has been studied in diverse assays and paradigms, some with questionable relevance to pathogenic mechanisms in PD. As discussed in other chapters, α-synuclein expression appears important for susceptibility to PD. Likewise, genetic and biochemical studies suggest loss of *PARKIN* expression is associated with increased susceptibility to PD, perhaps in an even more potent way than α-synuclein overexpression as evident by the earlier onset of *PARKIN* -linked disease in humans. Some evidence suggests that *PARKIN* can directly interact with rare posttranslation modified forms of α-synuclein, although the physiologic impact of the interaction is completely unknown (91). Therefore, a number of studies attempt to characterize a functional interaction between *PARKIN* and α-synuclein that are justified on a genetic and pathologic level even if the functions of either α-synuclein or *PARKIN* and how they might interact are not understood.

Genetic models of PD that recapitulate at least dopaminergic cell death involve viral transfer of mutant or wild type human α-synuclein into systems containing catecholaminergic neurons. Viral transduction by either adeno-associated virus or lentivirus can result in profound and progressive loss of TH immunoreactivity and cell loss in rats (92,93). When human wild-type *PARKIN* is introduced into this model via lentiviral transduction, TH immunoreactivity is significantly preserved thereby implicating *PARKIN* as protecting against α-synuclein-specific toxicity (94). Another study utilizing adeno-associated virus reported similar findings, but in both studies the effects of mutations linked to *PARKIN*-positive PD were not studied, and, instead, viral transduction was normalized to overexpressed fluorescent protein (95). In contrast, lentiviral transduction of human GDNF did not significantly protect against α-synuclein overexpression, perhaps implying a more specific role for *PARKIN*-mediated neuroprotection with implications in designing therapeutic strategies for PD (96).

In primary mouse midbrain cultures, HSV-mediated overexpression of α-synuclein resulted in catecholaminergic selective–cell death, and concomitant *PARKIN* expression afforded some protection from both α-synuclein and proteasome inhibition (97). Follow-up studies in cell lines suggest that the protection over-expressed *PARKIN* provides from overexpressed α-synuclein is independent of the proteasome, perhaps through activation of various proteases such as calpain that may metabolize overexpressed α-synuclein (98). In contrast, overexpression of *PARKIN* in SH-SY5Y cells protected from α-synuclein expression corresponding with the appearance of higher-molecular-weight (as opposed to cleaved) α-synuclein (99). Various in vitro studies have failed to identify a direct interaction between α-synuclein and parkin, as the two proteins cannot bind one another in most assays or influence protein turnover in an obvious way (100). In a genetic cross between *PARKIN*-knockout mice and α-synuclein overexpressing mice, the toxic-ity and phenotype associated with mutant α-synuclein was not affected by the loss of *PARKIN* (101). Indeed, little biochemical evidence suggests that the loss of *PARKIN* expression influences overexpressed α-synuclein toxicity as might be assumed from studies employing the reverse context, namely overexpressing both *PARKIN* and α-synuclein. The implication is that *PARKIN* may acquire novel (perhaps nonspecific) attributes when expressed at nonphysiologic concentra-tions. Additional studies concerning endogenous *PARKIN* seem required to understand a role in the largely unidentified α-synuclein toxicity pathway.

Versatile Neuroprotection

Loss of function mutations in human *PARKIN*, such as large deletions that span multiple *PARKIN* exons, can result in a phenotype highly reminiscent of idiopathic PD. Given this selectivity in pathology, specificity of *PARKIN*-mediated influence on a refined number of cellular pathways might be presumed. *PARKIN*-mediated protection from α-synuclein does not necessarily preclude the involvement of *PARKIN* in a number of biochemical processes, particularly since the pathways associated with α-synuclein toxicity are unknown. Therefore, a number of groups have studied the effect of *PARKIN* overexpression in cell line models challenged with a variety of stressors.

In *PARKIN*-inducible PC-12 cell lines, *PARKIN* significantly protected from mitochondrial swelling associated with ceramide or serum withdrawal, but no protection was observed with a variety of other inducers of oxidative stress or the unfolded protein response (102). Mitochondrial impairment, although not neces-sarily localized to the brain, has been implicated in a number of *PARKIN*-null animal models lending additional credibility that *PARKIN* may ultimately influence mitochondrial health through multiple unknown intermediaries (103,104). In pri-mary neuronal cultures, *PARKIN* overexpression was associated with protection from excitotoxicity caused by kainic acid exposure (87). In transiently transfected SH-SY5Y cells, *PARKIN* protected from manganese-induced cell death accompa-nied by a redistribution of *PARKIN* protein from a largely cytoplasmic configuration to concentration at the perinuclear region (105). Reorganization of overexpressed *PARKIN* into perinuclear concentrations or centrosomal localization also occurs in cells exposed to proteasome inhibitors, suggesting a general mechanism that impacts *PARKIN* localization and function during cell death (106,107). *PARKIN* also protects from cell death elicited by exposure to high concentrations of dopamine accompanied by activation of the c-Jun-terminal kinase (JNK) and caspase-3 pathways (108). Although these studies demonstrate *PARKIN* neuroprotection, they largely fail to provide a specific and physiologically proven molecular mechanism.

Some studies that attempt to dissect *PARKIN* function further show that *PARKIN* inhibits the JNK signaling pathway in an E3-activity-dependent manner and that JNK is activated in cells expressing mutant *PARKIN* (109). Although *PARKIN* E3 ligase activity may be required for *PARKIN*-mediated neuroprotection, the E3 ligase activity may not be associated with proteasome degradation pathways. *PARKIN* has been described in a number of cell lines to protect cells against death initiated by proteasome impairment (97,110). This paradox may best be rationalized by assuming that, at least in the case of delaying cell death associated with proteasome inhibition, physiologically relevant *PARKIN* function may be independent of the proteasome and protein degradation. This notion is supported by in vitro data suggesting that *PARKIN* typically forms ubiquitin linkages not recognized for degradation through the proteasome, as discussed in earlier in this chapter. In other studies that attribute a more generalized role for *PARKIN* protection, a *PARKIN*-inducible glial cell line showed that a reduction in induced *PARKIN* was accompanied by increased susceptibility to apoptotic and necrotic cell death with partial overlap to caspase-dependent pathways (111). However, on a more physiologically relevant *PARKIN*-null background, *PARKIN* knockout mice were subjected to acute MPTP treatment and proteasome inhibitors and dopaminergic cell death was comparable to wild type mice (Bobby Thomas, VLD and TMD, unpublished data). In this experimental paradigm, the loss of *PARKIN* function did not increase susceptibility to either proteasome inhibitors or acute MPTP treatment, thereby suggesting cell line models of *PARKIN* overexpression may not necessarily recapitulate in vivo experiments.

Finally, a number of studies attempt to compose a more complete hypothesis regarding the relationship of *PARKIN* to neurodegeneration by determining whether overexpression of *PARKIN* interacting substrates may be toxic to cells and whether *PARKIN* overexpression may alleviate the toxicity. Some evidence suggests that CDCrel-1 overexpression via viral transduction in rat brain may initiate degeneration specific to dopaminergic cells, and *PARKIN* overexpression in cell lines rescues cells from overexpressed CDCrel-1 (79,112). Similarly, overexpression of hypothesized *PARKIN* substrates Pael-R and AIMP2 causes dopaminergic-specific cell death in model systems (80,83). Other hypothesized substrates capable of inducing neurodegeneration include cyclin E and overexpression of both synphilin and α-synuclein (81,87). Lastly, *PARKIN* protects against and promotes the clearance of an expanded polygluatmine fragment (113). In most experiments, coexpression of *PARKIN* and the interacting substrate significantly protects against the toxicity associated with overexpression of the hypothesized substrate. It is difficult to reconcile a common biochemical pathway among the interacting substrates and there is no clear pre-existing genetic or biochemical data that might elevate a particular substrate to a more important status, with the possible exception of synphilin due to the robust interaction with α-synuclein. Also, the apparent specificity for dopaminergic neuronal toxicity for substrate-overexpression studies does not account for the degeneration occurring in other regions of the brain in human disease. Thus, *PARKIN* neuroprotection may be most relevant to PD in protecting against interacting substrates, but at this time none of the interacting substrates clearly falls into place in a mechanism crucial to susceptibility to PD.

Multiple lines of research suggest that *PARKIN* influences cell death at least in part through caspase-dependent pathways and JNK-dependent signaling. The disparate convergence of possible pathways of protection from such strikingly different stressors such as serum withdrawal, dopamine, ceramide, kainic acid or *PARKIN* -substrate overexpression suggests that either *PARKIN* affects some central pathway of cell death or that these studies are confounded by unanticipated variables that influence interpretation. Given the relatively narrow spectrum of cells affected in *PARKIN*-linked dysfunction in humans, it is improbable, although not impossible, that *PARKIN* is a critical factor in a pathway central to the life and death of cells. Rather, *PARKIN* may have off-target effects that influence what might be incorrectly understood as protection or death in cell lines or neurons. For example, *PARKIN* has been described with tumor suppressive properties, where overexpression of *PARKIN* slows the growth rate of some cell lines (114). Similarly, cell lines overexpressing *PARKIN* and transplanted to nude mice grew slower as solid tumors than cells not expressing *PARKIN* (115). *PARKIN* and other PD-related genes have been hypothesized to have a peripheral influence on the cell cycle (116), a feature perhaps exacerbated in some studies by overexpression of *PARKIN* in immortal cell lines. Therefore, in vitro studies attempting to dissect *PARKIN* neuroprotection should be approached with caution in lieu of a better understanding of *PARKIN* function in different cellular contexts, particularly when attempting to design more disease-relevant in vivo confirmation studies.

Modifiers of *PARKIN* Function

Since loss of function of *PARKIN* due either to mutation or loss of expression is associated with susceptibility to PD, the identification of factors that modulate *PARKIN* function may have therapeutic value. As such, studies have attempted to identify the specific factors that may regulate *PARKIN* enzymatic activity. In cell lines, activation of multiple caspase cascades serves to down regulate *PARKIN*, where both caspase-1 and -8 can directly cleave *PARKIN* at amino acid residue 126 (117). An interacting protein Nrdp1 may accelerate the degradation of *PARKIN* through a nonproteasome-dependent pathway, as Nrdp1 coimmunoprecipitates with *PARKIN* and decreases the half-life of overexpressed *PARKIN* (49). Another hypothesized negative regulator of *PARKIN* function, the 14-3-3eta chaperone-like protein, binds to *PARKIN* and abrogates intrinsic autoubiquitination activity, an effect alleviated by the overexpression of α-syuclein that might competitively bind 14-3-3eta (118).

PARKIN may interact with a number of chaperones in large protein complexes that help mediate the interaction of *PARKIN* with various substrates. HSP-70 expression promotes *PARKIN* ubiquitination of an expanded polyglutamine protein (113), while a member of the bcl-2-associated anthanogene family, BAG5, binds to *PARKIN* and HSP-70 as a complex and serves to down-regulate *PARKIN* E3-ubiquitin ligase and neuroprotective activity (119). The chaperone-like protein CHIP may bind to *PARKIN* and dissociate the interaction with HSP-70, resulting in increased ubiquitination and neuroprotective qualities of *PARKIN* (120). Numerous proteins may therefore regulate *PARKIN* function, although confirmation of a physiologically relevant interaction may depend on additional experiments with in vivo models of *PARKIN* function. As with the above interacting proteins, a number of post-translational modifications that serve to down regulate *PARKIN* function have been identified. Phosphorylated *PARKIN* has been described in a number of cell lines, associated with a decrease in autoubiquitination activity (121). S-nitrosylation of *PARKIN* was demonstrated in vivo in mouse and human brain, where S-nitrosylation serves to inhibit *PARKIN* E3 ligase and neuroprotection activity (110,122). S-nitrosylated protein generally appears increased in PD brains so that the impact of nitrosylation on other proteins and pathways important in PD warrants further examination (110).

Effect of Mutations

A common effect of pathogenic mutations on the *PARKIN* protein may reveal the pathogenic mechanisms related to *PARKIN* dysfunction and PD. For example, familial-linked Alzheimer's disease mutations in the amyloid precursor protein (APP) serve to increase production of the toxic Aβ-42 molecule. Hundreds of known mutations in the presenilin 1 and 2 gene also increase Aβ-42 production implicating a central role for Aβ-42 in Alzheimer's pathogenesis. As opposed to APP or presenilin mutations, *PARKIN* mutations range from single base pair substitutions to small deletions and splice site mutations, to deletions that span hundreds of thousands of nucleotides (12). Considering such diverse genetic variation, and assuming that most *PARKIN*-related PD arises from similar mechanisms, the simplest explanation is that *PARKIN* mutations serve to down-regulate normal *PARKIN* function in a loss of function model. This explanation is almost certain in *PARKIN*-linked PD where deletions span several exons, sometimes including exon 1, and even if truncated *PARKIN* mRNA was produced, nonsense-mediated decay would serve to destabilize the transcript and make sure no protein is expressed. Indeed, there is little evidence that truncated *PARKIN* protein is expressed in patients with exon deletions. However, more subtle point mutations that account for many *PARKIN*-linked PD cases warrant the effect of the substitutions on a biochemical level.

Many missense mutations appear to affect the solubility and stability of overexpressed *PARKIN* protein. In the most comprehensive study to date, more than half of the 22 missense/nonsense mutations in *PARKIN* studied produced alterations in solubility and localization in addition to affecting detergent extraction properties (123). Missense mutations in the first *PARKIN* RING domain resulted in the formation of large cytoplasmic and nuclear inclusions as compared with the normal diffuse cytoplasmic localization of wild-type *PARKIN* (124). Four missense mutations in the N-terminal UbL domain of *PARKIN* decrease the stability of *PARKIN* and induce a rapid proteasome-mediated degradation response, consistent with previous studies that suggest the UbL domain is critical for *PARKIN* stability (125). Moreover, the C-terminal end of *PARKIN* also appears to be a crucial regulator of proper folding of *PARKIN* protein, and mutations in this region act to destabilize the protein, an event associated with an increased propensity to aggregate (126). Therefore, a majority of point mutations associated with *PARKIN*-linked PD deleteriously affect *PARKIN* stability consistent with a loss-of-function model of disease pathogenesis.

In addition to mutations affecting protein stability, several missense mutations are used as controls in studies assessing the enzymatic and neuroprotective potential of *PARKIN*. In initial reports, E3 ligase activity appeared reduced or ablated in mutant *PARKIN* (54). In follow-up studies determining the effect of mutant *PARKIN* on substrate interaction, some mutants consistently demonstrate reduced E3 ligase activity in all assays, such as T240R, whereas other mutations such as R42P do not consistently affect E3 ligase activity but drastically affect stability. In addition, the overall effects of particular missense mutations may involve both a reduction in stability and E3 ligase activity. Conversely, some point mutations are not well described on a genetic basis and may represent rare nonsynonomous polymorphisms that are not associated with disease. Mutations that neither adversely affect *PARKIN* stability or activity are likely candidates for polymorphisms misassociated with susceptibility to PD.

CONCLUSION

Once considered the archetypal nongenetic neurodegenerative disorder, PD research has been revolutionized by the identification of genes, such as *PARKIN*, that contribute to a large number of familial-linked disease and some sporadic cases. Clinical, pathologic, and genetic studies suggest that loss of *PARKIN* function is associated with susceptibility to PD thereby focusing research on the normal function of *PARKIN* in health and disease. *PARKIN* is highly conserved and widely expressed in many organs, although in brain *PARKIN* is primarily expressed in neurons. *PARKIN* is localized to most membranous cellular structures in neurons, including the ER, golgi, lipid rafts, and vesicles, and endogenous *PARKIN* is largely excluded from the nucleus. Expression is restricted to postmitotic cells and neurons, and is up-regulated during the transition from growth to senescence. Protein domain structure implies a role in an ubiquitin-dependent pathway.

The UbL domain of *PARKIN* interacts with various proteasome subunits, but the physiologic consequence of this interaction is unknown. *PARKIN* overexpression provides neuroprotection from proteasome inhibition (among other stressors), implying that the primary mechanism of *PARKIN* neuroprotection is independent of proteasome-mediated degradation. Consistent with this notion is the biochemical dissection of *PARKIN*–E3 ligase activity where substrates can be monoubiquitinated or modified with lysine-63 chains. In all cases, *PARKIN* does not exact a robust and reproducible down-regulation in vivo of any substrate protein studied. Some candidates, such as AIMP2 and Pael-R, appear to accumulate in PD models and brains, but the exact consequence of this accumulation awaits the generation and description of more refined models such as transgenic animals. Taken together, the interacting proteins do not implicate *PARKIN* in a particular biochemical role, so that the next generation of research must describe how *PARKIN* mediates biologically significant pathways via substrate interaction.

Whether the neuroprotection mediated by *PARKIN* in various models of cell death is relevant in PD remains a matter of debate. The majority of studies utilize a nonphysiologic overexpression of *PARKIN* that would not necessarily recapitulate the condition in human disease where *PARKIN* expression is down regulated. Studies that examine the effect of *PARKIN* knock-down have not produced clear avenues of research but are likely vital toward understanding how *PARKIN* prevents PD in humans. The precedent for understanding even a portion of the endogenous function of a gene linked to human neurodegeneration, such as huntingtin, FMRI-1, APP, or presenilin, suggests several decades of research and hundreds of studies are required. Great strides have been made in a short time toward understanding *PARKIN*-linked PD, yet many fundamental aspects remain unclear. Future studies that address these fundamental aspects are most important in the ultimate goal of designing rational therapeutics for PD.

REFERENCES

1. Rao G, Fisch L, Srinivasan S, et al. JAMA 2003; 289(3):347–353.
2. Braak H, Del Tredici K, Bratzke H, Hamm-Clement J, Sandmann-Keil D, Rub U. J Neurol 2002; 249(Suppl 3):III1–III5.
3. Braak H, Del Tredici K, Rub U, de Vos RA, Jansen Steur EN, Braak E. Neurobiol Aging 2003; 24(2):197–211.
4. Spillantini MG, Schmidt ML, Lee VM, Trojanowski JQ, Jakes R, Goedert M. Nature 1997; 388(6645):839–840.
5. Melamed E, Offen D, Shirvan A, Ziv I. J Neurol 2000; 247(Suppl 2):II135–II139.
6. Maher NE, Golbe LI, Lazzarini AM, et al. Neurology 2002; 58(1):79–84.
7. Sveinbjornsdottir S, Hicks AA, Jonsson T, et al. N Engl J Med 2000; 343(24):1765–1770.
8. Langston JW. Neurotoxicology 2002; 23(4–5):443–450.
9. Langston JW, Tan LC. Eur J Neurol 2000; 7(5):465–466.
10. Matsumine H, Yamamura Y, Hattori N, et al. Genomics 1998; 49(1):143–146.
11. Kitada T, Asakawa S, Hattori N, et al. Nature 1998; 392(6676):605–608.
12. West AB, Maidment NT. Hum Genet 2004; 114(4):327–336.
13. West A, Periquet M, Lincoln S, et al. Am J Med Genet 2002; 114(5):584–591.
14. Lucking CB, Durr A, Bonifati V, et al. N Engl J Med 2000; 342(21):1560–1567.
15. Lohmann E, Periquet M, Bonifati V, et al. Ann Neurol 2003; 54(2):176–185.
16. Ohsawa Y, Kurokawa K, Sonoo, M, et al. Neurology 2005; 65(3):459–462.
17. Khan NL, Katzenschlager R, Watt H, et al. Neurology 2004; 62(7):1224–1226.
18. Broussolle E, Lucking CB, Ginovart N, Pollak P, Remy P, Durr A. Neurology 2000; 55(6):877–879.
19. Thobois S, Ribeiro MJ, Lohmann E, et al. Arch Neurol 2003; 60(5):713–718.
20. Khan NL, Brooks DJ, Pavese N, et al. Brain 2002; 125(Pt 10):2248–2256.
21. Khan NL, Scherfler C, Graham E, et al. Neurology 2005; 64(1):134–136.
22. Hilker R, Klein C, Hedrich K, et al. Neurosci Lett 2002; 323(1):50–54.
23. Hilker R, Klein C, Ghaemi M, et al. Ann Neurol 2001; 49(3):367–376.
24. Pal PK, Leung J, Hedrich K, et al. Mov Disord 2002; 17(4):789–794.
25. Ishikawa A, Takahashi H. J Neurol 1998; 245(11Suppl 3):P4–P9.
26. Hayashi S, Wakabayashi K, Ishikawa A, et al. Mov Disord 2000; 15(5):884–888.
27. van de Warrenburg BP, Lammens M, Lucking CB, et al. Neurology 2001; 56(4):555–557.
28. Mori H, Kondo T, Yokochi M, et al. Neurology 1998; 51(3):890–892.
29. Pramstaller PP, Schlossmacher MG, Jacques TS, et al. Ann Neurol 2005; 58(3):411–422.
30. Farrer M, Chan P, Chen R, et al. Ann Neurol 2001; 50(3):293–300.
31. Sasaki S, Shirata A, Yamane K, Iwata M. Neurology 2004; 63(4):678–682.
32. D'Agata V, Grimaldi M, Pascale A, Cavallaro S. Eur J Neurosci 2000; 12(10):3583–3588.
33. Gu WJ, Abbas N, Lagunes MZ, et al. J Neurochem 2000; 74(4):1773–1776.
34. Solano SM, Miller DW, Augood SJ, Young AB, Penney JB Jr. Ann Neurol 2000; 47(2):201–210.
35. Huynh DP, Scoles DR, Ho TH, Del Bigio MR, Pulst SM. Ann Neurol 2000; 48(5):737–744.
36. Kubo SI, Kitami T, Noda S, et al. J Neurochem 2001; 78(1):42–54.
37. Fallon L, Moreau F, Croft BG, Labib N, Gu WJ, Fon EA. J Biol Chem 2002; 277(1):486–491.
38. Pawlyk AC, Giasson BI, Sampathu DM, et al. J Biol Chem 2003; 278(48):48120–48128.
39. Shimura H, Hattori N, Kubo S, et al. Ann Neurol 1999; 45(5):668–672.
40. Bandopadhyay R, Kingsbury AE, Muqit MM, et al. Neurobiol Dis 2005; 20(2):401–411.
41. Schlossmacher MG, Frosch MP, Gai WP, et al. Am J Pathol 2002; 160(5):1655–1667.
42. Yu WP, Tan JM, Chew KC, et al. Gene 2005; 346:97–104.
43. West AB, Kapatos G, O'Farrell C, et al. J Biol Chem 2004; 279(28):28896–28902.
44. Greene JC, Whitworth AJ, Kuo I, Andrews LA, Feany MB, Pallanck LJ. Proc Natl Acad Sci USA 2003; 100(7):4078–4083.
45. Horowitz JM, Myers J, Vernace VA, Stachowiak MK, Torres G. Brain Res Dev Brain Res 2001; 126(1):31–41.
46. Kuhn K, Zhu XR, Lubbert H, Stichel CC. Brain Res Dev Brain Res 2004; 149(2):131–142.
47. West AB, Lockhart PJ, O'Farell C, Farrer MJ. J Mol Biol 2003; 326(1):11–19.

48. Mengesdorf T, Jensen PH, Mies G, Aufenberg C, Paschen W. Proc Natl Acad Sci USA 2002; 99(23):15042–15047.
49. Zhong L, Tan Y, Zhou A, Yu Q, Zhou J. J Biol Chem 2005; 280(10):9425–9430.
50. Choi P, Ostrerova-Golts N, Sparkman D, Cochran E, Lee JM, Wolozin B. Neuroreport 2000; 11(12):2635–2638.
51. Finney N, Walther F, Mantel PY, Stauffer D, Rovelli G, Dev KK. J Biol Chem 2003; 278(18):16054–16058.
52. Matsuda N, Kitami T, Suzuki T, Mizuno Y, Hattori N, Tanaka K. J Biol Chem 2006; 281: 3204–3209.
53. Li W, Lesuisse C, Xu Y, Troncoso JC, Price DL, Lee MK. J Neurosci 2004; 24(33): 7400–7409.
54. Shimura H, Hattori N, Kubo S, et al. Nat Genet 2000; 25(3):302–305.
55. Freemont PS. Curr Biol 2000; 10(2):R84–R87.
56. Capili AD, Edghill EL, Wu K, Borden KL. J Mol Biol 2004; 340(5):1117–1129.
57. Upadhya SC, Hegde AN. Trends Biochem Sci 2003; 28(6):280–283.
58. Hershko A, Ciechanover A. Annu Rev Biochem 1998; 67:425–479.
59. Schubert U, Anton LC, Gibbs J, Norbury CC, Yewdell JW, Bennink JR. Nature 2000; 404(6779):770–774.
60. Adams J. Nat Rev Cancer 2004; 4(5):349–360.
61. Aguilar RC, Wendland B. Curr Opin Cell Biol 2003; 15(2):184–190.
62. Hicke L. Nat Rev Mol Cell Biol 2001; 2(3):195–201.
63. Jenuwein T, Allis CD. Science 2001; 293(5532):1074–1080.
64. Goldknopf IL, Taylor CW, Baum RM, et al. J Biol Chem 1975; 250(18):7182–7187.
65. Pickar CM. Annu Rev Biochem 2001; 70:503–533.
66. Kuras L, Rouillon A, Lee T, Barbey R, Tyers M, Thomas D. Mol Cell 2002; 10(1):69–80.
67. Kaiser P, Flick K, Wittenberg C, Reed SI. Cell 2000; 102(3):303–314.
68. Adhikary S, Marinoni F, Hock A, et al. Cell 2005; 123(3):409–421.
69. Bres V, Kiernan RE, Linares LK, et al. Nat Cell Biol 2003; 5(8):754–761.
70. Imai Y, Soda M, Inoue H, Hattori N, Mizuno Y, Takahashi R. Cell 2001;105(7):891–902.
71. Zhang Y, Gao J, Chung KK, Huang H, Dawson VL, Dawson, TM. Proc Natl Acad Sci USA 2000; 97(24):13354–13359.
72. Doss-Pepe EW, Chen, L, Madura, K. J Biol Chem 2005; 280(17):16619–16624.
73. Lim KL, Dawson VL, Dawson TM. Neurobiol Aging 2005.
74. Dachsel JC, Lucking CB, Deeg S, et al. FEBS Lett 2005; 579(18):3913–3919.
75. Sakata E, Yamaguchi Y, Kurimoto E, et al. EMBO Rep 2003; 4(3):301–306.
76. Rankin CA, Joazeiro CA, Floor E, Hunter T. J Biomed Sci 2001; 8(5):421–429.
77. Peng XR, Jia Z, Zhang Y, Ware J, Trimble WS. Mol Cell Biol 2002; 22(1):378–387.
78. Periquet M, Corti O, Jacquier S, Brice A. J Neurochem 2005; 95(5):1259–1276.
79. Dong Z, Ferger B, Paterna JC, et al. Proc Natl Acad Sci USA 2003; 100(21):12438–12443.
80. Yang Y, Nishimura I, Imai Y, Takahashi R, Lu B. Neuron 2003; 37(6):911–924.
81. Chung KK, Zhang Y, Lim KL, et al. Nat Med 2001; 7(10):1144–1150.
82. Corti O, Hampe C, Koutnikova H, et al. Hum Mol Genet 2003; 12(12):1427–1437.
83. Ko HS, von Coelln R, Sriram SR, et al. J Neurosci 2005; 25(35):7968–7978.
84. Yang F, Jiang Q, Zhao J, Ren Y, Sutton MD, Feng J. J Biol Chem 2005; 280(17): 17154–17162.
85. Huynh DP, Scoles DR, Nguyen D, Pulst SM. Hum Mol Genet 2003; 12(20):2587–2597.
86. Choi P, Snyder H, Petrucelli L, et al. Brain Res Mol Brain Res 2003; 117(2):179–189.
87. Staropoli JF, McDermott C, Martinat C, Schulman B, Demireva E, Abeliovich A. Neuron 2003;37(5):735–749.
88. Um JW, Min DS, Rhim H, Kim J, Paik SR, Chung KC. J Biol Chem 2005.
89. Moore DJ, West AB, Dawson VL, Dawson TM. Annu Rev Neurosci 2005; 28:57–87.
90. Dawson TM, Dawson VL. Science 2003; 302(5646):819–822.
91. Shimura H, Schlossmacher MG, Hattori N, et al. Science 2001; 293(5528):263–269.
92. Lo Bianco C, Ridet JL, Schneider BL, Deglon N, Aebischer P. Proc Natl Acad Sci USA 2002; 99(16):10813–10818.
93. Klein RL, King MA, Hamby ME, Meyer EM. Hum Gene Ther 2002; 13(5):605–612.
94. Lo Bianco C, Schneider BL, Bauer M, et al. Proc Natl Acad Sci USA 2004; 101(50): 17510–17515.

95. Yamada M, Mizuno Y, Mochizuki H. Hum Gene Ther 2005; 16(2):262–270.
96. Lo Bianco C, Deglon N, Pralong W, Aebischer P. Neurobiol Dis 2004; 17(2):283–289.
97. Petrucelli L, O'Farrell C, Lockhart PJ, et al. Neuron 2002; 36(6):1007–1019.
98. Kim SJ, Sung JY, Um JW, et al. J Biol Chem 2003; 278(43):41890–41899.
99. Oluwatosin-Chigbu Y, Robbins A, Scott CW, et al. Biochem Biophys Res Commun 2003; 309(3):679–684.
100. Liani E, Eyal A, Avraham E, et al. Proc Natl Acad Sci USA 2004; 101(15):5500–5505.
101. von Coelln R, Thomas B, Andrabi SA, et al. J Neurosci 2006; 26(14):3685–3696.
102. Darios F, Corti O, Lucking CB, et al. Hum Mol Genet 2003; 12(5):517–526.
103. Pesah Y, Pham T, Burgess H, et al. Development 2004; 131(9):2183–2194.
104. Palacino JJ, Sagi D, Goldberg MS, et al. J Biol Chem 2004; 279(18):18614–18622.
105. Higashi Y, Asanuma M, Miyazaki I, Hattori N, Mizuno Y, Ogawa N. J Neurochem 2004; 89(6):1490–1497.
106. Junn E, Lee SS, Suhr UT, Mouradian MM. J Biol Chem 2002; 277(49):47870–47877.
107. Zhao J, Ren Y, Jiang Q, Feng J. J Cell Sci 2003; 116(Pt 19):4011–4019.
108. Jiang H, Ren Y, Zhao J, Feng J. Hum Mol Genet 2004; 13(16):1745–1754.
109. Cha GH, Kim S, Park J, et al. Proc Natl Acad Sci USA 2005; 102(29):10345–10350.
110. Chung KK, Thomas B, Li X, et al. Science 2004; 304(5675):1328–1331.
111. MacCormac LP, Muqit MM, Faulkes DJ, Wood NW, Latchman DS. Eur J Neurosci 2004; 20(8):2038–2048.
112. Son JH, Kawamata H, Yoo MS, et al. J Neurochem 2005; 94(4):1040–1053.
113. Tsai YC, Fishman PS, Thakor NV, Oyler GA. J Biol Chem 2003; 278(24):22044–22055.
114. Wang F, Denison S, Lai JP, et al. Genes Chromosomes Cancer 2004; 40(2):85–96.
115. Picchio MC, Martin ES, Cesari R, et al. Clin Cancer Res 2004; 10(8):2720–2724.
116. West AB, Dawson VL, Dawson TM. Trends Neurosci 2005; 28(7):348–352.
117. Kahns S, Kalai M, Jakobsen LD, Clark BF, Vandenabeele P, Jensen PH. J Biol Chem 2003; 278(26):23376–23380.
118. Sato S, Chiba T, Sakata E, et al. Embo J 2005.
119. Kalia SK, Lee S, Smith PD, et al. Neuron 2004; 44(6):931–945.
120. Imai Y, Soda M, Hatakeyama S, et al. Mol Cell 2002; 10(1):55–67.
121. Yamamoto A, Friedlein A, Imai Y, Takahashi R, Kahle PJ, Haass C. J Biol Chem 2005; 280(5):3390–3399.
122. Yao D, Gu Z, Nakamura T, et al. Proc Natl Acad Sci USA 2004; 101(29):10810–10814.
123. Wang C, Tan JM, Ho MW, et al. J Neurochem 2005; 93(2):422–431.
124. Cookson MR, Lockhart PJ, McLendon C, O'Farrell C, Schlossmacher M, Farrer MJ. Hum Mol Genet 2003; 12(22):2957–2965.
125. Henn IH, Gostner JM, Lackner P, Tatzelt J, Winklhofer KF. J Neurochem 2005; 92(1):114–122.
126. Winklhofer KF, Henn IH, Kay-Jackson PC, Heller U, Tatzelt J. J Biol Chem 2003; 278(47):47199–47208.

15 Mitochondrial Complex I Deficiency in Parkinson's Disease: A Mechanism for Oxidant-Based Pathogenesis

Tatyana V. Votyakova
Division of Immunogenetics, Department of Pediatrics, University of Pittsburgh, Pittsburgh, Pennsylvania, U.S.A.

Ian J. Reynolds
Neuroscience Drug Discovery, Merck Research Laboratories, West Point, Pennsylvania, U.S.A.

INTRODUCTION

There has been a steady accumulation of data that point to a role for mitochondria in the pathogenesis of Parkinson's disease (PD). In broad terms, it is evident that toxins that impair mitochondrial function produce lesions resembling PD in animals and humans, and that mitochondria may be a major source of reactive oxygen species (ROS) that could contribute to the oxidative damage evident in PD brains. It has also been suggested that there is a systemic impairment of mitochondrial function in patients with PD that extends beyond the central nervous system. In more specific terms, many of the proposed mechanisms that invoke mitochondrial dysfunction involve complex I of the electron transport chain, which is also known as the NADH: coenzyme Q oxidoreductase. A generous interpretation of these findings would lead to the conclusion that complex I impairment is the key early event in PD pathogenesis, and that this mechanism could initiate the loss of dopaminergic neurons that characterizes this disease. However, a more conservative interpretation raises a number of questions that need to be addressed before such conclusions can be considered reasonable. In particular, it is important to determine whether impaired complex I function is a characteristic of the disease, and also whether the proposed impairment can alter mitochondrial function in a manner that is mechanistically consistent with the putative consequence of excessive ROS production as a critical pathogenic event. Beyond these considerations, one must also evaluate the basis for any conclusions regarding ROS generation, because of the continuing evolution in experimental methods used in studies of mitochondrial function.

Accordingly, we will first review the methods used for measuring mitochondrial ROS generation, because the strengths and limitations of these methods have an important impact on the conclusions that can be reached. We will then consider the properties of complex I in the context of its function and putative mechanisms of ROS production. Finally, we will evaluate the claims of complex I impairment and the putative mechanisms that have been invoked and establish whether the suggested pathogenic mechanisms are reasonable based on the data supporting the claims.

METHODS FOR MEASURING MITOCHONDRIAL REACTIVE OXYGEN SPECIES PRODUCTION

The idea of mitochondrial production of free radicals as a byproduct of their respiratory chain activity first emerged after an observation that the inhibitor antimycin failed to completely suppress oxygen consumption as measured by an oxygen electrode (1). It was shown that approximately a fraction of 1% to 2% of molecular oxygen consumed by respiring mitochondria may be converted into some form of ROS (2). A rough estimate indicated that the concentration of ROS was in the picomolar range, which effectively sets the requirements for the sensitivity of an adequate monitoring method. Additionally, the ideal method should minimally interfere with mitochondrial function and should be specific for a particular form of ROS. Because the production of ROS by mitochondria is a dynamic process the ability to monitor production in real time would be considered an additional advantage.

The primary form of ROS produced by mitochondria is superoxide anion radical which is released into the matrix side of the inner membrane (3,4). Therein it is converted into hydrogen peroxide by the matrix Mn-superoxide dismutase, SOD2. Hydrogen peroxide easily penetrates through the membrane and can be detected outside of mitochondria. Thus, the task of investigation of mechanism ROS generated by mitochondria is limited to detection of either hydrogen peroxide or superoxide anion radical, or both.

The most common approach to monitoring hydrogen-peroxide release uses horseradish peroxidase (HRP)-based assay methods. HRP is a heme-containing enzyme, which performs two electron reduction of H_2O_2 by oxidation of a molecule of a hydrogen donor according to the following equation (5,6).

$HRP + H_2O_2 \rightarrow HRP\text{-}H_2O_2$ (Compound I)

Compound I + $SH_2 \rightarrow$ Compound II (one electron accepted) + $SH^\bullet$

Compound II + $SH^\bullet \rightarrow HRP + S + H_2O$

HRP is a promiscuous enzyme capable of oxidation of a wide range of substrates. Included in these substrates are some that change their fluorescence properties. Scopoletin, p-hydroxyphenylacetic acid (p-HPAA), p-hydroxy-3 methyl-phenylacetic acid or homovanillic acid (HVA), and Amplex red can be used as reporting dyes in the HRP-based assay, each of which have certain advantages and pitfalls. In general, however, advantages of the HRP-based method include the possibility to monitor H_2O_2 in real time, high selectivity to H_2O_2 and also high sensitivity with appropriate substrates.

HVA increases its fluorescence upon oxidation which is convenient as fluorescence rises directly along with accumulation of hydrogen peroxide. Its fluorescence (312 nm excitation/420 nm emission) does not overlap with that of mitochondrial constituents, and it gives a linear response for concentrations of hydrogen peroxide up to 5 µM (7). However, HVA should be considered as a low sensitivity dye since the fluorescence intensity yielded at a typical working concentration of 100 µM is five-fold less than that of 5 µM of scopoletin (7). Properties of p-HPAA with 320 nm excitation/400 nm emission wavelengths are in many respects similar to that of HVA. It is also a low-sensitivity dye as it is used in high concentrations [200 µM (8), 330 µM (9), 1 mM (10)].

Scopoletin has been used since the 1970s and numerous studies have been performed with this dye due to its higher quantum yield (6,11–15). The usual concentration of scopoletin is 1 to 3 µM. Two major shortcomings, however, are inherent to this dye. First, because it is fluorescent in its reduced form, accumulation of hydrogen peroxide can be monitored by the decrease of the fluorescent signal, which makes it less convenient. Second, its spectral characteristics overlap with that of pyridine nucleotides (340 nm excitation/460 nm emission). In practice, this has a relatively small impact into the overall fluorescent signal, typically comprising less than 5% of the total. Nonetheless, this obstacle makes precludes the simultaneous detection of NADH and the kinetics of ROS release by mitochondria.

Amplex red, which recently became commercially available, so far is the best choice among the indicators for hydrogen peroxide. It gains fluorescence upon oxidation, has highest sensitivity of all dyes in this class, responses linearly across a wide range of hydrogen peroxide concentrations, and has low background fluorescence. Additionally, due to longer excitation and emission wavelengths (560 nm/590 nm, respectively), the Amplex-red dye lacks interference with pyridine nucleotide fluorescence (16). A minor shortcoming of this dye that should be noticed is that resorufin, the product of Amplex-red oxidation, is a bright fluorescent compound which can be further oxidized to a nonfluorescent derivative in the presence of excess H_2O_2. This circumstance can be overcome by simply increasing the Amplex-red initial concentration. The presence of up to two-fold excess of the dye compared to the estimated maximal amount of accumulated H_2O_2 can avoid this problem (17). A variety of concentrations of Amplex red used in experiments with mitochondria have been reported in literature: 1 to 2 µM (18–20), 20 µM (21), 50 µM (22). We found that 2 µM of Amplex red give optimal results in experiments where 0.15 to 0.3 mg of rat brain mitochondria were employed (17).

HRP-based methods have a major disadvantage because HRP in some cases can act as an oxidase as well. For example, HRP can react with biological reductants like NADH or reduced glutathione and produce hydrogen peroxide and NAD^+ or GSSG (23). This reaction is substantially inhibited by SOD, indicating that superoxide anion is one of its intermediates (17). Thus, the addition of SOD to HRP-based assays can help to avoid aberrant signal detection, although this does result in limitations in the potential application of HRP-based assay approaches.

The complex formed by HRP with H_2O_2 (Compound II) as well as the complex of cytochrome c peroxidase (CCP) with H_2O_2 can be directly monitored by measuring their absorbance at 402 to 417 nm and 407 to 419 nm, respectively. According to Boveris et al. (12), detection of the CCP intermediate is a more efficient way of measuring hydrogen peroxide. These authors compared the detection of hydrogen peroxide using oxidation of scopoletin in the presence of HRP, and while also monitoring absorbencies of Compound II and CCP. They reported that CCP detected 100% of the H_2O_2 released in the reaction of glucose with glucose oxidase, while HRP-conjugated scopoletin oxidation or formation of Compound II assays yielded only 70% and 80% of H_2O_2 generated, respectively. Additionally, the kinetics of the signal obtained with CCP was more linear because this is a one-step reaction compared with the formation Compound II which goes in two steps, such that the former reflects the real rate of H_2O_2 generation more effectively (3,24). The comparison of scopoletin-HRP and CCP methods lead the authors to conclude that the broad specificity of HRP allowed it to react with other hydrogen donors instead of scopoletin, with the result that the scopoletin-HRP method may underestimate concentrations H_2O_2. However, CCP can accept electrons from cytochrome c as well. In experiments measuring mitochondrial ROS generation, there is always present a small fraction of mitochondria with damaged outer membrane. This in turn provides a possibility for overestimation of the production of hydrogen peroxide by the inadvertent detection of electrons donated by cytochrome c. The requirements of noncatalytic amounts of Compound II and CCP for the assay should be considered as a potential disadvantage of this approach.

Dichlorodihydrofluorescein diacetate (H_2-DCFDA) is commonly used to monitor ROS inside cells (25,26) and in whole tissues (27). It easily penetrates into cell and after cleavage of two ester bounds is partially trapped inside in the form of H_2-DCF. The latter is believed to have preference toward hydrogen peroxide. According to (28), H_2-DCF is not directly oxidized by either superoxide anion or by hydroxyl radical. However, these authors were cautious in regard to H_2-DCF specificity stating that "since DCFH oxidation may be derived from several reactive intermediates, interpretation of specific reactive oxygen species involved in biological systems should be approached with caution" and that it can be regarded rather as "a probe as an overall index of oxidative stress" (28).

H_2-DCFDA has been used in several studies with isolated mitochondria (29–31). For mitochondrial staining, the same procedure was used as for cells, e.g, mitochondria were preincubated with 10 to 20 µM of the dye, pelleted to remove extramitochondrial dye and resuspended in a fresh buffer, then presuming the detection of ROS reflected a signal derived from inside the mitochondrial matrix (29). However, if the dye is indeed trapped in the matrix it is very difficult to calibrate the signal effectively, and it is not possible to interrogate the signal using externally added SOD or catalase. In addition to that, there is some controversy in literature data obtained with this dye. Maciel et al. (29) reported an increase in succinate-supported ROS production by calcium monitored by H_2-DCFDA in rat brain mitochondria. However, in Starkov and Wallace (2002), where Amplex red + HRP assay was used, the reverse result was observed in similar experiments. These results were revisited in (30) where both assays were applied in the same experimental conditions with rat brain mitochondria. The authors reported that Ca^{2+} increased the H_2-DCFDA signal while decreasing that of Amplex red, thus confirming observations of each of the research groups. This may suggest that the assay systems detect different processes. However, as shown by Sousa et al. (31), Ca^{2+} addition to rotenone-inhibited rat brain mitochondria in the presence of NADH-linked substrates produced qualitatively similar results with H_2-DCFDA and the HRP-based method. The reason for these discrepancies remains obscure.

The main methods of superoxide anion radical detection are based on reporting dyes and its paramagnetic properties by the means of electron paramagnetic spectroscopy (EPR). As superoxide anion radical bears one negative charge, its diffusion through the hydrophobic lipid barrier is limited, which implies special requirements for its detection. It can be detected either in submitochondrial particles (SMP) which have an inside-out orientation of membrane, or in intact mitochondria using reporter molecules which are able to freely penetrate into the matrix space.

Boveris and Cadenas (4) introduced an assay to monitor superoxide anions which is based on one electron reduction of exogenously added cytochrome c according to the reaction (2):

$$\text{Cyt c}^{3+} + O_2^- \rightarrow \text{Cyt c}^{2+} + O_2$$

This reaction can be monitored by measuring absorbance of cytochrome c at 540 to 550 nm. SOD inhibits the reduction of cytochrome c in a competitive manner and that 4 µM of cytochrome and 0.3 µM of SOD c are optimal concentrations for the assay. It should be noted here that SMP represent a mixture of vesicles made of inner mitochondrial membrane fragments with normal and inverted orientation. Exogenously added cytochrome c can accept electrons from mitochondrial cytochrome b of the outside out-oriented vesicles. This circumstance necessitates the use of an SOD control for this assay in order to distinguish between cytochrome c reduction from superoxide anion and from respiratory chain.

The selectivity of the cytochrome c-based method of O_2^- detection can be increased by the use of the acetylated derivative of cytochrome c. As it was shown in (32) acetylation of 60% of lysine residues of cytochrome c almost completely diminished its ability to accept electrons from the reductases of mitochondrial respiratory chain preserving, none the less, its ability to be reduced by O_2^-. Though in model systems specificity of acetylated cytochrome c toward superoxide anion was considerably improved, in experiments with mitochondrial membranes its reduction was only 82% sensitive to SOD (32). Literature data on the specificity of acetylated cytochrome c for superoxide anion detection are rather controversial, though. Kang et al. developed a procedure for cytochrome c acetylation that Takeshige and Minakami (37) reported to be 100% SOD sensitive in experiments with isolated Complex I as well as with SMP, using NADH as a substrate. At the same time, according to Turrens et al. (33), cytochrome c as well its acetylated derivative in experiments with lung SMP and NADH as a substrate gave a very high signal which was insensitive to SOD. Apparently, selectivity of acetylated cytochrome c toward O_2^- depends on the portion of lysine residues of the polypeptide chain which have been modified. The concentration of acetylated cytochrome c used in this assay varies from 15 (34) to 50 µM (35) with SOD still as an essential control.

Misra and Fridovich (36) introduced a convenient method for monitoring superoxide anions by oxidation of epinephrine (synonym to adrenaline) to adrenochrome, which can be followed by change in absorbance at 485 to 575 nm. This assay can be considered as less sensitive since it requires higher concentration of the reporting molecule (1–1.2 mM vs. 4–50 µM of cytochrome c) (3,37–41). However, it is more specific than the cytochrome c-based assay because epinephrine does not interact directly with mitochondrial reductases. The SOD-sensitive component of adrenochrome formation in experiments with SMP was 90% to 94% depending on the pH (3,34), or depending on the substrate of oxidation (38). To confirm the assay specificity SOD should be added at the end of each experiment as in the case of cytochrome c.

Superoxide anion possesses one unpaired electron, which can be detected using EPR in the presence of spin traps. The latter helps to overcome the problem of short life time of superoxide anion radical. Due to the ability of some spin traps to penetrate through a hydrophobic barrier, EPR enables detection of O_2^- in mitochondria and SMP alike. This provides a relatively unambiguous method for detection of superoxide anion radicals in mitochondrial matrix. This approach, however, has several disadvantages. (*i*) it does not allow monitoring in real time; (*ii*) high concentrations of spin traps must be applied in order to get an EPR spectrum with a good resolution; and (*iii*) it is not possible to quantify the signal. A variety of spin traps were employed in experiments with mitochondria or SMP. The lowest concentration of 2 to 10 mM was mentioned for Tiron (42–44), while the concentration of other traps varied from 50 to 100 mM (45,46) and up to 160 mM (47). In the latter case, such a high concentration is likely to compromise osmotic properties of the media, not to mention potential interference inherent to chemical properties of the trap.

Measurements of chemiluminescence are less frequently employed in assays of mitochondrial oxidative events. Lucigenin (bis-*N*-methylacridinium) (46) and coelenterazine (or luceferin) were used as indicator molecules. Lucigenin can interact with H_2O_2 (48,49) and with O_2^- (50), while coelentarazine is believed to be more specific to O_2^- (51). The chemiluminescence method allows assessment of ROS in arbitrary units (light units/second) and cannot be considered as readily quantitative. According to Li et al. (52), lucigenin, which bears two positive charges, is accumulated inside mitochondria in a membrane potential-dependent manner. Five micromole of the dye is an adequate concentration to monitor mitochondrial production of ROS. At high concentrations (50 µM) lucigenin can undergo redox cycling accepting electrons from the mitochondrial electron transport chain and cause additional oxygen consumption (52,53). As it is shown in the detailed study by Yurkov et al. (53), lucigenin can accept electrons from Complex I and II and donate them to Complex III bypassing rotenone and TTFA inhibition of Complex I and II, respectively. Importantly, oxidation of reduced lucigenin by Complex III is accompanied by a massive production of superoxide anions (53). These observations illustrate a possible ambiguity in results obtained with lucigenin with respect to the source of the oxidant signal. Coelenterazine, another chemiluminescent compound, is a derivative from the aequorin luminescent protein from jellyfish; to monitor ROS signal it can be used in low concentrations (2.5 μM) (55).

To summarize, due to the high reactivity inherent in ROS by definition, the task of their monitoring and quantifying is not a trivial one. None of the methods used today could be considered as ideally answering to all requirements. However, the application of these methods, with careful consideration of their advantages and possible pitfalls, provides a number of useful approaches for the estimation of mitochondrial ROS generation.

COMPLEX I: STRUCTURE, FUNCTION, AND MECHANISMS OF ROS GENERATION

NADH-ubiquinone oxidoreductase, or Complex I, (EC 1.5.6.3) is the first and the largest complex in the chain of electron transporters of the inner mitochondrial membrane. Its function is to oxidize molecules of NADH produced in the Krebs cycle and to pass the yielded energy in the form of reduced quinone down the redox potential gradient to Complex III along with transferring protons ($n = 4$–5) across the inner membrane. Pumping protons from mitochondrial matrix creates the mitochondrial transmembrane electrical potential (55). Complex I consists of 43 subunits, seven encoded by the mitochondrial genome and 36 encoded in the nucleus, and thus represents the largest and the most complicated component of mitochondrial respiratory chain. The number of subunits is not the only reason why Complex I still remains the least studied part of respiratory chain. Many of subunits, including those encoded in mitochondrial genome, are highly hydrophobic making the task of isolation and reconstruction of Complex I extremely difficult.

Transferring electrons and protons is performed by a number of redox components. The enzyme possesses one noncovalently bound FMN (56) at least six Fe-S clusters (N1a, N1b, N2–N5) (57,58), and at least three distinct types of protein-bound quinones, called fast, slow, and very slow according to the rate of their spin relaxation (e.g., SQ_{Nf}, SQ_{Ns}, and SQ_{Nx}) (59,60). An important finding was that SQ_{Nf}, is $\Delta\mu H^+$-dependent and very sensitive to rotenone (18). By detecting the spin-spin interaction between SQ_{Nf} and the iron-sulfur cluster N2 their mutual distance was estimated to be 8–11 A. This generated the hypothesis that N2 and interacting ubisemiquinone species are spatially arranged within the hydrophobic domain of Complex I, allowing participation in vectorial proton translocation (60).

The amino acid sequences of flavin- and NADH-binding sites and those coordinating Fe-S clusters have been fully preserved in evolution and are functionally the same in prokaryotes and eukaryotes. The exact structural location of all redox components is still under investigation. However, they can be ranged according to their midpoint redox potentials (Em), a parameter derived from the EPR data. According to this range, electrons from NADH molecule are first accepted by FMN, and then the Fe-S cluster N1a, which is followed by four other clusters with similar

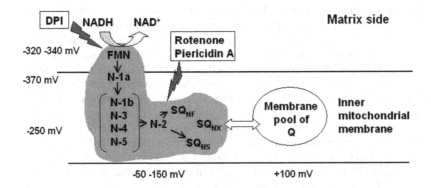

FIGURE 1 Structure of Complex 1. *Abbreviations*: DPI, diphenyleneiodonium; NADH, reduced form of nicotinamide adenine dinucleotide; NAD+, oxidized form of nicotinamide adenine dinucleotide.

Em (N1a, N3, N4, N5). The last one, the iron-sulfur cluster N2, has the highest redox potential and apparently donates electrons to semiquinones. The overall energy drop within the Complex I is 170 or 190 mV (from −320–340 mV to −50–150 mV) which is enough to make one molecule of ATP (55,61).

Free radical production by mitochondrial Complex I can be roughly divided into two mechanisms, one of which is regulated by the membrane potential, while the other is independent of it. $\Delta\Psi$-dependent ROS production is associated with the phenomenon of reverse electron transfer. This occurs when oxidation of succinate by Complex II results in donation of electrons not only downstream in the redox chain to Complex III, but also upstream to Complex I, reducing molecules of NAD+. The latter can be monitored spectrophotometrically. This phenomenon was observed on SMP supplemented with succinate and ATP + oligomycin for generation of membrane potential as well as KCN, which blocks the direct electron flow to Complex IV. In these very artificial conditions all redox centers upstream the cyanide block become highly reduced so that electrons from oxidation of succinate can be pumped against the redox potential to Complex I. Using this model Chance et al. (62) demonstrated the generation of hydrogen peroxide. They then established that this process can be inhibited by rotenone as well as uncoupler. The inhibitor of Complex III antimycin, however, had no effect. Based on these data authors concluded that a carrier in respiratory chain can donate electrons to oxygen as a result of reverse electron flow.

In intact mitochondria under more physiologic conditions reverse electron flow can be observed as well. To demonstrate reverse electron flow mitochondria must oxidize succinate and be tightly coupled to maintain a high membrane potential. Under these conditions succinate dehydrogenase, the fastest enzyme in the respiratory chain, is able to donate electrons to Complex III faster than the latter can send them downstream to Complex IV. As a result, some electrons can flow upstream to Complex I eventually reducing of NADH. In other words, the rapid kinetics of succinate dehydrogenase help to overcome energy barrier for electrons in their moving against the thermodynamic potential. The reverse electron transfer is tightly regulated by the value of membrane potential and is ceased when $\Delta\Psi$ drops below a certain threshold.

Working with intact heart mitochondria Chance, Loschen, and others (6,11) measured hydrogen-peroxide production supported by oxidation of succinate. They showed that succinate-driven ROS generation can be completely inhibited by an uncoupler and can be temporarily inhibited by ADP. The authors suggested as a tentative conclusion that the site of free radical production by uninhibited respiratory chain in the presence of succinate is located somewhere between Complex II and antimycin block in Complex III. However, they specifically mentioned that "the energy coupling mechanism is directly involved in mitochondrial H_2O_2 production" (11), giving a hint about a possible connection of this process to reverse electron transfer. Nevertheless, the main conclusion of these studies initially deflected attention of researches from Complex I as a possible source of ROS in intact mitochondria. Instead, the basic mechanisms of free radical generation by mitochondrial ETC were studied using SMP poisoned with antimycin and focused on the role of Q-cycle in ROS generation.

As the role of physiologic factors influencing free-radical production by respiratory chain was reexamined, the question about the membrane potential dependence of ROS production in intact mitochondria has been directly addressed (9,14,18). It was confirmed that the agents decreasing membrane potential, such as ADP, uncouplers and some inhibitors of respiratory chain, diminished the rate of ROS production. In a study by Korshunov et al. (14) the dilemma between membrane potential versus the rate of electron flow as factors responsible for ROS generation was resolved. Experiments with the Complex II inhibitor malonate showed decreased electron flow while an uncoupler increased flow. The results showed that both of these agents inhibited the rate of free radical generation along with depolarization of membrane. Hence, in the case of succinate-driven free-radical production the crucial factor is high membrane potential, but not the rate of overall electron flow.

The inhibition of succinate-supported ROS generation that results from a decrease in membrane potential is reversible. For example, upon restoration of membrane potential after the completion of phosphorylation of ADP (transition from metabolic state 3 to state 4) ROS production is resumed. Similar to that, inhibition ROS generation by ADP was reversed by stopping ATPase activity after addition of oligomycin or carboxyatractyloside (14,18). By titrating mitochondria with small increments of uncoupler it was found that the rate of ROS generation is a steep function of the value of $\Delta\Psi$ (18). Interestingly, the change in membrane potential induced by ADP is big enough to completely stop free radical generation by respiratory chain. This is the observation of physiologic importance, because it indicates that engagement of mitochondria in ATP synthesis will prevent ROS generation mediated by succinate oxidation (14,18). In the studies of Korshunov et al. (44) a direct correlation between the reverse electron transfer, estimated as a degree of reduction of NADH, membrane potential and the rate of hydrogen peroxide production was established.

The evidence that the site of ROS generation driven by the reverse electron transfer is located in Complex I comes from the fact that rotenone, which prevents reduction of the centers of Complex I, but does not cause depolarization of membrane, inhibited this process (9,14,18). Liu et al. (8) have used diphenyleneiodonium (DPI), which according to (63) in the absence of Cl^- ions can act as a specific inhibitor of Complex I. DPI decreased ROS generation by mitochondria respiring on succinate under conditions of reverse electron transfer, but did not affect ROS generated by Q-cycle observed in the presence of succinate and antimycin. The reason for the use of Cl^--free media is that DPI catalyses an exchange of chloride ions for hydroxyl ions across the inner membrane, which results in swelling mitochondria and inhibition of both Complex I and Complex II (63). It should be noted that antimycin and myxothiazol also decreased ROS generation resulting from reverse electron transfer, but this action results from a decrease in membrane potential. Myxothiazol, separate from its depolarizing effect, directly inhibits ROS generation in the Q-cycle, and thus has the most robust effect on succinate supported ROS generation in mitochondria (18).

It is believed that succinate is not a predominant mitochondrial substrate in vivo and that its concentration in cells is an order of magnitude less than is usually used in experiments with isolated mitochondria (9). Hansford (6) has shown that at physiological concentrations of succinate (0.5 mM or less) mitochondria do not produce a large free radical signal, apparently, because this concentration is not enough to sustain the reverse electron transfer. Thus, the mechanism of ROS generation connected with the reverse electron transfer may be more relevant to pathological circumstances. For example, it was suggested that the accumulation of succinate can occur in ischemia (64,65). Although substantial ROS generation can be demonstrated under reverse electron flow conditions, this mechanism is rarely realized in the cell.

The second mechanism of ROS generation by Complex I may be more relevant in vivo. It is associated with forward electron transfer from the substrate, reduced NADH, down the redox gradient to quinones of the Q-cycle and is independent of $\Delta\Psi$. Upon oxidation of NADH-linked substrates, mitochondria generate a small free radical signal, which comprises no more than 10% of that observed with succinate (18,66). However, blockade of electron flow within Complex I or lower in respiratory chain induces a profound rate of free radical release. This phenomenon was first observed on a simplified biological model of SMP, which offers several advantages in studying intricate mechanisms of free radical production, especially for studies of Complex I. Experiments with SMP enable the use of NADH, a direct substrate of Complex I that is normally nonpenetrable into intact mitochondria. This is more simple than the use of NADH-linked substrates of Krebs cycle, thus avoiding complications associated with regulation of the cycle being imposed upon mechanisms of radical generation. Additionally, it is possible to measure the release of superoxide radicals directly instead of measuring the product of its dismutation H_2O_2. Takeshige and Minokami (37) employing this approach have shown that rotenone induced generation of ROS by bovine heart SMP oxidizing NADH. The same result was obtained with isolated Complex I. Inhibitors of other sites of respiratory chain, antimycin and KCN, activated ROS generation of SMP but not of Complex I, proving that the effect of these inhibitors was connected with their specific sites downstream in the respiratory chain. In all experiments ROS release was 100% sensitive to superoxide dismutase. These observations were later confirmed by other researchers (38,40,67,68). Krishnamoorthy and Hinkle (40) suggested that reduced, bound pyridine nucleotide is the major source of O_2^- in rotenone-blocked Complex I. Ramsay and Singer (67) recorded the production of superoxide radicals induced by piericidin A and MPP$^+$, two other inhibitors of Complex I. The effect of the latter inhibitor is important because of its use in models of PD.

The increase of ROS generation after addition of rotenone or antimycin to intact brain mitochondria respired on NADH-linked substrates was qualitatively demonstrated in several studies (8,10,19, 69,70). Cino and Del Maestro (70) in their comprehensive study performed with several substrates and inhibitors of respiratory chain came to a conclusion, shared now by many that malfunctioning Complex I in brain mitochondria is a significant source of free radicals.

In the study by Votyakova and Reynolds (2001), the concentration dependence of rotenone-induced free radical production was addressed. It was found that the minimal concentration of rotenone causing noticeable increase of ROS generation in brain mitochondria was 20 nM or 100 pmoles/mg protein; at this point mitochondrial respiration is decreased by half. Two hundred nanomolar rotenone completely inhibited respiration and caused the maximal rate of ROS release. It should be noted that the rate of hydrogen peroxide release by mitochondria is not a linear function of the time, apparently, due to the presence of radical scavenging systems in matrix, which gradually become exhausted, as well as due to the kinetics of O_2^- dismutation. The maximal rate of H_2O_2 release is reached with a lag period after the introduction of stimuli. Experiments in vitro usually last no more than 20 minutes, but it might be anticipated that longer exposures of smaller concentrations of the inhibitor would cause a significant effect. Thus, with protracted inhibition, it is plausible that inhibition of Complex I activity less than 50% could result in a substantial accumulation of ROS in cell.

The low rate of ROS production upon oxidation of NADH-linked substrates in the absence of inhibitors (the basal rate of ROS generation supported by NADH-linked substrates) has a membrane potential-dependent component. As Starkov and Fiskum (66) reported, the basal rate can be diminished by 70% by an uncoupler. The authors also demonstrated the correlation between the basal rate of ROS generation, the redox level of NADH, and the value of $\Delta\Psi$. Since the redox state of pyridine nucleotides depends itself on mitochondrial potential, it is likely that $\Delta\Psi$ effects ROS production via the regulation of NADH redox state. Accumulation of some amount of succinate from the normal operation of the Krebs cycle and, consequently, reverse electron transfer from succinate oxidation by Complex II may be an alternative mechanism in this case. These findings suggest that ROS generation upon oxidation of NADH-linked substrates may fluctuate within physiological changes of membrane potential and redox status.

The question as to where, precisely, free radicals are generated within Complex I is still under debate. The data accumulated in literature suggest all three types of redox centers—FMN, iron-sulfur centers, and semiquinones—to be potential loci for electron leak to molecular oxygen. Additionally, as mentioned before, there is a possibility of radical generation outside of Complex I by molecule of NAD^+ bound to the enzyme, since the presence of NAD^+ substantially increased the rate of free radical generation during the reverse electron flow from succinate (40).

The role of FMN as a site for ROS generation was proposed by several groups (8,35,71). In experiments with rat brain mitochondria, diphenyleneiodonium (DPI), which is known as an inhibitor of flavoprotein in Complex I (63,72), and 1-chloro-2,4-dinitrobenzene (CDNB), which was suggested to directly and specifically increase production of ROS by Complex I in the conditions of reverse electron transfer (8), demonstrated that in Cl^--free media DPI-inhibited succinate-supported ROS induced by CDNB. In addition to that, chemical modification of thiol groups in two subunits located at the electron entry site of Complex I increased free-radical production (35). Covalent binding of oxidized glutathione (GSSG) to redox active thiols of 52-kDa and 75-kDa subunits of Complex I resulted in reversible loss of the enzyme activity which was associated with also reversible elevation of ROS generation. The fact that FMN is bound to the subunit 51 kDa and the 75 kDa is located close to it (73) is an important evidence in support of this hypothesis. Using tightly coupled, inside-out inverted submitochondrial particles and kinetic analysis (71) also suggested FMN as a locus of one electron reduction of molecular oxygen in Complex I.

Participation of different iron-sulfur clusters in ROS generation was also suggested by other findings. Takeshige (74) proposed that superoxide is produced between mercurial (*p*-chloromercuribenzoate)-sensitive and rotenone-sensitive sites in Complex I. Based on an analysis of an kinetics of superoxide formation, they also made a conclusion that at least two autoxidizable sites existed in NADH-dehydrogenase. This hypothesis is supported by findings of Genova et al. (68) who studied the effect of different types of Complex I inhibitors on the ability of SMP to produce free radicals in the presence of NADH and inhibitor of Complex III mucidin; the latter effectively prevents ROS generation in Q-cycle. Authors used *p*-hydroxy-mercuribenzoate (*p*HMB) known to inhibit at the level of iron-sulfur clusters (75) and three other inhibitors that act as quinone antagonists at different hydrophobic sites of Complex I: rolliniastatin at center A, rotenone at center B, and capsaicin at center C by nomenclature of Degli Esposti (76). Having found that *p*-HMB inhibited ROS production by Complex I, while all three quinone antagonists stimulated it, authors came to a conclusion that iron-sulfur center N2, which is located prior to the binding site of these quinone antagonists, donates electrons to molecular oxygen. The possibility that endogenous Complex I quinones could be the site of ROS production was ruled out since the extraction of quinones from SMP did not affect the rate of ROS generation. Kushnareva et al. (21) concluded, based on the results of redox titration, that the center N1a which has the most negative mid-point potential of all iron-sulfur centers of Complex I is the site of superoxide formation.

There is also a possibility that the quinones bound to Complex I ROS can contribute to ROS signal generated by Complex I. As mentioned above, the EPR signal from the fast relaxing pool of ubisemiquinones SQ_{Nf} is dependent of membrane potential and can be quenched by uncoupler (61). This mechanism may be responsible, at least in part, for the $\Delta\Psi$-dependent free radical production described by Starkov and Fiskum (66). However, the observation that rotenone, which blocks electron flow from N2 center to quinones, both quenches ubisemiquinone signal (60), but also induces ROS generation suggests that the majority of free radicals upon inhibition of Complex I originates in centers other than quinones.

It was suggested that the role of hydrophobic subunits of Complex I which are not involved into the enzyme catalytic activity is to protect the redox centers against a sporadic electron leak (61). Interestingly, Complex I in bacteria is much simpler, consisting only of 13 to 14 subunits, and lacks many structural subunits which were found in higher organisms. However, bacterial Complex I possesses the same number of redox centers and is functionally equivalent to its mammalian counterpart (77,55). Taking into account these facts, it is tempting to speculate that the evolution of Complex I design was directed toward an acquisition of additional structural subunits in order to decrease occasional free-radical release.

COMPLEX I IN PARKINSON'S DISEASE: EVIDENCE AND POTENTIAL MECHANISMS FOR IMPAIRMENT

The previous sections establish that complex I is clearly capable of generating ROS under appropriate experimental circumstances, and that excessive ROS generation is most likely to be associated with some level of inhibition of complex I activity. This section of the chapter will describe the mitochondrial impairment that has been reported in PD patients, and will also consider possible mechanisms underlying the impairment. Finally, we will consider whether this level of impairment is consistent with mitochondrial dysfunction being a key pathogenic mechanism in the disease.

Evidence for Complex I Impairment in Parkinson's Disease

Over the last 15 years there have been a number of reports of diminished complex I activity in tissues obtained from patients with Parkinson's disease. Decreased complex I activity has been reported in substantia nigra and striatum of PD brains, and has also been described in skeletal muscle and platelets (78,79), and such deficits are apparent before the onset of treatment (80). Typically, the reported decrease of complex I activity from these studies is approximately 30% to 40% when corrected for citrate synthase activity. Moreover, the defect in complex I activity appears to be relatively selective, in that complexes II to IV are usually found to be unaffected (78). It is important to note that there are also studies that have failed to find a decrease in either activity of complex I (81,82), or in the binding of [^{3}H]dihydrorotenone to complex I from platelets (83). A mechanism for this deficit has not been established, so that it remains unclear whether there is a decrease in the expression levels of one or more protein subunits from complex I, mutations in mtDNA that change activity of complex I, or some form of post-translational modification that alters complex I activity (78). Although each of these have been proposed, none have yet been rigorously supported by experimental evidence (see subsequently).

Potential Mechanisms for Complex I Inhibition

The concept that complex I inhibition could be a key pathogenic mechanism in PD is supported by the observation that systemic administration of complex I inhibitors results in injury to nigrostriatal dopaminergic neurons and a PD-like syndrome in rodents. This injury occurs as a result of accumulation and concentration of MPP+ in dopaminergic neurons following MPTP administration, which is necessary because MPP+ is not a potent complex I inhibitor (84). However, selective dopaminergic neuron damage is also the consequence of rotenone intoxication (85) as discussed elsewhere in this volume, which suggests that dopaminergic neurons may be especially vulnerable to complex I inhibition. Although there have been many suggestions of environmental toxins that could cause PD, we still lack a compelling "smoking gun" candidate toxin that could reasonably account for the disease. As an alternative, can we propose circumstances where dopaminergic neurons are at particular risk of complex I impairment?

Emerging evidence suggests that this may be possible. In particular, neurons that contain high concentrations of dopamine might be at particular risk from oxidative stress because of the oxidative metabolism of dopamine. This might place complex I in those neurons in harms way because it is clear that complex I can be inhibited by oxidants. For example, Zhang et al. (86) showed that hydrogen peroxide, superoxide, and hydroxyl radical can all inhibit complex I. More recent studies have shown that complex I subunits can be modified by peroxynitrite, S-nitrosation, glutathionylation, and formation of nitrotyrosine (87–89). The function of complex I could additionally be impaired if the supply of NADH is restricted, which could be the case following the oxidation of key tricarboxylic acid cycle enzymes like α-ketoglutarate dyhydrogenase (90,91). Glutathione depletion would be an anticipated consequence of an oxidative environment, and glutathione depletion results in complex I inhibition (92). It has additionally been shown that dopamine can contribute to the inhibition of mitochondrial function (93,94). Collectively, these studies illuminate a consistent theme, in that a variety of forms of oxidant burden, whether it is the production of oxidants, the failure to scavenge oxidants, or the reactive nature of the contents of dopaminergic neurons, can all result in the inhibition of complex I activity. Given that many of these mechanisms result in a persistent chemical modification of one or more complex I subunits, they represent the types of modification that should still be apparent after isolation and purification of mitochondria from affected tissues. Thus, oxidant modification of complex I appears to be a plausible mechanism to account for the impairment of complex I, and it would appear that mitochondria in dopaminergic neurons could be at particular risk.

Is Complex I Inhibited Enough?

It is still important to determine whether 30% to 40% inhibition of complex I presents significant pathogenic risk. As noted by Davey et al. (95), there are very different thresholds that have to be reached before inhibition of the individual complexes of the ETC result in decreased ATP synthesis in neuronal mitochondria. For example, complexes III and IV need to be inhibited by 80% and 70%, respectively, before ATP synthesis is impacted. In contrast, 25% inhibition of complex I was sufficient to impair energy production. Even so, 30% inhibition of complex I would not result in a robust energy deficit.

As discussed above, a similar threshold exists when the comparison is made between the inhibition of complex I and the release of hydrogen peroxide. As we demonstrated, complex I-derived ROS only becomes significant when the complex is inhibited >70%, which is far in excess of most estimates from postmortem tissue studies. Ostensibly, this argues against a mechanism in which an oxidative impairment of complex I activity in dopaminergic neurons then generates a feed-forward loop by increasing complex I-derived oxidant generation, because the extent of complex I impairment is too small. However, recent studies have illuminated circumstances where even this modest amount of inhibition could pose a significant risk. In particular, the interaction between calcium and mitochondria appears to increase the liability. Mitochondria are excellent calcium buffers, and glutamate receptor-mediated calcium loading results in calcium accumulation by neuronal mitochondria (96). Calcium-loaded neuronal mitochondria have impaired ADP-stimulated respiration (97), which argues that calcium might impair electron transport. In addition, we showed that calcium greatly increased the sensitivity of mitochondria to rotenone inhibition, such that substantial ROS generation could result with 30% to 40% inhibition of complex I by rotenone (19).

Collectively, these findings suggest a scenario that could make a significant contribution to the injury of dopaminergic neurons in PD. Firstly, the function of complex I is compromised by the oxidative environment found within dopaminergic neurons. This compromise could be exacerbated by environmental toxins that target complex I. Critically, the partially impaired complex I that results from the initial oxidative stress could then generate excess ROS when exposed to elevated intracellular calcium, such that even normal signaling events within neurons then become a liability. The excess ROS generated by mitochondria would then serve to further endanger the dopaminergic neuron. There are a number of other factors, including excess iron and glutathione depletion that could contribute either to the initial oxidative injury that damages complex I or else could exacerbate the down-stream events once mitochondria generate excess ROS, which might injure the neuron yet more.

CONCLUSIONS

Mitochondria are clearly an important potential source of ROS in neurons. However, it is critical to understand the mechanisms of ROS generation as well as have a solid appreciation of the methods used to dissect mechanisms. The analysis of mechanisms of ROS generation reveals several potential sources of oxidants, although we would conclude that the most efficacious oxidant-production pathway (succinate-driven reverse electron transport) is unlikely to be of major significance in either intact or injured neurons. Within the context of PD, it is intriguing to note several intersecting phenomena, including the generation of PD-like symptoms in animals treated with complex I inhibitors, the impairment of complex I activity in PD patients, and the increase in ROS generation when complex I is inhibited. We would speculate that these features together create the potential for a feed-forward mechanism to account for dopamine neuron death, whereby complex I inhibition results in increased oxidant generation in dopaminergic neurons, which then further inhibits complex I and enhances ROS production to a greater extent. While this speculation does not identify the initiating event in the cascade, it nevertheless provides a compelling mechanism for injury amplification, and suggests that abrogation of the oxidative stress could interrupt the progress of the disease.

SUMMARY

It is widely recognized that mitochondria are a significant source of reactive oxygen species in cells. As many neurodegenerative diseases have oxidative stress as a key phenotype, this leads to the conclusion that altered mitochondrial function could be a critical pathogenic mechanism. This is especially true in PD where it is possible to model the disease using mitochondrial inhibitors and where mitochondrial impairment has been described in PD patients. However, assessing the validity of the claim that mitochondria are at the center of PD pathogenesis requires a critical assessment of both the methods used for ROS detection and the putative mechanisms for ROS generation by these organelles. In this chapter we review the techniques commonly applied to ROS detection by mitochondria, and also describe the principle mechanisms by which mitochondria generate ROS. We conclude with a synthesis of the findings of mitochondrial impairment in PD, and suggest a self-amplifying mechanism for mitochondrial ROS generation that could underlie the loss of dopaminergic neurons in PD.

REFERENCES

1. Jensen PK. Antimycin-insensitive oxidation of succinate and reduced nicotinamide-adenine dinucleotide in electron-transport particles. I. pH dependency and hydrogen peroxide formation. Biochim Biophys Acta 1966; 122:157.
2. Boveris A, Chance B. The mitochondrial generation of hydrogen peroxide. General properties and effect of hyperbaric oxygen. Biochem J 1973; 134:707.
3. Loschen G, Azzi A, Richter C, Flohe L. Superoxide radicals as precursors of mitochondrial hydrogen peroxide. FEBS Lett 1974; 42:68.
4. Boveris A, Cadenas E. Mitochondrial production of superoxide anions and its relationship to the antimycin insensitive respiration. FEBS Lett 1975; 54:311.
5. Andreae WA. A sensitive method for the estimation of hydrogen peroxide in biological materials. Nature 1955; 175:859.
6. Loschen G, Flohe L, Chance B. Respiratory chain linked H(2)O(2) production in pigeon heart mitochondria. FEBS Lett 1971; 18:261.
7. Staniek K, Nohl H. H(2)O(2) detection from intact mitochondria as a measure for one-electron reduction of dioxygen requires a non-invasive assay system. Biochim Biophys Acta 1999; 1413:70.

8. Liu Y, Fiskum G, Schubert D. Generation of reactive oxygen species by the mitochondrial electron transport chain. J Neurochem 2002; 80:780.
9. Hansford RG, Hogue BA, Mildaziene V. Dependence of H2O2 formation by rat heart mitochondria on substrate availability and donor age. J Bioenerg Biomembr 1997; 29:89.
10. Kwong LK, Sohal RS. Substrate and site specificity of hydrogen peroxide generation in mouse mitochondria. Arch Biochem Biophys 1998; 350:118.
11. Loschen G, Azzi A, Flohe L. Mitochondrial H2O2 formation: relationship with energy conservation. FEBS Lett 1973; 33:84.
12. Boveris A, Martino E, Stoppani AO. Evaluation of the horseradish peroxidase-scopoletin method for the measurement of hydrogen peroxide formation in biological systems. Anal Biochem 1977; 80:145.
13. Patole MS, Swaroop A, Ramasarma T. Generation of H2O2 in brain mitochondria. J Neurochem 1986; 47:1.
14. Korshunov SS, Skulachev VP, Starkov AA. High protonic potential actuates a mechanism of production of reactive oxygen species in mitochondria. FEBS Lett 1997; 416:15.
15. Starkov AA, Fiskum G. Myxothiazol induces H(2)O(2) production from mitochondrial respiratory chain. Biochem Biophys Res Commun 2001; 281:645.
16. Mohanty JG, Jaffe JS, Schulman ES, Raible DG. A highly sensitive fluorescent microassay of H2O2 release from activated human leukocytes using a dihydroxyphenoxazine derivative. J Immunol Methods 1997; 202:133.
17. Votyakova TV, Reynolds IJ. Detection of hydrogen peroxide with Amplex Red: interference by NADH and reduced glutathione auto-oxidation. Arch Biochem Biophys 2004; 431:138.
18. Vinogradov AD, Sled VD, Burbaev DS, Grivennikova VG, Moroz IA, Ohnishi T. Energy-dependent Complex I-associated ubisemiquinones in submitochondrial particles. FEBS Lett 1995; 370:83.
19. Votyakova TV, Reynolds IJ. DeltaPsi(m)-Dependent and -independent production of reactive oxygen species by rat brain mitochondria. J Neurochem 2001; 79:266.
20. Starkov AA, Polster BM, Fiskum G. Regulation of hydrogen peroxide production by brain mitochondria by calcium and Bax. J Neurochem 2002; 83:220.
21. Kushnareva Y, Murphy AN, Andreyev A. Complex I-mediated reactive oxygen species generation: modulation by cytochrome c and NAD(P)+ oxidation-reduction state. Biochem J 2002; 368:545.
22. Chen Q, Vazquez EJ, Moghaddas S, Hoppel CL, Lesnefsky EJ. Production of reactive oxygen species by mitochondria: central role of complex III. J Biol Chem 2003; 278: 36027.
23. Halliwell B, Gutteridge JMC. Free radicals in biology and medicine, p 936. Oxford University Press, Oxford, UK. 2000
24. Boveris A, Oshino N, Chance B. The cellular production of hydrogen peroxide. Biochem J 1972; 128:617.
25. Rothe G, Valet G. Flow cytometric analysis of respiratory burst activity in phagocytes with hydroethidine and 2',7'-dichlorofluorescin. J Leukoc Biol 1990; 47:440.
26. Carter WO, Narayanan PK, Robinson JP. Intracellular hydrogen peroxide and superoxide anion detection in endothelial cells. J Leukoc Biol 1994; 55:253.
27. Tsuchiya M, Suematsu M, Suzuki H. In vivo visualization of oxygen radical-dependent photoemission. Methods Enzymol 1994; 233:128.
28. LeBel CP, Ischiropoulos H, Bondy SC. Evaluation of the probe 2',7'-dichlorofluorescin as an indicator of reactive oxygen species formation and oxidative stress. Chem Res Toxicol 1992; 5:227.
29. Maciel EN, Vercesi AE, Castilho RF. Oxidative stress in Ca(2+)-induced membrane permeability transition in brain mitochondria. J Neurochem 2001; 79:1237.
30. Brustovetsky N, Dubinsky JM, Antonsson B, Jemmerson R. Two pathways for tBID-induced cytochrome c release from rat brain mitochondria: BAK- versus BAX-dependence. J Neurochem 2003; 84:196.
31. Sousa SC, Maciel EN, Vercesi AE, Castilho RF. Ca2+-induced oxidative stress in brain mitochondria treated with the respiratory chain inhibitor rotenone. FEBS Lett 2003; 543:179.
32. Azzi A, Montecucco C, Richter C. The use of acetylated ferricytochrome c for the detection of superoxide radicals produced in biological membranes. Biochem Biophys Res Commun 1975; 65:597.

33. Turrens JF, Freeman BA, Levitt JG, Crapo JD. The effect of hyperoxia on superoxide production by lung submitochondrial particles. Arch Biochem Biophys 1982; 217:401.

34. Boveris A, Cadenas E, Stoppani AO. Role of ubiquinone in the mitochondrial generation of hydrogen peroxide. Biochem J 1976; 156:435.

35. Taylor ER, Hurrell F, Shannon RJ, Lin TK, Hirst J, Murphy MP. Reversible glutathionylation of complex I increases mitochondrial superoxide formation. J Biol Chem 2003; 278:19603.

36. Misra HP, Fridovich I. The purification and properties of superoxide dismutase from Neurospora crassa. J Biol Chem 1972; 247:3410.

37. Takeshige K, Minakami S. NADH- and NADPH-dependent formation of superoxide anions by bovine heart submitochondrial particles and NADH-ubiquinone reductase preparation. Biochem J 1979; 180:129–135.

38. Turrens JF, Boveris A. Generation of superoxide anion by the NADH dehydrogenase of bovine heart mitochondria. Biochem J 191:421.

39. Turrens JF, Freeman BA, Crapo JD. Hyperoxia increases H2O2 release by lung mitochondria and microsomes. Arch Biochem Biophys 1982a; 217:411.

40. Krishnamoorthy G, Hinkle PC. Studies on the electron transfer pathway, topography of iron-sulfur centers, and site of coupling in NADH-Q oxidoreductase. J Biol Chem 1988; 263:17566.

41. Arnaiz SL, Coronel MF, Boveris A. Nitric oxide, superoxide, and hydrogen peroxide production in brain mitochondria after haloperidol treatment. Nitric Oxide 1999; 3:235.

42. Ksenzenko M, Konstantinov AA, Khomutov GB, Tikhonov AN, Ruuge EK. Effect of electron transfer inhibitors on superoxide generation in the cytochrome bc1 site of the mitochondrial respiratory chain. FEBS Lett 1983; 155:19.

43. Ksenzenko M, Konstantinov AA, Khomutov GB, Tikhonov AN, Ruuge EK. Relationships between the effects of redox potential, alpha-thenoyltrifluoroacetone and malonate on O(2) and H2O2 generation by submitochondrial particles in the presence of succinate and antimycin. FEBS Lett 1984; 175:105.

44. Korshunov SS, Korkina OV, Ruuge EK, Skulachev VP, Starkov AA. Fatty acids as natural uncouplers preventing generation of O2- and H2O2 by mitochondria in the resting state. FEBS Lett 1998; 435:215.

45. Dykens JA. Isolated cerebral and cerebellar mitochondria produce free radicals when exposed to elevated CA2+ and Na+: implications for neurodegeneration. J Neurochem 1994; 63:584.

46. Morkunaite-Haimi S, Kruglov AG, Teplova VV, et al. Reactive oxygen species are involved in the stimulation of the mitochondrial permeability transition by dihydrolipoate. Biochem Pharmacol 2003; 65:43.

47. Han D, Williams E, Cadenas E. Mitochondrial respiratory chain-dependent generation of superoxide anion and its release into the intermembrane space. Biochem J 2001; 353:411.

48. Maskiewicz R, Sogah D, Bruice TC. Chemiluminescenct reactions of lucigenin.1. Reactions of lucigenin with hydrogen peroxide. Journal of American Chemical Society 1979; 101:5347–5354.

49. Malehorn CL, Riehl TE, Hinze WL. Improved determination of hydrogen peroxide or lucigenin by measurement of lucigenin chemiluminescence in organized assemblies. Analyst 1986; 3:941–948.

50. Li Y, Zhu H, Kuppusamy P, Roubaud V, Zweier JL, Trush MA. Validation of lucigenin (bis-N-methylacridinium) as a chemilumigenic probe for detecting superoxide anion radical production by enzymatic and cellular systems. J Biol Chem 1998; 273:2015–2023.

51. Lucas M, Solano F. Coelenterazine is a superoxide anion-sensitive chemiluminescent probe: its usefulness in the assay of respiratory burst in neutrophils. Anal Biochem 1992; 206:273–277.

52. Li Y, Stansbury KH, Zhu H, Trush MA. Biochemical characterization of lucigenin (Bis-N-methylacridinium) as a chemiluminescent probe for detecting intramitochondrial superoxide anion radical production. Biochem Biophys Res Commun 1999; 262:80.

53. Yurkov IS, Kruglov AG, Evtodienko YV, Yaguzhinsky LS. Mechanism of superoxide anion generation in intact mitochondria in the presence of lucigenin and cyanide. Biochemistry (Mosc) 2003; 68:1349.

54. Ohnishi T, Sled VD, Yano T, Yagi T, Burbaev DS, Vinogradov AD. Structure-function studies of iron-sulfur clusters and semiquinones in the NADH-Q oxidoreductase segment of the respiratory chain. Biochim Biophys Acta 1998; 1365:301.
55. Raha S, Myint AT, Johnstone L, Robinson BH. Control of oxygen free radical formation from mitochondrial complex I: roles for protein kinase A and pyruvate dehydrogenase kinase. Free Radic Biol Med 2002; 32:421.
56. Rao NA, Felton SP, Huennekens FM, Mackler B. Flavin mononucleotide: the coenzyme of reduced diphosphopyridine nucleotide dehydrogenase. J Biol Chem 1963; 238:449.
57. Ohnishi T, Salerno JC. Iron-sufur Proteins, Vol. 4. New-York: Willey, 1982:285–327.
58. Beinert H, Albracht SP. New insights, ideas, and unanswered questions concerning iron-sulfur clusters in mitochondria. Biochim Biophys Acta 1982; 683:245.
59. De Jong AM, Albracht SP. Ubisemiquinones as obligatory intermediates in the electron transfer from NADH to ubiquinone. Eur J Biochem 1994; 222:975.
60. Magnitsky S, Toulokhonova L, Yano T, et al. EPR characterization of ubisemiquinones and iron-sulfur cluster N2, central components of the energy coupling in the NADH-ubiquinone oxidoreductase (complex I) in situ. J Bioenerg Biomembr 2002; 34:193.
61. Vinogradov AD. Catalytic properties of the mitochondrial NADH-ubiquinone oxidoreductase (complex I) and the pseudo-reversible active/inactive enzyme transition. Biochim Biophys Acta 1998; 1364:169–185.
62. Hinkle PC, Butow RA, Racker E, Chance B. Partial resolution of the enzymes catalyzing oxidative phosphorylation. XV. Reverse electron transfer in the flavin-cytochrome beta region of the respiratory chain of beef heart submitochondrial particles. J Biol Chem 1967; 242:5169.
63. Holland PC, Clark MG, Bloxham DP, Lardy HA. Mechanism of action of the hypoglycemic agent diphenyleneiodonium. J Biol Chem 1973; 248:6050.
64. Hoyer S, Krier C. Ischemia and aging brain. Studies on glucose and energy metabolism in rat cerebral cortex. Neurobiol Aging 1986; 7:23.
65. Camici P, Marraccini P, Lorenzoni R, et al. Metabolic markers of stress-induced myocardial ischemia. Circulation 1991; 83:III8.
66. Starkov AA, Fiskum G. Regulation of brain mitochondrial H2O2 production by membrane potential and NAD(P)H redox state. J Neurochem 2003; 86:1101.
67. Ramsay RR, Singer TP. Relation of superoxide generation and lipid peroxidation to the inhibition of NADH-Q oxidoreductase by rotenone, piericidin A, and MPP+. Biochem Biophys Res Commun 1992; 189:47.
68. Genova ML, Ventura B, Giuliano G, et al. The site of production of superoxide radical in mitochondrial Complex I is not a bound ubisemiquinone but presumably iron-sulfur cluster N2. FEBS Lett 2001; 505:364.
69. Zoccarato F, Cavallini L, Deana R, Alexandre A. Pathways of hydrogen peroxide generation in guinea pig cerebral cortex mitochondria. Biochem Biophys Res Commun 1988; 154:727.
70. Cino M, Del Maestro RF. Generation of hydrogen peroxide by brain mitochondria: the effect of reoxygenation following postdecapitative ischemia. Arch Biochem Biophys 1989; 269:623.
71. Vinogradov AD, Grivennikova VG. Generation of superoxide-radical by the NADH: ubiquinone oxidoreductase of heart mitochondria. Biochemistry (Mosc) 2005; 70:120–127.
72. Ragan CI, Bloxham DP. Specific labelling of a constituent polypeptide of bovine heart mitochondrial reduced nicotinamide-adenine dinucleotide-ubiquinone reductase by the inhibitor diphenyleneiodonium. Biochem J 1977; 163:605.
73. Walker JE. The NADH: ubiquinone oxidoreductase (complex I) of respiratory chains. Q Rev Biophys 1992; 25:253.
74. Kang D, Narabayashi H, Sata T, Takeshige K. Kinetics of superoxide formation by respiratory chain. J Biochem (Tokyo) 1983; 94:1301.
75. Ruzicka FJ, Crane FL. Quinone interaction with the respiratory chain-linked NADH dehydrogenase of beef heart mitochondria. II. Duroquinone reductase activity. Biochim Biophys Acta 1971; 226:221.
76. Degli Esposti M. Inhibitors of NADH-ubiquinone reductase: an overview. Biochim Biophys Acta 1998; 1364:222.

77. Finel M. Organization and evolution of structural elements within complex I. Biochim Biophys Acta 1998; 1364:112.
78. Schapira AH. Evidence for mitochondrial dysfunction in Parkinson's disease—a critical appraisal. Mov Disord 1994; 9:125.
79. Shults CW. Mitochondrial dysfunction and possible treatments in Parkinson's disease-a review. Mitochondrion 2004; 4:641–648.
80. Haas RH, Nasirian F, Nakano K, et al. Low platelet mitochondrial complex I and complex II/III activity in early untreated Parkinson's disease. Ann Neurol 1995; 37:714–722.
81. Martin MA, Molina JA, Jimenez-Jimenez FJ, et al. Respiratory-chain enzyme activities in isolated mitochondria of lymphocytes from untreated Parkinson's disease patients. Grupo-Centro de Trastornos del Movimiento. Neurology 1996; 46:1343–1346.
82. Hanagasi HA, Ayribas D, Baysal K, Emre M. Mitochondrial complex I, II/III, and IV activities in familial and sporadic Parkinson's disease. Int J Neurosci 2005; 115:479–493.
83. Blandini F, Nappi G, Greenamyre JT. Quantitative study of mitochondrial complex I in platelets of parkinsonian patients. Mov Disord 1998; 13:11–15.
84. Ramsay RR, Salach JI, Singer TP. Uptake of the neurotoxin 1-methyl-4-phenylpyridine (MPP+) by mitochondria and its relation to the inhibition of the mitochondrial oxidation of NAD+-linked substrates by MPP+. Biochem Biophys Res Commun 1986; 134:743–748.
85. Betarbet R, Sherer TB, MacKenzie G, Garcia-Osuna M, Panov AV, Greenamyre JT. Chronic systemic pesticide exposure reproduces features of Parkinson's disease. Nat Neurosci 2000; 3:1301–1306.
86. Zhang Y, Marcillat O, Giulivi C, Ernster L, Davies KJ. The oxidative inactivation of mitochondrial electron transport chain components and ATPase. J Biol Chem 1990; 265:16330–16336.
87. Murray J, Taylor SW, Zhang B, Ghosh SS, Capaldi RA. Oxidative damage to mitochondrial complex I due to peroxynitrite: identification of reactive tyrosines by mass spectrometry. J Biol Chem 2003; 278:37223.
88. Beer SM, Taylor ER, Brown SE, et al. Glutaredoxin 2 catalyzes the reversible oxidation and glutathionylation of mitochondrial membrane thiol proteins: implications for mitochondrial redox regulation and antioxidant DEFENSE. J Biol Chem 2004; 279:47939–47951.
89. Brown GC, Borutaite V. Inhibition of mitochondrial respiratory complex I by nitric oxide, peroxynitrite and S-nitrosothiols. Biochim Biophys Acta 2004; 1658:44.
90. Tretter L, Adam-Vizi V. Inhibition of Krebs cycle enzymes by hydrogen peroxide: A key role of [alpha]-ketoglutarate dehydrogenase in limiting NADH production under oxidative stress. J Neurosci 2000; 20:8972.
91. Gibson GE, Kingsbury AE, Xu H, et al. Deficits in a tricarboxylic acid cycle enzyme in brains from patients with Parkinson's disease. Neurochem Int 2003; 43:129–135.
92. Hsu M, Srinivas B, Kumar J, Subramanian R, Andersen J. Glutathione depletion resulting in selective mitochondrial complex I inhibition in dopaminergic cells is via an NO-mediated pathway not involving peroxynitrite: implications for Parkinson's disease. J Neurochem 2005; 92:1091–1103.
93. Berman SB, Hastings TG. Dopamine oxidation alters mitochondrial respiration and induces permeability transition in brain mitochondria: implications for Parkinson's disease. J Neurochem 1999; 73:1127–1137.
94. Ben-Shachar D, Zuk R, Gazawi H, Ljubuncic P. Dopamine toxicity involves mitochondrial complex I inhibition: implications to dopamine-related neuropsychiatric disorders. Biochem Pharmacol 2004; 67:1965–1974.
95. Davey GP, Peuchen S, Clark JB. Energy thresholds in brain mitochondria. Potential involvement in neurodegeneration. J Biol Chem 1998; 273:12753–12757.
96. White RJ, Reynolds IJ. Mitochondria and Na+/Ca2+ exchange buffer glutamate-induced calcium loads in cultured cortical neurons. J Neurosci 1995; 15:1318–1328.
97. Kushnareva YE, Wiley SE, Ward MW, Andreyev AY, Murphy AN. Excitotoxic injury to mitochondria isolated from cultured neurons. J Biol Chem 2005; 280:28894–28902.
98. Votyakova TV, Reynolds IJ. Ca2+-induced permeabilization promotes free radical release from rat brain mitochondria with partially inhibited complex I. J Neurochem 2005; 93:526–537.

16 The Ubiquitin-Proteasome System in Parkinson's Disease

Leonidas Stefanis

Section of Basic Neurosciences, Foundation for Biomedical Research of the Academy of Athens, Athens, Greece

INTRODUCTION

Over the past few years, increasing evidence has linked the ubiquitin-proteasome system (UPS) to Parkinson's disease (PD) and related disorders. In particular, it has been posited that dysfunction of this system may underlie certain forms of PD (1). UPS dysfunction may also be involved in other neurodegenerative diseases. Whether this involvement is primary and plays a role in disease pathogenesis is a subject of debate (see 2). Primarily because of the existence of genetic data linking PD to the UPS, evidence for the involvement of this system is strongest for this particular neurodegenerative condition.

THE UBIQUITIN-PROTEASOME SYSTEM

The UPS is one of the main systems of intracellular protein degradation. Although for the purposes of this chapter, we will only address the potential involvement of the UPS in PD and related disorders, it is important to keep in mind that other protein degradation systems, such as the lysosomes, may also play a role in disease pathogenesis. Targets for degradation by the UPS include, but are not limited to, rapidly turning over, misfolded, damaged, or oxidatively modified proteins. In a typical cell, the majority of protein degradation may occur through this system. In most cases protein substrates are tagged with multiple adducts of a small molecule, ubiquitin, in order to be degraded through the UPS. The process of ubiquitination involves first the activation, in an Adenosine triphosphate (ATP)-dependent fashion, of ubiquitin by a universal E1 ubiquitin-activating–enzyme. Activated ubiquitin is then transferred to a member of the E2 ubiquitin conjugating enzyme (UBC) family, forming a high-energy intermediate. E2s then transfer the ubiquitin moiety to a complex formed between a member of the E3 ligase family and the particular protein substrate. The end result is the covalent attachment of ubiquitin to a lysine residue of the substrate, via the catalytic activity of the ligase. The cycle is then repeated to attach further ubiquitin moieties, thus forming a polyubiquitin chain on the substrate. In some cases, E4 enzymes are involved in the stacking of ubiquitin molecules on each other. E2s and, especially, E3s and E4s, unlike E1, are specific for a substrate or a group of substrates.

The polyubiquitinated proteins that are formed are subsequently recognized and degraded by the proteasome. Natively unfolded proteins may not need to be tagged by ubiquitin to be degraded by the proteasome, and thus ubiquitin-independent proteasomal degradation may also occur. The 26S proteasome contains a core catalytic component, the 20S proteasome, flanked on both sides by a 19S cap. Polyubiquitinated proteins signaled for degradation are recognized by and bind to components of the 19S cap. Four or more ubiquitin adducts are required for recognition. Following detachment of the polyubiquitin chain, substrates enter the cylindrical pore formed by the 20S proteasome, which is a barrel-like structure that consists of two identical outer rings of seven α subunits each and two identical inner rings of seven β subunits each. Within the 20S core, substrates are degraded by three sets of enzymes, with chymotrypsin-like, trypsin-like, and peptidylglutamyl-like activity. Proteasomal proteolysis is ATP-dependent and leads to the production of small peptides that are further degraded in the cytosol. The polyubiquitin chains are hydrolyzed to monomeric ubiquitin through the action of deubiquitinating enzymes, which include, among others, ubiquitin C-terminal hydrolases (UCHs). The released monomeric ubiquitin is reactivated by E1 in order to act on further substrates (2).

It should be noted that the structure of the proteasome is not always the same; it may differ depending on the cell type and the particular physiological state. Alternative structures apart from the 20S capped with two 19S particles include free 20S, 20S capped with only one 19S, or 20S capped with another regulatory subunit, PA28. Furthermore, the composition of the particular subunits of even the 20S proteasome may be variable. Proteolysis through isolated 20S proteasome or 20S proteasome linked to PA28 is ubiquitin independent.

Some technical notes about methods to assess UPS function are warranted here. The function of the proteasome is classically assessed by measuring the three enzymatic activities present within the 20S core. This is done by incubating cell lysates or tissue extracts with artificial fluorogenic substrates that are cleaved by the enzymatic activities, thus emitting signals that can be measured in a fluorimeter. Alternatively, the levels or, even better, the half-lives of particular substrate proteins that are known to be targeted to and degraded by the proteasome can be assessed. Such artificial substrates have been created and tagged to fluorescent proteins, so that their potential accumulation can be monitored in living cells. There are advantages and disadvantages to each approach: The enzymatic activity method measures directly proteasomal activity and is quite sensitive, but is performed in an artificial setting, after the cells have been lysed, and may not correlate with proteasomal activity in the cells. The fluorescent substrate method is not as sensitive as measurement of proteasomal enzymatic activity. Small differences may be hard to quantify by fluorescence imaging, although in some cases Western immunoblotting has been successfully used. This method may show impairment of the UPS that occurs at another level, and not at the proteasome, and it measures the activity of the UPS in a cellular context. Transgenic mice expressing fluorescent-tagged proteins that are artificial substrates could potentially be used to assess the function of the UPS in vivo. In terms of levels of substrate proteins, a method that can be used to assess them more globally is Western immunoblotting for ubiquitin. In the case of impairment of the proteasomal system, there should be accumulation of polyubiquitinated proteins. It is clear that every method has its merits, and ideally a combination should be used for more definitive results.

GENETIC DATA SUPPORTING A ROLE FOR UBIQUITIN-PROTEASOME SYSTEM INVOLVEMENT IN PARKINSON'S DISEASE

As mentioned, genetic data support the idea that defects in the UPS may lead to PD. Two proteins linked genetically to the disease, *PARKIN* and *UCH-L1*, are involved in the UPS. In many cases of early onset autosomal recessive PD affected individuals harbor mutations in the gene encoding for *PARKIN*. *PARKIN* has turned out to be an E3 ligase, and mutations in the gene lead to diminution or loss of this activity (reviewed in 3). The subject of *PARKIN* is discussed extensively elsewhere in this volume, but it is worth mentioning that *PARKIN* overexpression may ameliorate proteasomal function (4,5). Furthermore, *PARKIN* protected against proteasomal inhibition-induced death of cultured ventral midbrain dopaminergic neurons and other neuronal cells, and antisense-induced down regulation of the *PARKIN* expression in neuroblastoma cells led to inhibition of proteasomal-dependent protein clearance (6). In addition, *PARKIN* may act, through its binding to the molecular chaperone HSP70, as a general facilitator of the degradation of proteins that misfold in the endoplasmic reticulum or the cytosol (5). Consistent with this idea, the N-terminal ubiquitin-like domain of *PARKIN* binds directly to the 26S proteasome and enhances its degradative ability (5,7). Thus, the absence of *PARKIN*, apart from its effects on the build-up of its specific protein substrates, may lead to more generalized proteasomal defects. Whether such general defects exist in the affected regions of patients suffering from *PARKIN* -related neurodegeneration or in the brains of mice null for *PARKIN* has not been tested specifically.

A mutation in *UCH-L1*, I93M, has been found in one family with autosomal dominant PD (8). This mutation co-segregated with a Parkinsonian phenotype in this family, but the fact that it has not been encountered in multiple genetic studies around the world has cast doubt on its pathogenicity. Further genetic data regarding *UCH-L1* provide another link to PD. A meta-analysis from multiple data sets from different populations has shown that a relatively common polymorphism, S18Y, is negatively associated with the chance of developing PD (9). It should be noted however that an even more recent meta-analysis, that included a large number of cases from Britain, did not detect a correlation between the presence of S18Y and PD (10). Therefore, at this point, there are no definitive genetic data linking *UCH-L1* to PD. It is however likely that *UCH-L1* mutations or polymorphisms, and in particular the S18Y variant, may play a role in the PD development within specific populations. *UCH-L1* is an abundant neuronal-specific protein, which belongs to the family of UCHs (11). Although its exact cellular substrate(s) is unknown, it may act on linear poly-ubiquitin proteins, as they are produced during translation, or on polyubiquitinated proteins following their degradation by the proteasome to a small peptide bound to the polyubiquitin chain (11–14). *UCH-L1* may also function to maintain sufficient levels of free ubiquitin in the cell through direct binding and inhibition of the degradation of free ubiquitin in the lysosomes (15). Liu et al. (16) proposed an unexpected function of *UCH-L1*, as an aberrant E3 ligase, which binds to protein substrates such as α-synuclein and ubiquitinates them at an aberrant site, leading to their lack of recognition by the proteasome and consequent build-up in the cell. I93L confers a 50% decrease in the in vitro enzymatic activity of this protein as a deubiquitinating enzyme, leading to the hypothesis that in this particular case PD may be due to haploinsufficiency (8,17). This mutation also leads to an increase of the purported aberrant E3 ligase activity, suggesting instead a gain of function (16). The protective S18Y polymorphism leads to a slight increase of the in vitro deubiquitinating activity and to a decrease of the E3 ligase activity (16,17). Lack of *UCH-L1* in mice leads to sensory ataxia and axonal degeneration in the gracile nucleus. Such *gad* (gracile axonal dystrophy) mice show a marked decrease in the levels of free ubiquitin (15). In conjunction, it is clear that, despite the lack of consensus on the normal function of *UCH-L1* and on the changes conferred on this function by genetic alterations, this protein is somehow involved in the pathway of ubiquitination and subsequent proteasomal degradation. The notion that loss of function of *UCH-L1* is linked to PD pathogenesis is strengthened by studies in human post-mortem material, which have found decreased levels of *UCH-L1* in patients with PD and diffuse Lewy body disease (DLBD) (18,19). In one of these studies, extensive oxidative modifications were found on *UCH-L1*, likely leading to further loss of its function (18).

The proteins encoded by the two other genes linked to PD, *PINK-1* (20), and *DJ-1* (21), do not have an obvious link to the proteasome system of protein degradation, although *DJ-1* may subserve SUMOlation, a function akin to ubiquitylation. *PINK-1* overexpression led to protection from proteasomal inhibition-induced death (20), and *DJ-1* deficiency led to enhancement of death toward the same stimulus (22). It is likely that these effects are secondary to primary effects of these proteins at the levels of mitochondria and oxidative stress, but the possibility that there is a direct relationship with the UPS cannot be excluded.

α-SYNUCLEIN: RELATIONSHIP TO THE UBIQUITIN-PROTEASOME SYSTEM

The first gene found to be linked to PD encodes for the presynaptic protein α-synuclein (23), which turned out to be a major component of Lewy bodies (LBs) (24). Topics related to α-synuclein are reviewed elsewhere in this volume. We will only address here issues related to its possible relationship with the UPS. The first issue is whether α-synuclein is degraded by the UPS and whether it is ubiquitinated.

Initial reports (25,26) suggested that α-synuclein is ubiquitinated and degraded by the proteasome; however, others failed to find significant upregulation of overexpressed α-synuclein with the application of proteasomal inhibitors to cell lines (27,28). A subsequent study showed that α-synuclein has a long half-life and is not ubiquitinated, but is nevertheless degraded by the proteasome (29). Indeed, certain proteins with exposed hydrophobic domains or proteins present in a natively unfolded state, such as α-synuclein, do not need to be ubiquitinated to be degraded by the proteasome. In pathological specimens from patients with Lewy body diseases, although mono- and di-ubiquitination were noted, polyubiquitinated species were negligible (30,31). Mono- and di-ubiquitinated species would not be expected to be targeted for degradation by the proteasome. In our own hands, levels or half-life of endogenous rat α-synuclein were not increased following proteasomal inhibition in neuronal cell lines or primary neurons, including ventral midbrain dopaminergic neurons (32–34). Instead, we have recently presented evidence that α-synuclein is degraded in lysosomes via the specific active process of chaperone-mediated autophagy (CMA) (34). In particular, we have shown that purified α-synuclein is uptaken by isolated lysosomes through this mechanism. Degradation of α-synuclein occurred through lysosomes, but not through macroautophagy, in PC12 cells and ventral midbrain dopaminergic neurons, leading, by exclusion, to the notion that such degradation must occur through CMA (34). In a study that appears to reconcile opposing views, Webb et al. (35) used an inducible system of overexpression in naïve and neuronally differentiated PC12 cells, and found that α-synuclein was degraded not only by the proteasome but also by the mechanism of macroautophagy. The macroautophagy route of degradation was especially prominent for the mutant forms. Lee et al. (36) specifically assessed the degradation of oligomeric forms, and found that these were cleared by lysosomes, but not by macroautophagy, in neuroblastoma cells. Proteasomal inhibitors did not affect degradation of monomeric or oligomeric forms.

In view of the above conflicting data, it is fair to say that although the main route of α-synuclein degradation may be via CMA, alternative routes, such as macroautophagy or the UPS may play a role under physiologic or pathologic conditions. The manner of α-synuclein degradation may depend on the particular species, conformation and localization of α-synuclein, as well as the cellular context. Consistent with the importance of the particular species examined, recent results from our lab show that in PC12 cells stably transfected with A53T α-synuclein, application of a proteasomal inhibitor led to no change of total α-synuclein levels, but to a dramatic induction of specific SDS-collapsable oligomeric species that associate with the 26S proteasome (Evangelia Emmanouilidou, Kostas Vekrellis and Leonidas Stefanis, unpublished results). This indicates that only very specific oligomeric species of α-synuclein are degraded by the proteasome.

A number of laboratories, including our own, have shown that overexpression of mutant α-synuclein in neuronal cell lines leads to impairment of proteasomal activity (6,37–39). In another report, overexpression of WT α-synuclein was also associated with proteasomal impairment (40). A more recent study, however, failed to find significant impairment of proteasomal activity in PC12 cells' overexpressing fusion constructs of α-synuclein. Furthermore, there was no significant downregulation of proteasomal activity in the CNS of four-month-old transgenic mice expressing mutant A30P α-synuclein (41). It would be interesting to see if these mice develop proteasomal impairment at seven to eight months, when perikaryal accumulation of α-synuclein is first noted (42). In another recent study, there was a relative impairment of 20S proteasomal activity in the ventral midbrain of aged mice expressing double mutant (A30P and A53T) α-synuclein under the control of a tyrosine hydroxylase (TH) promoter compared to control animals (43). Overall, the weight of evidence suggests that overexpression of α-synuclein can be associated with UPS, and in particular proteasome, dysfunction. A critical question is at what time point this dysfunction occurs, and whether it contributes to the toxicity conferred by aberrant α-synuclein.

Purely in vitro studies have suggested a direct effect of α-synuclein on the proteasome. Purified α-synuclein was shown by Snyder et al. (40) to inhibit the function of the 26S proteasome. This effect was presumably mediated by direct binding to the S6' subunit of the 19S proteasome. The inhibitory effect was much stronger with fibrillar α-synuclein when compared to the native form (40). Of note, binding of α-synuclein to S6' had been previously reported by another group (44). Lindersson et al. (45) performed a similar study and also found that purified α-synuclein inhibited the proteasome. However, inhibition was confined to the chymotrypsin-like activity, and binding occurred almost exclusively with components of the 20S proteasome. Soluble oligomeric and not fully aggregated forms were primarily responsible for binding and inhibition. The authors suggested that experimental variables, and in particular differences in the purification procedures, may play a role in the differences observed between the two studies (45). Interestingly, β-synuclein prevented α-synuclein-induced proteasomal inhibition in this purified system (46). β-synuclein is known to antagonize the fibrillar components of α-synuclein. This therefore provides further support for the idea that fibrillar α-synuclein is the species involved in proteasomal inhibition in these in vitro studies.

The mechanism through which α-synuclein may induce proteasomal dysfunction is unclear, although the general principle of "clogging" of the proteasome by aggregates may apply. Lindersson et al. (45) proposed that allosteric modulation of the β5 subunit through binding of soluble oligomeric α-synuclein to its outer regions that are not facing the interior of the 20S may be responsible. In this case, one need not invoke degradation of α-synuclein by the proteasome to explain such inhibitory effects.

It is worth mentioning that in our own model where we found proteasomal inhibition by A53T α-synuclein in stably transfected PC12 cells, we had failed to detect obvious aggregation of mutant α-synuclein (37). In subsequent studies, we have observed soluble oligomers of α-synuclein that co-elute on gel filtration with the proteasome in these cells, adding further support to the idea that these may be the species involved in proteasomal inhibition. This notion is further strengthened by the fact that application of Congo Red removed these species from the proteasomal fraction and improved proteasomal function (Evangelia Emmanouilidou, Kostas Vekrellis, and Leonidas Stefanis, unpublished results).

STUDIES IN HUMAN PARKINSON'S DISEASE

Ubiquitin within LBs represents polyubiquitinated proteins (47), suggesting that, if there is dysfunction of the UPS in PD and related LB diseases, this should be at the level of the proteasome. A number of studies have directly assessed proteasomal activity in these disorders, using the method of cleavage of synthetic substrates by cell extracts from brain regions of patients and controls. McNaught and Jenner (48) measured enzymatic activities of the proteasome, and found a specific decrease of these activities in substantia nigra (SN) of PD patients compared to controls. This result has been confirmed by Tofaris et al. (29), who additionally found decreased proteasomal activity in the SN of DLBD patients. Other CNS regions showed normal activity in DLBD, except for frontal cortex, where activity was somewhat lower, without however reaching statistical significance. Furukawa et al. (49) also found normal proteasomal activity in extranigral regions of PD patients.

It therefore appears, based on these enzymatic assays, that if proteasomal dysfunction exists in LB diseases, it is relatively confined to the SN. It is worth adding here a technical note of caution. As mentioned earlier, enzymatic activities of the proteasome may be normal if a UPS deficit exists at another level, and not at the proteasome. In addition, this method is rather crude, and it is possible that proteasomal dysfunction exists within the cells, but is not observed when these cells are lysed, because the proteasome is studied outside its physiological context. For example, potential inhibitory factors may be removed during the lysis procedure. Furthermore, neurons represent only a subpopulation of the tissue classically sampled in these assays. Therefore, lack of proteasomal dysfunction measured by enzymatic assays in tissue homogenates cannot be construed as definitive evidence for a lack of UPS involvement. It is still possible, given the presence of polyubiquitinated proteins in LBs, that UPS dysfunction occurs in areas beyond the SN in LB diseases. It should be noted however that, based on a novel study, the presence of polyubiquitinated proteins need not necessarily signify UPS dysfunction. Mice lacking an essential macroautophagy gene specifically within the CNS-accumulated ubiquitinated aggregates and polyubiquitinated proteins, without any overt proteasomal dysfunction (50), suggesting that impairment of the lysosomal degradation pathway of macroautophagy is sufficient to cause this phenomenon.

In any case, it appears from the above studies that there is a regional impairment of enzymatic activity of the proteasome at the level of the SN in PD and DLBD patients. Again, caution is warranted, given that such impairment is observed in tissue that has markedly altered cellular composition, with loss of neurons, astrogliosis and microglial activation. Indeed, activation of neuronal cell death can lead to UPS dysfunction as a secondary phenomenon (51). It would be interesting in this regard to study proteasomal activity in the brains of patients with incidental LB disease, which is considered the prodrome of PD and is characterized by limited neuronal loss. It would also be interesting to look at other brain regions, such as the locus coeruleus, the dorsal motor nucleus of the vagus, and the nucleus basalis of Meynert, which have a heavy, early burden of synuclein pathology (52).

What could be the cause of such a decrease of proteasomal activity in the SN? It has been reported (53) that there is a dramatic decrease of labeling of α subunits of the 20S proteasome in melanized neurons of the SN of PD patients, whereas labeling for β subunits was normal. This study awaits replication, but raises the possibility of primary structural or biochemical defects of the proteasome in PD patients. Alternatively, other factors etiologically linked to PD, such as protein aggregation, aging, oxidative, nitrative or nitrosylative stress, or mitochondrial dysfunction may be responsible. All these factors have been shown to promote proteasomal dysfunction in certain settings. A case in point is a study in which chronic delivery of MPTP led to proteasomal impairment in mouse SN (54).

MODELS OF UBIQUITIN-PROTEASOME SYSTEM DYSFUNCTION IN CELL CULTURE

The co-existence of proteasomal dysfunction, at least in the SN, with obvious protein aggregation in the form of LBs raises the chicken and egg dilemma. As demonstrated by Bence et al. (55), protein aggregation can lead to UPS dysfunction. The studies of the effects of purified soluble or fully aggregated α-synuclein mentioned above support this idea. The question that ourselves and others have tried to tackle is whether the converse can also occur; that is whether proteasomal dysfunction can lead to a PD-like phenotype. To this end, we and others have applied selective pharmacological proteasomal inhibitors to cultured neuronal cells. Although these inhibitors are not entirely specific, they all appear to exert similar effects, and therefore such effects are thought to be due to proteasomal inhibition. We have found that such treatment leads to the formation of ubiquitinated inclusions and neuronal death in PC12 cells and cortical neurons (32,33). We have analyzed in more detail the antigenic components of these inclusions in cortical neuron cultures. They contain polyubiquitinated proteins and, in addition, α-synuclein, the early neurofilament-like protein α-internexin, β-tubulin, HSP70, and *PARKIN*, all components of LBs found in PD. Labeling with the histochemical marker Thioflavin S, which detects fibrillar, β-amyloid-like structures, was positive in about 60% of the inclusions (33).

As application of proteasomal inhibitors to neuronal cells led to features that are observed in LB diseases, namely, neuronal death and LB-like inclusion formation, we have performed a series of studies in which we have attempted to modulate these phenomena and to uncover their interrelationship. Whether inclusions are detrimental, protective, or incidental has been a subject of debate over the past few years. In our studies in PC12 cells and cortical neurons, we have found that caspase activation, p53 upregulation, and aberrant cell cycle activation are required for apoptotic death to occur, but not for inclusion formation (32,33,56,57). Furthermore, we were unable to identify a single apoptotic cortical neuron that simultaneously harbored an inclusion. Therefore, in a general sense, the two phenomena of inclusions and death can be dissociated, arguing that they represent parallel pathways.

The process through which LBs form in PD is essentially unknown, although the predominant theory is that abnormal conformations of α-synuclein are the instigating factor. Since the inclusions observed after proteasomal inhibition of primary neurons resembled LBs in some respects, we went on to examine the manner in which inclusions are formed in this model. We first evaluated the requirement for ubiquitination. To this end, we transduced cortical neuron cultures with a viral vector encoding a dominant-negative form of an E2 conjugating enzyme, Cdc34. This strategy had been previously utilized by Saudou et al. (58) to modulate inclusion formation induced by mutant Huntingtin overexpression. We found that expression of this dominant-negative construct completely abrogated inclusion formation in our cultures, arguing for a required role of ubiquitination in this process. Surprisingly, there was a concomitant increase in survival (33). We interpret this as a possible effect on cell cycle components, which are known to be degraded via this E2, but we cannot exclude the possibility that the formation of inclusions somehow influences survival, perhaps through a feed-forward loop of further proteasomal inhibition due to aggregation (55). Application of the transcriptional inhibitor actinomycin D provided another important clue to the process of inclusion formation. This agent completely abrogated inclusion formation in cortical and nigral neurons, without affecting overall levels of ubiquitination (33,59). Therefore, inclusion formation is dependent on novel or ongoing transcription. It is an active cellular process, and not simply the accumulation of nondigested protein material. Candidate genes involved in this process include molecular chaperones, accessory ubiquitin-like proteins and microtubule elements, which have been shown to be involved in "aggresome" formation (60). As expected, application of actinomycin D also prevented neuronal death, presumably by inhibiting other genes, such as transcription factors involved in death pathways (33,59).

Given the prominent presence of α-synuclein within LBs, its propensity to aggregate and its presumed role in LB formation, we have examined more closely its role in inclusion formation in our model. We first determined, using an in situ detergent-extraction protocol, that α-synuclein within the inclusions was present in part in an oligomeric conformation (61). Such oligomers were not present in soluble extracts. This raised the possibility that α-synuclein oligomerization, which is thought to be a prelude to its frank aggregation, occurred, so to speak, after the fact, after its incorporation within the inclusions. A mechanism that could account for this is molecular crowding, the high concentration of various proteins within the limited space of the inclusion. To examine this possibility, we utilized cortical neuron cultures derived from α-synuclein null mice. These neurons went on to develop insoluble ubiquitinated inclusions just like their wild-type counterparts. However, the fibrillar component, identified by Thioflavin S labeling, was absent. Neurons lacking α-synuclein showed no difference in death in response to proteasomal inhibition, arguing that the fibrillar nature of the inclusions does not influence survival, and thus providing further evidence for a dissociation between inclusions and death (61). In conjunction, these findings suggest that α-synuclein plays a role in the elaboration of the features of the inclusions, such as their fibrillization, but not in their initial formation. Furthermore, they suggest that oligomerization and subsequent aggregation of α-synuclein can occur within inclusions formed due to proteasomal inhibition.

Another issue that is interesting, and has received less attention, is that of inclusion dissolution. It is increasingly being recognized that at least certain forms of inclusions are dynamic structures that may exist in a tenuous equilibrium between

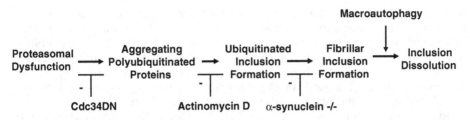

FIGURE 1 Pathway of inclusion formation and dissolution following proteasomal inhibition in primary neurons.

formation and dissolution. We had noted at later time points subsequent to the formation of inclusions in cortical neuron cultures the appearance of smaller ubiquitinated aggregates, many times in apoptotic neurons. This, in conjunction with the lack of correlation of apoptosis and inclusions at the single cell level, led us to suggest that inclusions may dissolve into smaller aggregates prior to cell death (33). To address this possibility, and to decipher the responsible mechanism, we modulated by pharmacological means the lysosomal macroautophagy pathway, which may be involved in the clearance of certain inclusions and protein aggregates in other settings (62). We found that macroautophagy and activation of the lysosomal pathway occurred following proteasomal inhibition of cortical neurons. An enhancer of macroautophagy diminished proteasomal inhibitor-induced inclusions and increased the small aggregates, whereas inhibitors of autophagy had the opposite effect (63). These data indicate that the large inclusions dissolve into smaller aggregates through the process of macroautophagy. Despite the marked effects on inclusions with the macroautophagy modulators, no effects were seen on survival, further arguing for a dissociation between inclusions and death.

The presumed pathway of inclusion formation and dissolution in this model is depicted in Figure 1. This is largely based on studies performed in cultured cortical neurons, but these findings, at least in part, have been replicated in dopaminergic VM neurons (59). It is important to state that it is unknown whether this represents events that actually occur in PD.

Various studies have attempted to answer the question of whether cultured dopaminergic neurons are selectively sensitive to death induced by proteasomal inhibition. McNaught et al. (64) and Petrucelli et al. (6) reported that the proteasomal inhibitors MG132 and lactacystin caused selective toxicity to dopaminergic neurons in ventral midbrain cultures. Kikuchi et al. (65) however failed to replicate this finding; in fact, they reported that dopaminergic neurons were relatively *resistant* to exposure to the selective proteasomal inhibitor epoxomicin. In an attempt to resolve this issue, we have also applied epoxomicin or lactacystin to ventral midbrain cultures. We found that dopaminergic neurons are selectively vulnerable to both these insults, as they underwent a significant degree of apoptosis, whereas GABAergic neurons in the same cultures did not (59). This is important because it indicates that the regional proteasomal impairment that occurs in the SN of PD patients could lead to selective degeneration of dopaminergic neurons. McNaught et al. (64,66) showed selective α-synuclein/ubiquitin-positive inclusions in dopaminergic neurons in ventral midbrain cultures. We also found such inclusions in our study; however, ubiquitinated inclusions were not confined to TH-positive neurons (59). It is possible that this reflects downregulation of the dopaminergic phenotype in these cells, but it may also indicate that nondopaminergic neurons develop such inclusions. Interestingly, in some dopaminergic neurons TH immunostaining was almost exclusively confined within the inclusions (59). This raises the possibility that TH may be sequestered in inclusions and thus be depleted from its normal sites of action. This could lead to functional impairment of the dopaminergic system in inclusion-bearing cells, since TH is the rate-limiting step in dopamine biosynthesis.

What could be the basis for this preferential vulnerability of cultured dopaminergic neurons to proteasomal inhibition? We have found that such neurons fail to up regulate the chaperone heat shock protein 70 (HSP70) in response to lactacystin application, whereas other cells in the cultures show a robust induction (59). Given the known protective effects of HSP70 in terms of protein folding and apoptosis, it is possible that this preferential lack of induction in dopaminergic neurons is a contributing factor for their selective vulnerability. Fornai et al. (67) reported that proteasomal inhibition-induced death of PC12 cells was dependent on dopamine biosynthesis, suggesting that oxidative products of dopamine metabolism may be causal in death in this setting.

MODELS OF UBIQUITIN-PROTEASOME SYSTEM DYSFUNCTION IN VIVO

Pharmacological proteasomal inhibitors have also been used in vivo in an attempt to model UPS dysfunction. Injection of lactacystin in rat SN induced death that was selective for neurons compared to glia. Accumulation of α-synuclein/ubiquitin in the form of some rather ill-defined inclusions was noted in the cytosol of nigral neurons (68). Injection of lactacystin or MG132 in rat striatum led to nigrostriatal fiber degeneration, loss of striatal dopamine, and death of nigral dopaminergic neurons, without affecting striatal neurons. Again, rather ill-defined α-synuclein-ubiquitin inclusions were noted by immunocytochemistry. Electronic micrographs were purported to confirm the presence of fibrillar structures, but in fact showed whorly membrane-bound vesicles, which likely represent lysosomal structures (67). Interestingly, and as in the PC12 cell model, this in vivo toxicity was dependent on dopamine biosynthesis, providing some explanation for the selective vulnerability of dopaminergic neurons. More recently, McNaught et al. (69) applied to rats epoxomicin and PSI, another proteasomal inhibitor, systemically, via the intraperitoneal (ip) route, over a period of two or more weeks. They report selective neuronal degeneration and ubiquitin/α-synuclein inclusion formation in the brainstem structures, including the SN, described by Braak et al. (52) as predominantly affected in PD. Inclusions stained positive with Thioflavin S, indicating that they were of fibrillar nature. Remarkably, no systemic toxicity seemed to occur, although no pathological studies were performed outside the CNS, and striatal or spinal cord neurons were not affected. There was an accompanying behavioral phenotype, with hypokinesia, rigidity and tremor that was partially reversed by apomorphine, as well as striatal dopamine depletion. Interestingly, in many CNS regions, that were not affected pathologically, proteasomal activity, measured with the enzymatic assays, did not decrease, and in fact showed an increase following systemic application of proteasomal inhibitors. In contrast, in the SN and lower brainstem proteasomal activity was substantially decreased. This further supports the idea that select brain regions, including the SN, may be especially vulnerable to proteasomal inhibition, perhaps because they do not have the reserve capacity to withstand such insults. This report raises the interesting notion that systemic exposure to natural proteasomal inhibitors may underlie certain forms of sporadic PD, since it appears to lead to these selective deficits in rats. However, a more detailed analysis of extra-neuronal tissues, as well as CNS regions purportedly not affected by the systemic administration of proteasomal inhibitors is warranted. The inclusions formed should be better characterized at the ultrastructural level.

Following the McNaught et al. report of this potential new model for PD based on systemic proteasomal inhibition, a number of groups have attempted to replicate this finding. A series of four articles related to the issue of reproducibility have appeared in the same issue of the *Annals of Neurology*. Three of these studies failed to reproduce the model, whereas in two studies a considerable loss of nigral dopaminergic neurons was found (70–74). It is fair to say that at this point, and until potential disparities between the studies are clarified, systemic proteasomal inhibition with PSI following the McNaught et al. protocol cannot be considered a reliable model for Parkinsonism.

CONCLUSIONS

Genetic, biochemical, and pathological data suggest that UPS dysfunction may underlie PD, or, at least, be an important feature of its pathogenesis. This notion is still a hypothesis. Future studies should address the issue of whether UPS dysfunction actually occurs in the early stages of PD pathogenesis and whether it plays an active pathogenetic role. If so, UPS dysfunction could be a target for therapeutic interventions in PD.

REFERENCES

1. McNaught K, Olanow CW, Halliwell B, Isacson O, Jenner P. Failure of the ubiquitin-proteasome system in Parkinson's disease. Nat Rev Neurosci 2001; 2:589–594.
2. Ciechanover A, Brundin P. The ubiquitin proteasome system in neurodegenerative diseases: sometimes the chicken, sometimes the egg. Neuron 2003; 40:427–446.
3. Hattori N, Mizuno Y. Pathogenetic mechanisms of parkin in Parkinson's disease. Lancet 2004; 364(9435):722–724.
4. Tsai YC, Fishman PS, Thakor NV, Oyler GA. Parkin facilitates the elimination of expanded polyglutamine proteins and leads to preservation of proteasome function. J Biol Chem 2003; 278(24):22044–22055.
5. Hyun DH, Lee M, Hattori N, et al. Effect of wild-type or mutant Parkin on oxidative damage, nitric oxide, antioxidant defenses, and the proteasome. J Biol Chem 2002; 277(32):28572–28577.
6. Petrucelli L, O'Farrell C, Lockhart PJ, et al. Parkin protects against the toxicity associated with mutant alpha-synuclein: proteasome dysfunction selectively affects catecholaminergic neurons. Neuron 2002; 36:1007–1019.
7. Sakata E, Yamaguchi Y, Kurimoto E, et al. Parkin binds the Rpn10 subunit of 26S proteasomes through its ubiquitin-like domain. EMBO Rep 2003; 4(3):301–306.
8. Leroy E, Boyer R, Auburger G, et al. The ubiquitin pathway in Parkinson's disease. Nature 1998; 395(6701):451–452.
9. Maraganore DM, Lesnick TG, Elbaz A, et al. UCHL1 is a Parkinson's disease susceptibility gene. Ann Neurol 2004; 55(4):512–521.
10. Healy DG, Abou-Sleiman PM, Casas JP, et al. UCHL-1 is not a Parkinson's disease susceptibility gene. Ann Neurol 2006; 59(4):627–633.
11. Chung CH, Baek SH. Deubiquitinating Enzymes: Their diversity and emerging roles. Biochem Biophys Res Com 1999; 266:633–640.
12. Pickart CM, Rose IA. Ubiquitin carboxyl-terminal hydrolase acts on ubiquitin carboxyl-terminal amides. J Biol Chem 1985; 260:7903–7910.

13. Larsen CN, Krantz BA, Wilkinson KD. Substrate specificity of deubiquitinating enzymes: Ubiquitin C-terminal hydrolases. Biochemistry 1998; 37:3358–3368.

14. Hegde AN, Inokuchi K, Pei W, et al. Ubiquitin C-terminal hydrolase is an immediate-early gene essential for long-term facilitation in Aplysia. Cell 1997; 89(1):115–126.

15. Osaka H, Wang YL, Takada K, et al. Ubiquitin carboxy-terminal hydrolase L1 binds to and stabilizes monoubiquitin in neuron. Hum Mol Genet 2003; 12(16):1945–1958.

16. Liu Y, Fallon L, Lashuel HA, et al. The UCH-L1 gene encodes two opposing enzymatic activities that affect alpha-synuclein degradation and Parkinson's disease susceptibility. Cell 2002; 111(2):209–218.

17. Nishikawa K, Li H, Kawamura R, et al. Alterations of structure and hydrolase activity of parkinsonism-associated human ubiquitin carboxyl-terminal hydrolase L1 variants. Biochem Biophys Res Commun 2003; 304(1):176–183.

18. Choi J, Levey AI, Weintraub ST, et al. Oxidative modifications and down-regulation of ubiquitin carboxyl-terminal hydrolase L1 associated with idiopathic Parkinson's and Alzheimer's diseases. J Biol Chem 2004; 279(13):13256–13264.

19. Barrachina M, Castano E, Dalfo E, et al. Reduced ubiquitin C-terminal hydrolase-1 expression levels in dementia with Lewy bodies. Neurobiol Dis 2006; 22(2):265–273.

20. Valente EM, Abou-Sleiman PM, Caputo V, et al. Hereditary early-onset Parkinson's disease caused by mutations in PINK1. Science 2004; 304(5674):1158–1160.

21. Bonifati V, Rizzu P, van Baren MJ, et al. Mutations in the DJ-1 gene associated with autosomal recessive early-onset parkinsonism. Science 2003; 299(5604):256–259.

22. Martinat C, Shendelman S, Jonason A, et al. Sensitivity to oxidative stress in DJ-1-deficient dopamine neurons: an ES- derived cell model of primary parkinsonism. PLoS Biol 2004; 2(11):e327.

23. Polymeropoulos MH, Lavedan C, Leroy E, et al. Mutation in the alpha-synuclein gene identified in families with Parkinson's disease. Science 1997; 276:2045–2047.

24. Duda JE, Lee VM, Trojanowski JQ. Neuropathology of synuclein aggregates. J Neurosci Res 2000; 61(2):121–127.

25. Bennett MC, Bishop JF, Leng Y, et al. Degradation of alpha-synuclein by proteasome. J Biol Chem 1999; 274(48):33855–33858.

26. Imai Y, Soda M, Takahashi R. Parkin suppresses unfolded protein stress-induced cell death through its E3 ubiquitin-protein ligase activity. J Biol Chem 2000; 276:35661–35664.

27. Ancolio K, Alves da Costa C, Ueda K, Checler F. Alpha-synuclein and the Parkinson's disease-related mutant Ala53Thr-alpha-synuclein do not undergo proteasomal degradation in HEK293 and neuronal cells. Neurosci Lett 2000; 285(2):79–82.

28. Paxinou E, Chen Q, Weisse M, et al. Induction of alpha-synuclein aggregation by intracellular nitrative insult. J Neurosci 2001; 21(20):8053–8061.

29. Tofaris GK, Layfield R, Spillantini MG. Alpha-synuclein metabolism and aggregation is linked to ubiquitin-independent degradation by the proteasome. FEBS Lett 2001; 509:22–26.

30. Sampathu DM, Giasson BI, Pawlyk AC, Trojanowski JQ, Lee VM. Ubiquitination of alpha-synuclein is not required for formation of pathological inclusions in alpha-synucleinopathies. Am J Pathol 2003; 163(1):91–100.

31. Tofaris GK, Razzaq A, Ghetti B, et al. Ubiquitination of alpha-synuclein in Lewy bodies is a pathological event not associated with impairment of proteasome function. J Biol Chem 2003; 278(45):44405–44411.

32. Rideout HJ, Larsen KE, Sulzer D, Stefanis L. Proteasomal inhibition leads to formation of ubiquitin/alpha-synuclein-immunoreactive inclusions in PC12 cells. J Neurochem 2001; 78(4):899–908.

33. Rideout HJ, Stefanis L. Transcription and ubiquitination are required for inclusion formation and death in proteasomal inhibitor-treated embryonic cortical neurons. Mol Cell Neurosci 2002; 21:223–238.

34. Cuervo AM, Stefanis L, Fredenburg R, et al. Impaired degradation of mutant alpha-synuclein by chaperone-mediated autophagy. Science 2004; 305(5688):1292–1295.

35. Webb JL, Ravikumar B, Atkins J, et al. Alpha-synuclein is degraded by both autophagy and the proteasome. J Biol Chem 2003; 278:25009–25013.

36. Lee HJ, Khoshaghideh F, Patel S, Lee SJ. Clearance of alpha-synuclein oligomeric intermediates via the lysosomal degradation pathway. J Neurosci 2004; 24(8):1888–1896.

37. Stefanis L, Larsen KL, Rideout HJ, et al. Expression of A53T mutant, but not wild type, α-synuclein in PC12 cells induces alterations of the ubiquitin-dependent degradation system, loss of dopamine release, and autophagic cell death. J Neurosci 2001; 21:9549–9560.
38. Tanaka Y, Engelender S, Igarashi S, et al. Inducible expression of mutant alpha-synuclein decreases proteasome activity and increases sensitivity to mitochondria-dependent apoptosis. Hum Mol Genet 2001; 10(9):919–926.
39. Smith WW, Jiang H, Pei Z, et al. Endoplasmic reticulum stress and mitochondrial cell death pathways mediate A53T mutant alpha-synuclein-induced toxicity. Hum Mol Genet 2005; 14(24):3801–3811.
40. Snyder H, Mensah K, Theisler C, et al. Aggregated and monomeric alpha-synuclein bind to the S6' proteasomal protein and inhibit proteasomal function. J Biol Chem 2003; 278(14):11753–11759.
41. Martin-Clemente B, Alvarez-Castelao B, Mayo I, et al. alpha-Synuclein expression levels do not significantly affect proteasome function and expression in mice and stably transfected PC12 cell lines. J Biol Chem 2004; 279(51):52984–52990.
42. Gomez-Isla T, Irizarry MC, Mariash A, et al. Motor dysfunction and gliosis with preserved dopaminergic markers in human alpha-synuclein A30P transgenic mice. Neurobiol Aging 2003; 24(2):245–258.
43. Chen L, Thiruchelvam MJ, Madura K, Richfield EK. Proteasome dysfunction in aged human alpha-synuclein transgenic mice. Neurobiol Dis 2006; 23(1):120–126.
44. Ghee M, Fournier A, Mallet J. Rat alpha-synuclein interacts with Tat binding protein 1, a component of the 26S proteasomal complex. J Neurochem 2000; 75(5):2221–2224.
45. Lindersson E, Beedholm R, Hojrup P, et al. Proteasomal inhibition by alpha-synuclein filaments and oligomers. J Biol Chem 2004; 279(13):12924–12934.
46. Snyder H, Mensah K, Theisler C, et al. Aggregated and monomeric alpha-synuclein bind to the S6' proteasomal protein and inhibit proteasomal function. J Biol Chem 2003; 278:11753–11759.
47. Iwatsubo T, Yamaguchi H, Fujimuro M, et al. Purification and characterization of Lewy bodies from the brains of patients with diffuse Lewy body disease. Am J Pathol 1996; 148:1517–1529.
48. McNaught KS, Jenner P. Proteasomal function is impaired in Substantia Nigra in Parkinson's disease. Neurosci Lett 2001; 297(3):191–194.
49. Furukawa Y, Vigouroux S, Wong H, et al. Brain proteasomal function in sporadic Parkinson's disease and related disorders. Ann Neurol 2002; 51(6):779–782.
50. Hara T, Nakamura K, Matsui M, et al. Suppression of basal autophagy in neural cells causes neurodegenerative disease in mice. Nature 2006; 441(7095):885–889.
51. Canu N, Barbato C, Ciotti MT, et al. Proteasome involvement and accumulation of ubiquitinated proteins in cerebellar granule neurons undergoing apoptosis. J Neurosci 2000; 20(2):589–599.
52. Braak H, Del Tredici K, Rub U, et al. Staging of brain pathology related to sporadic Parkinson's disease. Neurobiol Aging 2003; 24(2):197–211.
53. McNaught KS, Belizaire R, Jenner P, et al. Selective loss of 20S proteasome-subunits in the Substantia Nigra pars compacta in Parkinson's disease. Neurosci Lett 2002; 326(3):155–158.
54. Fornai F, Schluter OM, Lenzi P, et al. Parkinson-like syndrome induced by continuous MPTP infusion: Convergent roles of the ubiquitin-proteasome system and {alpha}-synuclein. Proc Natl Acad Sci USA 2005; 102(9):3413–3849.
55. Bence NF, Sampat RM, Kopito RR. Impairment of the ubiquitin-proteasome system by protein aggregation. Science 2001; 292(5521):1552–1555.
56. Rideout HJ, Wang Q, Park DS, Stefanis L. Cyclin dependent kinase activity is required for apoptotic death, but not inclusion formation in cortical neurons following proteasomal inhibition. J Neurosci 2003; 23:1237–1245.
57. Dietrich P, Rideout HJ, Wang Q, Stefanis L. Lack of p53 delays apoptosis, but increases ubiquitinated inclusions, in proteasomal inhibitor-treated cultured cortical neurons. Mol Cell Neurosci 2003; 24:430–441.
58. Saudou F, Finbeiner S, Devy D, et al. Huntingtin acts in the nucleus to induce apoptosis but death does not correlate with the formation of intranuclear inclusions. Cell 1998; 95:55–66.

59. Rideout HJ, Lang-Rollin ICJ, Savalle M, Stefanis L. Dopaminergic neurons in rat ventral midbrain cultures undergo selective apoptosis and form inclusions, but do not up-regulate iHSP70, following proteasomal inhibition. J Neurochem 2005; 93(5): 1304–1313.
60. Johnston JA, Ward CL, Kopito RR. Aggresomes: a cellular response to misfolded proteins. J Cell Biol 1998; 143(7):1883–1898.
61. Rideout HJ, Dietrich P, Wang Q, et al. alpha -synuclein is required for the fibrillar nature of ubiquitinated inclusions induced by proteasomal inhibition in primary neurons. J Biol Chem 2004; 279(45):46915–46920.
62. Ravikumar B, Duden R, Rubinsztein DC. Aggregate-prone proteins with polyglutamine and polyalanine expansions are degraded by autophagy. Hum Mol Genet 2002; 11(9): 1107–1117.
63. Rideout HJ, Lang-Rollin I, Stefanis L. Involvement of macroautophagy in the dissolution of neuronal inclusions. Int J Biochem Cell Biol 2004; 36:2551–2562.
64. McNaught KS, Mytilineou C, Jnobaptiste R, et al. Impairment of the ubiquitin-proteasome system causes dopaminergic cell death and inclusion body formation in ventral mesencephalic cultures. J Neurochem 2002; 81(2):301–306.
65. Kikuchi S, Shinpo K, Tsuji S, et al. Effect of proteasome inhibitor on cultured mesencephalic dopaminergic neurons. Brain Res 2003; 964(2):228–236.
66. McNaught KS, Shashidharan P, Perl DP, et al. Aggresome-related biogenesis of Lewy bodies. Eur J Neurosci 2002; 16(11):2136–2148.
67. Fornai F, Lenzi P, Gesi M, et al. Fine structure and biochemical mechanisms underlying nigrostriatal inclusions and cell death after proteasome inhibition. J Neurosci 2003; 23(26):8955–8966.
68. McNaught KS, Bjorklund LM, Belizaire R, et al. Proteasome inhibition causes nigral degeneration with inclusion bodies in rats. Neuroreport 2002; 13(11):1437–1441.
69. McNaught KS, Perl DP, Brownell AL, et al. Systemic exposure to proteasome inhibitors causes a progressive model of Parkinson's disease. Ann Neurol 2004; 56(1):149–1462.
70. Schapira AH, Cleeter MW, Muddle JR, et al. Proteasomal inhibition causes loss of nigral tyrosine hydroxylase neurons. Ann Neurol 2006; 60(2):253–255.
71. Bove J, Zhou C, Jackson-Lewis V, et al. Proteasome inhibition and Parkinson's disease modeling. Ann Neurol 2006; 60(2):260–264.
72. Kordower JH, Kanaan NM, Chu Y, et al. Failure of proteasome inhibitor administration to provide a model of Parkinson's disease in rats and monkeys. Ann Neurol 2006; 60(2):264–268.
73. Manning-Bog AB, Reaney SH, Chou VP, et al. Lack of nigrostriatal pathology in a rat model of proteasome inhibition. Ann Neurol 2006; 60(2):256–260.
74. Zeng BY, Bukhatwa S, Hikima A, et al. Reproducible nigral cell loss after systemic proteasomal inhibitor administration to rats. Ann Neurol 2006; 60(2):248–252.

17 Transgenic Models of α-Synucleinopathy

Michael K. Lee
*Department of Pathology, Johns Hopkins University School of Medicine,
Baltimore, Maryland, U.S.A.*

INTRODUCTION

Parkinson's disease (PD) is a common late-onset, progressive neurodegenerative disease characterized by selective loss of neuronal populations, including dopaminergic (DAergic) neurons of substantia nigra, pars compacta (SNpc), and presence of fibrillar, cytoplasmic inclusions called Lewy bodies (LBs) and Lewy neurites (LNs) (1). While degeneration of dopamine (DA) neurons is responsible for much of the motoric symptoms of PD, neuropathology in PD extends well beyond the DAergic systems (2,3). Significantly, non-DAergic pathology may precede DAergic pathology in PD (2,3).

While the causes of disease in most cases of PD are unknown, molecular genetic studies have identified disease causing mutations in the genes encoding α-Synuclein (α-Syn), *PARKIN*, *DJ-1*, and *Dardarin/LRRK* in a number of FPD pedigrees (4–10). Identification of disease-causing genetic lesions for PD has provided unparalleled opportunities to model features of PD in lower organisms. Among the genes implicated in PD, α-Syn abnormalities may have particular importance in understanding the pathogenesis of PD. In addition to the PD associated genetic abnormalities in the α-Syn gene (6,8,9), biochemical abnormalities of α-Syn are also found in more common sporadic PD and other related diseases. Specifically, α-Syn is the major fibrillar component of LBs and LNs, which are one of the key neuropathologic indicators of PD and dementia with LBs (11,12). Further, α-Syn aggregates form the glial cytoplasmic inclusions (GCIs) in multiple systems atrophy (MSA) and the cellular inclusions in neurodegeneration with brain iron accumulation type I (6,8,13–16). The disease with the common presence of α-Syn aggregates as a prominent pathologic feature is now collectively termed the α-synucleinopathies (13–16).

In the last several years, direct association between α-Syn abnormalities and neurodegeneration have been demonstrated in a variety of genetic models. For example, expression of either wild type or mutant human α-Syn (Huα-Syn) is associated with neurodegeneration in flies (17), transgenic mice (18–22), and Huα-Syn-virus infected rodents (23,24). These genetic models of α-synucleinopathies are valuable agents for gaining new insights the normal and abnormal physiology of α-Syn and the in vivo pathogenic mechanisms of α-synucleinopathies. This chapter will provide an overview of the various α-Syn transgenic mouse models that have contributed to understanding the in vivo role of α-Syn and the pathogenic processes that are relevant to human α-synucleinopthy.

SYNUCLEIN KNOCKOUT MICE: PROBING THE NORMATIVE FUNCTIONS OF SYNUCLEINS

α-Syn is a highly conserved protein of 140 amino acids belonging to a multigene family that includes β-Syn and γ-Syn (25). The synuclein family members contain a conserved N-terminal repeat region (100 amino acids) consisting of seven imperfect repeats of 11 amino acid residues (KTKEGV), a hydrophobic middle portion, and a less well conserved, negatively charged C-terminal region (26). Normally, α-Syn is predominantly expressed in neurons and is particularly at abundance in presynaptic terminals (25–29). Because of the predominant synaptic localization and the differential regulation of α-Syn during the period of synaptic plasticity (25), a role in synaptic plasticity has been proposed for α-Syn.

Synucleins as Modulators of Synaptic Function

To determine the in vivo functional roles of α-Syn, a number of groups have generated knockout mice lacking α-Syn expression (30–33). The results from α-Syn knockout mice indicate that α-Syn is not essential for the development and viability of the mice. The DAergic cell bodies, fibers, and synapses in the α-Syn knockout mice were not different from the wild type mice, indicating that loss of α-Syn function is not associated significant pathologic changes in the neuronal systems.

The first report of an α-Syn knockout mice showed that while the patterns of DA discharge and reuptake were unremarkable, DA terminals in α-Syn knockout mice were able to recover faster from the initial activation of transmitter release (30). These results were interpreted to indicate that α-Syn is a presynaptic, activity-dependent, negative regulator of DAergic neurotransmission. In addition, α-Syn knockout mice show reduced total striatal DA levels and reduced amphetamine-stimulated locomotion. While the bases for these latter phenotypes are not known, the first report of α-Syn knockout mice seems to support the notion that α-Syn is a presynaptic regulator of DA release, synthesis, and storage.

The initial conclusions regarding α-Syn as a presynaptic regulator of DA release appears to be supported by results from other groups that have independently analyzed mice lacking α-Syn expression (34,35). Ultrastructural and physiologic studies of hippocampal neurons from another α-Syn knockout mice revealed that the lack of α-Syn expression was associated with reduction in the reserve pool of synaptic vesicles and impaired synaptic response to high-frequency stimulation (34). Real-time voltametric monitoring of DA release in C57BL6 mice with the natural deletion of α-Syn gene (36) revealed that lack of α-Syn was associated with enhancement in the readily releasable pool (RRP) of DA at the expense of the storage pool (35). The increase in RRP in the α-Syn-null mice was ascribed to increase in the rate of refilling the RRP. However, one study has failed to find significant alterations in synaptic function in α-Syn knockout mice (31).

Modest phenotypes of the α-Syn knockout mice are unlikely due to some functional compensation by either β- and γ-synuclein. Double knockout mice lacking the expression of either α/β-Syn or α/γ-Syn are viable without obvious behavioral or synaptic abnormalities (31,37), confirming the view that the synucleins, in general, are not essential for the viability of the organisms. However, it is currently unknown if these combination knockout mice have more severe alterations in the DAergic neurotransmission.

Synucleins as Presynaptic Chaperones

In addition to regulating synaptic function, α-Syn may also act in concert with cysteine-string protein-α (CSPα) to maintain synaptic integrity and prevent neurodegeneration (38). CSPα is an abundant presynaptic protein containing a DNA-J chaperone domain, consisting of string of cystein residues. While CSPs are involved in a variety of cellular function, it appears that CSPα is important for maintaining normal neurotransmitter release in mice by acting as a presynaptic molecular chaperone. Mice lacking CSPα expression develop normally but develop lethal sensorimotor abnormalities associated with severe impairment in synaptic transmission and presynaptic degeneration (39). Significantly, mating of CSPα knockout mice with transgenic mice expressing human or mouse α-Syn under the Thy-1 promoter rescues the mice from CSPα knockout phenotype (38). Further, loss of endogenous α-Syn expression or combined loss of α/β-Syn expression exacerbates the CSPα knockout phenotype. While the mechanistic basis for this very interesting finding is not yet resolved, the chaperone-like activity of α-Syn (40) may allow for maintenance of synaptic function and synaptic integrity in absence of CSPα expression. Significantly, ability of α-Syn to associate with cellular membranes may be important for complementing CSPα phenotype since the A30P mutant Huα-Syn, which is known to be impaired in membrane association, is not able to rescue the mice from CSPα knockout phenotype (38).

Synucleins and Dopaminergic Toxins

In addition to acting as a modulator of synaptic function, DAergic neurons in the α-Syn knockout mice are almost completely protected from MPTP-dependent neurodegeneration (32). This result was quite surprising in light of the general findings that increased expression of α-Syn failed to increase vulnerability of DAergic neurons to MPTP (41). Further, DAergic neurons cultured from the α-Syn knockout mice are less sensitive to MPP+ toxicity while greater toxicity was observed with rotenone, another complex I inhibitor. Differential sensitivity of α-Syn knockout mice to MPP+ and rotenone does not appear to be due to the effects on MPP+ uptake sine the DA transporter and the vesicular monoamine transporter 2 activities, which would affect the accumulation of MPP+ in DAergic neurons, are not different between wild type and α-Syn knockout mice. Thus, it was concluded that MPTP-resistant phenotype of α-Syn is due to alterations in post-MPP+ uptake and precomplex I inhibition (32). However, the resistance of α-Syn knockout mice to degeneration induced by other mitochondrial toxins suggests that, at least in vivo, the resistance of α-Syn knockout mice to neurotoxins may also involve postmitochondrial processes (42). Further, there may be mouse strain–associated effects on how α-Syn modulates MPTP-sensitivity in mice (33). Significantly, it was later shown that lack of γ-Syn expression also protects DAergic neurons from MPTP toxicity in mice (37). Because β-Syn expression is increased in both α-Syn and γ-Syn knockout mice and because β-Syn can have neuroprotective effects, Buchman and colleagues have proposed that increase in β-Syn expression is mechanistically associated with the protection from MPTP toxicity (37). Thus, it would be of interest to determine if the β-Syn knockout mice exhibit increased vulnerability to MPTP toxicity. Given that α-Syn is required for vulnerability of DAergic neurons, it is puzzling that increased expression of human α-Syn does not seem to increase the vulnerability DAergic neurons to MPTP (41,43). The lack of increased MPTP toxicity with Huα-Syn overexpression is not because the Huα-Syn cannot function within the MPTP toxicity pathways since Huα-Syn can completely restore MPTP sensitivity in absence of mouse α-Syn expression (Thomas, Dawson, and Lee, Unpublished observation).

Finally, subsequent studies have revealed that α-Syn may have role in the normal development of DAergic neurons. Specifically, more detailed analysis revealed that α-Syn knockout mice have slightly fewer DAergic neurons than the wild type counterparts (37). The reduced number of DAergic neurons in α-Syn knockout mice appears to occur early during development and does not progress with aging.

TRANSGENIC MODELS OF α-SYNUCLEINOPATHY

With the identification that mutations in α-Syn gene are causative for familial PD, several groups have generated lines of transgenic mice expressing wild type of mutant Huα-Syn under the control of a variety of promoters have been generated (Table 1). In addition, viral vector mediated expression of Huα-Syn has shown Huα-Syn-dependent DAergic neurodegneration. While none of the Huα-Syn transgenic models fully recapitulate all features of PD, a number of these models exhibit significant α-synucleinopathy induced neurodegeneration, thus modeling characteristics of human α-synucleinopathies. Thus, some of these Huα-Syn transgenic models represent powerful tools to investigate the toxicity of α-Syn in vivo and factors that modulate in vivo aggregation of α-Syn.

Transgenic Mice Using "Pan-Neuronal" Promoters
PDGF-Huα-Syn Transgenic Mice
First demonstration of Huα-Syn-expression dependent neuronal abnormalities in transgenic mice was achieved by expressing wild type Huα-Syn using the PDGF-β promoter (20). Five lines of transgenic mice were produced that express different levels of wild type Huα-Syn and mice from highest expressing line (line D, about equal to the levels seen in human brain) exhibited motor deficits on rotarod performance. While the numbers of DAergic neurons were unchanged in line D, there was a modest reduction in striatal TH content. Subsequently, reduced striatal dopamine levels (25–50% at 12 months of age) and increased thigmotaxis was reported for the mice from line D (44).

Neuropathologically, PDGF-Huα-Syn transgenic mice develop nuclear and cytoplasmic inclusions that are immunoreative for Huα-Syn and, occasionally, for ubiquitin (20). Ultrastructurally, these inclusions are electron dense and composed of fine granular material. However, because they do not contain fibrillar elements, these inclusions appear distinct from LBs that are composed of α-Syn fibrils.

Thy1-Huα-Syn Transgenic Mice
Second lines of Huα-Syn transgenic mice used murine Thy-1 promoter to drive the expression of Huα-Syn harboring the A53T mutation (Thy1αSNA53T) (22). In these mice, the level of α-Syn expression in cortex was clearly higher in transgenic mice as compared to nontransgenic mice. Significantly, the Thy1αSNA53T mice develop progressive, early-onset motor deficits as indicated by decline in the rotating rod performance from 40 days of age to 200 days of age. However, it is not known whether these mice have shortened life span. Pathologically, affected mice show neuritic and neuronal α-Syn and ubiquitin accumulation, including in the spinal cord, the pons, and the cerebellar nuclei. Consistent with the motoric abnormalities,

TABLE 1 Summary of Huα-Syn Transgenic Mouse Models

Reference	Promoter	Huα-Syn *Affected	Motor deficit	Death	Neurodegeneration DAergic	Neurite	Cell Loss	Cellular inclusions Syn+	Ubiq+	Fibrillar	Biochemistry Insoluble	HMW
Masliah et al., 2000 (20); Hashimoto et al., 2003 (44)	PDGF-β	wt	Mild, ~12 months?	No	↓DA, TH	++	?	+	+	No	No	No
Van der Putten et al., 2000 (22)	mThy-1	wt, A53T	Moderate, ~2 months	?	No	++	?	++	++	No	?	?
Giasson et al., 2002 (18)	mPrp	wt, A30P, A53T*	Severe in homozygous lines, ~12 months	Yes	No	+++	?	+++	+++	Yes	Yes	Yes
Lee et al., 2002 (19); Martin et al., 2006 (46)	mPrp	wt, A30P, A53T*	Severe, ~11 months	Yes	No	+++	Yes (N)	+++	+++	Yes	Yes	Yes
Neumann et al., 2002 (21)	mThy-1	A30P	Severe in homozygous line, ~12 months	Yes	No	++	?	+++	+++	Yes	Yes	Yes
Gomez-Isla et al., 2003 (50)	Hamster Prp	wt, A30P*, A53T	Severe, ~11 months	Yes	No	?	?	No	No	No	No	No
Gispert et al., 2003 (51)	mPrp*	wt, A53T*	Mild, ~3–6 months	?	No	+	?	+/–	No	No	No	No
Chandra et al., 2005 (38)	mThy-1	mu and hu wt, A30P*, A53T*	Severe, ~8–12 months	Yes	No	?	Yes (N)	?	?	?	Yes	?
Matsuoka et al., 2001 (53)	Rat TH, 4.5 kb	wt, A30P, A53T	NR	No	No	No	No	No	No	No	No	No
Richfield et al., 2002 (54); Thiruchelvam et al., 2004 (55)	Rat TH, 9kb	wt, A30P + A53T*	Mild?	No	SNpc	+	Yes (DA)	No	No	No	No	No
Tofaris et al., 2006 (56)	Rat TH, 9kb	Truncated, 1–120	Mild, 3 months	?	↓DA	+	?	+	No	Yes	No	Yes
Kahle et al., 2002 (54)	Proteolipid	wt	None reported	No	?	?	?	+ (O)	No	No	Yes	Yes
Yazawa et al., 2005 (58)	pCNP	wt	Mild, 7–9 months	No	?	++	Yes (N, O)	++(O)	Yes	Yes	Yes	Yes
Shults et al., 2005 (59)	pMBP	wt	Moderate, ~6 months	?	↓TH	++	?	++(O)	Yes	Yes	Yes	Yes

Where multiple lines were examined, asterisk (*) indicates the lines with pathology. Neurodegeneration or pathology in neurons (N) or Oligodendrocytes (O) are indicated. (?) Indicates not examined or not reported.

these mice develop weakness related to motor endplate abnormalities and muscle denervation. While the inclusions were immunologically similar to LBs, they were not filamentous. In the same paper, it was also reported that transgenic mice expressing wild type Huα-Syn under the Thy1α-promoter also develop neuromuscular abnormalities. However, other groups have failed to observe significant pathology in transgenic mice expressing wild type Huα-Syn (18,19,38). In the Thy1αSNA53T transgenic mice, DAergic pathology was not observed (22).

Kahle and his colleagues used the Thy1α promoter to generate mice expressing high levels of Huα-Syn harboring the A30P mutation (45). Initial reports of mThy1-A30P transgenic mice shows α-Syn accumulation in neurons but overt neurodegenerative changes were not seen. However, subsequent analysis (21) revealed that mice at advanced ages (~24 months) develop α-Syn aggregates, as defined by the presence of proteinase-K resistant α-Syn immunoreactivity, in subcortical brain regions. Increased transgene dosage in the mice that are homozygous for the mThy1-A30P transgene develops pathology much earlier (~9 months of age). Aggregation of α-Syn was not present in the SNpc and the striatal DA levels were normal in the mThy1-A30P transgenic mice. It was later shown that the mThy1-A30P transgenic mice develop cognitive dysfunction, which may be related to the presence of proteinase-K resistant α-Syn in the amygdala (46).

PrP-Huα-Syn Transgenic Mice

Two groups have independently generated lines of transgenic mice expressing high levels of Huα-Syn using the murine prion promoter (PrP) (18,19). In both cases, mice from the lines expressing A53T mutant Huα-Syn develop adult onset, progressive motoric abnormalities characterized by reduced mobility, ataxia, and dystonia. The neurologic symptoms are first evident in mid-life adult mice (8–16 moths of age) with mice from higher expressing lines exhibiting earlier onset of neurologic phenotype. Following the initial onset, the disease rapidly progresses for two to three weeks, leading to complete paralysis and the reduced life-span of the MoPrp-Huα-Syn (A53T) transgenic mice. Significantly, mice expressing wild type Huα-Syn (18,19) or A30P Huα-Syn (19), at levels comparable or higher than the A53T α-Syn, do not develop neurologic phenotype. Thus, the A53T mutant Huα-Syn appears to have increased pathogenic potential than other human α-Syn variants in transgenic mice.

The fatal motoric phenotype in the MoPrp-Huα-Syn(A53T) transgenic mice is associated with abnormal neuronal accumulation of α-Syn and ubiquitin (18,19). The inclusions were widely distributed and particularly abundant in the subcortical regions, such as midbrain (red nucleus and colliculi), pons/medulla, cerebellar nuclei, and spinal cord. Immunoelectron microscopy (18) and Thioflavin-S staining (19) revealed that some of these inclusions were fibrils. Neuropathologic analysis of preclinical transgenic mice showed that abnormal neuronal accumulation of α-Syn and ubiquitin precedes development of severe motoric abnormalities (19). Other regions, such as cortex/hippocampus and striatum, despite high levels of transgene expression, were much less affected. Significantly, while Huα-Syn was expressed by DAergic neurons (19), no obvious pathology was observed in the SNpc and the neurochemical analysis showed normal striatal DA levels in the clinically affected A53T Huα-Syn transgenic mice (19). The regions containing abundant α-Syn and ubiquitin pathologies also exhibited prominent increase in the GFAP staining, indicating that neurodegeneration was present. A53T mutant Huα-Syn-dependent neurodegeneration was also indicated by the degeneration of myelinated axons in the ventral roots (18).

Subsequent study demonstrated the presence of overt neurodegeneration, as indicated by TUNEL-labeling, active caspase-3 immunoreactivity, and loss of neurons, in the PrP-Huα-Syn(A53T) transgenic mice (47). Significantly, this study also found that α-synucleinopathy in the transgenic mice is associated with significant mitochondrial abnormalities. Given that mitochondrial abnormalities are implicated in the pathogenesis of sporadic PD, it will be important to further define the in vivo pathologic link between α-Syn abnormalities and mitochondrial function.

Biochemical analysis shows that neuropathology in the MoPrP-Huα-Syn(A53T) transgenic mice was associated with increase in the levels of insoluble α-Syn. The α-Syn aggregates in the moPrP-αSyn(A53T) transgenic mice consists of full length α-Syn, truncated α-Syn, and higher molecular mass α-Syn in the transgenic mice. The overall pattern of the α-Syn variants deposited in mice is similar to that found in human α-synucleinopathies (18,48). Thus, the PrP-Huα-Syn transgenic mouse model appears to recapitulate many of the biochemical features of α-Syn aggregates associated with human α-synucleinopathies.

Subsequent analyses of the PrP-Huα-Syn transgenic mice have revealed additional features of this particular transgenic mouse model of α-synucleinopathy. Analysis of motoric activity revealed that transgenic mice expressing A53T mutant, but not wild type or A30P mutant, Huα-Syn develops significant hyperactivity (49). The hyperactivity phenotype is evident several months prior to onset of neuropathology. Significantly, studies with DA-receptor antagonist and agonist indicate that the hyperactivity in the PrP-Huα-Syn(A53T) transgenic mice is dependent on DAergic neurotransmission and is associated with increased sensitivity of D1-receptors. Finally, the levels of DA-transporter are decreased in the PrP-Huα-Syn(A53T) transgenic mice. Thus, while the overt DAergic pathology is not feature of the PrP-Huα-Syn transgenic mouse model, functional alterations of DAergic neurotransmission are present in these mice.

Two other variants of PrP were used to generate Huα-Syn transgenic mice. Expression of Huα-Syn using the hamster PrP promoter leads to generation of transgenic lines expressing very high levels of A30P mutant Huα-Syn (50). These mice develop fatal motoric abnormalities with the increased GFAP staining in the cortex and hippocampus. Despite the robust Huα-Syn expression in neurons, alterations in the solubility of α-Syn or specific neuropathologies were absent or not noted. As with the number of other Huα-Syn transgenic mice, DAergic markers were normal in the affected mice. In another variant of PrP-Huα-Syn transgenic mice, Huα-Syn expression was driven by a 3.5-kb promoter fragment from the mouse PrP gene (51), which is a truncated version of the previously used mouse PrP-cassett (52). While these mice do not develop overt aggregation of α-Syn, they develop deficits in vertical activity, grip strength, and rotarod performance.

Transgenic Mice Using Cell Type Specific Promoters

In addition to using promoters that drive expression of transgenes in a wide variety of neuronal populations, a number of transgenic lines expressing human α-Syn variants using a neuronal cell type specific promoter. Thus far, transgenic mice expressing α-Syn in DAergic neurons and in oligodendrocytes have been reported.

TH-Huα-Syn Transgenic Mice

First of these mice used a 4.8 kb rat tyrosine hydroxylase (TH) promoter was used to drive high levels of wild type and mutant (A30P and A53T) Huα-Syn expression in DAergic neurons (53). While the transgene derived protein accumulates in

DAergic cell bodies, inclusions do not develop in these mice. Further analysis showed that the number of DAergic neurons in the nigra, as well as the striatal DA level, is normal in the pTH-Huα-Syn transgenic mice.

More recently, a 9 kb rat TH promoter was used to express wild type (hwαSyn) or doubly mutated (harboring both A30P and A53T mutations, hm²αSyn) Huα-Syn (54). The mice expressing the doubly mutated hm²αSyn develop abnormal TH positive neurites that appear more beaded, dilated, and discontinuous. With aging, the hm²αSyn transgenic mice develop reduced locomotor activity and reduced striatal dopamine levels. The hm²αSyn mice also showed reduced sensitization to amphetamine and decreased response to apomorphine. The hm²αSyn transgenic mice were not more sensitive to MPTP toxicity than the hwαSyn transgenic mice. However, the DAergic neurons in the hm²αSyn were significantly more vulnerable to combined treatment of paraquat/Mn+-ethylenebisthiocarbamate (55).

Significantly, hm²αSyn mice show significant loss of DAergic neurons in SNpc (19% loss at 8.5 months and 55% loss at 18 months of age) (55). The loss of DAergic neurons in the hwαSyn transgenic mice expressing the wild type human α-Syn (13% loss at 18 months of age) was significantly less than in the hm²αSyn mice. It is also significant that the observed DAergic abnormalities in the hm²αSyn mice were not associated with overt aggregation of α-Syn in DAergic neurons. While the hm²αSyn transgenic mice do not develop full parkinsonian-like symptoms and do not develop LB-like inclusions, it is currently the only α-Syn transgenic mouse model where the progressive loss of DAergic neurons is reported.

More recently, α-Syn and DAergic abnormalities have been reported for transgenic mice expressing a carboxy-terminal truncation mutant, encoding the first 120 amino acids of α-Syn protein, under the transcriptional control of the 9 kb TH promoter (56). In this study, the TH9.0-α-Syn120 transgenic mice were bred into a strain of C57BL/6J mice with deletion of α-Syn gene (36). With aging, the TH9.0-α-Syn120 transgenic mice show abnormal accumulation of α-Syn120 in TH+ neurons of nigra and olfactory bulb (56). Immunoelectron microscopy and thioflavin S staining showed that some of the α-Syn120 accumulates as fibrils. The striatal dopamine level is normal at one month of age but is reduced at three months of age and remains reduced with aging. Further, the pTH9.0-α-Syn120 transgenic mice show normal response to amphetamine at six months of age but show reduced sensitivity to amphetamine at 18 months of age. However, the number of DA neurons in the SNpc of TH9.0-α-Syn120 transgenic mice was normal. While the basis for the apparent DAergic abnormalities in the pTH9.0-α-Syn120 transgenic mice remains to be determined, the pTH9.0-α-Syn120 transgenic mice seem to support the pathogenic importance of carboxy-terminal truncation of α-Syn (48).

Oligodendrocyte-Directed Expression of α-Syn in Transgenic Mice

While PD and LBD are associated with the presence of α-Syn aggregates in neurons, MSA is characterized by the presence of α-Syn aggregates in neurons and in oligodendrocytes. In order to study the in vivo consequence of α-Syn abnormalities in oligodendrocytes, transgenic mice expressing wild type Huα-Syn in oligodendrocyte were generated. The first of such mice used proteolipid promoter (PLP) to selectively drive the expression of wild type human α-Syn in oligodendrocytes of transgenic mice (57). The PLP-α-Syn transgenic mice develop α-Syn accumulation in oligodendendrocytes. The presence of serine129-phosporylated α-Syn in oligodendrocytes and the presence of detergent insoluble α-Syn indicate to overt aggregation of α-Syn in oligodendrocytes. Thus, the PLP-αSYN transgenic mice develop inclusions in oligodendrocytes that are similar to GCI's associated with MSA.

While the neuropathology was not evident in the PLP-αSYN transgenic mice, transgenic mice expressing of wild type Huα-Syn in oligodendrocytes using the 2′,3′-cyclic nucleotide 3′-phophodiesterase promoter (pCNP) develops MSA-like features, including motoric abnormalities and neurodegeneration (58). As with the PLP-α-Syn transgenic mice, the oligodendrocytes in the pCNP-α-Syn transgenic mice develop inclusions that are very similar to GCI's. In addition to the presence of α-Syn aggregates in oligodendrocytes and the presence of insoluble α-Syn, immuno-electron microscopy revealed fibrillar assembly α-Syn in oliogodendrocytes. Significantly, pCNP-α-Syn transgenic mice develop adult onset, progressive motoric abnormalities at seven to nine months of age, characterized by decline in rotarod performance, and reduced hanging time with wire hanging. Analysis of aged (24 months) transgenic mice showed significant brain atrophy, modest loss of spinal motor neurons, and the loss of oligodendrocytes. Moreover, neurodegeneration in the CNP-αSyn transgenic mice was associated with abnormal accumulation of endogenous mouse α-Syn in neuronal processes and synaptic terminals. The neurondegerative phenotype in the CNP-α-Syn transgenic mice, unlike the moPrp-αSyn transgenic mice, does not progress to lethality. The authors hypothesize that this is because neurodegeneration occurs at slower rate in CNP-α-Syn transgenic mice than in the moPrP-α-Syn transgenic mice because neurodegeneration is secondary to the degeneration of oligodendrocytes.

In addition to the CNP-α-Syn transgenic mice, expression of wild type Huα-Syn using a myelin basic protein promoter (MBP) (59). Like the above previous efforts, MBP-α-Syn transgenic mice develop GCI like α-Syn aggregates. Similar to the CNP-α-Syn transgenic mice, the MBP-α-Syn transgenic mice develop a variety of neuronal abnormalities, including axonal and dendritic atrophy and reduced DAergic terminals in the striatum. Unlike the CNP-α-Syn transgenic mice, mice from the highest expressing line show premature lethality.

The transgenic mice expressing wild type Huα-Syn in oligodendrocytes demonstrate that modest levels of α-Syn expression in oligodendrocytes are sufficient to drive abnormal aggregation of α-Syn in these cells. While the actual levels of α-Syn expression in oligodendrocytes are difficult to judge, the level of human α-Syn in oligodendrocytes does not appear to be very high, since the expression level of human α-Syn is significantly lower than that achieved with a pan-neuronal promoter (57), and the overall brain levels of total α-Syn do change in the CNP-α-Syn transgenic mice (58). Thus, oligodendrocytes seem to have lower threshold for developing α-Syn inclusions than in neurons. Another important implication of CNP-α-Syn and MBP-α-Syn transgenic mice is the demonstration that α-Syn abnormalities, even when limited to oligodendrocytes, can cause degeneration of oligodendrocytes and secondary neurodegeneration. Collectively, these lines of mice represent a significant advance for understanding the pathogenesis of MSA.

Viral, Vector-Based Models

In addition to the aforementioned transgenic mouse models, several groups have used viral vectors to directly express wild type and mutant Huα-Syn in rats (23,24) and nonhuman primates (60).

Kirik and his colleagues (23) used recombinant adeno associated virus (rAAV) vectors to express high levels of wild type and A53T mutant Huα-Syn in SNpc DAergic neurons of rats. The rAAV-Huα-Syn injected rats exhibited loss (~50%) of SNpc DA neurons and striatal DAergic innervation within eight weeks following viral transduction. There was only a trend toward abnormal motoric behavior.

While some neuron degenerative pathology was documented, there was clear evidence of significant Huα-Syn aggregation. Significantly, both wild type and A53T mutant Huα-Syn caused similar level of neurodegeneration. Transduction of adult marmosets with rAAV-Huα-Syn also leads to significant SNpc DAergic neurodegeneration (60). An interesting aspect of this study is that α-Syn pathology, such as abnormal accumulation of α-Syn in neurons, appears in SNpc to be more robust in the marmosets than in the rats.

Lo Bianco and his colleagues (24) used lentiviral vector to express wild type and mutant (A30P and A53T) Huα-Syn in rat SNpc. As with the rAAV-Huα-Syn model, significant loss (20–40%) of SNpc DA neurons and striatal DAergic terminals was observed within six weeks of transduction. There were no obvious differences in toxicity between the different Huα-Syn isoforms. However, expression of endogenous rat α-Syn did not lead to any toxicity, showing that Huα-Syn is qualitatively different from rodent α-Syn in terms of neurotoxicity. Despite the significant DAergic pathology, there were no obvious indications of α-Syn aggregation.

MECHANISTIC INSIGHTS INTO α-SYNUCLEINOPATHY FROM TRANSGENIC MODELS

Given the wide variety of phenotypes exhibited by the different α-Syn transgenic models, mechanistic conclusions from these models can be difficult for a casual observer. However, closer examinations of the transgenic mouse models do reveal significant mechanistic insights into the in vivo pathogenesis of α-synucleinopathy.

The most important implication of various α-Syn transgenic models is that we can conclude that α-Syn abnormalities cause neuronal dysfunction and neurodegeneration in vivo. Thus, even in diseases where the cause is not genetic mutations in the α-Syn gene, such as in most sporadic PD cases, the presence of α-Syn abnormalities indicates that these abnormalities are some how mechanistically linked to neurodegeneration in human disease. Further, α-Syn pathology in human α-synucleinopathies and the transgenic mouse models share significant biochemical and structural features. Thus, the transgenic mouse models of α-synucleinopathy can provide significant insights into the in vivo evolution of α-Syn abnormalities.

The main common feature of all transgenic models of α-synucleinopathy is that aging is required for expression of neurologic phenotype, neuropathology, and the aggregation of α-Syn. This is particularly true for the transgenic mouse models. In most transgenic mouse models, once the neurologic and/or neuropathologic phenotypes are expressed, they are progressive with aging. This progressive nature of the neurodegenerative phenotype is unknown for the viral, vector-based models. Regardless, the transgenic mouse models seem recapitulate the most significant risk factor for human α-synucleinopathy. It is significant that the effects of aging are one feature that is not easily reproduced in cellular models of α-Syn toxicity. Currently, it is not known what aspect of aging is responsible for promoting α-Syn-dependent neurodegeneration. Aging may lead to changes in the cell biology of α-Syn, promoting the pathologic conversion of α-Syn (61). For example, brain maturation and aging are associated with reduced rate of α-Syn degradation and increase in the accumulation of oxidatively modified α-Syn (61). Thus, aging may facilitate the formation and accumulation of toxic aggregates and oligomers of α-Syn. This may be a significant factor in the α-Syn transgenic mice using the pan-neuronal promoters since the onset of the disease phenotype appears to be temporally connected to onset of α-Syn aggregation in these mice. However, aging is not simply associated with the onset of α-Syn aggregation, since progressive loss of DAergic neurons in TH(9.0)-hm²αSyn transgenic mice occurs without signs of α-Syn aggregation in DAergic neurons. Thus, it is also likely that older neurons are more sensitive to any toxicity associated with α-Syn abnormalities.

Not surprisingly, the levels of transgene expression is a major factor in modeling α-synucleinopathy in these models. Despite the differences in clinical and pathologic features of various α-Syn transgenic models, neurologic abnormalities and neuropathology are clearly more severe with the higher levels of transgene expression. This aspect, together with the genetic data showing the pathogenic importance of gene dosage and promoter activity in human PD (9), is consistent with the view that α-Syn causes disease via dominant gain of deleterious property. The fact α-Syn knockout mice do not exhibit progressive neurodegenerative phenotype also supports this conclusion.

Another unique feature of the α-Syn transgenic mouse models is that differential pathogenic potentials of wild type and mutant human α-Syn can be demonstrated. In studies where transgenic mice expressing comparable levels of different Huα-Syn variants were generated by the same group, it is clear that the expression of mutant α-Syn can cause abnormalities more readily than the wild type α-Syn (18,19,39). Further, in one study where the A30P and A53T mutant α-Syn encoding transgenes were expressed at comparable levels in transgenic mice, it was clear that A53T mutant was more pathogenic than the A30P mutant (19). Since all Huα-Syn variants appear equally toxic in the invertebrate transgenic models and virally transduced models of α-synucleinopathy (17,23,24), apparent differences in the pathogenic potential of the Huα-Syn variants are one of the unique features of transgenic mouse models.

In all mammals, including humans, α-Syn is widely expressed in multiple neuronal populations. However, the fact that only a certain neuronal subset is more consistently affected by α-synucleinopthy in humans suggests that certain neuronal populations are more vulnerable to develop α-Syn abnormalities. Similarly, differential vulnerability of different neuronal populations in developing α-synucleinopathy is modeled by the α-Syn transgenic mouse models, where α-Syn expression is driven by the pan-neuronal promoters such as Thy1 and PrP (18,19). Both mouse Thy1 and PrP promoters drive very high levels of expression in most neuronal populations, particularly in cortex and hippocampus. However, the cortical regions are relatively spared from neuropathology in these mice. Thus, it is clear that relative resistance of human forebrain regions from developing α-synucleinopathy can be recapitulated in transgenic mice. Significantly, in transgenic mice where Huα-Syn transgene is expressed throughout the nervous system, the mice develop α-synucleinopathy in the overlapping populations of neurons (e.g., red nucleus, colliculi, deep cerebellar nuclei, pontine reticular nuclei, and spinal motor neurons). The fact that similar populations of neurons are affected in the lines of mice generated by multiple independent groups using two different promoters indicates that, in rodents, these neuronal populations are particularly vulnerable to developing α-synucleinopathy in mice. Even in viral vector-based models, where Huα-Syn causes neurodegeneration without significant α-Syn aggregation, there is a clear cell-type specificity in terms of toxicity. Specifically DAergic neurons in ventral tegmental area (62) and non-DAergic neurons in SN (24) are resistant to Huα-Syn induced neurodegeneration. Thus, defining the basis for this increased vulnerability may provide significant insights into the pathogenesis of α-synucleinopathy.

Another level of neural cell-type differences regarding the development of α-synucleinopathy is indicated by transgenic mouse models of MSA. As previously noted, α-Syn-dependent abnormality occurs in CNP-α-Syn transgenic mice with the modest levels of wild type α-Syn expression. Given that much higher levels of wild type Huα-Syn expression with the pan-neuronal promoter do not cause neuropathology in transgenic mice, an obvious implication is that oligodendrocytes are extremely vulnerable to developing α-synucleinopathy. Given the potential enhanced sensitivity of oligodendrocytes to α-synucleinopathy, defining the source of the oligodendrocyte α-Syn in human MSA is clearly warranted.

Despite the potential increased vulnerability of certain neuronal populations in developing α-synucleinopathy, the primary differences among the various promoters used may explain apparent variations in the distribution of neuropathology associated with various α-Syn transgenic mice. The effects of the promoter on the resulting neuropathology are obviously demonstrated by the transgenic mouse lines where α-Syn expression is limited to oligodendrocytes or TH-positive neurons. However, promoter-dependent effects may also effect pathology and phenotypes in transgenic mice generated with "pan-neuronal" promoters. For example, the difference in the pathology of Thy1αSyn/PrP-αSyn and PDGF-αSyn transgenic mice may be due to the fact that the human α-Syn expression in the PDGF-αSyn transgenic mice is more restricted than in the pThy-1-hαSyn transgenic mice (63). In particular, low transgene expression in subcortical regions with the PDGF-promoter is likely basis for the lack of brain stem pathology in the PDGF-αSyn transgenic mice. In addition, compared to the pThy1-promoter, PDGFβ-promoter drives significant amount human α-Syn expression in glial cells (63). Considering that relatively modest levels of wild type human α-Syn can cause neuropathology in the transgenic mouse models of MSA, the glial expression of hα-Syn in PDGF-hαSyn mice could contribute to neuronal dysfunction in these mice.

Thus far, it has been disappointing that none of the α-Syn transgenic mouse models recapitulate both α-Syn abnormalities and robust DAergic degeneration. It is not clear why most of the Huα-Syn transgenic mouse models have significant abnormalities in DAergic neurons, particularly in light of the dramatic pathologic changes in drosophila DAergic neurons (17), DA-dependent α-Syn toxicity in human neuronal cultures (64), and DAergic degeneration with viral transduction (23,24). It is important that in transgenic mouse models where DAergic degeneration is present, neurodegeneration is present without robust α-Syn aggregation (e.g., TH9.0-hm^{2}αSyn) and only at very advanced ages (>12 months of age) (54,55). Possibly, the aggressive onset and rapid progression of non-DAergic pathology with pan-neuronal expression of Huα-Syn may preclude development of DAergic pathology in the Thy-1 and the PrP promoter based transgenic mouse models. It should be noted that the currently used pan-neuronal promoters drive expression of α-Syn in neurons, such as motor neurons, that normally express relatively low levels of α-Syn. For example, lower endogenous levels of α-Syn expression in motor neurons may be a natural adaptation of these neurons. Thus, it is possible that the use of an alternative promoter that better reflects the endogenous pattern of α-Syn expression may provide a model with both progressive DAergic and non-DAergic phenotype.

It is also significant to note that DAergic neurodegeneration in a few transgenic mouse lines (PDGF and pTH9.0) and virally transduced rodents are rarely associated with obvious aggregation of α-Syn in DAergic neurons. In contrast, other transgenic mouse models of α-synucleinopathy, including the models of MSA, are always associated with robust aggregation of α-Syn. This difference suggests that DAergic neurons in rodents are relatively resistant to developing α-Syn aggregates. This idea is supported by the in vitro studies showing that DA and DA metabolites can inhibit α-Syn aggregation (65). The lack of α-Syn aggregates in DAergic neurons also suggests that the insoluble α-Syn aggregates may not be the primary toxic species responsible for DAergic neurodegeneration. Collectively, the observations with various α-Syn transgenic models suggest the possibility of two distinct pathways for α-Syn-dependent neurodegeneration. Specifically, α-Syn aggregates may cause neurodegeneration of nonDAergic neurons, whereas α-Syn-dependent DAergic neurodegeneration involve soluble α-Syn oligomer and other signaling pathways. This hypothesis is consistent with the proposal that α-Syn abnormalities in DAergic neurons are a relatively late event in PD pathogenesis (2,3).

MODULATION OF α-SYN AGGREGATION AND DISEASE IN α-SYN TRANSGENIC MODELS

With the availability of α-Syn transgenic mouse models of α-synucleinopathy, investigators are attempting to determine how α-synucleinopathy, particularly abnormal aggregation of α-Syn, could be modulated in vivo. Such experiments could potentially lead to novel therapeutic strategies.

In one of the first of such studies, it was shown that increased β-amyloid production could promote α-Syn aggregation. When PDGF-α-Syn transgenic mice were mated to transgenic mice overexpression human amyloid precursor protein, nonfibrillar α-Syn inclusions were converted to fibrillar inclusions (66). The increase in fibrillar α-Syn was associated with increased indices of synaptic degeneration and increased loss of DAergic markers in APP/α-Syn double Tg mice.

Another interesting endogenous factor that regulates α-Syn aggregation is β-Syn. In vitro studies have shown that β-Syn can inhibit formation of α-Syn fibrils (67). Expression of both human α-Syn (PDGF-α-Syn) and human β-Syn (Thy1-β-Syn) in mice leads to attenuated loss of striatal TH levels and improved rotarod performance over mice that only harbor PDGF-α-Syn transgene. Thus, β-Syn might function as an antiparkinsonian factor (68).

More recently, an α-Syn transgenic mouse model was used to demonstrate that α-Syn immunization could be used to attenuate α-synucleinopathy in vivo (66). In this study, Thy1-α-Syn transgenic mice were immunized with recombinant α-Syn for several months. The immunized mice generated antihuman α-Syn antibodies, and, in the brain, the antibodies localized to neuronal cells. Immunization was also associated with attenuated loss of synaptic terminals and reduced levels of oligomeric α-Syn. While this therapeutic approach clearly needs further analysis and development, the study demonstrates how the α-Syn transgenic model could be used to test novel and risky therapeutic approaches.

FUTURE OUTLOOK

As reviewed above, a variety of α-Syn transgenic models demonstrated that α-Syn abnormalities can cause neuronal dysfunction and degeneration. While animal studies have revealed significant new insights about the in vivo mechanisms of α-synucleinopathies, the differences among the models, as well as between the models and human disease, attest to the complexities of the question at hand. However, the insights provided by current models, combined with other genetic, pathologic, cell biologic, and biochemical studies, will allow for even deeper mechanistic understanding about PD and α-synucleinopathies.

Future efforts will clearly lead to additional refinement of current transgenic models, leading to better recapitulation of human PD pathology. For example, efforts to create α-Syn transgenic mice with endogenous pattern of α-Syn expression (e.g., using BAC-based transgenes) may lead to a pattern of neuropathology that more closely resembles human diseases. Further, with the availability of other transgenic models that are relevant to PD, it is now possible to test in vivo pathologic linkages between α-Syn abnormalities and other PD-linked genes. This is important since in vitro/cell culture studies do not always reflect in vivo interactions. For example, while in vitro studies have suggested a pathologic link between *PARKIN* dysfunction and α-Syn-toxicity (69), deleting *PARKIN* expression in mouse does not affect α-synucleinopathy in mouse (70). However, viral-based models do show that increased expression can protect SNpc DAergic neurons from Huα-Syn overexpression (71). In addition to better mechanistic understanding about the disease processes, the current and future mouse models of α-synucleinopathy will provide significant resources for testing novel therapeutic strategies.

REFERENCES

1. Fahn S, Przedborski S. Parkinsonism. In: Rowland LP, ed. Merritt's Neurology. New York: Lippincott, Williams & Wilkins, 2000:679–695.
2. Braak H, Del Tredici K, RubU, de Vos RA, Jansen Steur EN, Braak E. Staging of brain pathology related to sporadic Parkinson's disease. Neurobiol Aging 2003; 24:197–211.
3. Del Tredici K, Rub U, de Vos RA, Bohl JR, Braak H. Where does parkinson disease pathology begin in the brain? J Neuropathol Exp Neurol 2002; 61:413–426.
4. Bonifati V, Rizzu P, van Baren MJ, et al. Mutations in the DJ-1 gene associated with autosomal recessive early-onset parkinsonism. Science 2003; 299:256–259.
5. Kitada T, Asakawa S, Hattori N, et al. Mutations in the parkin gene cause autosomal recessive juvenile parkinsonism. Nature 1998; 392:605–608.
6. Kruger R, Kuhn W, Muller T, et al. Ala30Pro mutation in the gene encoding alpha-synuclein in Parkinson's disease. Nat Genet 1998; 18:106–108.
7. Paisan-Ruiz C, Jane S, Evan EW, et al. Cloning of the gene containing mutations that cause PARK8-linked Parkinson's disease. Neuron 2004; 44:595–600.
8. Polymeropoulos MH, Lavedan C, Leroy E, et al. Mutation in the alpha-synuclein gene identified in families with Parkinson's disease. Science 1997; 276:2045–2047.
9. Singleton AB, Farrer M, Johnson J, et al. Alpha-Synuclein locus triplication causes Parkinson's disease. Science 2003; 302:841.
10. Zimprich A, Biskup S, Leitner P, et al. Mutations in LRRK2 cause autosomal-dominant Parkinsonism with pleomorphic pathology. Neuron 2004; 44:601–607.
11. Spillantini MG, Crowther RA, Jakes R, Hasegawa M, Goedert M. Alpha-synuclein in filamentous inclusions of Lewy bodies from Parkinson's disease and dementia with lewy bodies. Proc Natl Acad Sci USA 1998; 95:6469–6473.
12. Spillantini MG, Schmidt ML, Lee VM, Trojanowski JQ, Jakes R, Goedert M. Alpha-synuclein in Lewy bodies. Nature 1997; 388:839–840.
13. Dickson DW. Alpha-synuclein and the lewy body disorders. Curr Opin Neurol 2001; 14:423–432.
14. Galvin JE, Lee VMY, Trojanowski JQ. Synucleinopathies. Arch Neurol 2001; 58:186–190.
15. Galvin JE, Uryu K, Lee VM, Trojanowski JQ. Axon pathology in Parkinson's disease and Lewy body dementia hippocampus contains alpha-, beta-, and gamma-synuclein. Proc Natl Acad Sci USA 1999; 96:13450–13455.
16. Goedert M, Spillantini MG. Lewy body diseases and multiple system atrophy as alpha-synucleinopathies. Mol Psychiatry 1998; 3:462–465.
17. Feany MB, Bender WW. A drosophila model of Parkinson's disease. Nature 2000; 404:394–398.

18. Giasson BI, Duda JE, Quinn SM, Zhang B, Trojanowski JQ, Lee VM. Neuronal alpha-synucleinopathy with severe movement disorder in mice expressing A53T human alpha-synuclein. Neuron 2002; 34:521–533.

19. Lee MK, Stirling W, Xu Y. Human alpha-synuclein-harboring familial Parkinson's disease-linked Ala-53 → Thr mutation causes neurodegenerative disease with alpha-synuclein aggregation in transgenic mice. Proc Natl Acad Sci USA 2002; 99:8968–8973.

20. Masliah E, Rockenstein E, Veinbergs I, et al. Dopaminergic loss and inclusion body formation in alpha-synuclein mice: implications for neurodegenerative disorders. Science 2000; 287:1265–1269.

21. Neumann M, Kahle PJ, Giasson BI, et al. Misfolded proteinase K-resistant hyperphosphorylated alpha-synuclein in aged transgenic mice with locomotor deterioration and in human alpha-synucleinopathies. J Clin Invest 2002; 110:1429–1439.

22. Van der Putten H, Wiederhold KH, Probst A, et al. Neuropathology in mice expressing human alpha-synuclein. J Neurosci 2000; 20:6021–6029.

23. Kirik D, Rosenblad C, Burger C, et al. Parkinson-like neurodegeneration induced by targeted overexpression of alpha-synuclein in the nigrostriatal system. J Neurosci 2002; 22:2780–2791.

24. Lo Bianco C, Ridet JL, Schneider BL. Alpha-synucleinopathy and selective dopaminergic neuron loss in a rat lentiviral-based model of Parkinson's disease. Proc Natl Acad Sci USA 2002; 99:10813–10818.

25. George JM. The synucleins. Genome Biol 2001; 3:reviews3002.1-3002.6.

26. Goedert M. The awakening of a-synuclein. Nature 1997; 388:232–233.

27. George JM, Clayton DF. Songbirds, synelfin, and neurodegenerative disease. Neurosci News 1998; 1:12–17.

28. Maroteaux L, Campanelli JT, Scheller RH. Synuclein: a neuron-specific protein localized to the nucleus and presynaptic nerve terminal. J Neurosci 1988; 8:2804–2815.

29. Ueda K, Fukushima H, Masliah E, et al. Molecular cloning of cDNA encoding an unrecognized component of amyloid in Alzheimer disease. Proc Natl Acad Sci USA 1993; 90:11282–11286.

30. Abeliovich A, Schmitz Y, Farinas I, et al. Mice lacking alpha-synuclein display functional deficits in the nigrostriatal dopamine system. Neuron 2000; 25:239–252.

31. Chandra S, Fornai F, Kwon HB, et al. Double-knockout mice for alpha- and beta-synucleins: effect on synaptic functions. Proc Natl Acad Sci USA 2004; 101:14966–14971.

32. Dauer W, Kholodilov N, Vila M, et al. Resistance of alpha-synuclein null mice to the parkinsonian neurotoxin MPTP. Proc Natl Acad Sci USA 2002; 99:14524–14529.

33. Schluter OM, Fornai F, Alessandri MG, et al. Role of alpha-synuclein in 1-methyl-4-phenyl-1,2,3,6-tetrahydropyridine-induced parkinsonism in mice. Neuroscience 2003; 118:985–1002.

34. Cabin DE, Shimazu K, Murphy D, et al. Synaptic vesicle depletion correlates with attenuated synaptic responses to prolonged repetitive stimulation in mice lacking alpha-synuclein. J Neurosci 2002; 22:8797–8807.

35. Yavich L, Tanila H, Vepsalainen S, Jakala P. Role of alpha-synuclein in presynaptic dopamine recruitment. J Neurosci 2004; 24:11165–11170.

36. Specht CG, Schoepfer R. Deletion of the alpha-synuclein locus in a subpopulation of C57BL/6J inbred mice. BMC Neurosci 2001; 2:11.

37. Robertson DC, Schmidt O, Ninkina N, Jones PA, Sharkey J, Buchman VL. Developmental loss and resistance to MPTP toxicity of dopaminergic neurones in substantia nigra pars compacta of gamma-synuclein, alpha-synuclein and double alpha/gamma-synuclein null mutant mice. J Neurochem 2004; 89:1126–1136.

38. Chandra S, Gallardo G, Fernandez-Chacon R, Schluter OM, Sudhof TC. Alpha-synuclein cooperates with CSPalpha in preventing neurodegeneration. Cell 2005; 123:383–396.

39. Fernandez-Chacon R, Wolfel M, Nishimune H, et al. The synaptic vesicle protein CSP alpha prevents presynaptic degeneration. Neuron 2004; 42:237–251.

40. Souza JM, Giasson BI, Lee VM, Ischiropoulos H. Chaperone-like activity of synucleins. FEBS Lett 2000; 474:116–119.

41. Rathke-Hartlieb S, Kahle PJ, Neumann M, et al. Sensitivity to MPTP is not increased in Parkinson's disease-associated mutant alpha-synuclein transgenic mice. J Neurochem 2001; 77:1181–1184.

42. Klivenyi P, Siwek D, Gardian G, et al. Mice lacking alpha-synuclein are resistant to mitochondrial toxins. Neurobiol Dis 2006; 21:541–548.
43. Dong Z, Ferger B, Feldon J, Bueler H. Overexpression of Parkinson's disease-associated alpha-synucleinA53T by recombinant adeno-associated virus in mice does not increase the vulnerability of dopaminergic neurons to MPTP. J Neurobiol 2002; 53:1–10.
44. Hashimoto M, Rockenstein E, Masliah E. Transgenic models of alpha-synuclein pathology: past, present, and future. Ann NY Acad Sci 2003; 991:171–188.
45. Kahle PJ, Neumann M, Ozmen L, et al. Subcellular localization of wild-type and Parkinson's disease-associated mutant alpha-synuclein in human and transgenic mouse brain. J Neurosci 2000; 20:6365–6373.
46. Freichel C, Neumann M, Ballard T, et al. Age-dependent cognitive decline and amygdala pathology in alpha-synuclein transgenic mice. Neurobiol Aging. In press.
47. Martin LJ, Pan Y, Price AC, et al. Parkinson's disease alpha-synuclein transgenic mice develop neuronal mitochondrial degeneration and cell death. J Neurosci 2006; 26:41–50.
48. Li W, West N, Colla E, et al. Aggregation promoting C-terminal truncation of {alpha}-synuclein is a normal cellular process and is enhanced by the familial Parkinson's disease-linked mutations. Proc Natl Acad Sci USA 2005; 102:2162–2167.
49. Unger EL, Eve DJ, Perez XA, et al. Locomotor hyperactivity and alterations in dopamine neurotransmission are associated with overexpression of A53T mutant human alpha-synuclein in mice. Neurobiol Dis 2006; 21:431–443.
50. Gomez-Isla T, Irizarry MC, Mariash A, et al. Motor dysfunction and gliosis with preserved dopaminergic markers in human alpha-synuclein A30P transgenic mice. Neurobiol Aging 2003; 24:245–258.
51. Gispert S, Del Turco D, Garrett L, et al. Transgenic mice expressing mutant A53T human alpha-synuclein show neuronal dysfunction in the absence of aggregate formation. Mol Cell Neurosci 2003; 24:419–429.
52. Borchelt DR, Davis J, Fischer M, et al. A vector for expressing foreign genes in the brains and hearts of transgenic mice. Genet Anal 1996; 13:159–163.
53. Matsuoka Y, Vila M, Lincoln S, et al. Lack of nigral pathology in transgenic mice expressing human alpha-synuclein driven by the tyrosine hydroxylase promoter. Neurobiol Dis 2001; 8:535–539.
54. Richfield EK, Thiruchelvam MJ, Cory-Slechta DA, et al. Behavioral and neurochemical effects of wild-type and mutated human alpha-synuclein in transgenic mice. Exp Neurol 2002; 175:35–48.
55. Thiruchelvam MJ, Powers JM, Cory-Slechta DA, Richfield EK. Risk factors for dopaminergic neuron loss in human alpha-synuclein transgenic mice. Eur J Neurosci 2004; 19:845–854.
56. Tofaris GK, Reitbock PG, Humby T, et al. Pathological changes in dopaminergic nerve cells of the substantia nigra and olfactory bulb in mice transgenic for truncated human alpha-synuclein (1–20): implications for Lewy body disorders. J Neurosci 2006; 26: 3942–3950.
57. Kahle PJ, Neumann M, Ozmen L, et al. Hyperphosphorylation and insolubility of alpha-synuclein in transgenic mouse oligodendrocytes. EMBO Rep 2002; 3:583–588.
58. Yazawa I, Giasson BI, Sasaki R, et al. Mouse model of multiple system atrophy alpha-synuclein expression in oligodendrocytes causes glial and neuronal degeneration. Neuron 2005; 45:847–859.
59. Shults CW, Rockenstein E, Crews L, et al. Neurological and neurodegenerative alterations in a transgenic mouse model expressing human alpha-synuclein under oligodendrocyte promoter: implications for multiple system atrophy. J Neurosci 2005; 25: 10689–10699.
60. Kirik D, Annett LE, Burger C, Muzyczka N, Mandel RJ, Bjorklund A. Nigrostriatal alpha-synucleinopathy induced by viral vector-mediated overexpression of human alpha-synuclein: a new primate model of Parkinson's disease. Proc Natl Acad Sci USA 2003; 100:2884–2889.
61. Li W, Lesuisse C, Xu Y, Troncoso JC, Price DL, Lee MK. Stabilization of alpha-synuclein protein with aging and familial parkinson's disease-linked A53T mutation. J Neurosci 2004; 24:9400–9409.

62. Maingay M, Romero-Ramos M, Carta M, Kirik D. Ventral tegmental area dopamine neurons are resistant to human mutant alpha-synuclein overexpression. Neurobiol Dis 2006; 23:522–532.
63. Rockenstein E, Mallory M, Hashimoto M, et al. Differential neuropathological alterations in transgenic mice expressing alpha-synuclein from the platelet-derived growth factor and Thy-1 promoters. J Neurosci Res 2002; 68:568–578.
64. Xu J, Kao SY, Lee FJ, Song W, Jin LW, Yankner BA. Dopamine-dependent neurotoxicity of alpha-synuclein: a mechanism for selective neurodegeneration in Parkinson disease. Nat Med 2002; 8:600–606.
65. Mazzulli JR, Mishizen AJ, Giasson BI. Cytosolic catechols inhibit alpha-synuclein aggregation and facilitate the formation of intracellular soluble oligomeric intermediates. J Neurosci 2006; 26:10068–10078.
66. Masliah E, Rockenstein E, Veinbergs I, et al. b-amyloid peptides enhance a-synuclein accumulation and neuronal deficits in a transgenic mouse model linking Alzheimer's disease and Parkinson's disease. Proc Natl Acad Sci USA 2001; 98:12245–12250.
67. Uversky VN, Li J, Souillac P, et al. Biophysical properties of the synucleins and their propensities to fibrillate: inhibition of alpha-synuclein assembly by beta- and gamma-synucleins. J Biol Chem 2002; 277:11970–11978.
68. Hashimoto M, Rockenstein E, Mante M, Mallory M, Masliah E. beta-Synuclein inhibits alpha-synuclein aggregation: a possible role as an anti-parkinsonian factor. Neuron 2001; 32:213–223.
69. Petrucelli L, O'Farrell C, Lockhart PJ, et al. Parkin protects against the toxicity associated with mutant alpha-synuclein: proteasome dysfunction selectively affects catecholaminergic neurons. Neuron 2002; 36:1007–1019.
70. von Coelln R, Thomas B, Andrabi SA, et al. Inclusion body formation and neurodegeneration are parkin independent in a mouse model of alpha-synucleinopathy. J Neurosci 2006; 26:3685–3696.
71. Lo BC, Schneider BL, Bauer M, et al. Lentiviral vector delivery of parkin prevents dopaminergic degeneration in an alpha-synuclein rat model of Parkinson's disease. Proc Natl Acad Sci USA 2004; 101:17510–17515.

18 Mouse Models of Recessive Parkinsonism

Matthew S. Goldberg and Jie Shen
Center for Neurologic Diseases, Brigham and Women's Hospital, Harvard Medical School, Boston, Massachusetts, U.S.A.

Recessively inherited mutations in the *PARKIN, DJ-1,* and *PINK1* genes have recently been linked to familial forms of parkinsonism, which are often clinically indistinguishable from Parkinson's disease (PD). Various mutant mice carrying a germline deletion in either the *PARKIN* or the *DJ-1* gene have been developed to study the normal functions of these gene products, which may provide insights into the pathogenic mechanisms underlying the selective degeneration of dopaminergic neurons. This chapter will summarize recent studies of these loss-of-function mutant mice and discuss their implications to the pathogenesis of PD.

The neuropathologic hallmarks of PD are progressive degeneration of dopaminergic neurons and the presence of Lewy bodies (LBs) in the substantia nigra pars compacta (SNpc). The loss of the dopaminergic innervation to the striatum is thought to be the primary cause of resting tremor, rigidity, and bradykinesia, which are the cardinal clinical features of PD. The discovery of autosomal-recessively inherited mutations in the *PARKIN* (1), *DJ-1* (2), and *PINK1* (3) genes associated with familial parkinsonism made it possible to study, through the generation and characterization of mutant mice mimicking the genetic alterations in familial patients, how these loss of function mutations cause the disease. Multiple groups have published the phenotypic characterization of their mutant mice carrying germline deletion mutations in either the *PARKIN* or *DJ-1* gene (Tables 1 and 2). The multidisciplinary analysis of these independently generated mutant mice are compared and summarized below.

PARKIN

PARKIN contains an ubiquitin-like domain and two really interesting new gene (RING) domains separated by an in-between ring (IBR) domain, and can function as E3 ubiquitin ligase (4,5). A number of *PARKIN* substrates identified in a variety of in vitro systems have been reported (4,6–11). However, the lack of accumulation of these substrate proteins in *PARKIN*-null mice raised the question of whether they are truly physiologic substrates of *PARKIN*. To study the normal physiologic role of *PARKIN*, four groups have generated independent knockout (KO) mice carrying distinct targeted germline deletions (12–15). Their independent findings and the distinctions among the knockout mice used will be summarized below.

Generation of Mutant Mice
In 2003, Itier et al. and Goldberg et al. reported their multidisciplinary analysis of two similarly generated *PARKIN* KO mice, in both of which exon 3 was targeted (12,13). The last 179 base pairs of exon 3 and the first 918 base pairs of intron 3 were replaced with a positive selection cassette encoding neomycin resistance

TABLE 1 Generation and Phenotypic Characterization of *PARKIN*-Deficient Mice. Ages Examined (in Months) are Shown in Parentheses

	Itier et al., 2003 (12)	Goldberg et al., 2003 (13)	von Coelln et al., 2004 (14)	Perez and Palmiter, 2005 (15)
Mutation	Δ exon 3	Δ exon 3	Δ exon 7	Δ exon 2
Targeting approach	Pgk-neo	Pgk-neo EGFP in-frame insertion	Cre-mediated deletion	Polr2a-neo
ES cell line	CK35	J1		AK18.1
Strain	B6x129	B6x129	B6x129	B6x129 & 129
Histology	No inclusions No nigral cell loss (15)	No inclusions No nigral cell loss (12,18,24)	Locus ceruleus cell loss (2,12,18) No nigral cell loss (2,12,18) No inclusions	No inclusions
Behavior	Reduced locomotor activity (5–6) Reduced locomotor response to amphetamine (6) Reduced alternance in T-maze (5)	More slips traversing a beam (2–4,7,18) Somatosensory deficits (2–4,7)	Reduced acoustic startle response (9)	No robust differences in 25 behavioral tests (18–22)
Neurochemistry	Increased DA and DOPAC in limbic system (11)	Increased extracellular DA in striatum (8,9)	Reduced NE in olfactory bulb and spinal cord (18)	No changes observed in NE, DA, DOPAC, HVA or 3-MT
Electrophysiology	Deficits in glutamate neurotransmission in hippocampus (13)	Decreased synaptic excitability of striatal neurons (6–9)	Not examined	Not examined
Biochemistry	Reduced DAT and VMAT2 in striatum Decreased DA uptake in cultured neurons Increased levels of reduced glutathione in striatum and cultured neurons	Normal abundance of PARKIN substrates Reduced levels of mitochondrial and antioxidant proteins in ventral midbrain	Not examined	Not examined

Abbreviations: DA, dopamine; DAT, DA transporter; DOPAC, 3,4-dihydroxyphenylacetic acid; HVA, homovanillic acid; NE, norepinephrine; VMAT2, vesicular monoamine transporter.

TABLE 2 Generation and Phenotypic Characterization of *DJ-1*-Deficient Mice. Ages Examined (in months) are Shown in Parentheses

	Goldberg et al., 2005 (38)	Kim et al., 2005 (39)	Chen et al., 2005 (40)
Mutation	Δ exon 2	exon 2 stop; Δ exons 3–5	Δ exons 1–5
Targeting approach	Pgk-neo	Pgk-neo	FRT-Pgk-neo-FRT
ES cell line	MKV6.5	E14K	E14Tg2A.4
Strain	B6x129	B6x129(B6N7)	B6x129
Histology	No inclusions No nigral cell loss (3,12)	Increased MPTP-induced nigral cell loss and DA nerve terminal loss (2)	No inclusions No nigral cell loss (6,11)
Behavior	Reduced locomotor activity (3) Reduced locomotor response to quinpirole	Reduced locomotor activity after challenge with amphetamine or MPTP (2)	Age-dependent reduction in locomotor activity (at 11 months but not 5,9) Somatosensory deficits (5,11)
Neurochemistry	Reduced evoked DA overflow in striatum consistent with increased DA reuptake (3)	Greater reduction in striatal DA following MPTP treatment (2)	Increased stimulated DA release and increased DA reuptake in the dorsal striatum (4) Increased striatal DA (6,11)
Electrophysiology	Reduced respon-siveness of nigral neurons to DA (1) Corticostriatal LTD deficits rescued by quinpirole (1)	Not examined	Not examined
Biochemistry	No changes in levels of TH, DAT, or D2 DA receptors	Increased sensitivity to cell death induced by oxidative stress in cultured neurons	No increase in oxidized proteins or levels of TH, DAT, or VMAT2

Abbreviations: DA, dopamine; DAT, DA transporter; ES, embryonic stem; LTD, long-term depression; MPTP, 1-methyl-4-phenyl-1,2,3,6-tetrahydropyridine; TH, tyrosine hydroxylase; VMAT, vesicular minoamine transporters.

(Pgk-*neo*^{r}) in the KO mouse generated by Itier et al. Northern analysis and RT-PCR followed by sequencing confirmed the skipping of exon 3 in the truncated mRNA found in *PARKIN* KO mice. This aberrant splicing results in a shift of the open reading frame after amino acid 57 and the occurrence of a premature stop codon at position 105, thus producing a truncated *PARKIN* protein lacking any of the RING or IBR domains, which were shown to be essential for *PARKIN*'s embryonic stem (ES) ubiquitin ligase activity (16).

Goldberg et al. replaced the last 128 base pairs of exon 3 and the first 306 base pairs of intron 3 with the coding sequence for enhanced green flourescent protein (EGFP) and a selection cassette (Pgk-*neo*^{r}). The coding sequence of EGFP was fused in-frame within the coding sequence of exon 3 of *PARKIN*, thus producing a chimeric protein consisting of the first 95 amino acids of *PARKIN* followed by EGFP. Similar to the results obtained by Itier et al., Northern analysis and RT-PCR followed by sequencing confirmed the presence of an additional mRNA lacking exon 3, which results in a reading frame shift after amino acid 57 and production of a drastically truncated protein.

The gene targeting approach used by von Coelln et al. (14) differed from the other three *PARKIN*-deficient mice reported to date. *PARKIN* mutant mice were purchased from Lexicon Genetics, in which a floxed exon 7 was removed upon breeding to *protamine-Cre* transgenic mice expressing the Cre recombinase in the male germ line. This results in the removal of exon 7 and the shift of the open reading frame thereafter, as exon 7 contains a nonintegral number of codons. This results in the translation of the first 243 amino acid residues of mouse *PARKIN* plus eight missense amino acid residues. It is theoretically possible that this truncated protein retains some residual function of *PARKIN*, even though it lacks the RING and IBR domains critical for its E3 ligase activity.

Perez and Palmiter (15) used the standard gene targeting approach to replace exon 2 and part of the surrounding introns with a selection cassette (*Polr2a-neo*). In theory, this would result in a 4 amino acid peptide, if exon 1 were to be spliced into exon 3, as exon 2 contains a nonintegral number of codons. However, if exon 1 were to be spliced to exon 4, the reading frame would be restored and a ~37 kDa protein that retains all of the IBR and RING domains would be produced. RT-PCR amplification of the region spanning exons 1–6 provided evidence that skipping of both exons 2 and 3 occurred in these mutant mice, as well as at detectable levels in WT mice, suggesting the existence of a previously unrecognized splice variant of *PARKIN* that could be functionally important. Furthermore, overexposed Western blots of WT and mutant mouse brains using the antihuman Parkin, clone 8 (PRK8) antibody specific for the C-terminus of *PARKIN* (17) revealed the presence of a protein with apparent molecular weight consistent with this splice variant. Although it is uncertain that this ~37kDa variant of *PARKIN* is truly functional in vivo, its presence may explain the absence of behavioral phenotypes reported for this mouse (see subsequently). It also remains to be determined whether this mouse exhibits any electrophysiologic phenotypes reported for the other *PARKIN*-deficient mice (12,13).

Neuropathologic Findings

All four independently generated *PARKIN*-deficient mice published to date are viable and fertile with no gross abnormalities. This is consistent with the absence of notable developmental abnormalities in humans bearing homozygous or compound heterozygous mutations in *PARKIN*. Given the profound loss of nigral dopaminergic neurons and consequent parkinsonism in humans bearing loss-of-function mutations in *PARKIN*, one might expect *PARKIN*-null mice to recapitulate these features, especially considering the very early age of disease onset of the disease in human patients. However, all four groups reported the lack of loss of dopaminergic neurons in the substantia nigra (SN) of *PARKIN*-null mice.

Itier et al. quantified the number of tyrosine hydroxylase (TH)-positive neurons in the substantia nigra pars compacta of mice at the age of 15 months and did not observe a significant difference between genotypes. Goldberg et al. used rigorous stereologic techniques to compare the number of TH-positive nigral neurons in wild type and *PARKIN*-deficient mice at ages 12, 18, and 24 months and did not find any statistically significant differences. Furthermore, Goldberg et al. quantified the size of nigral neurons and did not find any significant differences in morphology. Perez and Palmiter did not detect any gross neuropathologic or histologic abnormalities in their *PARKIN* KO mice, though stereologic neuron counting was not performed in their mice. von Coelln et al. counted the number of TH-positive and Nissl-positive neurons in the substantia nigra pars compact and the locus ceruleus of mice at ages 2, 12, and 18 months using rigorous stereologic techniques. Consistent with the previous results reported by Itier et al. and Goldberg et al., von Coelln et al. found no significant decrease in the number of nigral dopaminergic neurons at any age. However, they did observe a statistically significant reduction in the number of norepinephine neurons in the locus ceruleus in both young (two months) and aged (12 and 18 months) *PARKIN*-deficient mice compared to wild type controls. This is consistent with the loss of locus ceruleus neurons observed in postmortem examination of patients with *PARKIN* mutations (18–20).

Most of the reports of postmortem examinations of patients with *PARKIN* mutations have not identified LBs or other inclusions that are neuropathologic hallmarks of idiopathic PD. Consistent with the human findings, the absence of ubiquitinated aggregates of α-synuclein was specifically noted in all *PARKIN*-deficient mice.

Behavioral Deficits

The death of nigral dopaminergic neurons in humans with parkinsonism is presumably preceded by dysfunction and degeneration of these cells and their functional circuits. One of the primary benefits of modeling in mice loss-of-function mutations linked to recessive parkinsonism in humans is that it provides an opportunity to identify dysfunctions of the nigrostriatal pathway that occur in the absence of *PARKIN*. Many behavioral paradigms have been shown in rodents to be sensitive to impairments of the nigrostriatal pathway (21–26).

Goldberg et al. found that *PARKIN*-deficient mice at ages two to four months, seven months, and 18 months made significantly more slips while traversing a narrow beam compared to wild type mice. The two to four months and seven months old mice also exhibited significant somatosensory deficits as measured by the ability to sense and remove small adhesives placed on their fur. The difference between genotypes was not statistically significant at the age of 18 months largely due to the normal age-dependent decrease in somatosensory abilities of wild type mice. Goldberg et al. reported that mice at all age groups showed normal performance in the rotarod and open field tasks, indicating that both forced movements and spontaneous locomotor activity are not altered in the absence of *PARKIN*.

In contrast, Itier et al. reported that *PARKIN*-deficient mice at the age of 170 days have significantly reduced open field activity compared to wild type mice. They also reported a significantly reduced probability of 140-day-old *PARKIN*-deficient mice visiting the previously unknown arm of a T-maze, suggesting either working memory deficits or reduced exploratory activity in the absence of *PARKIN*. *PARKIN*-deficient mice were also observed to have a significantly altered response to the locomotor effects of 1 mg/kg and 5 mg/kg amphetamine compared to wild type mice, although the number of animals examined ($n = 5$ per group) was low and thus warrants further studies. Rotarod performance was not reported.

von Coelln et al. examined the rotarod performance, open field behavior and acoustic startle response of *PARKIN*-deficient mice. No differences were observed between genotypes in open field behavior or rotarod performance, consistent with the results of Goldberg et al. Interestingly, they found a significant decrease in acoustic startle response of nine month-old *PARKIN*-deficient mice compared to wild type mice, consistent with the decreased number of noradrenergic neurons in the locus ceruleus observed histologically. We have also found reduced acoustic startle response in our *PARKIN*-deficient mice at ages 12 to 17 months but not at ages three to six months, suggesting an age-dependent dysfunction of one or more pathways essential for acoustic startle response (Goldberg and Shen, unpublished data).

Perez and Palmiter conducted a large array of 25 behavioral tests on 18 to 22 months old *PARKIN*-deficient mice. These included tests of motor function, such as rotarod, general body function, and neurologic function, such as body weight and temperature, and tests of learning, memory and emotionality, such as Morris water maze, passive-avoidance, and elevated plus-maze. Mice at younger ages (three, six, or 12 months) were also examined for some of the motor tests. For those tests in which a statistically significant difference between genotypes was found at ages 18 to 22 months, *PARKIN* KO mice in 129 inbred strain were subsequently tested to examine the effect of genetic background.

Surprisingly, Perez and Palmiter concluded that *PARKIN*-deficient mice are not a robust model of parkinsonism because only 25 out of 442 statistical tests involving genotype showed a significant difference ($p < 0.05$), most of which were not reproducible on a pure 129 genetic background. Given such a large number of statistical tests, one would expect about 22 ($p < 0.05$) by chance. This is nearly as large as the 25 tests that were found to be statistically significant. However, this could also be a consequence of including an overly broad array of cognitive and behavioral tasks in their study, most of which are not known to be sensitive to dysfunction of the nigrostriatal pathway in rodents. It is worthwhile to consider the results of these tasks in more detail.

For the adhesive removal test, Goldberg et al. reported the largest size adhesive that could not be sensed and removed within a 60-second trial, averaged over each set of mice. In contrast, Perez and Palmiter reported the average latency to remove each size adhesive. Despite the difference in methodologies, the results obtained by Perez and Palmiter were consistent with the results previously reported by Goldberg et al. in that no difference between genotypes was observed in 18 to 19 months old mice. The results of Goldberg et al. indicate that the performance of this task decreases with age in wild type mice, such that 18 month-old mice score poorly regardless of genotype. Goldberg et al. found that younger wild type mice (ages two to four months and seven months) performed this task significantly better than *PARKIN*-deficient mice at the same age, suggesting somatosensory deficits in the absence of *PARKIN*. Perez and Palmiter did not report the results of mice tested at ages younger than 19 months.

For the beam traversal test, great care must be taken to score motor skills rather than other behaviors and emotions such as motivation, fear, and anxiety. Depending upon experimental design, the time it takes a mouse to traverse from one end of a beam to the other end can be more a measure of motivation than a measure of motor skills. In contrast, the number of slips while traversing the beam more purely reflects motor skills. However, even this can be more a measure of fear or anxiety if the beam is located too high above the work surface or bright lights are used to induce mice to traverse the beam. Goldberg et al. avoided the use of bright lights and kept the height of the beam as low as possible (about half the height as the beam used by Perez and Palmiter). This could possibly explain why Perez and Palmiter observed no difference between genotypes at the one age tested (19 months) while Goldberg et al. found that *PARKIN*-deficient mice made significantly more slips at all three sets of mice tested (ages two to four, seven, and 18 months). Furthermore, Goldberg et al.

found it to be important to overlay the beam with a 1 cm wire mesh grid to ensure that the task was much more a measure of motor skills than the numerous other behaviors and emotions that could otherwise predominate.

Catecholamine Measurements
All four groups with *PARKIN*-deficient mice measured brain catecholamine levels by high performance liquid chromotography (HPLC) with electrochemical detection. Itier et al. measured tissue levels of dopamine (DA) and its metabolites [3-methaxy tyramin (3-MT), 3-,4-dihydrophenyl acetic acid (DOPAC), and HVA], serotonin and its metabolite [5 hydroxy indol acetic acid (5-HIAA)], and norepinephrine (NE) in the striatum, diencephalon, brainstem, and limbic system. *PARKIN*-deficient mice had significant differences only in the limbic system, where the levels of DA and DOPAC were about 50% higher compared to wild type mice.

Goldberg et al. measured tissue levels of DA and its metabolites (DOPAC and HVA) in the dorsal striatum and found no differences between genotypes. This is consistent with the measurements of striatal DA reported by Itier et al. Goldberg et al. also measured the extracellular concentration of DA in the striatum of awake and freely moving mice using in vivo microdialysis. When dialysis membranes were stereotaxically implanted into the striatum of mice and perfused with artificial cerebrospinal fluid, the dialysate from *PARKIN*-deficient mice contained significantly more DA compared to wild type controls. This suggested that the extracellular concentration of striatal DA was higher in *PARKIN*-deficient mice. As a more direct measure of the extracellular concentration of DA, the no-net-flux method was employed to determine the DA concentration at which the levels in the dialysate exactly balanced the concentration of DA added to the perfusate. Using this method the concentration of extracellular DA was determined to be significantly higher in the striatum of *PARKIN*-deficient mice.

von Coelln et al. measured levels of DA and its metabolites (DOPAC and HVA) in the striatum and NE in the olfactory bulb, cortex, brainstem, and spinal cord. No changes in tissue levels of these biogenic amines were found in the striatum, cortex, or brainstem, consistent with the previous reports. Interestingly, they found significantly reduced levels of NE in the olfactory bulb and spinal cord of *PARKIN*-deficient mice compared to wild types, possibly as a result of the reduction in locus ceruleus neurons that was noted in their neuropathologic examinations.

Perez and Palmiter were the only other group to measure NE levels and they did not find a decrease in NE levels in the olfactory bulb or spinal cord of their *PARKIN* mutant mice. Given this discrepancy, quantification of NE levels in other *PARKIN*-deficient mice would be informative. Perez and Palmiter also measured striatal tissue levels of DA, DOPAC, HVA, NE, and 3-MT. No significant differences were detected between genotypes.

Electrophysiologic Deficits
Perhaps the most revealing data in terms of identifying the cellular function of *PARKIN* come from the analysis of the neuronal electrophysiology of mice lacking *PARKIN*. Two groups—Itier et al. and Goldberg et al.—have thus far examined *PARKIN*-deficient mice for electrophysiologic abnormalities. Itier et al. examined acute slices through the hippocampus of 64 to 68 weeks old *PARKIN*-deficient mice for electrophysiologic abnormalities and identified deficits in glutamatergic synaptic transmission. Specifically, the Schaeffer collateral-CA1 pathway

was examined for abnormalities in basal transmission, long-term potentiation (LTP), paired-pulse facilitation (PPF), and response to repetitive low-frequency stimulation.

Upon stimulation of the Schaeffer collateral-CA1 pathway, excitatory post-synaptic potentials (EPSPs) recorded from the extracellular field in slices from *PARKIN*-deficient mice showed similar shape but significantly smaller amplitude EPSPs compared to recordings in slices from wild type mice at the same stimulus intensities. The reduced EPSP amplitudes in *PARKIN* mutant mice could be due to alterations in presynaptic neurotransmitter release, postsynaptic events, or both. To examine presynaptic release, pairs of stimuli were applied in order to measure the well-known increase in EPSP amplitude in response to the second stimulation compared to the first pre pulse facilitation (PPF). A slight but statistically significant increase in PPF was observed in slices from *PARKIN*-deficient mice compared to slices from wild type mice. Itier et al. infered that this is due to decreased glutamate release because previous studies have indicated that decreased neurotransmitter release results in increased hippocampal PPF (27–29). This is consistent with the decreased EPSP amplitude in response to a single stimulus in the absence of *PARKIN*. In contrast, no deficits were observed in LTP, suggesting that postsynaptic events in this pathway are fully functional in the absence of *PARKIN*. Consistent with the increased PPF, the response to repetitive low-frequency stimulation was also significantly greater in slices from *PARKIN* mutant mice compared to wild type controls.

Goldberg et al. examined the synaptic responses of medium spiny neurons in the striatum of—six to nine months old mice by stimulation of corticostriatal afferents in acute coronal slices. Striatal medium spiny neurons are the primary targets of dopaminergic projections from the substantia nigra and receive glutamatergic input from the cortex. Upon stimulation of cortical afferents with a bipolar electrode placed in the corpus callosum, whole-cell recordings of medium spiny neurons showed that wild type and *PARKIN*-deficient neurons exhibited similar mean amplitudes and durations of evoked synaptic responses. However, significantly higher currents were needed to evoke the same response in *PARKIN*-deficient neurons relative to wild type neurons. This suggests that, in the absence of *PARKIN*, medium spiny neurons are less excitable synaptically. Consistent with this, the current required to evoke action potentials was also significantly greater in slices from *PARKIN*-deficient mice compared to wild types. This is also consistent with the increased extracellular striatal DA identified by in vivo microdialysis, which would be expected to decrease the excitability of striatal neurons. In contrast to the data reported by Itier et al. for the hippocampal Schaeffer collateral pathway, Goldberg et al. did not observed any alterations in PPF in the corticostriatal pathway. However, the decreased EPSP amplitude in response to a single stimulus observed by Itier et al. suggests that the hippocampal Schaeffer collateral pathway may also be less excitable synaptically in the absence of *PARKIN*.

Biochemical Studies

Although *PARKIN* is known to have E3 ubiquitin ligase activity, measurements of ubiquitin ligase activity were not reported for any of the *PARKIN*-deficient mice analyzed to date. This is in part due to the lack of a sufficiently sensitive or specific activity assay and further confounded by the large number of other E3 ubiquitin ligases in the brain. A number of proteins have been shown to be putative substrates of *PARKIN*'s E3 ligase activity, as these proteins can be ubiquitinated by *PARKIN* in vitro (4,6–11). However, Western analysis of proteins known to be substrates for *PARKIN*-mediated ubiquitinylation such as CDCrel-1, synphilin-1, and a glycosylated form of α-synuclein did not showed an accumulation of any of these proteins in the brains of *PARKIN*-deficient mice. This suggests that *PARKIN* is not critical for controlling the steady-state levels of these proteins under physiologic conditions, even though *PARKIN* may ubiquitinylate these proteins in vitro.

A few other biochemical abnormalities have also been reported in *PARKIN*-deficient mice. Itier et al. found reduced levels of DA transporter (DAT) and vesicular monoamine transporter (VMAT2) in the striatum of *PARKIN*-deficient mice compared to wild type mice based on Western analysis, although no difference was observed by immunohistochemical examination of DAT in 15 month-old mice. In vitro studies showed significantly decreased [^{3}H]-DA uptake in neuronal cultures from fetal midbrains of *PARKIN*-deficient mice, suggesting that DAT function is reduced as well as DAT protein levels. In vitro studies also showed a significant decrease in amphetamine-induced DA release. Levels of reduced glutathione were found to be increased selectively in the striatum of *PARKIN* mutant mice with no changes in the amount of oxidized glutathione. Interestingly, primary neuronal cultures derived from the ventral midbrain of embryonic *PARKIN*-deficient mice also showed increased levels of reduced glutathione compared to wild type cultures. This could be a compensatory or neuroprotective mechanism mitigating the effects of *PARKIN* deficiency. Goldberg et al. used radioligand binding assays to measure the maximal binding (Bmax) and dissociation constant (Kd) of D1- and D2-type dopamine receptors in homogenates of striatal tissue from wild type and *PARKIN*-deficient mice. No significant changes were found in DA receptor levels or binding affinities despite the alterations observed in extracellular striatal DA.

In an effort to identify the physiologic substrates of *PARKIN*'s E3 ligase activity, the same group used an unbiased proteomic approach to compare the relative abundance of the proteome in the ventral midbrain of *PARKIN*-deficient and control mice (30). Interestingly, rather than finding proteins that accumulate in the absence of *PARKIN*, which may be the physiologic substrates of *PARKIN*, the authors found 14 proteins that are decreased in the absence of *PARKIN*. Eight of the 14 proteins are involved in either mitochondrial respiration or antioxidant activities. Consistent with these results, *PARKIN*-deficient mice were found to have defects in mitochondrial respiration and age-dependent accumulation of markers of protein and lipid oxidation.

Mitochondrial Dysfunction

It has been proposed that mitochondrial dysfunction may play a key role in PD pathogenesis, based on postmortem studies showing mitochondrial impairment and oxidative damage in PD brains (31,32). This is further supported by observations that mitochondrial complex I inhibitors, such as MPTP, rotenone, and paraquat, can be used to produce a parkinsonian syndrome in experimental models and humans (33). The coexistence of mitochondrial dysfunction and nigral cell loss in these systems makes it difficult to establish whether mitochondrial dysfunction is causal or a secondary consequence of nigral degeneration. The fact that loss of *PARKIN* function in mice causes mitochondrial dysfunction and oxidative damage in the absence of neuronal degeneration seems to lend support for a causal role of mitochondrial dysfunction in nigral degeneration. How and whether *PARKIN* regulates mitochondrial function through its E3 ligase activity is less clear. None of the mitochondrial proteins was found to accumulate in the absence of *PARKIN*, suggesting that *PARKIN* does not regulate their abundance directly through its E3 ligase activity (13). In addition, none of the substrates identified for *PARKIN'S* E3 ligase activity has been implicated in mitochondrial function. However, it remains possible that physiologic substrates of *PARKIN'S* E3 ligase activity, which are yet to be identified, may be involved in the biogenesis of these mitochondrial proteins.

DJ-1

Before recessively inherited deletion and missense mutations in the *DJ-1* gene were linked to familial parkinsonism (PARK7) (2), *DJ-1* was identified independently as an oncogene (34), RNA binding protein (35), and contraception-associated protein (36,37). To understand how loss of *DJ-1* function can cause parkinsonian features, three laboratories have generated *DJ-1* null mice in an effort to elucidate the normal physiologic role of *DJ-1* at behavioral, cellular, and molecular levels and to reveal the consequences of its inactivation (38–40). Using a multidisciplinary approach, Goldberg et al. demonstrated that *DJ-1* plays essential roles in the dopaminergic system, especially in dopamine D2 receptor-mediated functions (38). The independent findings and the distinctions among the knockout mice generated by these three groups will be summarized and discussed.

GENERATION OF MUTANT MICE

Goldberg et al. (38) designed a targeting construct to replace exon 2 of the mouse *DJ-1* gene with a positive selection cassette encoding neomycin resistance [phosphoglycerate kinase neomycin (Pgk-*neo^r*)]. As exon 2 contains the ATG start codon for translation, removal of exon 2 would result in no protein translational initiation. If aberrant initiation of translation were to occur at one of the downstream in-frame ATGs in exons 3, 5, 6, or 7, radically truncated proteins would be produced. The embryonic stem cells (MKV6.5) targeted by Goldberg et al. were derived from C57BL/6;129 F1 hybrid mice and the studies were conducted on mice maintained on a C57BL/6;129/Sv hybrid genetic background. Western analysis using an antibody specific for the C-terminus of *DJ-1* verified the complete absence of *DJ-1* protein in the brains of homozygous mutant mice. Overloaded blots confirmed the absence of smaller *DJ-1* species indicating no aberrant internal initiation of translation at downstream ATGs. This targeted allele therefore represents a null mutation, which is a good model for human patients bearing loss of function mutations.

Kim et al. (39) designed a targeting construct to replace exons 3–5, with a neomycin selection cassette and to introduce a stop codon into the first coding exon (exon 2), resulting in the generation of a protein with only the first eight amino acid residues. Line E14K embryonic stem (ES) cells (derived from mouse strain 129/Ola) were transfected and successfully targeted. Chimeric mice were crossed with C57BL/6 mice to generate B6;129 hybrid F1 mice, which were backcrossed to C57BL/6 for seven generations. Northern analysis of RNA from embryonic fibroblasts confirmed the absence of *DJ-1* mRNA and Western analysis of protein from cortical neurons confirmed the absence of *DJ-1* protein in homozygous mutants.

Chen et al. (40) generated *DJ-1* mutant mice similarly by introducing a large deletion spanning exons 1–5. E14Tg2A.4 ES cells (derived from strain 129/Ola mice) were transfected with a targeting construct in which a 9.3 kb region encompassing mouse *DJ-1* exons 1–5 was replaced with a neomycin resistance cassette flanked by

FRT recombination sequences. Correctly targeted clones were injected into C57BL/6J blastocysts and chimeric mice were mated with C57BL/6J mice. Heterozygous mutants were intercrossed to yield B6;129 hybrid mice, which were used for analysis. RT-PCR and in situ hybridization were used to confirm the absence of *DJ-1* expression in homozygous mutants.

Neuropathologic Findings

Goldberg et al. used rigorous stereologic method to count the number of nigral TH-positive neurons at ages three and 12 months. At these ages, no decrease in the number of nigral neurons was observed in *DJ-1*-deficient mice compared to wild type mice. Careful examination of brains for inclusions immunoreactive for α-synuclein and ubiquitin, markers for LBs, showed no abnormalities in *DJ-1*-deficient mice.

Kim et al. assessed the number of TH immunoreactive or cresyl violet-stained neurons in the substantia nigra of 8 to 10 weeks old mice 14 days after treatment with MPTP or saline as a control. For the mice treated with saline, stereologic neuron counting revealed no decrease in the number of nigral neurons in *DJ-1*-deficient mice compared to wild type mice. In contrast, quantification of nigral neurons in mice treated with MPTP (30 mg/kg/day for five days) showed a significantly greater loss of these cells in *DJ-1* mutant mice compared to wild type mice. Nerve terminal projections from the substantia nigra to the dorsal striatum were examined by immunohistochemistry with antibodies to tyrosine hydroxylase (TH) and dopamine transporter (DAT) in coronal brain sections of the saline and MPTP-treated mice. Consistent with the significantly greater loss of nigral cell bodies, *DJ-1*-deficient mice treated with MPTP also had significantly greater loss of DAT and TH-positive nerve terminals in the striatum compared to MPTP treated wild type mice. This indicates that loss of *DJ-1* confers significantly increased sensitivity to MPTP toxicity in mice as assessed by nerve terminal density and by stereologic nigral neuron counts. Kim et al. further examined whether overexpression of *DJ-1* could protect wild type and *DJ-1*-deficient mice from MPTP-induced neurodegeneration. They engineered adenovirus vectors that expressed either wild type *DJ-1* or LacZ as a control in nigral neurons after injection into one hemisphere of the striatum. For both genotypes, the hemisphere overexpressing wild type *DJ-1* showed significantly less TH-positive neuronal cell loss upon MPTP treatment (seven days after adenoviral injections) compared to the uninjected hemisphere. In contrast the hemispheres overexpressing LacZ were not protected from MPTP-induced cell loss compared to uninjected hemispheres. No differences in TH-positive nigral neuron numbers were observed in virus-injected mice treated with saline instead of MPTP.

Chen et al. found no ubiquitin or α-synuclein immunoreactive or eosinophilic inclusions upon staining the brains of six-month and 11-month-old *DJ-1*-deficient mice, in contrast to what is observed in postmortem examinations of humans with PD. Immunohistochemical staining of sections through the substantia nigra of mice at these ages using antibodies specific for TH showed no decrease in the number of dopaminergic nigral neurons in the absence of *DJ-1* according to stereologic neuron counting.

Behavioral Deficits

Goldberg et al. assessed the locomotor abilities of *DJ-1*-deficient mice using several well-established behavioral tests. Observation of spontaneous movements during 15 minutes in an open field revealed a significant decrease in both horizontal and vertical (rearing) locomotor activity in *DJ-1*-deficient mice compared to wild type littermates at age three months (n = 18 per group). *DJ-1*-deficient mice were also less responsive to the locomotor behavioral effects of the D2 DA receptor agonist, quinpirole, compared to wild type mice. No deficits were observed in the ability of *DJ-1*-deficient mice to maintain their balance on a rotating rod (rotarod test) or to jump in response to loud acoustic stimuli (startle response test). Thus, forced movements seem to be relatively unaffected by the disruption of *DJ-1* function, while spontaneous, voluntary movements are significantly reduced.

Kim et al. examined open field locomotor behavior over a 24-hour period in the home cages of wild type and *DJ-1*-deficient mice at age eight weeks in a C57BL/6 genetic background and at age 13 months in a mixed background. In contrast to the significant decrease in locomotor activity in a novel environment reported in the other studies of *DJ-1*-deficient mice, Kim et al. found no significant differences in locomotor activity in the home cage environment averaged over 24 hours, although there was a strong trend toward decreased activity in the *DJ-1* mutant mice used in this study (6–10 animals per group). It is possible that this decrease in home cage locomotor activity would be statistically significant in a larger sample size, as was used for the novel environment locomotor activity measurements of Goldberg et al. (18 mice per group) and Chen et al. (12–16 mice per group). Kim et al. did not observe behavioral deficits in other tests conducted on aged *DJ-1*-deficient mice including the pole test, adhesive removal test, and novel environment test, although no details were provided regarding number of animals used. Because Kim et al. observed slightly lower basal activity of *DJ-1*-deficient mice, they sought to determine if this difference would be statistically significant if the dopaminergic system were challenged. Indeed, locomotor activity was statistically lower in *DJ-1* mutant mice compared to wild type mice when measured 14 days after treatment with MPTP (6–10 animals per group). Locomotor activity was also significantly lower in *DJ-1*-deficient mice compared to wild type mice following amphetamine challenge (2 mg/kg; four mice per group).

Chen et al. found age-dependent deficits in locomotor activity in *DJ-1* mutant mice. Motor function was assessed in the open field test in three different groups of mice at ages five, nine, and 11 months. Only the oldest group of *DJ-1*-deficient mice had a statistically significant reduction in open field path length and number of rearings. The younger groups showed slight reductions in path length and rearing activity compared to wild type mice, but the differences were not statistically significant in the groups tested (n = 15–16 per genotype). In the adhesive removal test, both groups of *DJ-1* mutants tested (ages five and 11 months) showed a significant reduction in the ability to sense and remove small adhesives taped to their heads. In contrast, neither of these age groups showed any decrease in the ability to remain on a rotating rod compared to wild type mice (the rotarod task).

Catecholamine Measurements

Goldberg et al. used HPLC with electrochemical detection to quantify the levels of DA in dissected striata. The total tissue content of DA in the dorsal striatum was similar in *DJ-1*-deficient mice compared to wild type mice, as were the levels of DOPAC and HVA. They further examined the rate of DA synthesis by injecting mice with the DOPA decarboxylase inhibitor NSD-1015 and measuring the accumulation of L-DOPA in the striatum. Similar levels were found in wild type and *DJ-1*-deficient mice, suggesting that DA synthesis rates are not altered in the absence of *DJ-1*. Goldberg et al. used carbon fiber electrode amperometry to measure evoked DA release in the dorsal striatum in acute slices from wild type and *DJ-1*-deficient mice. A significant decrease in evoked DA overflow was observed in the absence of *DJ-1*, which could be rescued by including the selective DA reuptake blocker, nomifensine, in the perfusion bath. This suggests increased reuptake of DA through DAT in the absence of *DJ-1*.

Kim et al. found no difference between genotypes in striatal tissue DA content, which was measured by HPLC with electrochemical detection. However, after treatment with MPTP, *DJ-1* mutant mice showed a greater reduction in striatal DA relative to wild type mice treated with MPTP, despite no difference in the amount of the toxic metabolite, MPP+, produced from MPTP.

Chen et al. used fast-scan cyclic voltammetry to measure DA release in the striatum and uptake kinetics of the DA transporter. In the dorsal striatum at four months of age, *DJ-1*-deficient mice showed increased stimulated DA release and faster DAT uptake kinetics compared to wild type mice. Interestingly, the same measurements in the ventral striatum and the nucleus acumbens showed no significant differences between genotypes. Given that the substantia nigra projects primarily to the dorsal striatum, this suggests defects specifically in the function of the nigrostriatal dopaminergic pathway in the absence of *DJ-1*. The faster DAT uptake kinetics are consistent with the results of Goldberg et al. showing reduced evoked DA release that could be rescued by blocking DAT. They also found that the total tissue content of DA in the striatum of six month and 11 month-old mice is greater in the striatum of *DJ-1*-deficient mice, in contrast to normal striatal DA levels found by the other two studies at either three or 13 months of age.

Electrophysiologic Deficits

Goldberg et al. examined the electrophysiologic responsiveness to DA in intracellular recordings of nigral neurons in acute midbrain slices from one month-old wild type and *DJ-1*-deficient mice. In *DJ-1* mutant mice, nigral neurons were observed to have a normal rhythmic firing of action potentials, indistinguishable from wild type. However, the well-established blockade of action potential firing by DA was significantly reduced in slices from *DJ-1*-deficient mice compared to wild type mice, suggesting reduced responsiveness to D2 autoreceptor activation in the absence of *DJ-1*. Similar results were obtained upon incubation of slices with the D2-specific DA receptor agonist quinpirole, further confirming that this phenotype is mediated through D2-type autoreceptors.

Because nigral cells project primarily to the striatum and modulate the activity of medium spiny neurons, Goldberg et al. also examined the electrophysiology of these cells in acute corticostriatal slices. Intracellular recordings of medium spiny neurons confirmed that the basic membrane properties were normal in *DJ-1* mutant mice. High-frequency stimulation of corticostriatal afferents produced the normal LTP of excitatory postsynaptic potentials in both genotypes. In contrast corticostriatal long-term depression (LTD) was absent in *DJ-1*-deficient striatal medium spiny neurons. Interestingly, LTD was restored in *DJ-1*-deficient slices upon application of the D2-like DA receptor agonist quinpirole. In contrast, the D1-specific agonist, SKF 38393, did not rescue the LTD deficits. Given that corticostriatal LTD is known to be dependent upon activation of both D1- and D2-type DA receptors, while corticostriatal LTP is known to be dependent upon activation of only D1-type DA receptors (41), the data from Goldberg et al. suggest a specific reduction in the responsiveness to activation of D2 receptors in the absence of *DJ-1* that can be compensated for by the agonist quinpirole.

Neither Chen et al. nor Kim et al. examined their *DJ-1*-deficient mice for electrophysiologic abnormalities.

Biochemical Studies

Goldberg et al. examined mRNA levels for TH, DAT, and the short and long isoforms of the D2 DA receptor (D2R) and found no changes in *DJ-1*-deficient mice. They further measured the maximal binding (Bmax) and dissociation constants (Kd) for DAT and D2R and found similar values in striatal membranes prepared from wild type and *DJ-1*-deficient mice.

Kim et al. examined whether *DJ-1* was involved in protecting cells against death induced by oxidative stress. Primary cortical neurons derived from wild type and *DJ-1*-deficient embryos were exposed to 30 μM hydrogen peroxide—one to two days after the initial plating. Homozygous mutant neurons showed a 20% increase in cell death compared to neurons cultured from wild type embryos. Heterozygous mutant neurons showed an intermediate increase in cell death suggesting that this increased susceptibility is dependent upon gene-dosage. Similar results were obtained upon exposing cultures to the mitochondrial inhibitor rotenone, which is known to increase reactive oxygen species. In contrast *DJ-1-/-*neurons were not more susceptible to nonoxidative stressors such as the topoisomerase I inhibitor camptothecin or the protein kinase inhibitor staurosporine.

Conversely, if wild type primary cortical cultures were transfected with adenoviral vectors expressing wild type *DJ-1* and GFP, these cells were significantly protected from cell death upon hydrogen peroxide exposure compared to the same cultures transfected with vectors expressing GFP alone or expressing the L166P mutant form of *DJ-1* linked to parkinsonism in humans (2). Similarly, cortical neuronal cultures derived from *DJ-1*-deficient embryos were significantly protected from hydrogen peroxide-induced cell death when they were transfected with wild type *DJ-1* and GFP but not GFP alone. The *DJ-1* expressing adenovirus was therefore able to partially rescue the hypersensitivity to hydrogen peroxide in neuronal cultures derived from *DJ-1*-deficient embryos. Together, this data suggest that overexpression of *DJ-1* can protect cells from oxidative stress while cells lacking *DJ-1* may be more sensitive to oxidative stress, as suggested by previous studies (42–46).

Chen et al. used a commercially available kit to measure protein carbonyl content in the brains of five- and 11-month-old *DJ-1* mutant mice as an indication of oxidative damage. No increase in carbonylated proteins was observed despite several publications suggesting a role for *DJ-1* in preventing oxidative damage or cell death (42–46). Western analysis showed normal levels of α-synuclein in the brains of five- and 11-month-old *DJ-1*-deficient mice compared to wild type controls. Surprisingly, western analysis also showed no changes in the protein levels of TH, DAT, or VMAT2 despite the significant increases in striatal DA, DA release, and DA uptake. Nevertheless, these results are consistent with the unchanged levels of TH and DAT mRNA and radioligand binding observed by Goldberg et al.

SUMMARY

Through the generation and analysis of *PARKIN*- and *DJ-1*-deficient mice, we have obtained a better understanding of how these proteins function in vivo, especially in the dopaminergic system, which is the most affected neural circuit in parkinsonian syndromes. For example, *PARKIN* appears to play an essential role in the maintenance of mitochondrial function and abundance of mitochondrial key components (30), even though the mechanistic link between its E3 ligase activity and mitochondrial proteins is still unclear. Furthermore, loss of *PARKIN* function also causes a number of behavioral deficits, including those that are indicative of function deficits in the nigrostriatal pathway (12–14). The detailed molecular and cellular mechanisms underlying these behavioral changes, however, are entirely unknown. Importantly, in the life span of mice, loss of *PARKIN* function is insufficient to cause significant loss of nigral dopaminergic neurons in all four independently generated *PARKIN*-null mice (12–15), though loss of Locus Coeruleus neurons was noted in one report (14). Neuropathologic analysis of *DJ-1*-null mice up to the age of 12 months similarly failed to detect a significant loss of dopaminergic neurons (38,39,40). Nevertheless, *DJ-1*-null mice exhibit a number of phenotypes indicative of dopaminergic dysfunction, such as decreased evoked dopamine overflow and increased dopamine reuptake, impaired D2 receptor-mediated functions in the nigral and striatal neurons, and reduced spontaneous activity, all of which are similarly exhibited by mice with one or no functional D2 receptor allele (38,40). However, how *DJ-1* regulates D2 receptor-mediated function is not yet known. Identification of the physiologic roles of these disease-linked gene products and elucidation of the cellular and molecular mechanisms by which these genes mediate their physiologic function will facilitate our understanding of the complex relationships between idiopathic PD and the recessive parkinsonian syndromes and eventually aid the development of novel therapeutic strategies combating the disease.

REFERENCES

1. Kitada T, Asakawa S, Hattori N, et al. Mutations in the PARKIN gene cause autosomal recessive juvenile parkinsonism. Nature 1998; 392(6676):605–608.
2. Bonifati V, Rizzu P, van Baren MJ, et al. Mutations in the DJ-1 gene associated with autosomal recessive early-onset parkinsonism. Science 2003; 299(5604):256–259.
3. Valente EM, Salvi S, Ialongo T, et al. PINK1 mutations are associated with sporadic early-onset parkinsonism. Ann Neurol 2004; 56(3):336–341.
4. Zhang Y, Gao J, Chung KK, et al. PARKIN functions as an E2-dependent ubiquitin-protein ligase and promotes the degradation of the synaptic vesicle-associated protein, CDCrel-1. Proc Natl Acad Sci USA 2000; 97(24):13354–13359.
5. Shimura H, Hattori N, Kubo S, et al. Familial parkinson disease gene product, parkin, is a ubiquitin-protein ligase. Nat Genet 2000; 25(3):302–305.
6. Staropoli JF, McDermott C, Martinat C, et al. PARKIN is a component of an SCF-like ubiquitin ligase complex and protects postmitotic neurons from kainate excitotoxicity. Neuron 2003; 37(5):735–749.
7. Imai Y, Soda M, Inoue H, et al. An unfolded putative transmembrane polypeptide, which can lead to endoplasmic reticulum stress, is a substrate of Parkin. Cell 2001; 105(7):891–902.
8. Shimura H, Schlossmacher MG, Hattori N, et al. Ubiquitination of a new form of alpha-synuclein by PARKIN from human brain: implications for Parkinson's disease. Science 2001; 293(5528):263–269.
9. Chung KK, Zhang Y, Lim KL, et al. PARKIN ubiquitinates the alpha-synuclein-interacting protein, synphilin-1: implications for Lewy-body formation in Parkinson disease. Nat Med 2001; 7(10):1144–1150.
10. Corti O, Hampe C, Koutnikova H, et al. The p38 subunit of the aminoacyl-tRNA synthetase complex is a PARKIN substrate: linking protein biosynthesis and neurodegeneration. Hum Mol Genet 2003; 12(12):1427–1437.
11. Ren Y, Zhao J, Feng J. PARKIN binds to alpha/beta tubulin and increases their ubiquitination and degradation. J Neurosci 2003; 23(8):3316–3324.

12. Itier JM, Ibanez P, Mena MA, et al. PARKIN gene inactivation alters behaviour and dopamine neurotransmission in the mouse. Hum Mol Genet 2003; 12(18):2277–2291.
13. Goldberg MS, Fleming SM, Palacino JJ, et al. Parkin-deficient mice exhibit nigrostriatal deficits but not loss of dopaminergic neurons. J Biol Chem 2003; 278(44):43628–43635.
14. Von Coelln R, Thomas B, Savitt JM, et al. Loss of locus coeruleus neurons and reduced startle in PARKIN null mice. Proc Natl Acad Sci USA 2004; 101(29):10744–10749.
15. Perez FA, Palmiter RD. Parkin-deficient mice are not a robust model of parkinsonism. Proc Natl Acad Sci USA 2005; 102(6):2174–2179.
16. Rankin CA, Joazeiro CA, Floor E, et al. E3 ubiquitin-protein ligase activity of PARKIN is dependent on cooperative interaction of RING finger (TRIAD) elements. J Biomed Sci 2001; 8(5):421–429.
17. Pawlyk AC, Giasson BI, Sampathu DM, et al. Novel monoclonal antibodies demonstrate biochemical variation of brain PARKIN with age. J Biol Chem 2003; 278(48):48120–48128.
18. Hayashi S, Wakabayashi K, Ishikawa A, et al. An autopsy case of autosomal-recessive juvenile parkinsonism with a homozygous exon 4 deletion in the PARKIN gene. Mov Disord 2000; 15(5):884–888.
19. Yamamura Y, Hattori N, Matsumine H, et al. Autosomal recessive early-onset parkinsonism with diurnal fluctuation: clinicopathologic characteristics and molecular genetic identification. Brain Dev 2000; 22(suppl 1):S87–S91.
20. Gouider-Khouja N, Larnaout A, Amouri R, et al. Autosomal recessive parkinsonism linked to PARKIN gene in a Tunisian family. Clinical, genetic and pathological study. Parkinsonism Relat Disord 2003; 9(5):247–251.
21. Garcia-Hernandez F, Pacheco-Cano MT, Drucker-Colin R. Reduction of motor impairment by adrenal medulla transplants in aged rats. Physiol Behav 1993; 54(3):589–598.
22. Dluzen DE, Gao X, Story GM, et al. Evaluation of nigrostriatal dopaminergic function in adult +/+ and +/- BDNF mutant mice. Exp Neurol 2001; 170(1):121–128.
23. Drucker-Colin R, Garcia-Hernandez F. A new motor test sensitive to aging and dopaminergic function. J Neurosci Methods 1991; 39(2):153–161.
24. Schallert T, Upchurch M, Lobaugh N, et al. Tactile extinction: distinguishing between sensorimotor and motor asymmetries in rats with unilateral nigrostriatal damage. Pharmacol Biochem Behav 1982; 16(3):455–462.
25. Schallert T, Upchurch M, Wilcox RE, et al. Posture-independent sensorimotor analysis of inter-hemispheric receptor asymmetries in neostriatum. Pharmacol Biochem Behav 1983; 18(5):753–759.
26. Schallert T, Fleming SM, Leasure JL, et al. CNS plasticity and assessment of forelimb sensorimotor outcome in unilateral rat models of stroke, cortical ablation, parkinsonism and spinal cord injury. Neuropharmacology 2000; 39(5):777–787.
27. Zucker RS. Short-term synaptic plasticity. Annu Rev Neurosci 1989; 12:13–31.
28. Creager R, Dunwiddie T, Lynch G. Paired-pulse and frequency facilitation in the CA1 region of the in vitro rat hippocampus. J Physiol 1980; 299:409–424.
29. Dunwiddie TV, Haas HL. Adenosine increases synaptic facilitation in the in vitro rat hippocampus: evidence for a presynaptic site of action. J Physiol 1985; 369:365–377.
30. Palacino JJ, Sagi D, Goldberg MS, et al. Mitochondrial dysfunction and oxidative damage in parkin-deficient mice. J Biol Chem 2004; 279(18):18614–18622.
31. Beal MF. Mitochondria, oxidative damage, and inflammation in Parkinson's disease. Ann N Y Acad Sci 2003; 991:120–131.
32. Jenner P. Oxidative mechanisms in nigral cell death in Parkinson's disease. Mov Disord 1998; 13(suppl 1):24–34.
33. Dauer W, Przedborski S. Parkinson's disease: mechanisms and models. Neuron 2003; 39(6):889–909.
34. Nagakubo D, Taira T, Kitaura H, et al. DJ-1, a novel oncogene which transforms mouse NIH3T3 cells in cooperation with ras. Biochem Biophys Res Commun 1997; 231(2):509–513.
35. Hod Y, Pentyala SN, Whyard TC, et al. Identification and characterization of a novel protein that regulates RNA-protein interaction. J Cell Biochem 1999; 72(3):435–444.
36. Wagenfeld A, Gromoll J, Cooper TG. Molecular cloning and expression of rat contraception associated protein 1 (CAP1), a protein putatively involved in fertilization. Biochem Biophys Res Commun 1998; 251(2):545–549.

37. Welch JE, Barbee RR, Roberts NL, et al. SP22: a novel fertility protein from a highly conserved gene family. J Androl 1998; 19(4):385–393.
38. Goldberg MS, Pisani A, Haburcak M, et al. Nigrostriatal dopaminergic deficits and hypo-kinesia caused by inactivation of the familial parkinsonism-linked gene DJ-1. Neuron 2005; 45(4):489–496.
39. Kim RH, Smith PD, Aleyasin H, et al. Hypersensitivity of DJ-1-deficient mice to 1-methyl-4-phenyl-1,2,3,6-tetrahydropyrindine (MPTP) and oxidative stress. Proc Natl Acad Sci USA 2005; 102(14):5215–5220.
40. Chen L, Cagniard B, Mathews T, et al. Age-dependent motor deficits and dopaminergic dysfunction in DJ-1 null mice. J Biol Chem 2005; 280(22):21418–21426.
41. Calabresi P, Pisani A, Mercuri NB, et al. The corticostriatal projection: from synaptic plasticity to dysfunctions of the basal ganglia. Trends Neurosci 1996; 19(1):19–24.
42. Martinat C, Shendelman S, Jonason A, et al. Sensitivity to oxidative stress in DJ-1-deficient dopamine neurons: an ES- derived cell model of primary parkinsonism. PLoS Biol 2004; 2(11):e327.
43. Takahashi-Niki K, Niki T, Taira T, et al. Reduced anti-oxidative stress activities of DJ-1 mutants found in Parkinson's disease patients. Biochem Biophys Res Commun 2004; 320(2):389–397.
44. Canet-Aviles RM, Wilson MA, Miller DW, et al. The Parkinson's disease protein DJ-1 is neuroprotective due to cysteine-sulfinic acid-driven mitochondrial localization. Proc Natl Acad Sci USA 2004; 101(24):9103–9108.
45. Taira T, Saito Y, Niki T, et al. DJ-1 has a role in antioxidative stress to prevent cell death. EMBO Rep 2004; 5(4):430.
46. Yokota T, Sugawara K, Ito K, et al. Down regulation of DJ-1 enhances cell death by oxidative stress, ER stress, and proteasome inhibition. Biochem Biophys Res Commun 2003; 312(4):1342–1348.

19 Drosophila Models of Parkinson's Disease

Leo J. Pallanck
Department of Genome Sciences, University of Washington, Seattle, Washington, U.S.A.

Alexander J. Whitworth
Department of Biomedical Sciences, University of Sheffield, Sheffield, U.K.

INTRODUCTION

Parkinson's disease (PD) remains a major challenge of modern medicine. Although PD is common and highly debilitating, the molecular mechanisms responsible for PD pathogenesis are poorly understood, and there are currently no effective preventative treatments for this disorder. Recently, linkage studies have begun to identify single-gene mutations responsible for rare, heritable forms of PD. While the identification of these genes has tremendous potential to provide insight into the mechanisms of PD and the interplay of genetics and environment in this disorder, we currently know very little about the biologic functions of the genes thus far identified and how their mutational alteration results in neuronal death. One promising approach to this problem involves the use of classical genetic analysis in the fruit fly *Drosophila melanogaster* to identify the genetic pathways leading to pathology in fly models of this disease. This review will describe the features that make Drosophila useful in studies of the genes implicated in heritable forms of PD, and how these studies have begun to contribute to our understanding of the pathogenesis of this disorder and the identification of potential treatment strategies for PD.

For nearly a century, studies of Drosophila genetic and molecular pathways have provided pivotal advances in our understanding of fundamental biological processes, such as chromosome structure and segregation, regulation of gene expression, and mechanisms of development (1). These studies, together with more recent genome sequencing efforts, have made it clear that gene sequence and gene function are highly conserved between flies and humans (2). This conservation has contributed enormously to our current understanding of human biology and the pathogenesis of particular human diseases. For example, the Drosophila counterparts to a number of tumor suppressor and proto-oncogenes (e.g., *wingless*, *Notch*, and *patched*) have provided a wealth of understanding about the pathways involved in cancer. While much of the insight into human disease mechanisms derived from genetic studies of Drosophila has been a byproduct of investigations of more fundamental biological questions, the increasing appreciation of the usefulness of Drosophila to address questions of human pathogenesis has led more recently to overt efforts to model specific human diseases. In particular, over the past seven years, significant effort has been invested in the development of Drosophila models of neurological diseases, such as polyglutamine diseases, Alzheimer's disease and PD (3). The extensive degree of conservation of neuronal function and development at the cellular level between Drosophila and higher vertebrates, coupled with the paucity of treatments for many neurological diseases, makes Drosophila an ideal system for advancement

TABLE 1   Putative Function of Human Genes Linked to Parkinson's Disease and Their Fly Homologs

PD locus	Gene/protein	Mode of inheritance	Fly homolog CG#	Fly homolog(s) identity, similarity	Putative function
PARK1 PARK4	SNCA/ α-synuclein	AD	No homolog	No homolog	Synaptic plasticity
PARK	UCH-L1	AD	Uch/CG4265	45%, 66%	Ubiquitin hydrolase/ ligase
PARK2	PARKIN	AR	PARKIN/CG10523	42%, 59%	E3 ubiquitin-protein ligase
PARK7	DJ-1	AR	DJ–1a/CG6646 DJ–1b/CG1349	56%, 70% and 52%, 69%	Oxidative stress sensor
PARK6	PINK1	AR	CG4523	32%, 50%	Mitochondrial kinase
PARK8	Dardarin/LRRK2	AD	CG5483	26%, 43%	Kinase

Abbreviations: AD, autosomal dominant; AR, autosomal recessive.

of our understanding of neurological disease mechanisms. Such advancement may ultimately yield preventative treatments for these disorders.

The completion and annotation of the genome sequence of *Drosophila melanogaster* (4) and the availability of internet accessible homology search algorithms make the identification of candidate Drosophila disease homologs relatively trivial. Use of these search algorithms indicates that the Drosophila genome encodes excellent homologs of five of the six currently identified PD-related genes (Table 1). In particular, the Drosophila genome encodes excellent homologs of the *Dardarin/ LRRK2, DJ-1, PARKIN, PINK1,* and *UCH-L1* genes (Table 1). There appears to be only a single Drosophila homolog of the *Dardarin/LRRK2, PARKIN, PINK1,* and *UCH-L1* genes, but there are two closely related *DJ-1* homologs in Drosophila. Only the human α*-synuclein* gene appears to lack a clear Drosophila counterpart. However, the dominant, toxic gain-of-function mechanism by which α-synuclein is thought to act in dopamine neuron death validates the use of a transgenic approach using the human α*-synuclein* gene to study α-synuclein pathogenesis in Drosophila (see below). The existence of Drosophila homologs of five of the six genes implicated in heritable forms of PD implies that the pathways regulated by these genes are also likely to be conserved in Drosophila.

TECHNIQUES AVAILABLE IN DROSOPHILA

Both mutational and transgenic approaches have been used to create and study Drosophila models of neurological disease. The mutational approach involves the generation of mutations in Drosophila counterparts of human disease genes, whereas the transgenic approach involves the introduction and expression of a human disease gene in Drosophila. The former approach is typically used when the corresponding human disease results from a loss-of-function mutation in a particular gene, whereas the latter approach is often used when the corresponding human disease appears to result from a dominant gain-of-function mechanism. In this section, we describe the methodology involved in the mutational and transgenic approaches.

Mutagenesis

There are a number of different techniques that can be employed to generate mutations in a particular Drosophila gene of interest. Many of the classical methods for recovering mutations in defined genes in Drosophila require a predictable phenotype that can be readily identified. However, there are now a number of methods available that allow the recovery of mutations in defined genes irrespective of the mutant phenotype. One particularly powerful approach involves the use of transposable elements. A number of specifically engineered transposons have been designed that can be used for insertional mutagenesis in Drosophila. These transposons are being utilized by the Berkeley Drosophila Genome Project in an effort to generate mutations in most *Drosophila* genes as a service to the Drosophila research community. Primarily as a result of these efforts it is currently estimated that >50% of the predicted *Drosophila* genes have associated transposon insertions (5). For those *Drosophila* genes that do not currently have associated transposon alleles, several methods can be used to selectively recover such alleles following mobilization of a transposon. One method involves using plasmid rescue in *E. coli* of genomic sequences flanking *P* element transposon insertions and testing these sequences for hybridization to a cDNA corresponding to the desired target gene (6). A second method selectively identifies desired *P* element insertions by using PCR primers specific to sequences within the *P* element and target gene (7). Only DNA from flies containing a *P* element insert in or near the gene of interest will be amplified. In this way, hundreds of flies bearing different inserts can be simultaneously screened to identify the rare individual with an appropriate insertion. Although frequencies of *P* element mutagenesis are somewhat locus dependent (8), recent estimates provided by the Berkeley Drosophila Genome Project indicate that the vast majority of genes in Drosophila can serve as targets for *P* element mutagenesis (9), and there are now a large number of examples of the successful use of transposon mutagenesis to selectively inactivate particular genes.

A more recently developed method to target genes for mutagenesis in Drosophila involves a homologous recombination methodology similar to that used in making mouse knockouts (10,11). Briefly, this method requires the generation of a targeting construct bearing an inactivating mutation in the gene of interest and a site for the rare cutting endonuclease *I-CreI* flanked by target sites for the yeast flp recombinase. Coexpression of *I-CreI* and flp recombinase in transgenic flies bearing the engineered targeting construct results in excision of the targeting construct as a linear extrachromosomal fragment which then recombines with the homologous chromosomal locus, possibly through a double strand break repair mechanism. A more recent iteration of gene-targeting, designated ends-out targeting (10), significantly simplifies the molecular engineering required to produce the targeting construct and should therefore make this methodology more attractive to Drosophila researchers.

Another approach that is being used with increasing frequency in place of traditional genetic analysis in Drosophila is RNA interference (RNAi) (13,14). This approach capitalizes on the finding that double-stranded RNA (dsRNA) molecules corresponding in sequence to endogenous transcripts can trigger the degradation of the endogenous transcript. This approach requires the construction of a transgenic construct bearing an inverted repeat sequence corresponding to the target transcript. Through the use of the GAL4 system (see below), targeted expression of the dsRNA in any desired tissue can be achieved simply by conducting the appropriate cross. One of the reasons this approach has become popular is the speed with which a transgenic line bearing an RNAi construct can be created relative to more traditional genetic approaches. However, it is clear from the many studies involving RNAi approaches that this method effects only partial gene inactivation. Thus, a phenotype resulting from RNAi is typically equivalent to a hypomorphic loss of function mutation [e.g., compare (15) and (16)]. This feature of RNAi can be an advantage or a limitation depending on the context of the experiment and the goals of the experimenter. Another potential concern with RNAi technology is the increasing evidence that RNAi can sometimes affect the abundance of unintended mRNA targets (17). Because it can be difficult to control for such "off-target" effects of RNAi the phenotypes resulting from RNAi must be interpreted with caution until a comparison with a traditional mutant allele can be made.

Transgenic Misexpression

One of the most powerful and versatile tools available in Drosophila is the ability to generate transgenic constructs that can be used to drive the expression of a chosen gene in a tissue specific manner by exploiting a yeast transcriptional activation mechanism. The GAL4/UAS system uses the yeast transcriptional activator protein, GAL4 expressed under the temporal and spatial control of endogenous Drosophila enhancer/promoter elements, to drive the expression of a specific GAL4-responsive transgene (18). The transgene is cloned in a vector containing a minimal promoter coupled with upstream activator sequences (UAS) that are specifically recognized by the GAL4 transcription factor. Upon binding of GAL4 to the UAS sites, expression of the transgene is induced in a tissue specific manner dependent on the endogenous enhancer/promoter elements controlling GAL4 expression. There are now many different GAL4 lines available that drive expression in a wide variety of tissues (e.g., nervous system, muscle tissue, ubiquitously, etc.). This technique has been used with great effect to determine the in vivo consequence of misexpression or overexpression of fly genes and has been adapted to study the ectopic expression of human genes and their disease causing aberrant forms.

Genetic Screening

Probably the single greatest advantage of using Drosophila to model human disease is the ability to conduct relatively unbiased genetic screens for mutations in other genes that suppress or enhance the phenotypes associated with the disease model. This approach has the potential to identify cellular factors that act in the same or parallel pathways to the disease gene and does not require any a priori knowledge of the function of the disease gene. The power of such screening approaches cannot be overstated; human counterparts corresponding to suppressors identified from screens using Drosophila define potential targets for therapeutic intervention. It is primarily the feasibility of conducting such high-throughput screens that sets Drosophila apart from vertebrate models of disease.

There are a large number of approaches available for conducting genetic modifier screens in Drosophila. One of the most commonly used approaches involves crossing a collection of 2,400 enhancer P (EP) element insertions (19) into a disease model background and investigating the effects of these insertions on the disease model phenotypes. The EP transposons have been engineered to drive overexpression of sequences flanking the transposon in a GAL4-dependent fashion. Thus, when used in conjunction with a particular GAL4 line, these transposons might suppress or enhance the disease model phenotype as a result of insertional inactivation of the genes they reside in or as a result of overexpression of flanking genes. These potential effects can be easily distinguished in subsequent studies. This modifier screening approach is compatible with a variety of phenotypes and could be used to identify modifiers of behavioral, morphological, or recessive lethal phenotypes. A particularly useful attribute of this screening method is that the insertion location of all of the EP lines has been determined and thus modifier genes are readily identified. Use of the *EP* collection in a modifier screening context has proven extremely valuable in studies to identify modifiers of polyglutamine, PD, and tau pathology in Drosophila (20–22).

Finally, a number of Drosophila cell lines are potentially available for cell biological studies of neurodegeneration. While there are also many vertebrate cell lines available for analysis, an advantage of many Drosophila cell lines is that they are highly amenable to RNAi manipulation. Highly efficient target transcript degradation can be achieved with many Drosophila cell lines by simply adding microgram quantities of dsRNA molecules ranging from 150 to 3000 bp directly to cell culture media (23–25). RNAi could potentially be used to create a Drosophila cell culture model of neurodegeneration, or to conduct a whole genome screen for dsRNA molecules that modify a cell culture phenotype. An RNAi screening center consisting of all of the necessary resources for conducting genome-wide screens in Drosophila cell lines was recently established at Harvard and is currently available for such screens (26).

THE NEUROANATOMY AND FUNCTION OF DOPAMINE NEURONS IN DROSOPHILA

Drosophila has a complex nervous system consisting of approximately 100,000 neurons including a subset of ~200 neurons that secrete the neurotransmitter dopamine (Fig. 1). The anatomical locations of all of the Drosophila dopamine producing neurons have been identified, and their development has been traced throughout the life cycle. Thus, genetic perturbations affecting the quantity, morphology, or locations of dopamine neurons in Drosophila can be readily identified. Although the anatomy of the fly brain and the distribution of dopamine neurons in the Drosophila central nervous system (CNS) differ from the vertebrate brain, previous work indicates that many fundamental cellular and molecular biological features of neuronal development and function are conserved between vertebrates and invertebrates (1). Recent work indicates that this conservation makes Drosophila a powerful system for cell biological studies of neuronal dysfunction.

During embryonic and larval brain development, dopamine is found to be expressed in approximately 80 cells in the CNS. Many of these cells are grouped together into three bilaterally symmetrical clusters in the two lobes of the brain, with the remaining dopamine neurons distributed singly along the length of the ventral ganglion. These dopamine neurons are retained in the CNS of adult flies and are primarily grouped together into six major clusters. These six clusters are arranged symmetrically about the midline with the neuronal cell bodies residing at the periphery of the brain and their axons projecting toward the center (Fig. 1). There are four additional clusters of dopamine neurons on the posterior side of the brain: two medial clusters, designated the protocerebral posterior medial (PPM) 2 and 3, and two lateral clusters, named the protocerebral posterior lateral (PPL) 1 and 2. The PPM2/3 and PPL2 clusters typically have five to eight neurons while the PPL1 cluster contains approximately 12 neurons (Fig. 1B). On the anterior side of the brain, there is a small cluster of approximately five dopamine neurons, designated the protocerebral anterior lateral (PAL), and a larger cluster

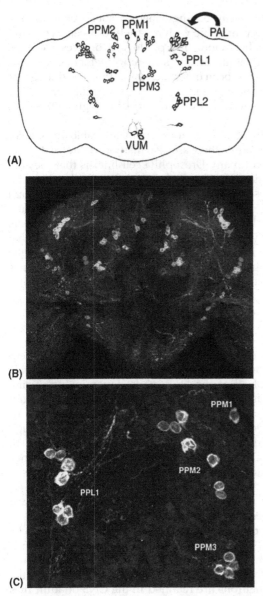

(A)

(B)

(C)

FIGURE 1 **(A)** Schematic representation of the distribution of dopaminergic neurons in the *Drosophila* adult brain. Dopaminergic neurons are grouped in small clusters arranged with bilateral symmetry. **(B)** Use of confocal microscopy to detect dopaminergic neurons in the adult drosophila brain. Expression of a GFP reporter (green) is induced by the endogenous tyrosine hydroxylase promoter and counter-stained with antityrosine hydroxylase antiserum (red) demonstrating significant but not complete overlap. Only neurons on the posterior side are shown in this view. **(C)** Detail of a projected Z-series of posterior clusters. Axons are revealed as punctate staining with antityrosine hydroxylase antiserum. *Abbreviations*: PAL, protocerebral anterior lateral; PPL, protocerebral posterior lateral; PPM, protocerebral posterior medial; VUM, ventral unpaired medial, GFP, green fluorescent protein.

of approximately 60 dopamine neurons with characteristically small cell bodies, designated the protocerebral anterior medial (PAM). In addition to these clusters, there are also a small number of dopamine neurons that are separate from the clusters, such as the PPM1, the deutocerebral 1 (D1), and the ventral unpaired medial (VUM) neurons.

To date, most studies of dopamine neuron integrity in Drosophila models of PD have used antisera against tyrosine hydroxylase (TH), an enzyme required for dopamine biosynthesis, to image dopamine neurons. However, several different immunocytochemical methods have been utilized to conduct these imaging studies. Most of the studies conducted to date have used thick sections of paraffin-embedded central nervous system (CNS) samples in conjunction with light microscopy to analyze dopamine neuron integrity. More recently, confocal microscopy of whole mount brain samples has been applied to image the CNS dopamine neurons. Although both of these methods are in routine use, recent work indicates that the confocal microscopic imaging approach is more sensitive in detecting dopamine neurons than the methodology employing paraffin sections and light microscopy (see below) thus confocal microscopy is emerging as the technique of choice. Another potential advantage of confocal microscopy relative to the methodology employing paraffin sections is that this technique allows a better visualization of the three-dimensional arrangement of the neurons within the intact brain. Thus, this methodology might facilitate studies of more subtle aspects of dopamine neuron dysfunction, such as axonal projection and synaptic defects (Fig. 1C).

In addition to the spatial distribution of dopamine neurons in Drosophila, the functional effects of dopamine depletion and dopamine neuron perturbation have also been studied. Genetic or pharmacologic depletion of dopamine in Drosophila results in a variety of characteristic phenotypes. Mutations affecting the *Dopa decarboxylase* gene result in decreased learning ability, while mutations in the TH encoding gene *pale* cause a dose-dependent loss of general locomotor ability (27,28). The systemic administration of chemical inhibitors of TH synthesis, such as 3-iodo-tyrosine, resulted in developmental delay, decreased fertility, and inhibition of a simple learning paradigm (29,30). However, it is unclear from these studies whether these phenotypes result from loss of dopamine signaling in the nervous system or from a non-neuronal requirement for dopamine. The Drosophila *pale* gene encodes two alternatively spliced isoforms of TH; one isoform is neuronally expressed while the other is expressed in the developing mesoderm and required for cuticle hardening and pigmentation (31,32).

Several recent studies have utilized the GAL4/UAS system to address the behavioral effects of perturbation of dopamine neuron signaling in the Drosophila nervous system. In one report, investigators expressed tetanus toxin in TH-expressing neurons to block dopamine neuron signaling (33). Tetanus toxin cleaves the synaptic vesicle protein synaptobrevin, and this cleavage has been previously shown to block evoked neurotransmitter release in Drosophila (34). Flies expressing tetanus toxin in TH-positive neurons are viable, display normal locomotion, and have a wild type appearance (33). However, these flies exhibit a hyperexcitable response to a startle stimulus. Vigorous tapping of vials containing flies expressing tetanus toxin in dopamine neurons causes the flies to fall and whirl erratically, failing to immediately right themselves. Another study in Drosophila made use of a transgene encoding an adenosine triphosphate (ATP)-gated calcium channel in conjunction with a photo-labile caged version of ATP to depolarize and thereby activate neuron signaling (35). Expression of this transgene in dopamine neurons followed by photostimulation of the caged ATP produced differing effects dependent on the locomotor state of the flies preceding photostimulation. One population of flies with low locomotor activity prior to photostimulation exhibited an increased frequency of locomotion and an alteration in the routes traversed following photostimulation. Photostimulation of a second population of flies with high locomotor activity prior to photostimulation was found to result in a transient locomotor arrest. Together, these results demonstrate that a function of dopamine signaling in the Drosophila nervous system is to regulate locomotor behavior.

THE α-SYNUCLEIN TRANSGENIC DROSOPHILA MODEL OF PARKINSON'S DISEASE
Generation and Characterization
The first gene shown to be associated with a heritable form of PD, α-synuclein, was also the first of the PD-related genes to be studied in Drosophila. Although mutations of the α-synuclein gene appear to be an extremely rare cause of PD, the finding that α-synuclein is a component of the Lewy body protein inclusions observed in patients with the sporadic form of the disease implies that this factor is a causative agent in most forms of PD (36,37). Thus, insight gleaned from studies aimed at the mechanism by which α-synuclein induces neuronal loss could lead to the development of treatment strategies impacting most cases of PD.

While most of the human genes that have been implicated in PD have Drosophila counterparts (Table 1), there appears to be no Drosophila ortholog of the α-synuclein gene. However, because both missense mutations and increased dosage of the α-synuclein gene confer dominant forms of parkinsonism (38,39), Feany and Bender (40) generated transgenic flies bearing the human α-synuclein gene with the rationale that aberrantly high levels of α-synuclein protein are toxic to dopamine neurons. α-synuclein transgenic constructs containing either the wild type sequence or the A30P and A53T familial mutations were placed under the transcriptional control of a GAL4–responsive UAS element. These lines were crossed to existing transgenic fly lines that express the GAL4 transcription factor in the nervous system to induce expression of α-synuclein in the fly brain. Antiserum against TH was used to stain thick sections of paraffin imbedded fly heads from α-synuclein expressing flies to assess the effects of α-synuclein expression on dopamine neuron integrity. Remarkably, this analysis revealed progressive loss of TH-staining restricted primarily to the PPM1/2 cluster of dopamine neurons (also called the dorsomedial cluster). Similar results were obtained from the expression of wild type (WT) α-synuclein and the A30P and A53T mutationally altered forms of α-synuclein.

To investigate whether the loss of TH-staining represents loss of dopamine neurons and not simply loss of TH expression, additional experiments were carried out with transgenic lines coexpressing α-synuclein and β-galactosidase. Results of these experiments revealed that β-galactosidase and α-synuclein staining was also absent in a subset of dopamine neurons from aged flies relative to controls, leading the authors to conclude that α-synuclein expression induces the death of a subset of dopamine neurons in the CNS (41). The number of serotonergic neurons and gross brain morphology in α-synuclein expressing flies were reportedly unaffected, indicating that the toxic effects of α-synuclein expression are relatively specific to dopamine neurons in the CNS. However, expression of α-synuclein in the Drosophila compound eye was found to induce a retinal degeneration phenotype, demonstrating that α-synuclein toxicity is not entirely restricted to dopamine neurons (41).

Pan-neuronal expression of α-synuclein in the Drosophila CNS was also found to result in the appearance of neuronal protein aggregates crudely resembling the Lewy bodies seen in postmortem tissue from idiopathic PD patients, and an accompanying locomotor defect (41). While young α-synuclein expressing flies displayed a normal geotactic response, quickly climbing to the top of a vial after being tapped down, climbing ability attenuated significantly in older α-synuclein expressing flies. Climbing ability also decayed in aged wild type flies, but the rate of decay was found to be significantly accelerated in all of the α-synuclein-expressing flies tested. The appearance of this motor defect paralleled the loss of dopamine neurons and the onset of aggregate formation, suggesting a mechanistic connection among aggregate formation, neuron loss, and motor dysfunction. This initial work provided the foundation for subsequent studies of α-synuclein pathogenesis in Drosophila.

Applications of the Drosophila α-Synuclein Model

The coincidence of neuronal loss and the formation of α-synuclein positive aggregates in α-synuclein-expressing flies prompted several studies of the possible involvement of aggregate formation in dopamine neuron loss. The first study in Drosophila to investigate this matter demonstrated that overexpression of the chaperone, HSP70, abrogated the α-synuclein-induced loss of TH-positive neurons without detectably influencing the appearance of Lewy body-like aggregates (42). Furthermore, feeding α-synuclein transgenic flies the chaperone inducing compound geldanamycin was found to phenocopy, the protective effect of HSP70 expression (43). Consistent with these findings, coexpression of a dominant-negative form of HSP70 was found to enhance the loss of TH-staining resulting from α-synuclein expression (42). Interestingly, expression of this dominant-negative form of HSP70 in flies completely lacking α-synuclein expression was also found to induce dopamine neuron loss. Together, these findings demonstrated that the formation of large α-synuclein-containing aggregates is not sufficient for neuronal loss and that HSP70 induction is protective from the harmful effects of α-synuclein.

These results suggest several possible models by which HSP70 exerts its protective effect. First, the finding that HSP70 overexpression suppresses α-synuclein toxicity without detectably influencing aggregate formation raises the possibility that soluble monomeric or oligomeric forms of α-synuclein rather than large aggregates are the true toxic entities and that HSP70 acts to prevent these species from assuming a toxic conformation. An alternative model, consistent with the effect of reduced HSP70 activity on dopamine neuron integrity in the complete absence of α-synuclein is that α-synuclein toxicity ensues from titration of HSP70 into an inactive form, possibly by sequestration into inclusions. Consistent with this model, the authors of this study also showed that Lewy bodies from human postmortem tissue stain positively for the presence of molecular chaperones (44). Finally, these findings are also consistent with a general effect of HSP70 on dopamine neuron viability that is independent of any interaction between HSP70 and α-synuclein. Regardless of the mechanism by which HSP70 acts to suppress α-synuclein toxicity, the finding that feeding flies geldanamycin is able to suppress the loss of TH positive cells suggests a possible treatment strategy for PD.

In another study to explore the relationship of α-synuclein aggregate formation to dopamine neuron loss, investigators analyzed the effects of post-translational modifications of α-synuclein on aggregate formation and neuronal viability. Previous work showed that α-synuclein is extensively phosphorylated in the brains of PD individuals, particularly at serine residue 129, and that the phosphorylation status of α-synuclein influences its propensity to form aggregates in vitro (45,46). Interestingly, the phosphorylation of α-synuclein at Ser129 appears to be conserved in Drosophila (47). To explore the consequence of Ser129 phosphorylation on aggregate formation and neuronal integrity Chen and Feany (48) generated mutationally altered α-synuclein transgenic constructs consisting of a Ser129 to Ala (S129A) mutation to prevent phosphorylation and a Ser129 to Asp (S129D) mutation to mimic the phosphorylated state. They expressed these transgenic constructs in the Drosophila nervous system and compared the extent and timing of pathology in these lines to flies expressing WT α-synuclein. In agreement with previous work, WT α-synuclein protein was found to be phosphorylated at Ser129, whereas the mutationally altered α-synuclein proteins lacked this modification. Further studies demonstrated that expression of the S129D construct accelerated the onset of loss of TH-positive neurons, increased retinal degeneration, and reduced the amount of α-synuclein in aggregates relative to WT α-synuclein. In contrast, expression of the S129A construct resulted in reduced loss of TH-positive neurons and increased the total load of aggregated α-synuclein protein relative to WT α-synuclein. These results suggest that phosphorylation of Ser129 maintains α-synuclein in a nonaggregated but more toxic conformation. Furthermore, these findings suggest that an increase in α-synuclein aggregates correlate with decreased cellular toxicity, implying that Lewy body formation is a neuronal detoxification response.

The studies of Chen and Feany have several potential therapeutic implications. First, the evidence that inclusion formation is protective challenges current therapeutic strategies for preventing inclusion formation. Second, the finding that phosphorylation enhances α-synuclein toxicity suggests that the kinases responsible for phosphorylation might represent therapeutic targets for small-molecule inhibitors. However, a number of important issues will need to be addressed in order for the latter strategy to be viable. For example, while several protein kinases have been identified that can phosporylate α-synuclein in vitro (46,49) and in flies, it is unclear which, if any, of these kinases act to phosphorylate α-synuclein in the human brain. Thus, it will be important to identify the appropriate kinase targets for therapeutic intervention. However, the biologically relevant kinase(s) may not prove to be viable drug targets, since they may be involved in multiple critical biological processes. Perhaps more importantly, the main findings of Chen and Feany appear to conflict with previous work showing that the phosphorylation of α-synuclein enhances inclusion formation in cell culture, and that highly phosphorylated α-synuclein is primarily found in Lewy bodies (45,50). Further work will be required to resolve these conflicts.

Investigators have also begun to explore the model that the genetic factors responsible for monogenic heritable forms of PD act in a common pathway influencing the abundance, toxicity, and/or aggregate formation properties of α-synuclein. In one such study, Yang et al. analyzed the effects of overexpression of the E3 ubiquitin-protein ligase, PARKIN, on α-synuclein pathogenesis, and aggregate formation in Drosophila (51). Loss-of-function mutations of the PARKIN gene result in an early onset form of autosomal recessive parkinsonism and previous work has shown that PARKIN can bind to and ubiquitinate a glycosylated form of α-synuclein in vitro (52,53). To study the possible involvement of PARKIN in α-synuclein pathogenesis Yang et al. generated transgenic flies bearing a copy of the human PARKIN gene under the transcriptional control of a GAL4-responsive UAS element. Coexpresssion of human PARKIN and α-synuclein was found to result in significantly reduced loss of TH positive neurons relative to flies expressing α-synuclein protein alone. Moreover, *PARKIN* overexpression also suppressed the formation of α-synuclein-containing aggregates, but without detectably affecting the overall abundance of α-synuclein protein. Further studies showed that overexpression of a Drosophila *PARKIN* ortholog also suppressed the α-synuclein-induced retinal degeneration and climbing phenotypes and that RNAi mediated attenuation of Drosophila *PARKIN* expression resulted in enhanced loss of dopamine neurons in α-synuclein transgenic flies (51,54).

While the findings of Yang et al. are consistent with the model that *PARKIN* is responsible for the degradation of α-synuclein aggregates or their precursors, and that α-synuclein aggregates are the toxic species responsible for dopamine neuron degeneration, this model conflicts with other work on *PARKIN* and α-synuclein. In particular, the results of Yang et al. appear contradictory to the observation that most cases of PD resulting from loss of *PARKIN* function do not display α-synuclein positive Lewy body aggregates. If *PARKIN* acts to degrade, or otherwise prevent the formation of α-synuclein positive inclusions, then one might expect to see Lewy bodies in great abundance in humans with PD resulting from loss of *PARKIN* function. The work of Yang et al. also appears to conflict with the findings of Chen and Feany on the effects of phosphorylation of α-synuclein, which suggest that aggregate formation is neuroprotective. Finally, the findings of Yang et al. contrast with our recent work demonstrating that Drosophila *PARKIN* null mutants display dopamine neuron loss in the absence of human α-synuclein, or an apparent Drosophila counterpart, indicating that α-synuclein is not obligate in the pathogenesis resulting from loss of *PARKIN* function (see below). Further work will be required to resolve these discordant findings and to establish whether the O-glycosylated form of α-synuclein that is believed to be the substrate of *PARKIN* is produced in Drosophila and is a direct target of the *PARKIN* ubiquitin-protein ligase activity in this organism.

Another application of Drosophila models of PD is to use these models in genomic studies to identify pathways involved in pathogenesis. A recent genomic study of the α-synuclein transgenic fly model of PD identified 51 Drosophila transcripts that displayed an altered abundance relative to control flies (55). Importantly, these transcripts were unaffected in transgenic flies expressing the neurodegeneration-inducing tau protein, indicating that the abundance of these 51 transcripts are specifically altered in response to α-synuclein expression. The 51 transcripts that display altered abundance in the α-synuclein transgenic flies encode proteins involved in lipid metabolism, energy production, and membrane transport, potentially implicating these pathways in α-synuclein pathogenesis. Interestingly, a recent study of α-synuclein pathogenesis in yeast identified lipid metabolism and vesicle transport components as a major category of genetic modifiers of α-synuclein toxicity (56). Together, these two studies suggest an evolutionarily conserved pathway of PD pathogenesis involving lipid metabolic and vesicle trafficking defects. Additional work will be required to validate the functional significance of these pathways to dopamine neuron degeneration.

Caveats of the Drosophila α-Synuclein Model

While the remarkable degree with which the phenotypes associated with PD appear to be recapitulated in α-synuclein-expressing transgenic Drosophila have made this an attractive model for studies of PD pathogenesis, it is important to point out that several key features of this disease model have not been reliably replicated. One of the earliest conflicts concerns the locomotor defect of α-synuclein expressing flies. At present, only half of the studies that have examined locomotor ability in α-synuclein transgenic flies were able to detect a climbing defect associated with α-synuclein expression (41,44,57,58). While these conflicts are not easily reconciled, several possible explanations can be offered. One potential source of variation in studies examining climbing behavior in flies relates to methodology. The finding that dopamine neuron dysfunction results in a hyperexcitable or startle phenotype upon vigorous mechanical disturbance of flies raises the possibility that the intensity of tapping flies to the bottom of a vial may impact the outcome of a climbing assay (33). Thus, the results of a climbing assay may vary among individual researchers because vigorous tapping of vials might induce a startle response that would manifest as a climbing defect in response to dopamine neuron loss, whereas milder handling might fail to induce the startle response. Another possible source of variation in climbing behavior relates to recent work demonstrating that apparently homogeneous fly populations consist of subpopulations with either "high" or "low" locomotor activity (35). Failing to account for this phenomenon could result in situations in which there are an excess of α-synuclein expressing flies in the low locomotor activity state relative to the control population.

Recently, a more concerning challenge to the α-synuclein transgenic model was raised in a report by Pesah et al. (58) which failed to detect evidence of loss of dopamine neurons. These investigators were also unable to document retinal degeneration despite using the same WT α-synuclein transgenic lines reported by other investigators to cause neuronal loss. The inability of these investigators to detect neuron loss is independently supported by our own work with these same α-synuclein transgenic lines. Moreover, we also find that an A30P mutationally altered α-synuclein transgenic line fails to induce loss of TH-positive neurons (Table 2).

A recent study by Auluck et al. (59) strongly suggests that the conflicting results of dopamine neuron analysis in α-synuclein transgenic flies are likely explained by differences in the methodology used to analyze dopamine neurons. While all of the studies that documented neuronal loss in α-synuclein-expressing flies utilized paraffin embedded sectioning and light microscopy techniques to visualize: TH-positive neurons, the conflicting studies of Pesah et al. (and our own work) involved the use of confocal microscopy of whole-mount brains to detect TH-positive neurons. Thus, one possible explanation for these conflicting results is

TABLE 2 The Number of Dopamine Neurons in the PPM2 Cluster of α-Synuclein-Expressing Flies as Determined by Anti-TH Immunostaining and Whole Mount Confocal Analysis

Age (days)	Genotype	#PPM2 neurons
35	Wild type	6.6 ± 0.5
35	elav–GAL4; UAS-α-synuclein	6.8 ± 0.2
50	Wild type	6.0 ± 0.5
50	elav–GAL4; UAS-α-synuclein	6.2 ± 0.4
23	Wild type	6.0 ± 0.4
23	ddc–GAL4; UAS-α-synuclein (A30P)	6.1 ± 0.3
45	Wild type	6.7 ± 0.6
45	ddc–GAL4; UAS-α-synuclein (A30P)	5.8 ± 0.6

Abbreviations: PPM, protocerebral posterier medial; TH, tyrosine hydroxylase.

that the different methods employed to identify TH-positive neurons may differ in their sensitivity of detection. Auluck et al. directly addressed this possibility and demonstrated that the subpopulation of dopamine neurons reported to degenerate in α-synuclein expressing flies could still be detected by confocal analysis of whole-mount brains from flies expressing α-synuclein. Further, they demonstrated that this same cell population generally stains less intensely than those in clusters reportedly unaffected by α-synuclein expression [(59), supplementary data]. These findings indicate that the loss of TH-staining previously reported in α-synuclein transgenic flies reflects reduced TH levels rather than overt cell loss. While the reduced TH expression conferred by α-synuclein expression suggests that these cells are dysfunctional, whether this phenotype reflects an early stage leading to the death of these neurons, as proposed by Auluck et al. (59), remains an open question. Additional characterization of the α-synuclein transgenic model is warranted given the recent results with this model.

LOSS OF FUNCTION MODELS OF PARKINSON'S DISEASE
Functional Analysis of a Drosophila *PARKIN* Ortholog
In contrast to the dominant toxic gain-of-function of α-synuclein mutations, at least three of the six known genes associated with heritable forms of PD appear to involve loss-of-function mutations (Table 1). Insight into the mechanisms by which these loss-of-function mutations cause PD will require detailed knowledge of the biological functions of the corresponding genes and the pathways regulated by these genes. One of the most powerful approaches to address these issues involves the use of classical genetic analysis in a simple model organism such as Drosophila to explore the biological functions of evolutionarily conserved homologs of these genes. This approach has recently been used to analyze the biological functions of Drosophila *PARKIN*, *DJ-1*, and *PINK1* homologs.

To explore the biological role of *PARKIN*, we and others generated a series of mutations in the Drosophila ortholog of *PARKIN*, including deletion, nonsense, and missense mutations. Flies lacking the *PARKIN* gene are semiviable and display reduced longevity, motor deficits, and male sterility (60,61). The motor deficit of *PARKIN* mutants is associated with a dramatic and widespread apoptotic degeneration of muscle tissue, and the male-sterility derives from a late defect in spermatid formation in the germline. Ultrastructural studies indicate that mitochondrial dysfunction is the earliest manifestation of muscle degeneration in *PARKIN* mutants, suggesting a role for *PARKIN* in mitochondrial integrity (60). This conclusion is further underscored by the finding that late spermatids in *PARKIN* mutants manifest dramatic structural alterations in the mitochondrial derivatives known as Nebenkern that are responsible for the energy production required for sperm motility (62). While humans and mice with *PARKIN* mutations do not appear to manifest similar muscle and germline phenotypes, mitochondrial defects are a common characteristic of sporadic PD and a conserved feature in all organisms with *PARKIN* mutations, including humans (63,64). These observations suggest that *PARKIN* may act, either directly or indirectly, to regulate mitochondrial integrity and that mitochondrial dysfunction is a triggering feature of dopamine neuron death in humans lacking *PARKIN* function. The mitochondrial dysfunction observed in *PARKIN* mutants may also explain the reported sensitivity of mutant flies to oxidative stress inducing agents (61). However, our unpublished work indicates that *PARKIN* mutants are

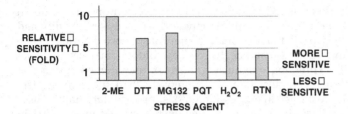

FIGURE 2 Drosophila *PARKIN* mutants are sensitive to a wide variety of different chemical agents. The sensitivity of *PARKIN* mutants and an isogenic wild type control-line to chemical agents was determined by identifying the LD_{50} values of each chemical following a 48-hour exposure. Relative sensitivity refers to the ratio of LD_{50} values of WT controls and *PARKIN* mutants. Values greater than one indicate greater sensitivity of *PARKIN* mutants. Results for each chemical tested represent the average LD_{50} value from three independent experiments involving 50 flies each. *Abbreviations*: DTT, dithiothreitol 2-ME, 2-mercaptoethanol; MG132, a proteasome inhibitor; PQT, paraquat RTN rotenone.

similarly sensitive to a variety of chemical insults, including those that induce ER stress and proteosomal inhibition (Fig. 2).

All of the initial studies of Drosophila *PARKIN* mutants failed to detect dopamine neuron loss, fueling speculation that the lack of evolutionary conservation in Drosophila of putatively pathogenic *PARKIN* substrates, such as α-synuclein and Pael-R, might be responsible for the observed lack of effect of *PARKIN* mutations on dopamine neuron integrity in this organism. However, recent work from our laboratory indicates that a subset of dopamine neurons restricted to the PPL1 cluster do indeed degenerate in *PARKIN* mutants (65). Importantly, the loss of dopamine neurons in the PPL1 cluster was detected in blinded studies involving confocal microscopy, the more sensitive of the methods available for analyzing dopamine neuron integrity in Drosophila. The inability of previous work to detect neuron loss in *PARKIN* mutants is likely explained by technical limitations of the approaches used (62,65) and the simple fact that most of these studies focused exclusively on the PPM1/2 cluster (51,61,66) owing to the reported effects of α-synuclein expression on this neuronal cluster.

In addition to the degeneration of neurons in the PPL1 cluster, *PARKIN* mutants also manifest reduced TH-staining in the PPM1/2 cluster and significantly reduced dopamine content in the brain (66,62). Feeding *PARKIN* mutants the dopamine precursor, L-DOPA, partially rescues a motor deficit associated with loss of *PARKIN* function, suggesting that this phenotype arises in part from the loss of dopamine neuron signaling (66). No cell loss was detected in any of the serotonergic neuronal clusters and overall brain integrity appeared to be intact in *PARKIN* mutants, indicating that neuronal cell loss is restricted to the PPL1 cluster of dopamine neurons (65). The dopamine neuron loss in *PARKIN* mutants is largely rescued by ectopic expression of wild type *PARKIN* protein in dopamine neurons, indicating that *PARKIN* plays a cell autonomous role in dopamine neuron integrity (65).

Our finding that Drosophila *PARKIN* mutants exhibit neuron loss further suggests that the mechanisms responsible for neuron loss in humans lacking *PARKIN* function are conserved in Drosophila. Moreover, this finding potentially bears on models of *PARKIN* pathogenesis. In particular, the apparent absence of α-synuclein and Pael-R homologs in Drosophila indicates that these factors are not obligate in *PARKIN*-mediated pathogenesis. While previous work indicates that

PARKIN can regulate the pathogenesis of these factors in Drosophila (51,57), and it remains possible that these factors contribute to the magnitude and/or severity of pathogenesis in humans lacking *PARKIN* function, our findings suggest that other pathogenic substrates of *PARKIN* exist. Although further work will be required to identify these pathogenic substrates, the recent finding that Drosophila *PARKIN* suppresses the activation of the JNK pathway indicates that JNK pathway components represent candidate targets of *PARKIN* (66).

In an ongoing effort to elucidate the pathogenic mechanism resulting from loss of *PARKIN* function in Drosophila we recently conducted a genetic screen for mutations in other genes that either enhance or suppress a *PARKIN* phenotype (67). While, ideally we would like to conduct screens for genetic modifiers of the dopamine neuron loss phenotype of *PARKIN* mutants, this phenotype is not amenable to high-throughput analysis. Thus, we chose to use the partial lethality of Drosophila *PARKIN* mutants as a surrogate phenotype in screens for mutations in genes that enhanced or suppressed this lethality. This work revealed a number of factors that influence the partial lethality of *PARKIN* mutants, including genes involved in the oxidative stress pathway. The most potent enhancer of the *PARKIN* recessive lethal phenotype recovered from our screen was a loss-of-function allele of the *glutathione S-transferase S1* (*GstS1*) gene. The glutathione S-transferase family of polypeptides is thought to act in cellular detoxification pathways and by regulating the cellular redox balance in a number of ways, such as covalently coupling glutathione to a variety of products of oxidative damage, including 4-hydroxynonenol, or by maintaining the correct redox state of protein thiol groups (68). Another Drosophila glutathione S-transferase family member (*GstE1*) was found to be induced early in the timecourse of *PARKIN* pathogenesis and genetic studies of this factor showed that it exhibits a dominant synthetic lethal interaction with *PARKIN* (28).

In an initial effort to test the relevance of genetic factors that influence the viability of *PARKIN* mutants to the dopamine neuron loss phenotype of *PARKIN* mutants, we explored the effect of altered *GstS1* dosage on dopamine neuron integrity in *PARKIN* mutants (65). Results of this analysis demonstrated that reduced *GstS1* activity enhanced neuron loss in *PARKIN* mutants while transgenic overexpression of *GstS1* significantly suppressed the loss of dopamine neurons in *PARKIN* mutants (69). The implications of these results are threefold. First, these findings demonstrate that the partial lethality of *PARKIN* mutants can effectively serve as a surrogate phenotype for neuronal loss, and supports the validity of further screening. Second, because previous work suggests that defective glutathione metabolism and oxidative stress are important contributory factors to sporadic PD (70) our work suggests that the causes of neuronal loss resulting from loss of *PARKIN* function are mechanistically related to the loss of dopamine neurons in sporadic PD. Third, and most importantly, since there are several dietary components and drugs that are able to induce the expression of glutathione S-transferase activity and glutathione production in vertebrates (71), our findings suggest that these compounds should be tested as potential therapeutics in preventing PD.

Mutational Analysis of the Drosophila *DJ-1* Gene Family

Drosophila has also proven useful in dissecting the role of the *DJ-1* gene. Similar to *PARKIN*, loss-of-function mutations in *DJ-1*, a small protein of unknown function with homology to proteases, kinases, and small heat shock proteins, result in parkinsonism in humans (72). The Drosophila genome encodes two homologs of the human *DJ-1* gene, designated as *DJ-1a* and *DJ-1b* (Table 1). The *DJ-1b* gene appears to be ubiquitously expressed whereas *DJ-1a* expression is largely, or exclusively, restricted to testes (73–75). To explore the biological roles of *DJ-1a* and *DJ-1b*, we and others have used traditional genetics and RNAi to perturb the functions of these genes (75–78). The results of studies involving traditional mutant alleles of the *DJ-1* genes indicate that flies lacking one or both of the *DJ-1* genes are fully viable, fertile, and display no evidence of dopamine neuron loss. However, further studies of these mutants revealed that *DJ-1b* single mutants and *DJ-1a; DJ-1b* double mutants display a striking sensitivity to particular stress-inducing agents, including paraquat and rotenone—chemicals which have been epidemiologically linked to PD (75,77). Unlike *PARKIN* mutants, this sensitivity is unique to chemical agents that induce oxidative stress and is not manifest by chemical agents that induce other types of cellular stress implicated in PD, including ER stress and proteasome inhibition. Moreover, treatment of WT flies with these oxidative stress-inducing chemical agents results in a modification of *DJ-1b* protein electrophoretic mobility that can be detected by Western blot analysis or isoelectric focusing, suggesting that *DJ-1b* is a direct target of an oxidative modification as has been seen with vertebrate *DJ-1*. *DJ-1a* mutants manifest no apparent sensitivity to these same oxidative stress-inducing agents, although transgenic expression of either *DJ-1a* or *DJ-1b* is able to rescue the chemical sensitivity of *DJ-1b* and *DJ-1a; DJ-1b* double mutants.

In contrast to these findings, work by Menzies et al. (76), using independently generated alleles of the *DJ-1b* gene, found that these mutants were less sensitive to paraquat exposure than wild type flies. Moreover, Menzies et al. found that *DJ-1b* mutants exhibit delayed age-dependent reduction of TH-staining in the central nervous system. The authors ascribe these two phenotypes to a compensatory induction of *DJ-1a* expression in response to loss of *DJ-1b* function, and provide expression and transgenic data in support of this model. Even more surprisingly, a recent study of the *DJ-1a* gene by Yang et al. (78) found that ubiquitous knockdown of the *DJ-1a* transcript with RNAi resulted in larval lethality in contrast to our previous finding that *DJ-1a* null mutants are fully viable and exhibit no apparent phenotype. Moreover, these investigators found that targeted knockdown of *DJ-1a* expression in the compound eye results in photoreceptor cell loss, and that knock-down of *DJ-1a* expression in the nervous system results in the progressive loss of TH-positive neurons in the PPM1/2 cluster (documented using the paraffin sectioning/light microscopy methodology) and reduced dopamine content in fly heads. Cultured neurons from *DJ-1a* RNAi treated animals also displayed an increased production of reactive oxygen species and increased sensitivity to oxidative stress-inducing agents. Further genetic studies by Yang et al. showed that signaling through the phosphatidylinositol 3-kinase/Akt pathway suppressed the *DJ-1a* RNAi-induced eye and dopaminergic neuron phenotypes, possibly by reducing the production of reactive oxygen species.

While all four studies of the Drosophila *DJ-1* gene family reached similar conclusions, a disconcerting feature of this work involves the stark phenotypic differences reported in the individual studies. Although further work will be required to explain these discrepancies, there are several likely sources. One potential source of the discordant results is methodologic. In particular, while our work and the work of Park et al. (75), made use of definitive null alleles of the Drosophila *DJ-1* gene family, the alleles used by Menzies et al. may well be hypomorphic in nature, and the work of Yang et al. involved RNAi. Thus, the compensatory effects of *DJ-1a* in response to reduced *DJ-1b* activity reported by Menzies et al. may reflect a feature of the *DJ-1a* gene that is only manifest in a *DJ-1b* hypomorphic animal. In contrast, the more severe phenotypes resulting from RNAi-mediated knockdown of *DJ-1a* activity reported by Yang et al. relative to our null alleles of *DJ-1a* cannot readily be explained by a hypomorphic effect of RNAi. These conflicting results are better explained by a possible developmental compensation to loss of *DJ-1a* in null animals relative to the acute loss of *DJ-1a* activity in RNAi treated animals later in development, or to an unexpected off-target effect of the *DJ-1a* RNAi constructs. While Yang et al. performed several experiments in an effort to control for the specificity of the *DJ-1a* RNAi effects, these experiments do not definitively exclude an off-target effect of RNAi and it is difficult to envision how perturbation of a gene that is predominantly or exclusively expressed in the male germline could result in loss of viability and neuronal integrity. An alternative explanation for the discordant results reported in these three studies involves the possible influence of genetic background. While our study of the *DJ-1a* and *DJ-1b* genes involved comparisons to isogenic control flies, the work of Menzies et al. and Park et al. involved studies comparing *DJ-1b* mutants against unrelated wild type lines and the studies of Yang et al. likely involved studies with fly strains that are genetically unrelated to those used in the other two studies of *DJ-1* function in Drosophila. Thus, the different outcomes reported in these studies may be explained by the influence of modifier loci in some of these studies.

Regardless of the explanations for the discordant results of studies of the Drosophila *DJ-1* gene family, all of these studies support the increasing body of evidence linking *DJ-1* to the oxidative stress response pathway. An important challenge of future work will be to discern between the myriad biological functions ascribed to this protein family to define the mechanism by which loss of *DJ-1* function results in neuronal loss. Clues should emerge from the application of classical genetic methods to identify suppressors of the *DJ-1* chemical sensitivity phenotype.

Functional Analysis of a Drosophila *PINK1* Ortholog

Three recent papers described the effects of perturbation of a Drosophila homolog of the *PINK1* gene (79–81). The human *PINK1* gene encodes a putative protein kinase that is upregulated in cancer cells by the tumor-suppressor PTEN (82). The presence of a putative mitochondrial targeting sequence in *PINK1* coupled with its predominant localization to mitochondria (83,84) strongly suggested that loss-of-function mutations in *PINK1* somehow compromise mitochondrial integrity. This prediction is born out in the three studies conducted in flies (79–81). Two of the three papers show that null mutations of the Drosophila *PINK1* ortholog result in degeneration of indirect flight muscles and defective spermatid formation (79,80). Using a combination of ultrastructural and biochemical assays these papers further report that mitochondrial defects accompany both of these phenotypes. The third paper reports equivalent findings using an RNAi approach to target the *PINK1* gene, although phenotypes are only documented in the indirect flight muscle, presumably because the GAL4 line chosen for this study is not expressed in the male germline (81). Two of these studies also report dopamine neuron loss upon perturbation of *PINK1* function (80,81). Interestingly, one of these three studies also reported mitochondrial swelling in dopamine neurons of *PINK1* mutants, suggesting that the pathogenic mechanisms responsible for muscle degeneration, spermatid defects, and dopamine neuron loss all involve mitochondrial dysfunction (80). The observation that human *PINK1* expression in the male germline is able to partially rescue the spermatid developmental defect of drosophila *PINK1* mutants (79) strongly suggests that the findings reported in these three studies have direct relevance to the biological function of the human *PINK1* gene.

While the finding that Drosophila *PINK1* mutants display mitochondrial defects advances our knowledge, the real surprise of these three papers is the finding that *PARKIN* appears to act downstream from *PINK1* in a common pathway influencing mitochondrial integrity. Specifically, the authors of these three studies show that overexpresssion of either Drosophila or human *PARKIN* are able to rescue the *PINK1* phenotypes, but conversely *PINK1* overexpression does not detectably influence the *PARKIN* phenotypes (79–81). Although a caveat of this finding is that *PARKIN* overexpression can generally be protective, Park et al. (80) showed that *PARKIN* overexpression is unable to suppress the toxicity of several other cellular insults, demonstrating at least some specificity in this interaction. These papers also show that *PINK1*, *PARKIN* double mutants are phenotypically indistinguishable from the respective single mutants (79,80). Indeed, the strikingly similar phenotypes of Drosophila *PINK1* and *PARKIN* mutants, both of which include flight muscle degeneration, germline defects, and mitochondrial pathology, alone argue that these two genes act in a common pathway. In contrast, the phenotypes of Drosophila *DJ-1* mutants are phenotypically quite different from *PARKIN* and *PINK1* mutants, and our own unpublished findings have failed to detect genetic interactions between the *PARKIN*, *DJ-1a*, and *DJ-1b* genes, suggesting that these genes influence different pathways. The current findings parallel recent work showing that *PINK1* and *PARKIN* mutations confer similar symptoms in humans (85). These findings also suggest that other unique features of parkinsonism resulting from *PARKIN* mutations, such as absence of Lewy body inclusions, will be manifest in *PINK1* patients.

Given the findings reported in these papers, how can we explain the nature of the pathway regulated by *PINK1* and *PARKIN*? The simplest interpretation of the data is that *PINK1* regulates *PARKIN* abundance or activity. This mode of regulation could involve a transcriptional or post-transcriptional effect of *PINK1* on *PARKIN* expression or, alternatively, *PINK1* may phosphorylate *PARKIN* and directly influence its ubiquitin-ligase activity. Indeed, Yang et al. (81) reported decreased *PARKIN* expression in flies with reduced *PINK1* expression, consistent with the model that *PINK1* regulates the expression of *PARKIN*. However, we have been unable to replicate this finding using *PINK1* null mutants, so further work will be required to test this model. Moreover, a problem with the model that *PINK1* directly phosphorylates *PARKIN* to regulate its activity is that most data suggest that *PINK1* protein resides primarily in mitochondria and that *PARKIN* lies outside of mitochondria. Nevertheless, it remains possible that the localization of either *PARKIN* or *PINK1* changes upon stress and there are several reports, including the one by Park et al. that have argued that at least some *PARKIN* associates with mitochondria. It is also possible that *PINK1* regulates the activity of *PARKIN* in an indirect fashion involving additional unknown signaling components.

Another model to explain the current findings, that is consistent with many other pathways regulated by protein degradation, is that phosphorylation of specific mitochondrial targets by *PINK1* serves as a recognition signal for subsequent ubiquitination by *PARKIN*. Although previous work indicates that mitochondrial protein turnover occurs through a nonproteosomal pathway and mitochondrial proteomic studies have thus far largely failed to detect proteosome pathway components, the possibility that some mitochondrial proteins are exported to the cytoplasm (as occurs in the endoplasmic reticulum stress pathway) and ultimately degraded through a proteosomal mechanism has not been rigorously excluded.

PINK1, perhaps in conjunction with *PARKIN* could serve the role of tagging such proteins for export.

Finally, it remains possible that *PARKIN* plays a functional role in mitochondria that does not involve its ubiquitin-ligase activity. Although there is substantial evidence in vitro that *PARKIN* can function as an ubiquitin-ligase, few of the reported substrates of *PARKIN* have been validated in vivo. Future experiments to address the mechanism of the *PINK1/PARKIN* pathway promise to clarify the mechanisms underlying mitochondrial dysfunction in PD and should also shed new light on some very basic questions of mitochondrial biology.

CONCLUSION

The fruit fly *Drosophila melanogaster* has proven itself to be an invaluable model system in basic studies of genetics and biology for nearly 100 years. Given the remarkable degree of genetic, molecular, and cell biological conservation between flies and mammals that has been revealed over the decades, *Drosophila* remains a valid model system in which to address novel biological questions in the future, including those relevant to human health. Indeed, work aimed at an understanding of the genes involved in heritable forms of PD has already made significant contributions to our understanding of this debilitating disease. Moreover, these studies have begun to define small molecule compounds that could potentially impinge on the pathways implicated in PD (Table 3). While these compounds offer real potential as therapeutic strategies, Drosophila models also lend themselves directly to unbiased high-throughput screening of small molecule libraries in the search for novel compounds that are able to prevent pathogenesis. EnVivo Pharmaceuticals has taken such an approach by developing an automated platform for in vivo screening of compound libraries in a variety of Drosophila neurodegenerative disease models and has begun to move several positive hits forward in the drug discovery process (86).

TABLE 3 Summary of Key Features and Potential Therapeutic Strategies Revealed by Analysis of Drosophila Models of Parkinson's Disease

Genetic model	Associated phenotypes	Potential therapeutic
α-synuclein	DA neuron dysfunction[a] Locomotor deficits[a] Retinal degeneration[a] Lewy body-like protein aggregates	Induction of heat shock factors/ chaperones (e.g., geldanomycin) Modulation of α-synuclein phosphorylation
PARKIN	DA neuron loss Mitochondrial pathology Locomotor deficits Sensitivity to multiple stress agents	Induction of phase II detoxifying enzymes (e.g., sulphoraphane) Induced expression of antioxidant enzymes
DJ-1	Sensitivity to oxidative stress Modification of *DJ–1*	Induced expression of antioxidant enzymes
PINK1	DA neuron loss[a] Mitochondrial pathology Locomotor deficits Sensitivity to multiple stress agents	Induction of phase II detoxifying enzymes (e.g., sulphoraphane) Induced expression of antioxidant enzymes

[a]Conflicting findings have been reported for these phenotypes.

While the Drosophila system has enormous potential for studies aimed at a mechanistic understanding of PD, it is also important to point out that PD modeling in Drosophila is still relatively new and that the reagents and methodologies for conducting these studies are evolving. In particular, important priorities of future work should be to define the most appropriate methods for analyzing dopamine neuron integrity and to resolve conflicts in studies of some of the current Drosophila models of PD. It is also imperative that we have realistic expectations from these models. For example, at present the phenotypes of the loss-of-function Drosophila models of PD do not precisely match the phenotypes of humans with mutations in the corresponding genes. While these findings may be of concern, phenotypic differences resulting from mutations in orthologous genes in different species often believe significant underlying molecular pathway conservation. Indeed, the weight of evidence suggests that the phenotypes associated with the Drosophila *PARKIN* and *DJ-1* models, which include sensitivity to oxidative stress agents and mitochondrial dysfunction, are directly relevant to the mechanisms implicated in PD. We have only just begun to tap the insight that modeling PD in Drosophila can potentially provide. This insight will only be fully realized if we focus our efforts on understanding what the phenotypes of these models are telling us and take full advantage of the power of genetics to lead us down unexpected, and even unintuitive, paths.

REFERENCES

1. Ashburner M, Novitski E. The Genetics and Biology of Drosophila. London: Academic Press, 1976.
2. Rubin GM, Yandell MD, Wortman JR, et al. Comparative genomics of the eukaryotes. Science 2000; 287:2204–2215.
3. Bilen J, Bonini NM. Drosophila as a model for human neurodegenerative disease. Annu Rev Genet 2005; 39:153–171.
4. Adams MD, Celniker SE, Holt RA, et al. The genome sequence of Drosophila melanogaster. Science 2000; 287:2185–2195.
5. Hiesinger PR, Bellen HJ. Flying in the face of total disruption. Nat Genet 2004; 36:211–212.
6. Hamilton BA, Palazzolo MJ, Chang JH, et al. Large scale screen for transposon insertions into cloned genes. Proc Natl Acad Sci USA 1991; 88:2731–2735.
7. Ballinger DG, Benzer S. Targeted gene mutations in Drosophila. Proc Natl Acad Sci USA 1989; 86:9402–9406.
8. Engels W. Mobile DNA. Washington, DC: American Society of Microbiology, 1989.
9. Spradling AC, Stern D, Beaton A, et al. The Berkeley Drosophila Genome Project gene disruption project: single P-element insertions mutating 25% of vital Drosophila genes. Genetics 1999; 153:135–177.
10. Gong WJ, Golic KG. Ends-out, or replacement, gene targeting in Drosophila. Proc Natl Acad Sci USA 2003; 100:2556–2561.
11. Rong YS, Golic KG. Gene targeting by homologous recombination in Drosophila. Science 2000; 288:2013–2018.
12. Kalidas S, Smith DP. Novel genomic cDNA hybrids produce effective RNA interference in adult Drosophila. Neuron 2002; 33:177–184.
13. Lee YS, Carthew RW. Making a better RNAi vector for Drosophila: use of intron spacers. Methods 2003; 30:322–329.
14. Andrews HK, Zhang YQ, Trotta N, Broadie K. Drosophila sec10 is required for hormone secretion but not general exocytosis or neurotransmission. Traffic 2002; 3:906–921.
15. Murthy M, Garza D, Scheller RH, Schwarz TL. Mutations in the exocyst component Sec5 disrupt neuronal membrane traffic, but neurotransmitter release persists. Neuron 2003; 37:433–447.
16. Sarov M, Stewart AF. The best control for the specificity of RNAi. Trends Biotechnol 2005; 23:446–448.

17. Brand AH, Perrimon N. Targeted gene expression as a means of altering cell fates and generating dominant phenotypes. Development 1993; 118:401–415.
18. Rorth P. A modular misexpression screen in Drosophila detecting tissue-specific phenotypes. Proc Natl Acad Sci USA 1996; 93:12418–12422.
19. Fernandez-Funez P, Nino-Rosales ML, de Gouyon B, et al. Identification of genes that modify ataxin-1-induced neurodegeneration. Nature 2000; 408:101–106.
20. Greene JC, Whitworth AJ, Andrews LA, Parker TJ, Pallanck LJ. Genetic and genomic studies of Drosophila parkin mutants implicate oxidative stress and innate immune responses in pathogenesis. Hum Mol Genet 2005; 14:799–811.
21. Shulman JM, Feany MB. Genetic modifiers of tauopathy in Drosophila. Genetics 2003; 165:1233–1242.
22. Boutros M, Kiger AA, Armknecht S, et al. Genome-wide RNAi analysis of growth and viability in Drosophila cells. Science 2004; 303:832–835.
23. Clemens JC, Worby CA, Simonson-Leff N, et al. Use of double-stranded RNA interference in Drosophila cell lines to dissect signal transduction pathways. Proc Natl Acad Sci USA 2000; 97:6499–6503.
24. Lum L, Yao S, Mozer B, et al. Identification of Hedgehog pathway components by RNAi in Drosophila cultured cells. Science 2003; 299:2039–2045.
25. Echeverri CJ, Perrimon N. High-throughput RNAi screening in cultured cells: a user's guide. Nat Rev Genet 2006; 7:373–384.
26. Pendleton RG, Rasheed A, Sardina T, Tully T, Hillman R. Effects of tyrosine hydroxylase mutants on locomotor activity in Drosophila: a study in functional genomics. Behav Genet 2002; 32:89–94.
27. Tempel BL, Livingstone MS, Quinn WG. Mutations in the dopa decarboxylase gene affect learning in Drosophila. Proc Natl Acad Sci USA 1984; 81:3577–3581.
28. Neckameyer WS, White K. Drosophila tyrosine hydroxylase is encoded by the pale locus. J Neurogenet 1993; 8:189–199.
29. Neckameyer WS. Dopamine and mushroom bodies in Drosophila: experience-dependent and -independent aspects of sexual behavior. Learn Mem 1998; 5:157–165.
30. Neckameyer WS. Dopamine modulates female sexual receptivity in Drosophila melanogaster. J Neurogenet 1998; 12:101–114.
31. Birman S, Morgan B, Anzivino M, Hirsh J. A novel and major isoform of tyrosine hydroxylase in Drosophila is generated by alternative RNA processing. J Biol Chem 1994; 269:26559–26567.
32. Neckameyer WS. Multiple roles for dopamine in Drosophila development. Dev Biol 1996; 176:209–219.
33. Friggi-Grelin F, Coulom H, Meller M, Gomez D, Hirsh J, Birman S. Targeted gene expression in Drosophila dopaminergic cells using regulatory sequences from tyrosine hydroxylase. J Neurobiol 2003; 54:618–627.
34. Sweeney ST, Broadie K, Keane J, Niemann H, O'Kane CJ. Targeted expression of tetanus toxin light chain in Drosophila specifically eliminates synaptic transmission and causes behavioral defects. Neuron 1995; 14:341–351.
35. Lima SQ, Miesenbock G. Remote control of behavior through genetically targeted photostimulation of neurons. Cell 2005; 121:141–152.
36. Polymeropoulos MH, Lavedan C, Leroy E, et al. Mutation in the alpha-synuclein gene identified in families with Parkinson's disease. Science 1997; 276:2045–2047.
37. Spillantini MG, Schmidt ML, Lee VM, Trojanowski JQ, Jakes R, Goedert M. Alpha-synuclein in Lewy bodies. Nature 1997; 388:839–840.
38. Bennett MC. The role of alpha-synuclein in neurodegenerative diseases. Pharmacol Ther 2005; 105:311–331.
39. Eriksen JL, Przedborski S, Petrucelli L. Gene dosage and pathogenesis of Parkinson's disease. Trends Mol Med 2005; 11:91–96.
40. Feany MB, Bender WW. A Drosophila model of Parkinson's disease. Nature 2000; 404:394–398.
41. Feany MB, Bender WW. A Drosophila model of Parkinson's disease. Nature 2000; 404:394–398.
42. Auluck PK, Chan HY, Trojanowski JQ, Lee VM, Bonini NM. Chaperone suppression of alpha-synuclein toxicity in a Drosophila model for Parkinson's disease. Science 2002; 295:865–868.

43. Auluck PK, Bonini NM. Pharmacological prevention of Parkinson disease in Drosophila. Nat Med 2002; 8:1185–1186.
44. Auluck P, Chan H, Trojanowski J, Lee V, Bonini NM. Chaperone suppression of alpha-synuclein toxicity in a Drosophila model for Parkinson's disease. Science 2002; 295: 809–810.
45. Fujiwara H, Hasegawa M, Dohmae N, et al. Alpha-synuclein is phosphorylated in synucleinopathy lesions. Nat Cell Biol 2005; 4:160–164.
46. Okochi M, Walter J, Koyama A, et al. Constitutive phosphorylation of the Parkinson's disease associated alpha-synuclein. J Biol Chem 2000; 275:390–397.
47. Takahashi M, Kanuka H, Fujiwara H, et al. Phosphorylation of alpha-synuclein characteristic of synucleinopathy lesions is recapitulated in alpha-synuclein transgenic Drosophila. Neurosci Lett 2003; 336:155–158.
48. Chen L, Feany MB. Alpha-synuclein phosphorylation controls neurotoxicity and inclusion formation in a Drosophila model of Parkinson disease. Nat Neurosci 2005; 8:657–663.
49. Pronin AN, Morris AJ, Surguchov A, Benovic JL. Synucleins are a novel class of substrates for G protein-coupled receptor kinases. J Biol Chem 2000; 275:26515–26522.
50. Smith WW, Margolis RL, Li X, et al. Alpha-synuclein phosphorylation enhances eosinophilic cytoplasmic inclusion formation in SH-SY5Y cells. J Neurosci 2005; 25:5544–5552.
51. Yang Y, Nishimura I, Imai Y, Takahashi R, Lu B. Parkin suppresses dopaminergic neuron-selective neurotoxicity induced by Pael-R in Drosophila. Neuron 2003; 37:911–924.
52. Kitada T, Asakawa S, Hattori N, et al. Mutations in the parkin gene cause autosomal recessive juvenile parkinsonism. Nature 1998; 392:605–608.
53. Shimura H, Schlossmacher MG, Hattori N, et al. Ubiquitination of a new form of alpha-synuclein by parkin from human brain: implications for Parkinson's disease. Science 2001; 293:263–269.
54. Haywood AF, Staveley BE. Parkin counteracts symptoms in a Drosophila model of Parkinson's disease. BMC Neurosci 2004; 5:14–26.
55. Scherzer CR, Jensen RV, Gullans SR, Feany MB. Gene expression changes presage neurodegeneration in a Drosophila model of Parkinson's disease. Hum Mol Genet 2003; 12:2457–2466.
56. Willingham S, Outeiro TF, DeVit MJ, Lindquist SL, Muchowski PJ. Yeast genes that enhance the toxicity of a mutant huntingtin fragment or alpha-synuclein. Science 2003; 302:1769–1772.
57. Haywood AF, Staveley BE. Parkin counteracts symptoms in a Drosophila model of Parkinson's disease. BMC Neurosci 2004; 5:14.
58. Pesah Y, Burgess H, Middlebrooks B, et al. Whole-mount analysis reveals normal numbers of dopaminergic neurons following misexpression of alpha-synuclein in Drosophila. Genesis 2005; 41:154–159.
59. Auluck PK, Meulener MC, Bonini NM. Mechanisms of suppression of {alpha}-synuclein neurotoxicity by geldanamycin in Drosophila. J Biol Chem 2005; 280:2873–2878.
60. Greene JC, Whitworth AJ, Kuo I, Andrews LA, Feany MB, Pallanck LJ. Mitochondrial pathology and apoptotic muscle degeneration in Drosophila parkin mutants. Proc Natl Acad Sci USA 2003; 100:4078–4083.
61. Pesah Y, Pham T, Burgess H, et al. Drosophila parkin mutants have decreased mass and cell size and increased sensitivity to oxygen radical stress. Development 2004; 131:2183–2194.
62. Greene JC, Whitworth AJ, Kuo I, Andrews LA, Feany MB, Pallanck LJ. Mitochondrial pathology and apoptotic muscle degeneration in Drosophila parkin mutants. Proc Natl Acad Sci USA 2003; 100:4078–4083.
63. Muftuoglu M, Elibol B, Dalmizrak O, et al. Mitochondrial complex I and IV activities in leukocytes from patients with parkin mutations. Mov Disord 2004; 19:544–548.
64. Palacino JJ, Sagi D, Goldberg MS, et al. Mitochondrial dysfunction and oxidative damage in parkin-deficient mice. J Biol Chem 2004; 279:18614–18622.
65. Whitworth AJ, Theodore DA, Greene JC, Benes H, Wes PD, Pallanck LJ. Increased glutathione S-transferase activity rescues dopaminergic neuron loss in a Drosophila model of Parkinson's disease. Proc Natl Acad Sci USA 2005; 102:8024–8029.
66. Cha GH, Kim S, Park J, et al. Parkin negatively regulates JNK pathway in the dopaminergic neurons of Drosophila. Proc Natl Acad Sci USA 2005; 102:10345–10350.

67. Greene JC, Whitworth AJ, Andrews LA, Parker TJ, Pallanck LJ. Genetic and genomic studies of Drosophila parkin mutants implicate oxidative stress and innate immune responses in pathogenesis. Hum Mol Genet 2005; 14:799–811.

68. Hayes JD, Flanagan JU, Jowsey IR. Glutathione transferases. Annu Rev Pharmacol Toxicol 2005; 45:51–88.

69. Whitworth AJ, Theodore DA, Greene JC, Benes H, Wes PD, Pallanck LJ. Increased glutathione S-transferase activity rescues dopaminergic neuron loss in a Drosophila model of Parkinson's disease. Proc Natl Acad Sci USA 2005; 102:8024–8029.

70. Bharath S, Hsu M, Kaur D, Rajagopalan S, Andersen JK. Glutathione, iron and Parkinson's disease. Biochem Pharmacol 2002; 64:1037–1048.

71. Nguyen T, Sherratt PJ, Pickett CB. Regulatory mechanisms controlling gene expression mediated by the antioxidant response element. Annu Rev Pharmacol Toxicol 2003; 43:233–260.

72. Bonifati V, Rizzu P, van Baren MJ, et al. Mutations in the DJ-1 gene associated with autosomal recessive early-onset parkinsonism. Science 2003; 299:256–259.

73. Menzies FM, Yenisetti SC, Min KT. Roles of Drosophila DJ-1 in survival of dopaminergic neurons and oxidative stress. Curr Biol 2005; 15:1578–1582.

74. Meulener M, Whitworth AJ, Armstrong-Gold CE, et al. Drosophila DJ-1 mutants are selectively sensitive to environmental toxins associated with Parkinson's disease. Curr Biol 2005; 15:1572–1577.

75. Park J, Kim SY, Cha GH, Lee SB, Kim S, Chung J. Drosophila DJ-1 mutants show oxidative stress-sensitive locomotive dysfunction. Gene 2005; 361:133–139.

76. Menzies FM, Sarat CY, Min K-T. Roles of Drosophila DJ-1 in survival of dopaminergic neurons and oxidative stress. Curr Biol 2005; 15:1578–1582.

77. Meulener MC, Whitworth AJ, Armstrong-Gold CE, et al. Drosophila DJ-1 mutants are selectively sensitive to environmental toxins associated with Parkinson's disease. Curr Biol 2005; 15:1572–1577.

78. Yang Y, Gehrke S, Haque ME, et al. Inactivation of Drosophila DJ-1 leads to impairments of oxidative stress response and phosphatidylinositol 3-kinase/Akt signaling. Proc Natl Acad Sci USA 2005; 103:10793–10798.

79. Clark IE, Dodson MW, Jiang C, et al. Drosophila pink1 is required for mitochondrial function and interacts genetically with parkin. Nature 2006; 441:1162–1166.

80. Park J, Lee SB, Lee S, et al. Mitochondrial dysfunction in Drosophila PINK1 mutants is complemented by parkin. Nature 2006; 441:1157–1161.

81. Yang Y, Gehrke S, Imai Y, et al. Mitochondrial pathology and muscle and dopaminergic neuron degeneration caused by inactivation of Drosophila Pink1 is rescued by Parkin. Proc Natl Acad Sci USA 2006; 103:10793–10798.

82. Unoki M, Nakamura Y. Growth-suppressive effects of BPOZ and EGR2, two genes involved in the PTEN signaling pathway. Oncogene 2001; 20:4457–4465.

83. Silvestri L, Caputo V, Bellacchio E, et al. Mitochondrial import and enzymatic activity of PINK1 mutants associated to recessive parkinsonism. Hum Mol Genet 2005; 14:3477–3492.

84. Valente EM, Abou-Sleiman PM, Caputo V, et al. Hereditary early-onset Parkinson's disease caused by mutations in PINK1. Science 2004; 304:1158–1160.

85. Zadikoff C, Rogaeva E, Djarmati A, et al. Homozygous and heterozygous PINK1 mutations: considerations for diagnosis and care of Parkinson's disease patients. Mov Disord 2006; 21:875–879.

86. Brokars J. Fly Fishing on the Brain. In Bio-IT World, 2002.

20

Caenorhabditis elegans Models of Parkinson's Disease

Garry Wong

Department of Neurobiology, A.I. Virtanen Institute and Department of Biochemistry, Kuopio University, Kuopio, Finland

INTRODUCTION

The use of *Caenorhabditis elegans* as an animal model has its historical roots in the laboratory of Sydney Brenner during the early 1960s. Together with members of his laboratory, which included John Sulston and Robert Horvitz, these pioneers found and exploited the many advantageous features of the nematode as a model system. Initially, the idea was to find a system suitable for studying the fields of development and neuroscience. The model needed to be simple enough to manipulate genetically, yet sufficiently complex to probe deep questions relevant to higher organisms. Later, a few features of the nematode, which now seem obvious in hindsight, proved to be critical. First, the organism was transparent, which was essential to study cell-division, -proliferation, and -death within a living animal. Second, the organism had a reproductive cycle of three days, which allowed for extremely fast and convenient genetic analysis. Third, a point which is often overlooked by the scientific community, is that Sydney Brenner and his early colleagues encouraged a culture of sharing resources and information that has benefited not only the worm research community, but also has served as a model for many later, large scale scientific efforts, including the human genome sequencing project. These efforts culminated in the Nobel prize being awarded to these three early pioneers. Their legacy, however, may be better signified by the enormous collection of worm mutants, clones, sequences, and techniques that are utilized and shared by the worm research community which will be described in the following section.

CAENORHABDITIS ELEGANS GENETICS
Genomics
The entire *C. elegans* genome was sequenced and reported in 1998 (1). It was the first animal genome to be sequenced, and it provided insights into the number and variety of genes necessary to encode an entire multicellular organism. The 19,099 predicted genes turned out to be surprisingly close to the estimated 27,000 genes in humans. Moreover, the redundancy in gene families, when compared to the partially completed genomes of other organisms, suggested a stark resemblance and conservation between all animals, despite their diverse morphologies. This includes genes encoding neurotransmitter synthesis, storage, use, and signaling pathways (2). The gene sequence data itself now provide a firm source from which genetic approaches can be taken. Thus, genes can be knocked out or ectopically expressed from *C. elegans*, and, based on the function of the gene in *C. elegans*, the results can be interpreted and extrapolated to humans.

A major difference between *C. elegans* and human genomes is the compactness. Thus, the 19,099 predicted genes are spread through a genome size of 97 million

TABLE 1   Summary of Genetic Approaches Used in *C. elegans* Parkinson's Disease Models

C. elegans genetic approach	Description	References
Transgenics	Targeted deletion of genes (null mutants) or over expression of ectopic proteins	(3,4)
Forward genetic screens	Random mutagenesis of worm populations followed by selection of lines based on phenotypic criteria	(5)
RNA interference	Feeding, soaking, or microinjection of double stranded RNA to knock down expression of corresponding transcript	(7–9)
Microarrays	Profile of expression levels of RNA transcripts on a genome level	(11)

nucleotides, whereas the human genome of 27,000 genes occurs in a 3.1 billion sized genome. *C. elegans* genes are then about 20-fold more compact than human genes and span, on average, 5000 nucleotides in total. The actual total size for the gene might be more if coding on both strands taken in to account. The *C. elegans* genome also contains many poly-cistronic operons; thus more than one transcript can be expressed from a single promoter. The impact of a densely packed genome is not trivial. Since ectopic expression is driven by promoters, it has made it possible to collect and experimentally define promoters for thousands of genes. Indeed, it has led to a "promoterome" project where among the goals are the identification, cloning, and affordable distribution of all promoters of *C.elegans*. The genome of *C. elegans* ultimately provides a foundation from which the other experimental approaches rest (Table 1).

Transgenic and Knockout Lines

Production of *C. elegans* transgenic models is a streamlined process. In comparison with the production of mouse transgenic models, the steps required are considerably less involved. Expression vectors are composed of promoters a few thousand nucleotides in length located upstream of a copy DNA (cDNA) construct (3). The cDNA can be a *C. elegans* gene or a human gene. Polyadenosine signals and introns are also included in the construct. In the case of human genes, specific mutations or alleles can be incorporated into the cDNA portion of the construct. This DNA material is propagated by conventional cloning methods and purified. The DNA is then introduced directly into the gonad arms containing developing embryos of larvae stage 4 or young adult hermaphrodite worms by microinjection. Equipment for transgenic microinjection is identical to those used for mice. Worms are allowed to recover from injection and to continue develop to and lay eggs. The eggs from injected worms hatch within the next two to three days and are scored for transgenesis by a coinjection marker. The markers cause rescue of a mutant phenotype in the adult or a visible phenotype, such as movement. Green fluorescent protein (GFP) is also used as an easy to detect visible transgenic injection marker. Skilled laboratory personnel can inject, obtain, and confirm transgenic worms within a week of injection. The injected DNAs form extrachromosomal arrays and do not integrate into the genome except under very rare cases (<1%) of recombination. Nonintegrated transgenes are carried to the next generation at 10% to 90% transmission efficiency and thus need to be continually selected. For important transgenic worm lines, integration of the transgene can be accomplished by X- or γ-irradiation treatment followed by selection over many generations. Stable integrants are backcrossed into the wild type line and are necessary to remove extraneous random mutations caused by radiation.

The isolation of specific null-mutant alleles can be obtained by random mutagenesis of the entire *C. elegans* genome followed by polymerase chain reaction (PCR) analysis of individual pools (4). Up to 1000 genomes representing 500 different mutagenized worm lines can be pooled and screened at a time in a single PCR reaction in order to detect a single mutant. Successive dilution of pools and repeated PCR screening are performed until recovery of a single worm line with the mutation is identified. Although on the surface, this method appears laborious, a desired null-mutant allele can be isolated after 200–400 PCR reactions. Strategies to pool in multiple dimensions and multiplex PCR reactions permit even more efficient and faster screening of genomes. Because of the simple but large scale and highly repetitive nature of null-mutant screens, these methods are mostly carried out by core facilities.

A more classic method for mutagenesis screening relies on forward genetic principles. Here, populations of *C. elegans* are randomly mutagenized and allowed to propagate to the F2 generation (5). This is necessary to isolate homozygous recessive null alleles. Next, the mutagenized F2 *C. elegans* populations are screened for specific phenotypes. These phenotypes include movement disorders, morphologic changes, or resistance to toxins. Once isolated, the *C. elegans* mutant lines that continue to breed with the desired phenotype are then crossed to mapping strains of *C. elegans*. Segregation of the phenotype to a specific chromosome location marker eventually yields the approximate location of mutation that underlies the phenotype. Further experiments that include rescue of the phenotype by a candidate gene and sequencing of the gene in the mutant eventually lead to the identity of the gene causing the phenotype. These classic approaches, while laborious, have nonetheless linked particular genes to phenotypes. As one of the most powerful genetic tools available, it has provided the identity of genes and their encoded products that regulate processes such as apoptosis, cell specification, and neurotransmitter signalling, and memory among many others.

RNA Interference and Microarrays

A more recent approach to determine the effect of a gene on a phenotype is RNA interference (RNAi) (6). The accidental finding that RNA administration can decrease the number of complementary RNA molecules in the organism has created new opportunities to study the function of genes in a model system. Current knowledge suggests that double stranded RNA of 22–25 nucleotides in length are optimal in eliciting the RNAi effect (7). In *C. elegans*, several methodologic factors in how RNAi can be applied have brought this as a model to the forefront. *C. elegans* is sensitive to the effects of double stranded RNA whether it is administered by microinjection, soaked in the material, or fed *E. coli* that synthesizes in vivo the RNA. *E. coli* is the standard laboratory diet of *C. elegans*, so eating a different strain of bacteria producing the double stranded RNA is a routine procedure (8). The RNA is produced in the bacteria by a vector containing an RNA polymerase promoter that can be induced by chemical treatment. Since bacterial clones can be grown separately, each clone can represent a single *C. elegans* gene. Once ingested, the double-stranded RNA is chopped into 22–25 nucleotide pieces by the enzyme dicer, transported, and then amplified to its sites of action by a still yet poorly understood mechanism. Thus, it is possible to screen the entire genome of *C. elegans* simply by separately feeding

19,000 different bacterial cultures and scoring the phenotype after each feeding. Since *C. elegans* has the ability to live both on agar plates or in liquid culture, has a small size, and can ingest the bacteria, screening can be performed in 96 or 384 well plates, further streamlining the process (8,9). Several types of RNAi screens can be performed. One type of screen searches for the effect of a family of genes on a phenotype (again this can be movement, cell development, etc). A more powerful screening method utilizes a transgenic *C. elegans* model, such as a human disease model, that is fed different candidate RNAs. The knockdown of genes can enhance or suppress a phenotype in the model (10). Genes identified in this manner can be inferred to be involved in the expression of the phenotype as an enhancer or suppressor depending upon the effect of the RNAi molecule.

Microarrays are the most recent genomic approach that has been used to understand *C. elegans* as a model organism (11). Microarrays are spatially addressable microscope slides containing oligonucleotides or cDNAs of genes of interest. Hybridization onto the array of labeled cDNA or cRNA probes derived from a population of mRNAs provides a quantitative profile of the presence and levels of individual RNA transcripts within an organism transcriptome. Commercially available microarrays cover the entire *C. elegans* genome and thus provide a comprehensive picture of the state of each gene at a given time under a given condition. As a model organism, results from *C. elegans* microarray hybridizations can be compared between different transgenic models or after drug treatments. Comparisons can also be made between *C. elegans* models and other models in compendium studies. A large-scale study comparing gene expression profiles of humans, yeast, flies, and worms during aging showed conserved expression modules (12). These modules confirm common expression programs that indicate the validity of extrapolating microarray results across species. A major difference with *C. elegans* as a model is its small size and thus limited amount of RNA obtainable as experimental material. It has only recently been possible to perform microarray experiments with single worms and the method is not currently routine practice (13).

The transparency of *C. elegans* permits the visual analysis and inspection of all cells of the animal during its entire lifetime. Indeed, this ability to follow the fate of each cell and to establish its cell lineage is one of the strengths of this model organism (14). The adult hermaphrodite produces 1090 cells during its lifetime of which 131 undergoe programmed cell death to leave 959 cells total. The male produces 1179 cells of which 148 undergoe programmed cell death to leave 1031. In the adult hermaphrodite 302 cells are neurons. Approximately 200 of these neurons are located in the head region and arranged in a pattern called the nerve ring. Cells are named with a three or four letter abbreviation indicating their location and function. Adult hermaphrodites have eight dopaminergic neurons: two anterior deirid, four cephalic, and two posterior deirid neurons (15,16). Males have an additional five ray neurons. All of these neurons are easily visible under low power microscopy using either formaldehyde-induced fluorescence or by transgenic overexpression of GFP. Since their presence is easy to visualize, their deterioration or loss is also straightforward to score (17,18). Previous studies have used laser ablation to eliminate dopaminergic cells within the living and developing animal. Animals without dopaminergic neurons are still viable, but they have deficits in adjusting their rate of movement when foraging for food (19). There also appears to be deficits in the ability of males to mate with hermaphrodites. The typical mating "ritual" for *C. elegans* involves the male locating a hermaphrodite, and then sensing the vulva using its tail ray. The tail ray will feel along the entire body of the hermaphrodite until the vulva is located and will then insert its spicules for transfer of its genetic material. In *C. elegans*, the dopaminergic neurons are important for sensing the external environment. In addition, the dopaminergic neurons are also important as a modulator of muscular function such as in determining the rate of egg laying. *C. elegans* also uses neurotransmitters common in higher organisms such as serotonin, glutamate, gamma-aminobutyric acid (GABA), and acetylcholine. The use of histamine, adenosine, and glycine, norepinephrine or epinephrine as neurotransmitters has not yet been fully established in *C. elegans*.

CAENORHABDITIS ELEGANS MODELS
Mutant Lines
Early forward genetic screens of *C. elegans* mutants took advantage of the ability to detect various monoamines using formaldehyde-induced fluorescence. After random mutagenesis, worm lines were isolated and bred that displayed deficits in the amounts of dopamine, serotonin, or both. Gene mapping later identified these mutant lines as having mutations in the vesicular monoamine transporter (*cat-1*) (20), tyrosine hydroxylase (*cat-2*) (21), aromatic 1-aminoacid decarboxylase (*bas-1*) (22–23), and GTP cyclohydrolase 1 (*cat-4*) (22). These mutant lines have significantly less dopamine, <10%, compared to wild types and may also have less serotonin (*cat-1* and *cat-4*). Cat-1 and *cat-2* mutants move well although they have deficits in dopamine mediated sensory behaviors including rate of movement while grazing. Cat-4 mutants are sluggish and move slowly with diminished sine wave amplitude and distance traveled for a period of time. Dopamine receptor mutants have also been isolated using a directed mutagenesis strategy as well as by homology searches (24,25). Mutants of the *C. elegans* ortholog for human dopamine D-1 receptors (*dop-1*) also have deficits in dopamine mediated sensory responses while grazing but otherwise seem to move normally (26). These early mutant models highlight the robustness of *C. elegans* as a model system. With limited amounts of neurotransmitters, the animals remain viable and therefore amenable to genetic manipulation. The *C. elegans* orthologs for catechol-o-methyl transferase and monoamine oxidase have been identified. Null mutant allelles for these will eventually be available and should be useful for exploring the pharmacologic effects of anti-Parkinson's disease agents.

Transgenic Models
The production of transgenic *C. elegans* lines has been aimed to explore the pathology of disease progression in an experimental system. Many lines have been produced that are aimed at different stages or aspects of the disease (Table 2). One of the principle diagnostic criteria of Parkinson's disease is the loss of dopaminergic neurons from the substantia nigra. While it is known that neuronal loss occurs, symptoms of the disease are not normally seen until 80% of the neurons have been lost. Moreover, it is extraordinarily difficult to access loss of these neurons until autopsy. As *C. elegans* has only eight total dopaminergic neurons in the hermaphrodite, and these can be visualized through the transparent body using microscopy, a model of the neurodegeneration aspect of the pathology of the disease can be useful since the neurons can be visualized in the living animal (Fig. 1). A study by Nass and coworkers were able to mark all *C. elegans* dopaminergic neurons in living animals by transgenic overexpression of GFP using the *C. elegans* dopamine transporter (*dat-1*) promoter (27,28). Next, they were able to cause degeneration of these

TABLE 2 Summary of *Caenorhabditis elegans* Models Useful for Parkinson's Disease Studies

C. elegans model	Description	References
Isolated mutants	Worm lines from forward genetic screens lacking dopamine and other neurotransmitters.	(20–23)
Targeted null mutants	Worm lines from null mutant screens lacking dopamine receptors, or *PARKIN*.	(24–26,44)
Neurotoxic	Worms treated with neurotoxins coupled to transgenic GFP lines.	(28,42)
Transgenic	Worm lines over expressing genes, which lead to Parkinson's disease like pathology.	(28,31,41–43,46–52)

Abbreviation: GFP, green fluorescent protein.

neurons by treatment with the neurotoxin 6-hydroxydopamine. This loss of dopaminergic neurons could be seen quickly (within 30 minutes). Ultrastructural studies using electron microscopy revealed that the degeneration had properties consistent with apoptosis. The model was then used to address the question of whether there was a role for dopamine in the degeneration of the neurons (29). By crossing their GFP transgenic line with a line lacking a dopamine transporter (*dat-1*) they were able to show that a dopamine transporter was necessary for cell perturbations. They then crossed their GFP transgenic line with a line lacking cell death abnormality-3 (CED-3) and CED-4, both molecules crucial for mediating apoptosis driven cell pathways. These genes were not seen as necessary for dopaminergic cell death in this model, suggesting that the 6-hydroxydopamine–induced cell death had aspects of apoptosis that did not follow a classical death pathway. Other neurotoxins used to destroy dopaminergic neurons such as 1-methyl-4-phenyl-1,2,3,6-tetrahydropyridine (MPTP), rotanone, and mitochondrial function inhibitors have been suggested and could also be used in this approach. Since *C. elegans* grows in liquid culture, it would be possible to screen compounds in a high-throughput format. The approach would be then to combine neurotoxin with candidate neuroprotective agents and score for protection from degeneration of specific neuronal subtypes. *C. elegans* would be convenient in this respect since hundreds of animals could live for days in liquid culture in a 96 well plate format. Indeed the attraction of this approach is that it is an in vivo model, which would also incorporate other

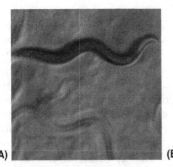 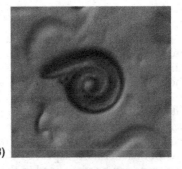

(A)   **(B)**

FIGURE 1 Movements of living wild type and transgenic *Caenorhabditis elegans*. The adult wild type worm (**A**) has an S-shaped posture and moves in a sigmatactic motion across an agar plate. A transgenic worm (**B**) overexpressing human α-synuclein A53T mutation in all neurons displays an abnormal coiled posture and moves irregularly. Photo is courtesy of Vuokko Aarnio.

aspects of drug screening such as absorption, distribution, metabolism, and excretion (30). With respect to drug metabolism, although *C. elegans* does not have a liver, it has nearly 100 putative cytochrome P-450 molecules that would prove valuable in a whole animal screening system that takes into account pharmacodynamic and pharmacokinetic properties.

A *C. elegans* transgenic model of human Parkinson's disease has been produced by overexpression of human α-synuclein (31). Mutations in α-synuclein cause a rare but highly penetrant form of Parkinson's disease that follows a dominant mode of inheritance (32). α-Synuclein is also found as the principle component of Lewy bodies and Lewy neurites, a primary neuropathologic feature of Parkinson's disease (33). Both the wild type and mutant forms of α-synuclein were overexpressed using different *C. elegans* promoters. α-Synuclein was overexpressed in dopaminerigic neurons using the *dat-1* promoter, in motor neurons using the acetylcholine receptor promoter, and in most visible neurons using a pan-neuronal promotor (27,34–35). *C. elegans* that overexpressed either wild type or mutant (alanine to threonine at position 53; A53T) α-synuclein showed loss of dopaminergic neurons when the transgene was expressed in those cells. When α-synuclein was overexpressed in most neurons or in motor neurons, the worms showed deficits in normal movement consisting of curling instead of the smooth and regular sine wave movement of nontransgenic worms. There was no evidence that worms had unilateral movement deficits: transgenic worms were able to turn both left and right. The amplitude of the sine wave was, however, attenuated, suggesting inability to fully contract its bilateral muscles. Worms also traveled less overall distance within a specific amount of time. Consistent with the role of dopaminergic neurons in *C. elegans* as a modulator of movement, rather than a direct effector, trangenic *C. elegans* overexpressing α-synuclein in dopaminergic neurons had movement scores similar to nontransgenic worms.

Several features of this transgenic model distinguish it from models in other organisms (36–40). First, the loss of dopaminergic neurons was seen at the young adult stage (four days) and did not show steady progression during aging, even up to 16 days, which is a substantial portion of the normal three weeks lifespan for *C. elegans*. Transgenes expressed under the *C. elegans* dopamine transporter are expressed already during the embryo stage, and transgenic animals can even be seen via the GFP coexpression marker while developing as an in vivo embryo. Controlled expression of the transgene under an inducible promoter can help to discern the timing of neurodegeneration, as well as to more finely control the expression of the transgene. Second, aggregates of α-synuclein in cells for which the transgenes were expressed were rare. This could be due to missing proteins necessary for aggregation in *C. elegans* or to the technical limitations of the study as neurons are smaller than many other cells in *C. elegans*. To solve this issue, it would be necessary to overexpress the transgene in nonneuronal cells that provide easier visual inspection of aggregate formation, such as the much larger body wall cells. Third, there seemed to be no difference in perturbations in the transgenic *C. elegans*, behavioural, or neuropathologic, depending upon whether the transgene was the wild type or mutant version of the gene. It should be noted that the overwhelming majority of Parkinson's disease cases arise sporadically with disease pathology marked by Lewy bodies containing wild type α-synuclein aggregates. Thus, this wild type α-synuclein *C. elegans* model might better describe the sporadic form rather than the mutant form.

Similar and more detailed findings were established by another research group producing overexpressing human transgenic α-synuclein in dopaminergic neurons (41). In their set of studies, wild type (WT) and mutant A30P and A53T transgenic worms showed dopaminergic neuron dendritic loss, which was more prominent in the mutants. Accompanied by this loss was the decrease in locomotor rate in response to food, a behavior mediated in *C. elegans* by dopaminergic neurons. These worms also displayed decreases in dopamine content, and exogenously added dopamine could rescue the behavioral phenotype.

Another group has investigated mitochodrial vulnerability in transgenic worms overexpressing α-synuclein (42). Transgenic worms overexpressing both WT and mutant alanine to threonine substitution at position 53 (A53T), as well as RNAi knockdown of the *C. elegans* PARKIN ortholog, showed increased vulnerability to several mitochondrial compex I inhibitors including rotonone. These lines were partially rescued by a mitochondrial complex II activator. Increased aggregation of α-synuclein could also be demonstrated in the overexpressing mutant A53T line when compared to WT, and this effect was even more pronounced when the worms were treated with rotonone. Interestingly, the WT and mutant A53T line did not show any changes in lifespan compared to nontransgenic animals while the *PARKIN* RNAi knockdown showed a significant decrease. In contrast, another study has shown increased lifespan in both WT and mutant A53T overexpressing lines that is independent of the *daf-2* insulin like receptor signalling pathway (43). Differences in the lifespan results between these two studies might be due to the different transgenic promoters used, but other technical explanations are possible.

PARKIN is another human PD protein that has a recessive mode of inheritance in man and a worm ortholog. A series of genetic deletion mutants have been obtained in *C. elegans* (44). While the initial phenotypic characterization of most loss of function mutants revealed no obvious phenotypes in reproduction, morphology, or lifespan; an in-frame deletion variant displayed increased sensitivity to proteotoxic stress. Moreover, in a genetic background consisting of overexpressing human α-synuclein A53T, the in-frame *PARKIN* deletion variant worms had severe developmental defects and displayed a temperature sensitive lethal phenotype. In contrast, these abnormal phenotypes were absent in an overexpressing human WT α-synuclein background. The *C. elegans* PARKIN in-frame deletion variant protein itself aggregates when expressed in cell culture, and this is enhanced by coexpression of A53T and not WT human α-synuclein. Finally, this *PARKIN* variant protein maintains the ability to interact with its ubiquitylation coenzymes.

Protein Aggregation Models

Protein aggregation has become an important unifying theme in the study of neuropathology of neurodegenerative diseases. Aggregation is believed to be a defining step in the formation of pathologic hallmarks from Lewy bodies in Parkinson's disease to amyloid placques in Alzheimer's disease. The inability to correctly fold, process, or eliminate proteins leads to aggregation. Among these proteins, polyglutamine lengths in the huntingtonin protein are correlated with disease outcome in Huntington's disease. The polyglutamine length has also been shown experimentally to directly correlate with aggregate formation. As a model to study protein aggregation in vivo, transgenic overexpressing *C. elegans* have been produced with varying lengths of glutamine (45–48). Only longer stretches of glutamine (>30 Q) are sufficient to form protein aggregates in vivo. Aggregates can easily be visualized in living worms since the glutamine stretches are fused to a fluorescent protein, either GFP or yellow fluorescent protein (YFP) in the transgenic construct. Transgenic

C. elegans overexpressing polyglutamines also display movement deficits such as paralysis. These models demonstrate that *C. elegans* can be used to model some of the features of human diseases.

Another transgenic *C. elegans* model, with direct relevance to the aggregation of α-synuclein has been produced that overexpresses torsin. Torsin dystonia is a human movement disorder characterized by twisting contortions and involuntary muscle contractions. An autosomal dominant form of the disease is linked to deletions in the human torsin-A gene. *C. elegans* has three torsin homologs related to the human gene. One of these, torsin-2, was overexpressed in *C. elegans* both in the presence and absence of an 82 residue polyglutamine stretch (Q82) fused to GFP. Using both a human wild type and mutant torsin-2 changed in residue 368, it was shown that the human wild type version could suppress aggregation whereas the mutant version could not (49). More importantly, overexpression of torsins in *C. elegans* and other model systems can reduce the formation of aggregates of human α-synuclein (50–51).

Another transgenic model produced overexpresses the human wild type and mutant tau (52). Tau protein is found to accumulate as aggregates in neuronal and glial fibrillary tangles. It is seen in neurodegenerative diseases including Alzheimer's disease. Mutations in human tau underly frontotemporal dementia with parkinsonism. The transgenic animals in this study displayed movement deficits, loss of neurons, and accumulation of insoluble aggregates of tau. The model also demonstrated that the behavioral phenotype, uncoordinated movement, as well as pathologic hallmarks, such as latency to tau accummulation, and severity of axonal degeneration were greater in transgenic lines expressing the human mutant versions (P301L and V337M) than the wild type.

A more open screening approach using RNAi has been implemented to identify suppressors and enhancers of polyglutamine aggregation. Different length stretches of glutamine (Q0–40) were fused to YFP and transgenic animals with the integrated constructs produced. The transgenes were expressed in muscle cells to aid visualization using fluorescence microscopy. Whereas worms overexpressing up to Q24 showed diffuse YFP expression in muscle cells, those with Q40 or longer show punctate localization (47–8). These animals were grown in 96 well liquid culture plates containing *E. coli* producing double stranded RNA. In the whole genome screen 10–15 transgenic worms synchronized to the L1 developmental stage expressing Q24 or Q33 were grown in each well containing *E. coli* producing a *C. elegans* double stranded RNA representing a single gene. After three days of growth in these plates, worms were scored for suppression of aggregates (10). The screen revealed 186 genes which corresponded to five principle classes: RNA synthesis and processing, 38 genes; protein synthesis, 53 genes; protein folding, 10 genes; protein transport, 25 genes; protein degradation 14 genes; and other, 46 genes. These results suggest a common protein pathway from synthesis to degradation that participates in the handling of protein. These proteins are important regulators of polyglutamine aggregation in *C. elegans* and may be important regulators of protein aggregation in general. Since the screen was designed to find novel enhancers of protein aggregation, their identification should open up new strategies for interrupting this important neuropathologic process.

Finally, a microarray study on transgenic *C. elegans* overexpressing human α-synuclein has been performed (53). Both WT and mutant A53T worm lines were profiled and >400 upregulated genes and ~170 downregulated common genes were found. The genes fell into several categories, but the most prominent groups of upregulated genes were involved in mitochondrial function and the proteasomal pathway. The microarray study suggests that such functional genomic approaches may validate previous biochemical and cell biology investigations. Among the downregulated genes were genes involved in nuclear function. This is rather curious since the nucleous is the subcellular organelle, in addition to the synapse, where α-synuclein is abundant and from where the protein has derived its name.

CONCLUSIONS

In summary, the creation of several *C. elegans* models to understand pathology of Parkinson's disease has been shown. Basic overexpressing transgenic lines have been produced that recapitulate some of the aspects of the human disease. While the primary weakness of these models may be the inability to mimic some of the cardinal features of the disease that includes resting tremor, rigidity, postural instability, and bradykinesia, many of the neuropathologic features can be observed. Deficits in motor function could also be observed in some of these models. The extent to which these uncoordinated movements correlate to human movement remains to be determined. On the cell level, degeneration of dopaminergic neurons that are characterized by perturbations in cell body and axonal morphology can be seen in several models. On the biochemical level, these include the formation of protein aggregates.

Transgenic *C. elegans* models using human cDNAs have only been applied to a limited number. In addition, knockouts or knockdowns of particular human genes genetically linked to Parkinson's disease have still to be created and reported. These would include genes that have known *C. elegans* orthologs such as *PARKIN*, ubiquitin hydrolase (*UCH-L1*), and *DJ-1* (54–56). The generation of a transgenic or neurochemical *C. elegans* model of Parkinson's disease, as it is with other animal models, is only the beginning. The models that have already been produced can be exploited by means of functional genomic approaches to gain deeper understanding into disease pathogenesis. Follow-up studies that utilize crosses to preexisting mutant lines, whole genome RNAi screening for supressors or enhancers, and microarray analysis, as a whole should provide new clues and identify novel protein interactions that are critical for progression toward biochemical and cellular pathology. Such information, when coupled to data obtained from other model systems, such as those in mice, drosophila, and zebrafish, could provide an overall concept of the conserved changes common in all living systems. Exploitation of the information obtained using bioinformatics should further help to unravel new possible players in the disease and thus lead to novel therapeutic approaches.

It should be emphasized that while most of these approaches work backward from a neuropathologic perspective, the initial events and etiology of Parkinson's disease in the majority of cases remain enigmatic. The role of molecules that are involved in development and specification of dopaminergic neurons such as Nurr1, LIM homeodomain transcription factor Lmx1b, and Pitx3, all of which have orthologs in elegans remains to be explored (57–60). The cloning of these genes and transgenic over expression, or knockdown by RNAi in *C. elegans* models should be relatively straighforward to perform experimentally yet provide broad insights into an important part of the developmental process of dopaminergic neurons.

Finally, *C. elegans* has already been proven to be a model that produces dramatic insights into such fundamental biology processes as development, aging, and behavior. In the future, the availability of current high throughput genome-level approaches and their implementation should provide in the future such large amounts of data that the probability of breakthroughs in the understanding of Parkinson's disease pathobiology is assured.

REFERENCES

1. *C. elegans* Sequencing Consortium. Genome sequence of the nematode *Caenorhabditis elegans*: a platform for investigating biology. Science 1998; 282:2012–2018.
2. Miller KG, Alfonso A, Nguyen M. A genetic selection for *Caenorhabditis elegans* synaptic transmission mutants. Proc Natl Acad Sci USA 1996; 93:12593–12598.
3. Mello C, Fire A. DNA transformation Methods. Cel Biol 1995, 48:451–482.
4. Jansen G, Thijssen KL, Werner P, et al. The complete family of genes encoding G proteines of *Caenorhabditis elegans*. Nature Genet 1999; 21:414–419.
5. Jorgensen EM, Mango S. The art and design of genetic screens: *Caenorhabditis elegans*. Nature Rev Genet 2002; 3:356–369.
6. Fire A, Xu S, Montgomery, et al. Potent and specific genetic interference by double stranded RNA in *Caenorhabditis elegans*. Nature 1998; 391:806–881.
7. Meister G, Tuschl T. Mechanisms of gene silencing by double-stranded RNA. Nature 2004; 431:343–349.
8. Kamath RS, Martinez-Campos M, Zipperlen P, et al. Effectiveness of specific RNA-mediated interference through ingested double-stranded RNA in *Caenorhabditis elegans*. Genome Biol 2001; 2:1–10.
9. Kamath RS, Fraser AG, Dong Y, et al. Systemic functional analysis of the *Caenorhabditis elegans* genome using RNAi. Nature 2003; 421:231–237.
10. Nollen EAA, Garcia SM, van Haaften G, et al. Genome-wide RNA interference screen identifies previously undescribed regulators of polyglutamine aggregation. Proc Natl Acad Sci USA 2004; 101:6403–6408.
11. Reinke V. Functional exploration of the *C. elegans* genome using DNA microarrays. Nat Genet 2002; 32(suppl):541–546.
12. McCarroll SA, Murphy CT, Zou S, Comparing genomic expression patterns across species identifies shared transcriptional profile in aging. Nat Genet 2004; 36:197–204.
13. Golden TR, Melov S. Microarray analysis of gene expression with age in individual nematodes. Aging Cell 2004; 3:111–124.
14. White JG, Southgate E, Thomson JN, et al. The structure of the nervous system of the nematode *Caenorhabditis elegans*. Philos Trans R Soc Lond B Biol Sci 1986; 314:1–340.
15. Sulston J, Dew M, Brenner S. Dopaminergic neurons in the nematode *C. elegans*. J Comp Neurol 1975; 163:215–226.
16. Nass R, Blakely RD. The *Caenorhabditis elegans* dopaminergic system: opportunities for insights into dopamine transport and neurodegeneration. Annu Rev Pharmacol Toxicol 2003; 43:521–544.
17. Crittenden SL, Kimble J. Confocal methods for *Caenorhabditis elegans*. Methods Mol Biol 1999; 122:141–151.
18. Miller DM, Shakes DC. Immunofluorescence microscopy. Methods Cell Biol 1995; 48:365–394.
19. Sawin ER. Genetic and cellular analysis of modulated behaviors in *Caenorhabditis elegans*. 1996. PhD thesis, Massachusetts Institute of Technology.
20. Duerr JS, Frisby DL, Gaskin J, et al. The *cat-1* gene of *Caenorhabditis elegans* encodes a vesicular monoamine transporter required for specific monoamine-dependent behaviors. J Neurosci 1999; 19:72–84.
21. Lints R, Emmons SW. Patterning of dopaminergic neurotransmitter identity among *Caenorhabditis elegans* ray sensory neurons by a TGFβ family signaling pathway and a *Hox* gene. Development 1999; 126:5819–5831.
22. Loer CM, Kenyon CJ. Serotonin-deficient mutants and male mating behavior in the nematode *Caenorhabditis elegans*. J Neurosci 1993; 13:5407–5417
23. Wintle RF, Van Tol HH. Dopamine signaling in *Caenorhabditis elegans*-potential for parkinsonism research. Parkinsonism Rel Dis 2001; 7:177–183.
24. Suo S, Sasagawa N, Ishiura S. Identification of a dopamine receptor from *Caenorhabditis elegans*. Neurosci Lett 2002; 319:13–16.

25. Suo S, Sasagawa N, Ishiura S. Cloning and characterization of a *Caenorhabditis elegans* D2-like dopamine receptor. J Neurochem 2003; 86:869–878.
26. Sanyal S, Wintle RF, Kindt KS, et al. Dopamine modulates the plasticity of mechanosensory responses in *Caenorhabditis elegans*. EMBO J 2004; 23:473–482.
27. Jayanthi LD, Apparsundaram S, Malone MD, et al. The *Caenorhabditis elegans* gene T23G5.5 encodes an antidepressant- and cocaine-sensitive dopamine transporter. Mol Pharmacol 1998; 54:601–609.
28. Nass R, Hall DH, Miller DM 3rd, et al. Neurotoxin-induced degeneration of dopamine eurons in *Caenorhabditis elegans*. Proc Natl Acad Sci USA 2002; 99:3264–3269.
29. Lee FJS, Liu F, Pristupa ZB, et al. Direct binding and functional coupling of α-synuclein to the dopamine transporters accelerate dopamine-induced apoptosis. FASEB J 2001; 15:916–926.
30. Baumeister R, Ge L. The worm in us—*Caenorhabditis* as a model of human disease. Trends Biotech 2002; 20:147–148.
31. Lakso M, Vartiainen S, Moilanen AM, et al. Dopaminergic neuronal loss and motor deficits in *Caenorhabditis elegans* overexpressing human α-synuclein. J Neurochem 2003; 86:165–172.
32. Polymeropoulos MH, Lavedan C, Leroy E, et al. Mutation in the α-synuclein gene identified in families with Parkinson's disease. Science 1997; 276:2045–2047.
33. Spillantini MG, Schmidt ML, Lee VM, et al. α-Synuclein in Lewy bodies. Nature 1997; 388:839–840.
34. Hallam S, Singer E, Waring D, et al. The *C. elegans* NeuroD homolog cnd-1 functions in multiple aspects of motor neuron fate specification. Development 2000; 127:4239–4252.
35. Iwasaki K, Staunton J, Saifee O, et al. aex-3 encodes a novel regulator of presynaptic activity in *C. elegans*. Neuron 1997; 18:613–622.
36. Masliah E, Rockenstein E, Veinbergs I, et al. Dopaminergic loss and inclusion body formation in α-synuclein mice: implications for neurodegenerative disorders. Science 2000; 287:1265–1268.
37. Feany MB, Bender WW. A Drosophila model of Parkinson's disease. Nature 2000; 404:394–398.
38. van der Putten H, Wiederhold KH, Probst A, et al. Neuropathology in mice expressing human α-synuclein. J Neurosci 2000; 20:6021–6029.
39. Kirik D, Rosenblad C, Burger C, et al. Parkinson-like neurodegeneration induced by targeted over expression of α-synuclein in the nigrostriatal system. J Neurosci 2002; 22:2780–2791.
40. Lee MK, Stirling W, Xu Y, et al. Human α-synuclein-harboring familial Parkinson's disease-linked Ala-53 → Thr mutation causes neurodegenerative disease with α-synuclein aggregation in transgenic mice. Proc Natl Acad Sci USA 2002; 99:8968–8973.
41. Kuwahara T, Koyama A, Gengyo-Ando K, et al. Familial Parkinson mutant alpha-synuclein causes dopamine neuron dysfunction in transgenic Caenorhabditis elegans. J Biol Chem 2006; 281:334–340.
42. Ved R, Saha S, Westlund, et al. Similar patterns of mitochondrial vulnerability and rescue induced by genetic modification of alpha-synuclein, parkin, and DJ-1 in Caenorhabditis elegans. J Biol Chem 2005; 280:42655–42668.
43. Vartiainen S, Aarnio V, Lakso M, et al. Increased lifespan in transgenic Caenorhabditis elegans overexpressing human alpha-synuclein. Exp Gerontol 2006; 41:871–876.
44. Springer W, Hoppe T, Schmidt E, et al. A Caenorhabditis elegans Parkin mutant with altered solubility couples alpha-synuclein aggregation to proteotoxic stress. Hum Mol Genet 2005; 14:3407–3423.
45. Faber PW, Alter JR, MacDonald ME, et al. Polyglutamine-mediated dysfunction and apoptotic death of a *Caenorhabditis elegans* sensory neuron. Proc Natl Acad Sci USA 1999; 96:179–184.
46. Parker JA, Connolly JB, Wellington C, et al. Expanded polyglutamines in *Caenorhabditis elegans* cause axonal abnormalities and severe dysfunction of PLM mechanosensory neurons without cell death. Proc Natl Acad Sci USA 2001; 98:13318–13323.
47. Morley JF, Brignull HR, Weyers JJ, et al. The threshold for polyglutamine-expansion protein aggregation and cellular toxicity is dynamic and influenced by aging in *Caenorhabditis elegans*. Proc Natl Acad Sci USA 2002; 99:10417–10422.

48. Satyal SH, Schmidt E, Kitagawa N, et al. Polyglutamine aggregates alter protein-folding homeostasis in Caenorhabditis elegans. Proc Natl Acad Sci USA 2000; 97:5750–5755.
49. Caldwell GA, Cao S, Sexton EG, et al. Suppression of polyglutamine-induced protein aggregation in Caenorhabditis elegans by torsin proteins. Hum Mol Genet 2003; 12:307–319.
50. McLean PJ, Kawamata H, Shariff S, et al. TorsinA and heat shock proteins act as molecular chaperones: suppression of α-synuclein aggregation. J Neurochem 2002, 83:846–854.
51. Caldwell GA, Cao S, Izevbaye I, et al. Use of C. elegans to model human movement disorders. In: LeDoux M, ed. Animal Model of Movement Disorders, 1st ed. Burlington, MA: Elsevier Academic Press, 2004:111–126.
52. Kraemer BC, Zhang B, Leverenz JB, et al. Neurodegeneration and defective neurotransmission in a Caenorhabditis elegans model of tauopathy. Proc Natl Acad Sci USA 2003; 100:9980–9985.
53. Vartiainen S, Pehkonen P, Lakso M, et al. Identification of gene expression changes in transgenic C. elegans overexpressing human alpha-synuclein. Neurobiol Dis 2006; 22: 477–486.
54. Lucking CB, Durr A, Bonifati V, et al. Association between early-onset Parkinson's disease and mutations in the parkin gene. French Parkinson's disease genetics study group. N Engl J Med 2000; 342:1560–1567.
55. Leroy E, Boyer R, Auburger G, et al. The ubiquitin pathway in Parkinson's disease. Nature 1999; 395:451–452.
56. Bonifati V, Rizzu P, van Baren MJ, et al. Mutations in the DJ-1 gene associated with autosomal recessive early-onset Parkinsonism. Science 2003; 299:256–259.
57. Zetterstrom RH, Solomin L, Jansson L, et al. Dopamine neuron agenesis in Nurr1-deficient mice. Science 1997; 276:248–250.
58. Smidt MP, Asbreuk CH, Cox JJ, et al. A second independent pathway for development of mesencephalic dopaminergic neurons requires Lmx 1b. Nat Neuroscience 2000; 3:337–341.
59. Van den Munckhof P, Luk KC, Ste-Marie L, et al. Pitx3 is required for motor activity and for survival of a subset of midbrain dopaminergic neurons. Development 2003; 130:2535–2542.
60. Nunes I, Tovmasian LT, Silva RM, et al. Pitx3 is required for development of substantia nigra dopaminergic neurons. Proc Natl Acad Sci USA 2003; 100:4245–4250.

21

The MPTP Model of Parkinson's Disease

Serge Przedborski

Department of Neurology, Pathology, and Cell Biology and Center for Motor Neuron Biology and Disease, Columbia University, New York, New York, U.S.A.

INTRODUCTION

In his monograph "The case of the frozen addicts," William Langston reported the story of six patients, who, in 1982, in California, developed mysterious symptoms provoked by 1-methyl-4-phenyl-1,2,3,6-tetrahydropyridine (MPTP) that were reminiscent of Parkinson's disease (PD). Since that time, MPTP has been recognized as a highly selective neurotoxin; in reality, this compound has a much longer history (1). Apparently, the synthesis of MPTP was first reported by Ziering and his colleagues in 1947 as part of a series of papers on meperidine derivatives (2), and, using these methods, it was shown that piperidols may be acylated with a propionic group to produce MPPP (1-methyl-4-phenyl-4-propionoxypiperidine), a compound 25 times more potent than morphine in the rat (2,3). Since then, MPTP has been used extensively as a synthetic intermediate in meperidine chemistry and has become commercially available (Aldrich Chemical Company, Milwaukee, Wisconsin) for this purpose long before it had been identified as a potent neurotoxin.

Early studies involving MPTP received little attention and were probably not even published. Ironically, MPTP was first investigated in the early 1950s as an antiparkinsonian agent (3a). Rats treated with MPTP failed to develop any neurological problems, while two monkeys given a single dose of MPTP (0.5 mg/kg subcutaneously) developed severe limb rigidity less than two days after the injection. Two other monkeys given a higher dose of MPTP (2 mg/kg) became extremely rigid and totally immobile by the third day after the injection; both were dead by the end of the second and third weeks. Despite these reported findings in monkeys, investigators did not come to the conclusion that MPTP administration caused behavioral changes resembling parkinsonism. As part of the same investigation, MPTP was administered to six parkinsonian patients in doses ranging from 50 to 300 mg/kg daily for three weeks. Two of these patients died during or shortly after the trial presumably from uremia, pancreatitis, cholecystitis, and congestive heart failure. Following this observation, MPTP was abandoned because of its toxicity. No further details regarding these patients had been collected.

The first published case of MPTP-induced toxicity in humans involved a graduate student who succeeded in producing MPPP for his personal consumption using Zeiring's method (4). After several months of MPPP abuse, he apparently decided to increase the reaction temperature and to abandon the purification step to reduce the preparation time of the compound. Unfortunately, the amount of MPPP produced by this method was markedly dependent upon experimental conditions and drastic conditions, such as those caused by using excess acid or higher reaction temperatures dramatically increased the amount of MPTP generated. Not surprisingly shortly after he altered the protocol, he became severely parkinsonian. His symptoms were well controlled by levodopa/carbidopa and large doses of bromocriptine. Less than two years after the onset of illness, the patient was found dead of an overdose. Neuropathological changes were characterized mainly by a loss of nigrostriatal dopaminergic neurons (see MPTP-induced parkinsonism in humans below for details).

Four years later, in Vancouver, another young drug addict attempted to synthesize MPPP using the Schimdle and Mansfield formula. After he snorted his home-synthesized meperidine analog daily for seven days, he was admitted to the hospital in an immobile, mute state (5). This addict was first diagnosed as having an acute psychotic episode with catatonia and was treated with neuroleptics for about a year without any significant improvement. At that time, the patient was admitted to another institution, where he was found to present severe bradykinesia, stooped posture, shuffling gait, excessive drooling, and severe dysarthria. He was diagnosed as having parkinsonism and was started on levodopa/carbidopa, to which he responded dramatically. About 20 months after the onset of the illness, he died in a drowning accident. The delay between the death and autopsy was too long, and thus no appropriate examination of the basal ganglia or the substantia nigra could be done. A definite identification was not made, even though in these first two cases MPPP or an intermediate compound was the suspected damaging agent.

The next case found in the literature of possible MPTP toxicity in humans is of particular interest since it may represent an example of cutaneous absorption or vapor inhalation (6). In 1964, an organic chemist working for a major pharmaceutical company began synthesizing many compounds, which required repeated preparation of MPTP (he synthesized more than 3 kg MPTP). There were many opportunities for cutaneous contact or inhalation of MPTP, which was purified by vacuum distillation, since no evidence of intravenous exposure to MPTP could be found. In 1970, when the patient was 37 years old, he began experiencing coordination difficulty in his left hand and, within a year, he was diagnosed as having PD. There has been some progression of his symptoms since that time, with generalized cogwheel rigidity, bradykinesia, facial hypomimia, and stooped posture; no tremor was present. In 1991, he was reported as taking levodopa/carbidopa, and had an excellent clinical response to this therapy (6a).

Recognition that MPTP, a by-product of MPPP synthesis, was toxic finally occurred after MPPP was again produced for illicit use in northern California during 1982 (6b). This time, however, it was destined for mass distribution. In the early spring and summer of 1982, several young drug addicts mysteriously developed a profound parkinsonian syndrome after the intravenous use of street preparations of meperidine analogs sold as heroin, synthetic heroin, Mexican brown heroin ("organic heroin"), and "china white" (high-grade heroin from southeast Asia). After tracking down samples of the "heroin" for analyses and searching for additional cases, it became evident that MPTP was most likely the offending agent (7). In addition, this view was further supported by the fact that the "epidemic" started not long after contaminated batches of MPPP containing MPTP (one contained almost pure MPTP) began appearing on the street (6b).

MPTP-INDUCED PARKINSONISM IN HUMANS

It is estimated that more than 400 drug addicts might have been exposed to MPTP (7a). However, among these only a small number have been interviewed and examined. Therefore, it is important to emphasize that the epidemiologic data available on MPTP-induced parkinsonism in humans derived from studies performed on a limited number of affected individuals (8,9).

Index Cases

Case histories of the seven individuals discovered in 1982 as having MPTP-induced parkinsonism have been reviewed by Ballard et al. (9). In four of the seven cases, samples of the drug they had been using were analyzed and were found to contain a high proportion of MPTP. All of the seven patients displayed a characteristic clinical syndrome involving two stages: an acute phase followed by a chronic phase.

During the acute stage, all patients noted a burning sensation when the drug was injected intravenously. The immediate subjective effect included a heroin-like euphoria, but more dream-like. Disorientation, blurred vision, visual delusions, or hallucinations were also noted by some patients. The initial motor symptoms included intermittent, jerking movements of the limbs, increasing slowness, or both. Jerking movements generally disappeared within a few days, to be followed by slowness and stiffness, difficulty in speaking and swallowing, and in some cases, tremor. This progressed over several days to three weeks. By the time they reached the chronic stage of the disease, patients displayed most of the hallmarks of PD (Table 1). There was no autonomic impairment, cerebellar, or pyramidal signs. Six of these patients were also studied to assess intellectual functions (10). The authors found a slight but significant difference between the MPTP group and healthy controls in the level of general intellectual function on the modified mini-mental status examination, which was due to poor performance by the MPTP group on orientation, naming presidents, and construction subtests. MPTP patients also exhibited a significantly poorer performance on tests of construction (Rosen Drawing Test), verbal fluency (Category Naming), and executive function (Stroop Word-Color Test). Although patients with MPTP-induced parkinsonism performed less effectively than controls on these tasks, none met criteria for dementia. Performance on attention tests (reaction time and continuous performance tests), memory, attention, digit span, calculation, and overall language test (other than verbal fluency) was comparable in the two groups. Interestingly, the authors observed that the tasks on which the MPTP group exhibited a poorer performance than controls were comparable to the pattern of neuropsychological deficits seen in PD (11). Spinal fluid analyses performed in six of the patients showed that homovanillic acid (HVA) levels, the major metabolite of dopamine, were markedly reduced, whereas the levels of the serotonin metabolite, 5-hydroxyindoleacetic acid, and 3-methoxy-4-hydroxyphenylethylene glycol, the major metabolite of norepinephrine, were normal and elevated, respectively, compared to the levels measured in six healthy subjects (12). In all seven patients, the administration of levodopa/carbidopa alone or with dopamine agonists resulted in dramatic improvement. However, all developed early side effects to the treatment such as "wearing-off" effect, "peak-dose" dyskinesias, or "on–off" fluctuations.

Other MPTP-Exposure Cases in Humans

Ruttenber et al. (9) described the results of interviews and physical examinations of 83 individuals who allegedly were exposed to MPTP. Among these, 80% had at least one of the following clinical signs of parkinsonism and 60% had two or more: lack of facial expression, "en bloc" turning, action tremor, bradykinesia, impairment in rapid alternative movements, seborrhea, or resting tremor. In addition, 49% had increased tone and 64% had cogwheel rigidity in at least one limb. Although the acute and chronic symptoms of these patients were similar to those found in the index cases, they were less severe. This finding supports the hypothesis that the index cases received a heavy exposure to MPTP (9).

TABLE 1 Signs of Parkinson's Disease in MPTP Patients

Features of idiopathic Parkinson's disease	Severity in untreated MPTP patients						
	1	2	3	4	5	6	7
Bradykinesia	+++	+++	+++	+++	+++	+	++
Rigidity	+++	++	+++	++	+++	+	++
Resting tremor	0	++	0	0	++	+++	+++
Flexion posture	++	++	+++	++	++	++	++
Loss of postural reflexes	++	+	+++	++	+++	+	++
Loss of associated movements	+++	++	+++	++	+++	++	++
Shuffling, *petit pas* gait	++	++	+++	++	+++	+	++
En bloc turning	++	++	+++	++	+++	+	++
Difficulty initiating movements	++	++	+++	++	+++	+	++
Cogwheeling	++	++	+	+	+++	+++	+++
Loss of finger dexterity	++	++	+++	++	+++	++	++
Micrographia	++	++	+++	++	+++	+	+
Masked facies	+++	++	+++	++	+++	++	++
Reduced blink rate	+++	+++	+++	++	+++	++	++
Widened palpebral fissure	+++	+++	+++	++	+++	++	+
Limitation of upward gaze	++	+	++	++	0	0	0
Glabellar sign	+++	++	+++	++	+++	++	+
Hypophonia	+++	++	+++	++	+++	++	+
Drooling	++	++	+++	++	+++	++	+
Difficulty swallowing	++	++	+++	+	+++	++	0
Freezing	#	#	#	#	#	0	#
Kinesia paradoxical	#	#	#	#	#	0	0
Seborrhea	+	+++	+	+	+++	++	0
Diaphoresis	0	0	0	0	0	++	0
Hoehn and Yahr score[a]	V	V	V	IV	V	IV	IV

Note: 0, absent; +, mild; ++, moderate; +++, severe; #, present but not rated.
[a]Score: IV = severe disability; still able to walk or stand unassisted; V = wheelchair bound or bedridden unless aided.
Abbreviation: MPTP, 1-methyl-4-phenyl-1,2,3,6-tetrahydropyridine.
Source: From Ref. 8.

Another group of MPTP-affected individuals was described by Tetrud et al. (13). In their study, the authors compared 22 individuals with mild parkinsonism resulting from MPTP exposure to 130 patients with early, untreated PD and 51 intravenous narcotic users not exposed to MPTP. The MPTP-exposed group was highly comparable to the patients with early PD, except for a lower prevalence of resting tremor. Interestingly, intravenous narcotic users not exposed to MPTP had no signs of parkinsonism, suggesting that drug abuse alone does not cause these neurological manifestations.

The parkinsonian syndrome induced by MPTP in humans is clinically indistinguishable from PD except for a few features. First, after onset, parkinsonism worsens slowly in PD patients, but much faster in MPTP-intoxicated individuals. Second, whether an acute exposure to MPTP causes a progressive neurodegeneration like in PD remains a debatable issue. Indeed, Burns and collaborators reported the case of a young chemist who developed parkinsonism after substantial laboratory exposure to MPTP and who failed to show any evidence of worsening of his neurological condition over several years (14). Yet, positron emission tomography (PET) performed twice, seven years apart, on 10 individuals exposed to MPTP, revealed worsening of striatal [^{18}F]fluorodopa uptake in these patients (15). Moreover, postmortem studies in three individuals who survived 3 to 16 years after exposure to MPTP (16) and in six monkeys that survived 5 to 14 years after exposure to MPTP (17) showed evidence of extracellular neuromelanin and activated microglia in the substantia nigra, two neuropathological features consistent with an ongoing degenerative process. Third, dementia has not been documented in individuals with MPTP-induced parkinsonism either.

Brain pathology is another aspect upon which PD and MPTP are somewhat divergent. At autopsy, brains from PD patients exhibit a severe loss of large neuromelanin-containing neurons in the substantia nigra. This cell loss is associated with characteristic eosinophilic intracytoplamic inclusions called Lewy bodies. Other areas showing degenerative changes include the locus coeruleus, the dorsal motor nucleus of the vagus, and the basal nucleus of Meynert; these changes are also accompanied by the presence of Lewy bodies. In the four known brains from MPTP-intoxicated individuals who underwent neuropathological examination (4,16), there was a marked neuronal loss and gliosis limited to the pars compacta of the substantia nigra and minor changes in the locus coeruleus. The other pigmented nuclei did not show pathological changes nor could any compelling evidence of Lewy body in the diseased areas be found, and that in contrast to the situation encountered typically in PD. The fact that the dopaminergic system in MPTP-exposed individuals is affected has been further documented by using PET with [^{18}F]-fluorodopa to label the dopaminergic neurons in vivo (18). The study demonstrated that the striatal uptake of 6-fluorodopa was markedly reduced in all six MPTP-exposed individuals compared to normal controls (18). Subsequently, the pattern of striatal loss of [^{18}F]-fluorodopa uptake was compared between nine MPTP-exposed individuals with parkinsonism and six PD patients (19). This study demonstrated that there was an equal degree of reduction of dopaminergic function in the caudate and putamen in the MPTP group, whereas there was the typical greater putaminal than caudate loss in the PD group (19). These findings suggest that while MPTP damages the nigrostriatal pathway, the injury may be too harsh or acute to elicit the PD-like putaminal/caudate gradient of loss. Consistent with this view is the work of Moratalla and collaborators (20), which demonstrates that the regional pattern of dopaminergic loss seen in the striatum of PD patients could be recapitulated in monkeys only if the intoxication was achieved with low doses of MPTP.

MPTP-INDUCED PARKINSONISM IN ANIMALS

Shortly after MPTP was found to provoke a parkinsonian syndrome in humans, researchers were prompted to test MPTP toxicity in a variety of animal species including monkeys, dogs, cats, and rodents (21,22). These investigations showed that most of the vertebrates and invertebrates tested were sensitive to the neurotoxic effects of MPTP (21,22), but with marked differences among species. Among mammals, monkeys, for example, were by far the most sensitive to MPTP whereas rats and guinea pigs were resistant and mice were of intermediate susceptibility.

Behavioral Effects

All species of monkeys tested thus far (i.e., rhesus, squirrel, and cynomegalus monkeys, marmoset and baboons) exhibit the motor features of PD (23) with the exception of resting tremor. MPTP induces a resting tremor with a frequency of 4–5 hertz indistinguishable from that of PD only in the African Green monkey (24), whereas mainly action and postural tremor were observed in other species.

Levodopa and dopamine agonists alleviated the behavioral deficits induced by MPTP in all monkeys (25) and the chronic use of levodopa in these animals is, as in PD, accompanied with motor side effects such as dyskinesias (25). This fact has made the MPTP monkey the preclinical model *par excellence* to better understand the pathophysiology of levodopa-induced dyskinesia (26) and to develop effective pharmacological strategies to alleviate this disabling problem (27). In addition to monkeys, MPTP has also been reported to induce a paucity of spontaneous motor activity resembling bradykinesia in sheep (28), dog (29), and cat (30).

In mice, the notion that MPTP administration induces behavioral manifestations reminiscent of PD is more controversial. Most studies claiming to see motor abnormalities in MPTP-intoxicated mice refer to reduced spontaneous motor activity and exploratory behavioral within the first days post-MPTP (31). From our experience, within the first 24 to 48 hours post-MPTP mice will often exhibit episodes of generalized shivering (or seizure) and unsteady gait, resembling cerebellar ataxia. During that time, mice are usually markedly hypothermic and hypotensive, especially if they were injected with the typical high doses of MPTP. Again, in our hand, these arrays of motor abnormalities—abusively labeled PD-like symptoms—never responded to levodopa or apomorphine and disappear spontaneously (if the animal survives) in a few days even in the presence of more than 90% depletion in striatal dopamine. It is our experience that irrespective of MPTP regimen, mouse strain, or degree of striatal dopamine depletion, MPTP-intoxicated mice appear normal, with respect to their spontaneous motor behavior, by seven to 14 days after the last injection of the toxin. It has always been our assertion that the aforementioned acute behavioral abnormalities seen in mice injected with MPTP do not reflect dysfunction of the nigrostriatal dopaminergic system but rather a state of generalized toxicosis. Supporting this view are the observations of depressed cardiac contractility (32), damaged spleen with defective immunoresponsiveness (33), and altered blood chemistry consistent with liver dysfunction (23) in animals soon after MPTP administration. It is thus advisable to remain highly circumspect about the PD relevance of such *acute* motor manifestations in MPTP mice. That said some other studies, including some of our own, have evidenced motor abnormalities in MPTP mice with devices such as rotarod more than seven days post-MPTP injections (34,35). Yet, these abnormalities, which can be reversed by levodopa administration, are often subtle and only observed in animals with extreme nigrostriatal damage. Perhaps behaviors that involve striatal function, such as habituation to a novel environment or the ability to learn a stimulus-response paradigm, may prove to be more fruitful and reliable for assessing the striatal dopaminergic function in MPTP mice.

Neurochemical Effects of MPTP

PD neurochemical alterations not only involve dopamine, but also other monoaminergic and nonmonoaminergic systems including acetylcholine and several neuropeptides (36). Although following MPTP administration, changes in a number of neurotransmitter and neuromodulator systems have also been documented especially in monkeys, the most consistent and significant alterations occur in the dopaminergic systems (21). Overall, it is fair to say that among the different species sensitive to MPTP, regional biochemical changes were observed mainly in the caudate-putamen and the substantia nigra and, to variable extent, in the nucleus accumbens, the olfactory tubercle, the ventral tegmental area, the locus coeruleus, and the hypothalamus (21). Inconsistently, monoaminergic changes were found in the cerebral cortex.

Acute increases in striatal levels of dopamine were observed in monkeys (37) and mice (38) with marked reduction in dopamine's main metabolites, HVA and 3,4-dihydroxyphenylacetic acid soon after the administration of the toxin. The observations that MPTP causes acute release of dopamine was subsequently confirmed in live animals by microdialysis in rats (39). This massive release of dopamine seems to be mediated by MPTP's toxic metabolite, 1-methyl-4-phenylpyridinium (MPP^+), as pretreatment with monoamine oxidase-B (MAO-B) inhibitor prevents this release. This acute effect also stimulated the release of norepinephrine and serotonin (37,38). Unexpectedly, the effect does not seem to be restricted to the monoaminergic systems, since the acute rise in striatal acetylcholine has also been demonstrated in mice after MPTP administration (40). It is surprising that while this phenomenon has been recognized for so many years, so little is still known about the pathophysiology of this acute neurotransmitter response to MPTP.

Chronic effects of MPTP on monoaminergic systems have been studied more extensively. In the monkey, striatal dopamine and metabolite levels are dramatically reduced after 10 days and remain low even after one year (37,41–43). A similar situation has been reported in other animal species, although in both cat and mice some studies have documented striking recovery of striatal dopamine levels over time (44,45). In addition to caudate-putamen, MPTP-induced dopamine depletion occurs also in substantia nigra (46,47) and to a lesser extent in nucleus accumbens (46,48) and olfactory tubercle (46,48). Dopamine depletion has been occasionally found in regions such as the hypothalamus, frontal cortex, or ventral tegmental area (49). Chronic effects on norepinephrine and serotonin are more controversial. Striatal norepinephrine levels have been reported to be reduced as much as dopamine at five weeks in mice (50). A different image is found in the cat, where initially norepinephrine levels were dramatically reduced in the caudate-putamen and the nucleus accumbens, but, after five months, striatal levels were increased, while the levels in the accumbens remained low (30). In the monkey (21) and the dog (51) MPTP produces a chronic depletion of serotonin in the caudate-putamen, while no chronic effects on this monoamine have been reported in mice (44). It is interesting to note that an effect on the serotonergic system appears to parallel a species susceptibility to MPTP. Increases in number of striatal dopamine D2 receptors (52,53) and in enkephalin mRNA (54) have also been observed in monkeys and in rodents after MPTP administration. Because these elements are located postsynaptically to dopaminergic cells, these changes can be explained by a secondary adaptative mechanism to the deficit in dopamine. No similar increases were seen in striatal dopamine D1 receptors (52,55,56), cholecystokinin receptors (55), or substance P concentrations (57), although these elements are also postsynaptically located. Finally, no consistent changes in glutamic acid decarboxylase or choline acetyltransferase activities or muscarinic receptor densities have been observed suggesting that MPTP most likely does not affect GABAergic or cholinergic neurons (58,59).

Neuropathological Effects of MPTP

In the MPTP-treated monkey, the major neuropathological finding is a profound loss of pigmented neurons within the substantia nigra (1,37,60) with some gliosis (17,61). The tyrosine hydroxylase-positive neurons of the substantia nigra are extensively destroyed or damaged, as demonstrated by immunohistochemistry (1,37,60).

The pattern of substantia nigra cell death in MPTP-treated monkeys is similar to that following knife cuts in the nigrostriatal pathway. Cells in the centrolateral area of the pars compacta are damaged more extensively than those in the medial portion (62), which resembles the pattern seen in PD. In the mouse, neuronal loss in the substantia nigra after MPTP injection is not uniformly obtained as this depends on the regimen used. Following the administration of four times 20 mg/kg of free base MPTP in one day at two hours apart, there is a massive loss of the nigral neurons. Degenerating neurons are already detectable by 12 hours post-MPTP, reach a maximum between 24 and 48 hours, and are no longer detected by five days (63). With this regimen, the morphology of dying neurons is nonapoptotic (63). Conversely, upon administration of 30 mg/kg once a day for five consecutive days, not only is the degeneration of dopaminergic neurons more protracted up to 21 days after MPTP, but also the morphology is apoptotic (64). In rats, the systemic administration of MPTP is rarely used, and the vast majority of studies involve the stereotaxic infusion of MPP$^+$ (65–69). In contrast to the substantia nigra, there is no noticeable loss of intrinsic neurons in the caudate nucleus and putamen of MPTP-treated monkeys or mice, despite dramatic decrements in TH-activity (70,71), [^{3}H]-dopamine uptake capacity (72), and [^{3}H]-mazindol binding (73), all indicative of a loss of dopaminergic terminals. Other dopamine-containing neuronal nuclei, like the ventral tegmental area, which is adjacent to the substantia nigra, show limited and variable neuronal lesions. In young primates treated with MPTP, there is no observable damage to this structure (37,58,60,74), while in the mouse, a small but definite neuronal loss was found after high-dose MPTP (49,75). The locus coeruleus has also been the subject of several investigations because of its involvement in PD. Histological studies in monkeys sacrificed during the acute phase of MPTP intoxication demonstrated involvement of locus coeruleus, but studies conducted in animals investigated six weeks after administration of the toxin, lesions of the locus coeruleus were found only in the oldest monkeys (5–20 years). In addition, a positive correlation between the dose of the toxin injected and the extent of the lesion was seen in the locus coeruleus in mice after administration of MPTP (49). The authors also identified substantial loss in TH-positive neurons in the hypothalamus of these animals. It is also worthnoting that both in monkeys and in mice, the nigrostriatal lesion produced by MPTP is consistently detectable earlier and more profound at the level of the fiber terminals than over the cell bodies. In light of this finding, several researchers have raised the possibility that the degenerative process in the MPTP model occurs, at least in part, by a dying-back process (43,76). The fact that an intrastriatal delivery of antioxidant mitigates the loss of nigral dopaminergic neurons in mice injected systemically with MPTP (76) provides strong support for the concept that damage to the terminals does indeed govern, to some extent, the fate of the intoxicated neurons. It is also important to mention that, like as in monkeys, the death of dopaminergic neurons in mice is accompanied by a robust glial response composed of primarily astrocytes and microglia whose time course parallels that of neuronal degeneration (77–81). As discussed below (see Secondary Events), this glial reaction appears to be more than a housekeeping event, as it seems to play a real pathogenic role in the MPTP model.

Although its significance is unknown, Lewy body is another important feature of the pathology of PD. Eosinophilic intraneuronal inclusion bodies have been found in the brain of aged monkeys (15–20 years) after prolonged administration of MPTP (82). The inclusion bodies bear some resemblance to Lewy bodies at the light microscopic level, although they do not exhibit the dense central core that is typical of brainstem Lewy bodies under electron microscope examination. The authors of this description speculated that these MPTP-induced inclusions could represent a form of immature Lewy body. It is of interest to note that these eosinophilic inclusions have been identified in the medulla, nucleus basalis of Meynert, substantia nigra, locus coeruleus, and dorsal raphe nucleus, areas in which typical Lewy bodies are found in PD. In only one report was the presence of Lewy body-like inclusions shown in MPTP monkeys (83); contained alpha-synuclein (83). In mice intoxicated with MPTP, it seems that the formation of proteinaceous inclusions can only be elicited by administering the toxin for an extended period, which can be achieved by either serial subcutaneous injections of MPTP in association with probenecid (84) or by chronic infusion using osmotic minipumps (85).

Because of the close relationship between the rate of energy metabolism and local functional activity, it is of interest to report the results on cerebral glucose metabolism in MPTP monkeys (86). The authors of this work have found significant reductions in glucose metabolism in areas of cell loss such as the substantia nigra and the ventral tegmental area. In contrast, they found significant increases in glucose metabolism in the caudate-putamen, the external segment of the globus pallidus, the subthalamic nucleus, the ventral anterior nucleus of the thalamus, and the premotor cortex, regions which are all involved in the production of movement and maintenance of posture.

Toxicokinetics of MPTP
Systemic Metabolism of MPTP and Its Penetration in the Brain
Following its systemic administration, MPTP, which, as indicated by its octanol/water partition coefficient of 15.6 (87), is highly lipophilic, is able to readily permeate all lipid bilayer membranes, and accumulates in virtually all organs. That said, not all organs are capable of either activating this protoxin into its actual toxic derivative (see below) or catabolizing it. For instance, organs such as the lung and the kidney seem to play a minor role in the conversion of MPTP to inactive metabolites (88). On the other hand, the biotransformation of MPTP by liver enzymes like cytochrome P-450 and flavin mono-oxygenase (88) seem to be more instrumental in this regard as inhibition of either enzymes enhance the neurotoxicity of MPTP (88,89). Corroborating this view is the demonstration that the anticonvulsants diphenylhydantoin and phenobarbital, which are known inducers of these liver enzymes, mitigate MPTP-induced dopamine depletion in mice (90).

After a certain amount of injected MPTP has been catabolized by the liver and possibly other organs, the remaining protoxin quickly gains access to the brain since it readily crosses the blood-brain barrier (Fig. 1). The rapidity with which MPTP reaches the central nervous system is remarkable, and Markey et al. (91) were the first to show that one minute after its intraperitoneal injection, MPTP can be measured in the brain of monkeys and mice by high-performance liquid chromatography (HPLC).

Bioactivation of MPTP by Monoamine Oxidase
Once in the brain parenchyma, MPTP is rapidly converted into its toxic metabolite MPP^+ by a two-step process (Fig. 2). First, MPTP undergoes a two electron oxidation, catalyzed by MAO-B that yields the intermediate 1-methyl-4-phenyl-2,3-dihydropyridinium ($MPDP^+$) (92). Second, the produced $MPDP^+$, which is an unstable molecule, readily undergoes spontaneous disproportionation to MPP^+ and MPTP (93,94) as depicted in Figure 2.

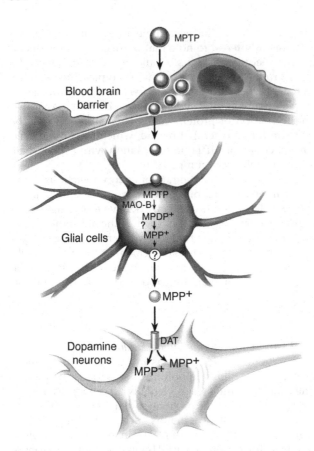

FIGURE 1 Schematic representation of MPTP metabolism. After systemic administration, MPTP crosses the blood-brain barrier. Once in the brain, MPTP is converted to MPDP$^+$ by MAO-B within nondopaminergic cells, such as glial cells and serotonergic neurons (not shown), and then to MPP$^+$ by an unknown mechanism (?). Thereafter, MPP$^+$ is released, again by an unknown mechanism (?), into the extracellular space. MPP$^+$ is concentrated within dopaminergic neurons via the dopamine transporter. *Abbreviation*: DAT, dopamine transporter; MAO-B, monoamine oxidase-B; MPDP$^+$, 1-methyl-4-phenyl-2,3-dihydropyridinium, MPP$^+$, 1-methyl-4-phenyl-pyridinium; MPTP, 1-methyl-4-phenyl-1,2,3,6-tetrahydropyridine. *Source*: From Ref. 165.

Independent of the MPTP story, MPP$^+$, presented in the early 1970s as a powerful new herbicide (Cyperquat™; has never been commercialized), was recognized as a potent toxin. Thus, based on the fact that MPP$^+$, a major metabolite of MPTP and a known potent cytotoxin, was found in the brains of monkeys for several days after MPTP administration when MPTP itself was not longer detectable, led to the idea that MPP$^+$ or the process of MPP$^+$ formation had to be linked to MPTP-induced toxicity (91).

Crude mitochondrial preparations from rat brains have been shown to transform MPTP to MPP$^+$ (92). Since pargyline (a nonselective MAO inhibitor) and deprenyl (a selective MAO-B inhibitor) but not clorgyline (a selective MAO-A inhibitor) block the formation of MPP$^+$, MAO-B was implicated as the enzyme involved in the metabolism of MPTP. The importance of MAO-B-mediated

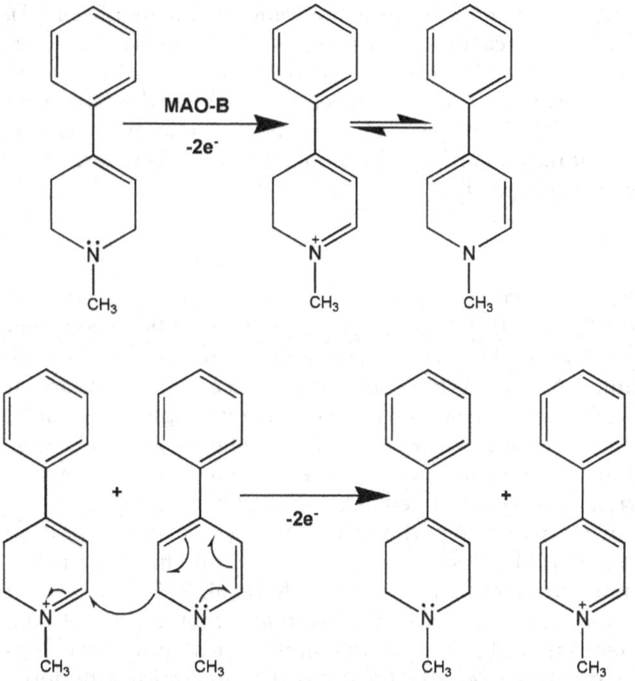

FIGURE 2 Proposed mechanism of biotransformation of MPTP to MPP⁺. This reaction occurs in two phases. First, MPTP undergoes a two electron oxidation catalyzed by MAO-B that yields MPDP⁺ (and its conjugated base MPDP). Then, the disproportionation of MPDP⁺ proceeds through a reaction in which its conjugated base serves as a hybrid donor molecule and MPDP⁺ as a hybrid acceptor molecule. Based on this event, the reduction of MPTP⁺, which involves the transfer of one proton from its conjugated base, results in the formation of MPTP while the concomitant oxidation of MPDP⁺ results in the formation of MPP⁺. *Abbreviation*: MAOB, monoamine oxidase-B; MPDP⁺, 1-methyl-4-phenyl-2,3-dihydropyridinium, MPP⁺, 1-methyl-4-phenyl-pyridinium; MPTP, 1-methyl-4-phenyl-1,2,3,6-tetrahydropyridine. *Source*: From Ref. 94.

bioactivation of MPP⁺ in the toxicity of MPTP has been established by the demonstration that the inhibition of MAO-B by pretreatment with pargyline, deprenyl, or other MAO-B inhibitors not only blocks the formation of MPP⁺ but also prevents dopamine depletion in the brains of mice (91,95) and protects against the development of MPTP-induced parkinsonism in monkeys (96). An important aspect of MPTP-induced toxicity is the demonstration that MAO-B is localized in nondopaminergic cells, such as astrocytes and serotonergic neurons (97,98). Thus, it appears that MAO-B catalyzes MPTP conversion to MPP⁺ outside of dopaminergic neurons (Fig. 1), a view which is consistent with the findings that animals with substantial loss in serotonergic neurons (99) or astroglial ablation (100) are more resistant to MPTP.

MAO-B has also been identified in blood vessel walls of some species. If MAO-B is present in sufficiently high enough concentrations in capillary or blood vessel walls outside of the blood-brain barrier, then the conversion of MPTP to MPP⁺ at this site might limit entry of the toxin into the brain, as MPP⁺ does not readily enter the brain. It was found that arterial walls accumulated [³H]-MPTP as densely as did the caudate-putamen 24 hours after its intravenous injection to monkeys (91). In other species, MAO-B may have a real protective effect as Harik and his colleagues (101) attribute the resistance of rats to the toxic effects of the systemically injected MPTP to an enzymatic barrier resulting from high levels of MAO-B in the capillaries of rat brain. They found that MPTP oxidation by rat cerebral microvessels was 30-fold more rapid than by human microvessels; mouse microvessels were intermediate in their MPTP-oxidizing capacity.

Neuronal Uptake of MPP+

Thus far, the mechanism by which MPP+ is released from serotonergic neurons and astrocytes remains unclear (Fig. 1). MPP+ has an octanol/water partition coefficient of 0.09 (87), which indicates that, while being a lipophilic cation, it is far less lipophilic than MPTP. Thus, unlike MPTP, MPP+ is not expected to easily diffuse across cellular lipid bilayer membranes, and there is no evidence that it simply leaks out by killing the cell within which it has been formed. Instead, it is believed that the release of MPP+ from its intracellular sites of formation and entry into adjacent neurons depend on specialized carriers whose nature remains to be determined (Fig. 1).

A second important event, which in part may explain the selectivity of MPTP for dopaminergic neurons, is that MPP+ is actively transported into the dopaminergic neurons by the dopamine uptake system (Fig. 1). Javitch et al. (102) have shown that the kinetic parameters for the uptake of MPP+ into crude preparations of striatal synaptosomes from rats were similar to those for dopamine. These authors (102) as well as others (38,103) have demonstrated that the pretreatment of mice with dopamine uptake inhibitors prevents MPTP-induced dopaminergic toxicity as does the genetic ablation of the dopamine transporter (104). These findings indicate that the dopamine uptake system plays a critical role in MPTP dopaminergic neurotoxicity (Fig. 1). What remains unclear, however, is why other dopaminergic neurons such as the mesolimbic dopaminergic neurons with presumably a similar uptake system, are much less affected by MPTP than nigrostriatal dopaminergic neurons. Nor is it understood why noradrenergic and serotonergic neurons are only minimally or not at all affected by MPTP, even though MPP+ has an equally high affinity for norepinephrine and serotonin uptake sites and is readily transported into these cells (105,106). As reviewed in (107), there are wide variations in the vulnerability of catecholamines in mice to MPTP toxicity. Striatal dopamine levels in C57BL/6 mice were found to be more affected by MPTP than were those of Swiss-Webster mice. Differences in vulnerability of striatal dopamine levels among Swiss-Webster mice obtained from different suppliers have also been reported. Age, route of MPTP administration, and gender have also been demonstrated as additional factors in determining the effect of MPTP in monkeys as well as in mice. Thus, while the uptake of MPP+ into dopaminergic neurons appears to be necessary for MPTP toxicity, it does not fully explain the specificity for the dopaminergic neurons.

Mitochondrial and Synaptic Vesicle Uptake of MPP+

As illustrated in Figure 3, once inside neurons, MPP+ rapidly accumulates in the mitochondrial matrix (108), not via a specific carrier but by being passively transported (109,110) by a mechanism relying on the mitochondrial transmembrane potential gradient ($\Delta\Psi$) of -150 to -170 mV (108–111). As with other lipophilic cations, the higher the concentration of intramitochondrial MPP+, the lower the $\Delta\Psi$ and, consequently, the slower the uptake of extramitochondrial MPP+

(109,110). The demonstration that the ion-pairing agent tetraphenylboron anion increases both the rate and the extent of MPP$^+$ uptake in isolated mitochondria (112) further supports this concept. Remarkably, energized mitochondria incubated with 0.5 mM MPP$^+$ reach matrix concentrations of more than 24 mM after only 10 minutes (111). This fast and avid uptake suggests that most of the cytosolic MPP$^+$ would eventually accumulate in the mitochondrial matrix after the systemic injection of MPTP.

As shown in Figure 3, MPP$^+$ can also bind to the vesicular monoamine transporters (VMAT), whereby it is translocated into synaptosomal vesicles (113). The vesicular accumulation of MPP$^+$ appears to protect cells from MPTP-induced neurodegeneration by sequestering the toxin and preventing it from accessing mitochondria, its probable main site of action (Fig. 3). The importance of the vesicular sequestration of MPP$^+$ is demonstrated by the fact that cells transfected to express a greater density of VMAT are converted from MPP$^+$-sensitive to MPP$^+$-resistant cells (113). Conversely, mutant mice heterozygous for a VMAT null mutation are significantly more sensitive to MPTP-induced dopaminergic neurotoxicity compared to their wild type littermates (114). These findings indicate that there is an inverse relationship between the capacity to sequester MPP$^+$ in synaptic vesicles and the magnitude of MPTP neurotoxicity (Fig. 3).

Brain Elimination of MPP$^+$ and Role of Neuromelanin

MPTP rapidly disappears from the mouse brain. Two hours after a single intraperitoneal injection of 10 mg/kg of MPTP, it can no longer be detected in brain extracts by HPLC, likely because it has been effectively converted into MPP$^+$. Interestingly, a similar situation is found for MPP$^+$ after approximately eight hours (115), despite the fact that there is no evidence that MPP$^+$ is further metabolized. Of note, the

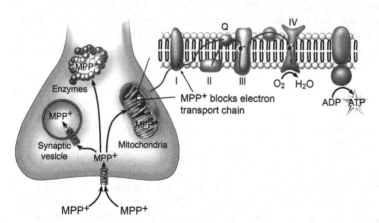

FIGURE 3 Schematic representation of MPP$^+$ intracellular pathways. Inside dopaminergic neurons, MPP$^+$ can follow one of three routes: (*i*) concentration into mitochondria through an active process (toxic); (*ii*) interaction with cytosolic enzymes (toxic); (*iii*) sequestration into synaptic vesicles via the *vesicular monoamine transporters* (protective). Within the mitochondria, MPP$^+$ blocks complex I (X), which interrupts the transfer of electrons from complex I to ubiquinone (Q). This perturbation enhances the production of reactive oxygen species (not shown) and decreases the synthesis of ATP. *Abbreviations*: ADP, adenosine diphosphate; ATP, adenosine triphosphate; IV, intravenous; MPP$^+$, 1-methyl-4-phenyl-pyridinium. *Source*: From Ref. 165.

half-life of MPP+ in the monkey brain is much longer (±48 to 100 hours), which is more than 10 times longer than the half-life determined in mice [approximately four hours; (116)]. This marked difference in the retention or the disposition of MPP+ is most likely a major contributing factor in the large interspecies variation in MPTP susceptibility. Regardless of species differences in MPP+ biodisposition, it remains enigmatic how this poorly lipophilic molecule exits the brain. Whether it is secreted into the CSF or succeeds in crossing the blood–brain barrier with the help of an organic cation transporter is a possibility that needs to be investigated.

Neuromelanin is the pigment responsible for the dark color of the substantia nigra in primates and several other vertebrates and whose formation relies on the oxidation of dopamine and other catechols (117). MPP+ was found to bind to neuromelanin with relative high affinity (Kd = 28–32 nM) (118), and thus it can be imagined that a slow release of MPP+ into the cytoplasm from this intracellular depot might maintain toxic levels in the neuron sufficiently long enough to cause irreversible neuronal damage and death. This hypothesis is further supported by the observation that inhibition of the binding of MPP+ to neuromelanin by the antimalarial drug chloroquine partially protects monkeys against MPTP toxicity (119). No such effect was seen in mice (119), which lack brain neuromelanin. The view that neuromelanin might be instrumental in MPTP-induced dopaminergic neurotoxicity has been challenged, however, by Herkenham et al. (43) who failed to find in monkeys any significant relationship between the content of neuromelanin in neurons the amount MPP+ accumulated in neurons and their respective vulnerability.

HOW DOES MPTP KILL NEURONS?

The prevailing view of the macular basis of MPTP-induced dopaminergic neurotoxicity is that following MPTP administration and its accumulation within dopaminergic neurons, a cascade of multiple deleterious events is set in motion. Based on a large body of literature, those pathogenic events can be divided into early and late neuronal perturbations and secondary alterations. Each of these, to a variable degree and at different stages of the degenerative process, participates in the ultimate demise of dopaminergic neurons.

Early Events
Energy Crisis
As discussed above, soon after its entry into dopaminergic neurons, MPP+ accumulates in the mitochondria (Fig. 3). Once in the mitochondria, MPP+ impairs oxidative phosphorylation by inhibiting nicotinamide adenine dinucleotide (NADH)-ubiquinone reductase activity (120) which, as shown by photoaffinity labeling, is due to the binding of MPP+ to the PSST subunit of complex I (121). In so doing MPP+ interrupts the flow of electrons along the chain of cytochromes and provokes an acute failure in adenosine triphosphate (ATP) formation. It appears, however, that complex I activity should be reduced by >70% to cause a significant depletion of ATP in nonsynaptic mitochondria (122) and that, in contrast to in vitro, in vivo MPTP causes only a transient 20% reduction in mouse striatal and midbrain ATP levels (123). Still, it is likely that this transient perturbation does contribute to the cell death process since different strategies aimed at boosting cellular energy stores, such as beta-hydroxybutyrate or creatine do attenuate MPTP-induced dopaminergic neurodegeneration in mice (34,124). Nonetheless, it is legitimate to

wonder whether MPP$^+$-mediated ATP deficit is the sole factor underlying MPTP-induced dopaminergic neuronal death or rather one of the contributors to a multifactorial pathogenic cascade.

Oxidative Stress

Consistent with this multifactorial concept is the fact that another consequence of complex I inhibition by MPP$^+$ is an increased production of reactive oxygen species (ROS), especially of superoxide radical (125,126). It seems that early ROS production can also occur in the MPTP model from the auto-oxidation of dopamine resulting from an MPP$^+$-induced massive release of vesicular dopamine to the cytosol (127). The importance of MPP$^+$-related ROS production in the dopaminergic toxicity process in vivo is demonstrated by the fact that transgenic mice with increased brain activity of copper/zinc superoxide dismutase (SOD1), a key ROS scavenging enzyme, are significantly more resistant to MPTP-induced dopaminergic toxicity than their nontransgenic littermates (128). However, superoxide is poorly reactive, and it is the general consensus that this radical does not cause serious direct injury. Instead, superoxide is believed to exert many or most of its toxic effects through the generation of secondary oxidants with much stronger reactivity such as the hydroxyl radical, whose oxidative properties can ultimately kill cells. MPTP does stimulate the formation of hydroxyl radicals in vivo, as evidenced by the increase in the hydroxyl radical-dependent conversion of salicylate to 2,3- and 2,5-dihydroxybenzoates (129,130). However, there is no compelling evidence that the produced hydroxyl radical actually contributes to the oxidative stress in the MPTP model (131).

Superoxide can also react with nitric oxide (NO) to produce peroxynitrite, another potent oxidant. Supporting the relevance of this chemical reaction in the MPTP neurotoxic process is the demonstration that inhibition of neuronal NO synthase (nNOS) attenuates, in a dose-dependent fashion, MPTP-induced striatal dopaminergic loss in mice (129,132). Of note, nNOS has, thus far, not been identified inside of dopaminergic neurons in rodents. Yet, dopaminergic structures are surrounded by nNOS-expressing fibers and cell bodies in the striatum, and, to a much lesser extent, in the substantia nigra pars compacta (133,134). NO is uncharged and lipophilic; hence it is able to travel away from its site of synthesis and inflict remote cellular damage without the need for any export mechanism. Because several lines of evidence (135) support the notion that a molecule of NO can cover a distance many times greater than the diameter of a dopaminergic neuron, it can be speculated that the NO production involved in MPTP toxicity takes place in nondopaminergic cells present in the vicinity of dopaminergical structures. As discussed elsewhere (135), under physiologic conditions, while copious amounts of NO are likely constantly produced, concentration of superoxide is low; hence a minimal formation of peroxynitrite likely occurs. Conversely, in pathological situations as caused by MPTP, superoxide formation increases, which consequently may lead to the generation of appreciable amounts of peroxynitrite. Supporting the participation of peroxynitrite in the MPTP model is the demonstration that MPTP significantly increases striatal levels of both free and protein-bound nitrotyrosine in mice (129,131), which is a marker of peroxynitrite damage to proteins. Aside from being a marker, nitrotyrosine exerts toxic effects in its own right as shown by the fact that stereotaxic injection of nitrotyrosine causes striatal neurodegeneration in vivo (136). Furthermore, TH (137), α-synuclein (138), and *PARKIN* (139) are all post-translationally damaged by a NO-based process.

DNA Damage and PARP Activation

Thus far, the lion's share of attention has been given to the effects of reactive species produced after MPTP administration on proteins. However, most of the reactive species, like peroxynitrite, that are implicated in the MPTP model can damage, through oxidative processes, many vital cellular elements other than proteins. Among these, DNA is of unique importance, because it is the repository for genetic information and is present in single copies. In light of the proposed oxidant species involved in MPTP neurotoxicity, all of the aforementioned DNA modifications can possibly occur in this model, as well as in PD. Consistent with this view is the quantitative polymerase chain reaction (PCR) finding that MPTP administration to mice produced damage in both mitochondrial and nuclear DNA of the substantia nigra, while there was no damage in either mitochondria or nuclei in the cerebellum, which was used as a negative control (140). Although all DNA modifications are potentially mutagenic and thus harmful, strand breakage is especially deleterious because of its link to poly [adenosine diphosphate (ADP)-ribose] polymerase (PARP). The activation of PARP, by synthesizing poly(ADP-ribose) polymer, can rapidly deplete intracellular stores of NAD^+ which may impair glycolysis, mitochondrial electron transport chain activities, and, consequently, ATP formation. In the case of the MPTP model, the production of ATP in substantia nigra pars compacta dopaminergic neurons is already compromised due to the inhibition of the mitochondrial complex I by MPP^+ and thus activation of PARP may exacerbate the energy crisis. Corroborating the significance of PARP activation in the MPTP acute neurotoxic process in vivo is our demonstration that PARP is intensely activated following MPTP administration and that mutant mice deficient in PARP are more resistant to MPTP-induced dopaminergic neuronal death (141).

Late Events

Surprisingly, when one compares the time course of ATP depletion, ROS production, and PARP activation to that of SNpc dopaminergic neuronal loss, it clearly appears that the former alterations precede the actual neuronal demise (63). This suggests that the early alterations discussed above probably do not provoke the death of many dopaminergic neurons per se, but instead activate molecular pathways, which are the real executioners of the majority of dopaminergic neurons. Among the multiplicity of death-related cellular pathways, mounting evidence implicates the recruitment of the apoptotic molecular machinery in the demise of dopaminergic neurons after MPTP administration. As reviewed in (142), the proapoptotic protein Bax appears instrumental in this toxic model (143); in contrast, Bak, which cooperates with Bax to initiate apoptosis in response to activation of cell-surface death receptors, is dispensable in MPTP-mediated neuronal death (144). Overexpression of the antiapoptotic Bcl-2 also protects dopaminergic cells against MPTP-induced neurodegeneration (145,146). Similarly, adenovirus-mediated transgenic expression of the X-chromosome-linked inhibitor of apoptosis protein (XIAP), an inhibitor of executioner caspases such as caspase-3, also blocks the death of dopaminergic neurons in the substantia nigra pars compacta following the administration of MPTP (147,148). Additional caspases are also activated in MPTP-intoxicated mice such as caspase-8 (149), which is a proximal effector of the tumor necrosis factor receptor (TNFr) family death pathway. Interestingly, however, in the MPTP mouse model it is possible that caspase-8 activation is consequent to the recruitment of the mitochondrial-dependent apoptotic pathway and not, like in many other pathological settings, to the ligation of TNFr (150). Other observations supporting a role for apoptosis in the MPTP neurotoxic process include the demonstration of the resistance to MPTP of mutant mice deficient in p53 (151), a cell cycle control molecule involved in programmed cell death, mice with pharmacological or genetic inhibition of c-Jun N-terminal kinases (152–154) or mice that received a striatal adeno-associated virus vector delivery of an Apaf-1-dominant negative inhibitor (155). Collectively, these data show that during the degenerative process the apoptotic pathways are activated and contribute to the actual death of intoxicated neurons in the MPTP model.

Secondary Events

The loss of dopaminergic neurons in the MPTP mouse model is associated with a glial response composed mainly of activated microglial cells and, to a lesser extent, of reactive astrocytes and T-cells (156). In the MPTP mouse model, the astrocyte activation appears secondary to the death of neurons and not the reverse since the blockade of MPP+ uptake into dopaminergic neurons prevents not only substantia nigra pars compacta dopaminergic neuronal death but also Glial fibrillary acidic protein (GFAP) upregulation (80). Yet, activation of microglia, which is also quite strong in the MPTP mouse model (77,78), occurs earlier than that of astrocytes and, more importantly, reaches a maximum before the peak of dopaminergic neurodegeneration (157). In light of the MPTP data presented above, it can be surmised that the response of both astrocytes and microglial cells in the substantia nigra pars compacta clearly occurs within a timeframe allowing these glial cells to participate in the demise of dopaminergic neurons in the MPTP mouse model and possibly in PD. Activated microglial cells can produce a variety of noxious factors including ROS, reactive nitrogen species, proinflammatory cytokines, and prostaglandins. Observations showing that blockade of microglial activation mitigates nigrostriatal damage caused by MPTP (158,159) supports the notion that microglia participate in MPTP-induced neurodegeneration. Among the specific factors that could mediate the deleterious actions of microglia on dopaminergic neurons, nicotinamide adenine dinucleotide phosphate (NADPH)-oxidase, and inducible nitric oxide synthase (iNOS) have emerged as potentially critical. Using mutant mice deficient in these respective enzymes, it was shown that both NADPH-oxidase (76) and iNOS (157) do contribute to MPTP-induced neurodegeneration. However, ablation of either of these enzymes did provide profound protection, thus suggesting that to abate microglial-mediated deleterious effects many factors must be targeted simultaneously. Previous studies have shown that the type of action mediated by neuroinflammation could be modified by vaccination. Based on this findings, it was recently demonstrated that adoptive transfer of copolymer-1 immune cells to MPTP recipient mice led to T-cell accumulation within the substantia nigra pars compacta, suppression of microglial activation, and increased local expression of glial-derived neurotrophic factor (GDNF) (33).

CONCLUSION

Despite some neuropathological shortcomings, the monkey MPTP model is the gold standard for the assessment of novel strategies and agents for treatment of PD symptoms. For example, electrophysiologic studies of MPTP monkeys revealed that hyperactivity of the subthalamic nucleus is a key factor in the genesis of PD motor dysfunction (160). This seminal discovery led to the targeting of this structure using chronic high-frequency stimulation procedures (also called deep brain stimulation) to effectively ameliorate the motor function of PD patients whose symptoms cannot be further improved with medical therapy (161). In addition, MPTP-treated monkeys (162,163) were used to demonstrate that the delivery of GDNF both significantly limits MPTP-induced nigrostriatal dopaminergic neurodegeneration and can lead to behavioral recovery when given to previously lesioned animals (163). These studies form the basis for current attempts to use GDNF in PD patients (164). Because of practical considerations, MPTP monkeys have not generally been used to explore the molecular mechanisms of dopaminergic neurodegeneration; the MPTP mouse model is typically used for such studies. As summarized in this chapter, over the year a large number of cellular and molecular investigations have been performed in mice following the administration of MPTP and have led to a wealth of information regarding the mechanisms involved in the death of dopaminergic neurons. Because of the close similarity between PD and the MPTP model, it can be asserted that a cascade of deleterious events similar to that elucidated in animals intoxicated with MPTP underlies the death of dopaminergic neurons in PD.

ACKNOWLEDGMENTS

The author thanks Mr. Matthew Lucas for his assistance in preparing this manuscript and is supported by NIH/NINDS Grants RO1 NS42269, P50 NS38370, and P01 NS11766, NIH/NIA RO1 AG21617, NIH/NIEHS R21 ES013177, the US Department of Defense Grant DAMD 17-03-1, the Parkinson Disease Foundation (New York, USA), and the Muscular Dystrophy Association Wings over Wall Street.

REFERENCES

1. Langston JW, Langston EB, Irwin I. MPTP-induced parkinsonism in human and non-human primates—clinical and experimental aspects. Acta Neurol Scand 1984; 70(suppl 100):49–54.
2. Ziering A, Berger L, Heineman SD, Lee J. Piperidine derivatives. Part III. 4-Arylpiperidines. J Org Chem 1947; 12:894–903.
3. Janssen PAJ, Eddy NB. Compounds related to pethidine-IV. New general chemical methods of increasing the analgesic activity of pethidine. J Med Pharma Chem 1960; 2:31–45.
3a. Sorter, personal communication, 1983.
4. Davis GC, Williams AC, Markey SP, et al. Chronic parkinsonism secondary to intravenous injection of meperidine analogs. Psychiatry Res 1979; 1:249–254.
5. Wright JM, Wall RA, Perry TL, Patty DW. Chronic parkinsonism secondary to the intranasal administration of a product of meperidine-analogue synthesis. N Engl J Med 1984; 310:325.
6. Langston JW, Ballard P. Parkinson's disease in a chemist working with 1-methyl-4-phenyl-1,2,5,6-tetrahydropyridine (MPTP). N Engl J Med 1983; 309:310.
6a. Côté, personal communication, 1991.
6b. Heagy, DEA Western Regional Laboratory, San Francisco, personal communication, 1982.
7. Langston JW, Ballard P, Irwin I. Chronic parkinsonism in humans due to a product of meperidine-analog synthesis. Science 1983; 219:979–980.
7a. Langston, personal communication, 1994.
8. Ballard P, Tetrud JW, Langston JW. Permanent human parkinsonism due to 1-methyl-4-phenyl-1,2,3,6-tetrahydropyridine (MPTP): 7 cases. Neurology 1985; 35:949–956.
9. Ruttenber AJ, Garbe PL, Kalter HD, et al. Meperidine analogue exposure in California narcotics abusers: initial epidemiologic findings. In: Markey SP, Castagnoli N Jr,

Trevor AJ, Kopin IJ, eds. MPTP: A Neurotoxin Producing a Parkinsonian Syndrome. New York: Academic Press, 1986.
10. Stern Y, Langston JW. Intellectual changes in patients with MPTP-induced parkinsonism. Neurology 1985; 35:1506–1509.
11. Stern Y, Mayeux R. Intellectual impairement in Parkinson's disease. Adv Neurol 1986; 45:405–408.
12. Burns RS, LeWitt PA, Ebert MH, Pakkenberg H, Kopin IJ. The clinical syndrome of striatal dopamine deficiency. Parkinsonism induced by 1-methyl-4-phenyl-1,2,3,6-tetrahydropyridine (MPTP). N Engl J Med 1985; 312:1418–1421.
13. Tetrud JW, Langston JW, Garbe PL, Ruttenber AJ. Mild parkinsonism in persons exposed to 1-methyl-4-phenyl-1,2,3,6-tetrahydropyridine (MPTP). Neurology 1989; 39:1483–1487.
14. Burns RS, Pakkenberg H, Kopin IJ. Lack of progression of MPTP-induced parkinsonism during long-term treatment with L-DOPA. Ann Neurol 1985; 18:117.
15. Vingerhoets FJ, Snow BJ, Tetrud JW, Langston JW, Schulzer M, Calne DB. Positron emission tomographic evidence for progression of human MPTP-induced dopaminergic lesions. Ann Neurol 1994; 36:765–770.
16. Langston JW, Forno LS, Tetrud J, Reeves AG, Kaplan JA, Karluk D. Evidence of active nerve cell degeneration in the substantia nigra of humans years after 1-methyl-4-phenyl-1,2,3,6-tetrahydropyridine exposure. Ann Neurol 1999; 46:598–605.
17. McGeer PL, Schwab C, Parent A, Doudet D. Presence of reactive microglia in monkey substantia nigra years after 1-methyl-4-phenyl-1,2,3,6-tetrahydropyridine administration. Ann Neurol 2003; 54:599–604.
18. Calne DB, Langston JW, Martin WR, et al. Observations relating to the cause of Parkinson's disease: PET scans after MPTP. Nature 1985; 317:246–248.
19. Snow BJ, Vingerhoets FJ, Langston JW, Tetrud JW, Sossi V, Calne DB. Pattern of dopaminergic loss in the striatum of humans with MPTP induced parkinsonism. J Neurol Neurosurg Psychiat 2000; 68:313–316.
20. Moratalla R, Quinn B, DeLanney LE, Irwin I, Langston JW, Graybiel AM. Differential vulnerability of primate caudate-putamen and striosome-matrix dopamine systems to the neurotoxic effects of 1-methyl-4-phenyl-1,2,3,6-tetrahydropyridine. Proc Natl Acad Sci USA 1992; 89:3859–3863.
21. Kopin IJ, Markey SP. MPTP toxicity: implication for research in Parkinson's disease. Annu Rev Neurosci 1988; 11:81–96.
22. Jakowec MW, Petzinger GM. 1-methyl-4-phenyl-1,2,3,6-tetrahydropyridine-lesioned model of parkinson's disease, with emphasis on mice and nonhuman primates. Comp Med 2004; 54:497–513.
23. Petzinger GM, Langston JW. The MPTP-lesioned non-human primate: a model for Parkinson's disease. In: Marwah J, Teiltelbaum H, eds. Advances in Neurodegenerative Disorders. Parkinson's Disease. Scottsdale: Prominent Press, 1998.
24. Tetrud JW, Langston JW, Redmond DE Jr, Roth RH, Sladek JR, Angel RW. MPTP-induced tremor in human and non-human primates. Neurology 1986; 36(suppl 1):308.
25. Crossman AR, Clarke CE, Boyse S, Robertson RC, Sambrook MA. MPTP-induced parkinsonim in the monkey: neurochemical pathology, complications of treatment and pathophysiological mechanisms. Can J Neurol Sci 1987; 14:428–435.
26. Blanchet PJ, Calon F, Morissette M, et al. Relevance of the MPTP primate model in the study of dyskinesia priming mechanisms. Parkinsonism Relat Disord 2004; 10:297–304.
27. Bezard E, Ferry S, Mach U, et al. Attenuation of levodopa-induced dyskinesia by normalizing dopamine D3 receptor function. Nat Med 2003; 9:762–767.
28. Hammock BD, Beale AM, Work T, et al. A sheep model for MPTP induced Parkinson-like symptoms. Life Sci 1989; 45:1601–1608.
29. Parisi JE, Burns RS. MPTP-induced parkinsonism in man and experimental animals. J Neuropathol Exp Neurol 1985; 44:325.
30. Schneider JS, Yuwiler A, Markham CH. Production of a Parkinson-like syndrome in the cat with N-methyl-4-phenyl-1,2,3,6,-tetrahydropyridine (MPTP): behavior, histology, and biochemistry. Exp Neurol 1986; 91:293–307.
31. Sedelis M, Schwarting RK, Huston JP. Behavioral phenotyping of the MPTP mouse model of Parkinson's disease. Behav Brain Res 2001; 125:109–125.

32. Ren J, Porter JE, Wold LE, Aberle NS, Muralikrishnan D, Haselton JR. Depressed contractile function and adrenergic responsiveness of cardiac myocytes in an experimental model of Parkinson disease, the MPTP-treated mouse. Neurobiol Aging 2004; 25:131–138.

33. Benner EJ, Mosley RL, Destache CJ, et al. Therapeutic immunization protects dopaminergic neurons in a mouse model of Parkinson's disease. Proc Natl Acad Sci USA 2004; 101:9435–9440.

34. Tieu K, Perier C, Caspersen C, et al. D-beta-hydroxybutyrate rescues mitochondrial respiration and mitigates features of Parkinson disease. J Clin Invest 2003; 112:892–901.

35. Rozas G, López-Martín E, Guerra MJ, Labandeira-García JL. The overall rod performance test in the MPTP-treated-mouse model of Parkinsonism. J Neurosci Meth 1998; 83:165–175.

36. Agid Y, Javoy-Agid F, Ruberg M. Biochemistry of neurotransmitters in Parkinson's disease. In: Marsden CD, Fahn S, eds. Movement Disorders 2. London: Butterworths, 1987.

37. Burns RS, Chiueh CC, Markey SP, Ebert MH, Jacobowitz DM, Kopin IJ. A primate model of parkinsonism: selective destruction of dopaminergic neurons in the pars compacta of substantia nigra by N-methyl-4-phenyl,1,2,3,6-tetrahydropyridine. Proc Natl Acad Sci USA 1983; 80:4546–4550.

38. Pileblad E, Carlsson A. Catecholamine-uptake inhibitors prevent the neurotoxicity of 1-methyl-4-phenyl-1,2,3,6-tetrahydropyridine(MPTP) in mouse brain. Neuropharmacology 1985; 24:689–692.

39. Rollema H, Damsma G, Horn AS, De Vries JB, Westerink BH. Brain dialysis in conscious rats reveals an instantaneous massive release of striatal dopamine in response to MPP+. Eur J Pharmacol 1986; 126:345–346.

40. Hadjiconstantinou M, Cavalla D, Anthoupoulou E, Laird HE, Neff NH. N-Methyl-4-phenyl-1,2,3,6-tetrahydropyridine increases acetylcholine and decreases dopamine in mouse striatum: both responses are blocked by anticholinergic drugs. J Neurochem 1985; 45:1957–1959.

41. Jenner P, Rupniak NM, Rose S, et al. 1-Methyl-4-phenyl-1,2,3,6-tetrahydropyridine-induced parkinsonism in the common marmoset. Neurosci Lett 1984; 50:85–90.

42. Cohen G, Pasik P, Cohen B, Leist A, Mytilineou C, Yahr MD. Pargyline and deprenyl prevent the neurotoxicity of 1-methyl-4-phenyl-1,2,3,6-tetrahydropyridine (MPTP) in monkeys. Eur J Pharmacol 1985; 106:209–210.

43. Herkenham M, Little MD, Bankiewicz K, Yang SC, Markey SP, Johannessen JN. Selective retention of MPP+ within the monoaminergic systems of the primate brain following MPTP administration: an in vivo autoradiographic study. Neuroscience 1991; 40:133–158.

44. Heikkila RE, Sieber BA, Manzino L, Sonsalla PK. Some features of the nigrostriatal dopaminergic neurotoxin 1-methyl-4-phenyl-1,2,3,6-tetrahydropyridine (MPTP) in the mouse. Mol Chemic Neuropathol 1989; 10:171–183.

45. Schneider JS, Rothblat DS. Neurochemical evaluation of the striatum in symptomatic and recovered MPTP-treated cats. Neuroscience 1991; 44:421–429.

46. Melamed E, Rosenthal J, Globus M, Cohen O, Frucht Y, Uzzan A. Mesolimbic dopaminergic neurons are not spared by MPTP neurotoxicity in mice. Eur J Pharmacol 1985; 114:97–100.

47. Bradbury AJ, Costall B, Jenner P, Kelly ME, Marsden CD, Naylor RJ. The neurotoxic actions of 1-methyl-4-phenylpyridinium (MPP+) are not prevented by deprenyl treatment. Neurosci Lett 1985; 58:177–181.

48. Gupta M, Felten DL, Felten SY. MPTP alters monoamine levels in systems other than the nigrostriatal dopaminergic system in mice. In: Markey SP, Castagnoli N Jr, Trevor AJ, Kopin IJ, ed. MPTP: a neurotoxin producing a parkinsonian syndrome. New York: Academic Press, 1986.

49. Seniuk NA, Tatton WG, Greenwood CE. Dose-dependent destruction of the coeruleus-cortical and nigral-striatal projections by MPTP. Brain Res 1990; 527:7–20.

50. Hallman H, Olson L, Jonsson G. Neurotoxicity of the meperidine analogue N-methyl-4-phenyl-1,2,3,6-tetrahydropyridine on brain catecholamine neurons in the mouse. Eur J Pharmacol 1984; 97:133–136.

51. Johannessen JN, Chiueh CC, Bacon JP. Neurchemical effects of MPTP in the dog: effects of pargyline pretreatment. Soc Neurosci Abstr 1985; 11:631.

52. Graham WC, Clarke CE, Boyce S, Sambrook MA, Crossman AR, Woodruff GN. Autoradiographic studies in animal models of hemi-parkinsonism reveal dopamine D2

but not D1 receptor supersensitivity. II. Unilateral intra-carotid infusion of MPTP in the monkey (Macaca fascicularis). Brain Res 1990; 514:103–110.

53. Przedborski S, Kostic V, Jackson-Lewis V, Cadet JL, Burke RE. Effect of unilateral perinatal hypoxic-ischemic brain injury in the rat on dopamine D1 and D2 receptors and uptake sites: a quantitative autoradiographic study. J Neurochem 1991; 57:1951–1961.

54. Augood SJ, Emson PC, Mitchell IJ, Boyce S, Clarke CE, Crossman AR. Cellular localisation of enkephalin gene expression in MPTP-treated cynomolgus monkeys. Brain Res Mol Brain Res 1989; 6:85–92.

55. Beresford IJ, Davenport AP, Sirinathsinghji DJ, Hall MD, Hill RG, Hughes J. Experimental hemiparkinsonism in the rat following chronic unilateral infusion of MPP+ into the nigrostriatal dopamine pathway—II. Differential localization of dopamine and cholecystokinin receptors. Neuroscience 1988; 27:129–143.

56. Przedborski S, Jackson-Lewis V, Popilskis S, et al. Unilateral MPTP-induced parkinsonism in monkeys: a quantitative autoradiographic study of dopamine D1 and D2 receptors and re-uptake sites. Neurochirurgie 1991; 37:377–382.

57. Ogawa N, Mizukawa K, Hirose Y, Kajita S, Ohara S, Watanabe Y. MPTP-induced parkinsonian model in mice: biochemistry, pharmacology and behavior. Eur Neurol 1987; 26(suppl 1):16–23.

58. Garvey J, Petersen M, Waters CM, et al. Administration of MPTP to the common marmoset does not alter cortical cholinergic function. Mov Disord 1986; 1:129–134.

59. Jenner P, Taquet H, Mauborgne A, et al. Lack of change in basal ganglia neuropeptide content following subacute 1-methyl-4-phenyl-1,2,3,6-tetrahydropyridine treatment of the common marmoset. J Neurochem 1986; 47:1548–1551.

60. Kitt CA, Cork LC, Eidelberg F, Joh TH, Price DL. Injury of nigral neurons exposed to 1-methyl-4-phenyl-1,2,3,6-tetrahydropyridine: a tyrosine hydroxylase immunocytochemical study in monkey. Neuroscience 1986; 17:1089–1103.

61. Forno LS, Langston JW, DeLanney LE, Irwin I, Ricaurte GA. Locus ceruleus lesions and eosinophilic inclusions in MPTP-treated monkeys. Ann Neurol 1986; 20:449–455.

62. Gibb C, Willoughby J, Glover V, et al. Analogues of 1-methyl-4-phenyl-1,2,3,6-tetrahydropyridine as monoamine oxidase substrates: a second ring is not necessary. Neurosci Lett 1987; 76:316–322.

63. Jackson-Lewis V, Jakowec M, Burke RE, Przedborski S. Time course and morphology of dopaminergic neuronal death caused by the neurotoxin 1-methyl-4-phenyl-1,2,3,6-tetrahydropyridine. Neurodegeneration 1995; 4:257–269.

64. Tatton NA, Kish SJ. In situ detection of apoptotic nuclei in the substantia nigra compacta of 1-methyl-4-phenyl-1,2,3,6-tetrahydropyridine-treated mice using terminal deoxynucleotidyl transferase labelling and acridine orange staining. Neuroscience 1997; 77: 1037–1048.

65. Storey E, Hyman BT, Jenkins B, et al. 1-Methyl-4-phenylpyridinium produces excitotoxic lesions in rat striatum as a result of impairment of oxidative metabolism. J Neurochem 1992; 58:1975–1978.

66. Giovanni A, Sieber B-A, Heikkila RE, Sonsalla PK. Studies on species sensitivity to the dopaminergic neurotoxin 1-methyl-4-phenyl-1,2,3,6-tetrahydropyridine. Part 1: Systemic administration. J Pharmacol Exp Ther 1994; 270:1000–1007.

67. Giovanni A, Sonsalla PK, Heikkila RE. Studies on species sensitivity to the dopaminergic neurotoxin 1-methyl-4-phenyl-1,2,3,6-tetrahydropyridine. Part 2: Central administration of 1-methyl-4-phenylpyridinium. J Pharmacol Exp Ther 1994; 270:1008–1014.

68. Staal RG, Sonsalla PK. Inhibition of brain vesicular monoamine transporter (VMAT2) enhances 1-methyl-4-phenylpyridinium neurotoxicity in vivo in rat striata. J Pharmacol Exp Ther 2000; 293:336–342.

69. Staal RG, Hogan KA, Liang CL, German DC, Sonsalla PK. In vitro studies of striatal vesicles containing the vesicular monoamine transporter (VMAT2): rat versus mouse differences in sequestration of 1-methyl-4-phenylpyridinium. J Pharmacol Exp Ther 2000; 293:329–335.

70. Mayer RA, Walters AS, Heikkila RE. 1-Methyl-4-phenyl-1,2,3,6-tetrahydropyridine (MPTP) administration to C57-black mice leads to parallel decrement in nigrostriatal dopamine content and tyrosine hydroxylase activity. Eur J Pharmacol 1986; 120: 375–377.

71. Sundstrom E, Stromberg I, Tsutsumi T, Olson L, Jonsson G. Studies on the effect of 1-methyl-4-phenyl-1,2,3,6-tetrahydropyridine (MPTP) on central catecholamine neurons in C57BL/6 mice. Comparison with three other strains of mice. Brain Res 1987; 405:26–38.

72. Heikkila RE, Hess A, Duvoisin RC. Dopaminergic neurotoxicity of 1-methyl-4-phenyl-1,2,3,6-tetrahydropyridine in mice. Science 1984; 224:1451–1453.

73. Javitch JA, D'Amato RJ, Strittmatter SM, Snyder SH. Parkinsonism-inducing neurotoxin, N-methyl-4-phenyl-1,2,3,6-tetrahydropyridine: uptake of the metabolite N-methyl-4-phenylpyridine by dopamine neurons explains selective toxicity. Proc Natl Acad Sci USA 1985; 82:2173–2177.

74. Langston JW, Forno LS, Rebert CS, Irwin I. Selective nigral toxicity after systemic administration of 1-methyl-4-phenyl-1,2,3,6-tetrahydropyridine (MPTP) in squirrel monkey. Brain Res 1984; 292:390–394.

75. Muthane U, Ramsay KA, Jiang H, et al. Differences in nigral neuron number and sensitivity to 1-methyl-4-phenyl-1,2,3,6-tetrahydropyridine in C57/bl and CD-1mice. Exp Neurol 1994; 126:195–204.

76. Wu DC, Teismann P, Tieu K, et al. NADPH oxidase mediates oxidative stress in the 1-methyl-4-phenyl-1,2,3,6-tetrahydropyridine model of Parkinson's disease. Proc Natl Acad Sci USA 2003; 100:6145–6150.

77. Czlonkowska A, Kohutnicka M, Kurkowska-Jastrzebska I, Czlonkowski A. Microglial reaction in MPTP (1-methyl-4-phenyl-1,2,3,6-tetrahydropyridine) induced Parkinson's disease mice model. Neurodegeneration 1996; 5:137–143.

78. Kohutnicka M, Lewandowska E, Kurkowska-Jastrzebska I, Czlonkowski A, Czlonkowska A. Microglial and astrocytic involvement in a murine model of Parkinson's disease induced by 1-methyl-4-phenyl-1,2,3,6-tetrahydropyridine (MPTP). Immunopharmacology 1998; 39:167–180.

79. Liberatore GT, Jackson-Lewis V, Vukosavic S, et al. Inducible nitric oxide synthase stimulates dopaminergic neurodegeneration in the MPTP model of Parkinson disease. Nat Med 1999; 5:1403–1409.

80. O'Callaghan JP, Miller DB, Reinhard JF. Characterization of the origins of astrocyte response to injury using the dopaminergic neurotoxicant, 1-methyl-4-phenyl-1,2,3,6-tetrahydropyridine. Brain Res 1990; 521:73–80.

81. OCallaghan JP. Quantification of glial fibrillary acidic protein: comparison of slot-immunobinding assays with a novel sandwich ELISA. Neurotoxicol Teratol 1991; 13:275–281.

82. Forno LS, Langston JW, DeLanney LE, Irwin I. An electron microscopic study of MPTP-induced inclusion bodies in an old monkey. Brain Res 1988; 448:150–157.

83. Kowall NW, Hantraye P, Brouillet E, Beal MF, McKee AC, Ferrante RJ. MPTP induces alpha-synuclein aggregation in the substantia nigra of baboons. Neuroreport 2000; 11:211–213.

84. Meredith GE, Totterdell S, Petroske E, Santa CK, Callison RC Jr, Lau YS. Lysosomal malfunction accompanies alpha-synuclein aggregation in a progressive mouse model of Parkinson's disease. Brain Res 2002; 956:156–165.

85. Fornai F, Schluter OM, Lenzi P, et al. Parkinson-like syndrome induced by continuous MPTP infusion: Convergent roles of the ubiquitin-proteasome system and {alpha}-synuclein. Proc Natl Acad Sci USA 2005.

86. Palombo E, Porrino LJ, Bankiewicz KS, Crane AM, Sokoloff L, Kopin IJ. Local cerebral glucose utilization in monkeys with hemiparkinsonism induced by intracarotid infusion of the neurotoxin MPTP. J Neurosci 1990; 10:860–869.

87. Riachi NJ, LaManna JC, Harik SI. Entry of 1-methyl-4-phenyl-1,2,3,6-tetrahydropyridine into the rat brain. J Pharmacol Exp Ther 1989; 249:744–748.

88. Chiba K, Kubota E, Miyakawa T, Kato Y, Ishizaki T. Characterization of hepatic microsomal metabolism as an in vivo detoxication pathway of 1-methyl-4-phenyl-1,2,3,6-tetrahydropyridine in mice. J Pharmacol Exp Ther 1988; 246:1108–1115.

89. Smith MT, Ekstrom G, Sandy MS, Di Monte D. Studies on the mechanism of 1-methyl-4-phenyl-1,2,3,6-tetrahydropyridine cytotoxicity in isolated hepatocytes. Life Sci 1987; 40:741–748.

90. Melamed E, Martinovits G, Pikarsky E, Rosenthal J, Uzzan A. Diphenylhydantoin and phenobarbital suppress the dopaminergic neurotoxicity of MPTP in mice. Eur J Pharmacol 1986; 128:255–257.

91. Markey SP, Johannessen JN, Chiueh CC, Burns RS, Herkenham MA. Intraneuronal generation of a pyridinium metabolite may cause drug-induced parkinsonism. Nature 1984; 311:464–467.
92. Chiba K, Trevor A, Castagnoli N Jr. Metabolism of the neurotoxic tertiary amine, MPTP, by brain monoamine oxidase. Biochem Biophys Res Commun 1984; P 574–P 578.
93. Chiba K, Peterson LA, Castagnoli KP, Trevor AJ, Castagnoli N Jr. Studies on the molecular mechanism of bioactivation of the selective nigrostriatal toxin 1-methyl-4-phenyl-1,2,3,6-tetrahydropyridine. Drug Metab Dispos 1985; 13:342–347.
94. Peterson LA, Caldera PS, Trevor A, Chiba K, Castagnoli N Jr. Studies on the 1-methyl-4-phenyl-2,3-dihydropyridinium species 2,3-MPDP+, the monoamine oxidase catalyzed oxidation product of the nigrostriatal toxin 1-methyl-4-phenyl-1,2,3,6-tetrahydropyridine (MPTP). J Med Chem 1985; 28:1432–1436.
95. Heikkila RE, Manzino L, Cabbat FS, Duvoisin RC. Protection against the dopaminergic neurotoxicity of 1-methyl-4-phenyl-1,2,3,6-tetrahydropyridine by monoamine oxidase inhibitors. Nature 1984; 311:467–469.
96. Langston JW, Irwin I, Langston EB, Forno LS. Pargyline prevents MPTP-induced parkinsonism in primates. Science 1984; 225:1480–1482.
97. Levitt P, Pintar JE, Breakefield XO. Immunocytochemical demonstration of monoamine oxidase B in brain astrocytes and serotonergic neurons. Proc Natl Acad Sci USA 1982; 79:6385–6389.
98. Westlund KN, Denney RM, Kochersperger LM, Rose RM, Abell CW. Distinct monoamine oxidase A and B populations in primate brain. Science 1985; 230:181–183.
99. Melamed E, Pikarski E, Goldberg A, Rosenthal J, Uzzan A, Conforti N. Effect of serotonergic, corticostriatal and kainic acid lesions on the dopaminergic neurotoxicity of 1-methyl-4-phenyl-1,2,3,6-tetrahydropyridine (MPTP) in mice. Brain Res 1986; 399:178–180.
100. Takada M, Li ZK, Hattori T. Astroglial ablation prevents MPTP-induced nigrostriatal neuronal death. Brain Res 1990; 509:55–61.
101. Harik SI, Mitchell MJ, Kalaria RN. Human susceptibility and rat resistance to systemic 1-methy-4-phenyl-1,2,3,6-tetrahydropyridine (MPTP) neurotoxicity correlate with blood brain barrier monoamine oxidase B activity. Neurology 1987; 37:338–339.
102. Javitch JA, Snyder SH. Uptake of MPP+ by dopamine neurons explains selectivity of parkinsonism-inducing neurotoxin, MPTP. Eur J Pharmacol 1984; 455–456.
103. Sundstrom E, Goldstein M, Jonsson G. Uptake inhibition protects nigro-striatal dopamine neurons from the neurotoxicity of 1-methyl-4-phenylpyridine (MPP+) in mice. Eur J Pharmacol 1986; 131:289–292.
104. Bezard E, Gross CE, Fournier MC, Dovero S, Bloch B, Jaber M. Absence of MPTP-induced neuronal death in mice lacking the dopamine transporter. Exp Neurol 1999; 155:268–273.
105. Javitch JA, D'Amato RJ, Strittmatter SM, Snyder SH. Parkinsonism-inducing neurotoxin, N-methyl-4-phenyl-1,2,3,6-tetrahydropyridine: uptake of the metabolite N-methyl-4-phenylpyridinium by dopamine neurons explain selective toxicity. Proc Natl Acad Sci USA 1985; 82:2173–2177.
106. Brooks WJ, Jarvis MF, Wagner GC. Attenuation of MPTP-induced dopaminergic neurotoxicity by a serotonin uptake blocker. J Neural Transm 1988; 71:85–90.
107. Przedborski S, Jackson-Lewis V, Naini A, et al. The parkinsonian toxin 1-methyl-4-phenyl-1,2,3,6-tetrahydropyridine (MPTP): a technical review of its utility and safety. J Neurochem 2001; 76:1265–1274.
108. Ramsay RR, Dadgar J, Trevor A, Singer TP. Energy-driven uptake of N-methyl-4-phenylpyridine by brain mitochondria mediates the neurotoxicity of MPTP. Life Sci 1986; 39:581–588.
109. Hoppel CL, Grinblatt D, Kwok HC, et al. Inhibition of mitochondrial respiration by analogs of 4-phenylpyridine and 1-methyl-4-phenylpyridinium cation (MPP+), the neurotoxic metabolite of MPTP. Biochem Biophys Res Commun 1987; 148:684–693.
110. Davey GP, Tipton KF, Murphy MP. Uptake and accumulation of 1-methyl-4-phenylpyridinium by rat liver mitochondria measured using an ion-selective electrode. Biochem J 1992; 288:439–443.
111. Ramsay RR, Singer TP. Energy-dependent uptake of N-methyl-4-phenylpyridinium, the neurotoxic metabolite of 1-methyl-4-phenyl-1,2,3,6-tetrahydropyridine, by mitochondria. J Biol Chem 1986; 261:7585–7587.

112. Aiuchi T, Shirane Y, Kinemuchi H, Arai Y, Nakaya K, Nakamura Y. Enhancement by tetraphenylboron of inhibition of mitochondrial respiration induced by 1-methyl-4-phenylpyridinium ion (MPP+). Neurochem Int 1988; 12:525–531.

113. Liu Y, Roghani A, Edwards RH. Gene transfer of a reserpine-sensitive mechanism of resistance to N-methyl-4-phenylpyridinium. Proc Natl Acad Sci USA 1992; 89: 9074–9078.

114. Takahashi N, Miner LL, Sora I, et al. VMAT2 knockout mice: heterozygotes display reduced amphetamine-conditioned reward, enhanced amphetamine locomotion, and enhanced MPTP toxicity. Proc Natl Acad Sci USA 1997; 94:9938–9943.

115. Irwin I, DeLanney LE, Di Monte D, Langston JW. The biodisposition of MPP+ in mouse brain. Neurosci Lett 1989; 101:83–88.

116. Irwin I, Langston JW. Safety and handling of MPTP. Neurology 1985; 35:619–619.

117. Zecca L, Tampellini D, Gerlach M, Riederer P, Fariello RG, Sulzer D. Substantia nigra neuromelanin: structure, synthesis, and molecular behaviour. Mol Pathol 2001; 54:414–418.

118. D'Amato RJ, Lipman ZP, Snyder SH. Selectivity of the parkinsonian neurotoxin MPTP: toxic metabolite MPP+ binds to neuromelanin. Science 1986; 231:987–989.

119. D'Amato RJ, Alexander GM, Schwartzman RJ, Kitt CA, Price DL, Snyder SH. Evidence for neuromelanin involvement in MPTP-induced neurotoxicity. Nature 1987; 327: 324–326.

120. Nicklas WJ, Vyas I, Heikkila RE. Inhibition of NADH-linked oxidation in brain mitochondria by MPP+, a metabolite of the neurotoxin MPTP. Life Sci 1985; 36:2503–2508.

121. Schuler F, Casida JE. Functional coupling of PSST and ND1 subunits in NADH:ubiquinone oxidoreductase established by photoaffinity labeling. Biochim Biophys Acta 2001; 1506:79–87.

122. Davey GP, Clark JB. Threshold effects and control of oxidative phosphorylation in nonsynaptic rat brain mitochondria. J Neurochem 1996; 66:1617–1624.

123. Chan P, DeLanney LE, Irwin I, Langston JW, Di Monte D. Rapid ATP loss caused by 1-methyl-4-phenyl-1,2,3,6-tetrahydropyridine in mouse brain. J Neurochem 1991; 57:348–351.

124. Matthews RT, Ferrante RJ, Klivenyi P, et al. Creatine and cyclocreatine attenuate MPTP neurotoxicity. Exp Neurol 1999; 157:142–149.

125. Hasegawa E, Takeshige K, Oishi T, Murai Y, Minakami S. 1-Mehtyl-4-phenylpyridinium (MPP+) induces NADH-dependent superoxide formation and enhances NADH-dependent lipid peroxidation in bovine heart submitochondrial particles. Biochem Biophys Res Commun 1990; 170:1049–1055.

126. Cleeter MW, Cooper JM, Schapira AH. Irreversible inhibition of mitochondrial complex I by 1-methyl-4-phenylpyridinium: evidence for free radical involvement. J Neurochem 1992; 58:786–789.

127. Lotharius J, O'Malley KL. The parkinsonism-inducing drug 1-methyl-4-phenylpyridinium triggers intracellular dopamine oxidation. A novel mechanism of toxicity. J Biol Chem 2000; 275:38581–38588.

128. Przedborski S, Kostic V, Jackson-Lewis V, et al. Transgenic mice with increased Cu/Zn-superoxide dismutase activity are resistant to N-methyl-4-phenyl-1,2,3,6- tetrahydropyridine-induced neurotoxicity. J Neurosci 1992; 12:1658–1667.

129. Schulz JB, Matthews RT, Muqit MMK, Browne SE, Beal MF. Inhibition of neuronal nitric oxide synthase by 7-nitroindazole protects against MPTP-induced neurotoxicity in mice. J Neurochem 1995; 64:936–939.

130. Teismann P, Schwaninger M, Weih F, Ferger B. Nuclear factor-kappaB activation is not involved in a MPTP model of Parkinson's disease. Neuroreport 2001; 12:1049–1053.

131. Pennathur S, Jackson-Lewis V, Przedborski S, Heinecke JW. Mass spectrometric quantification of 3-nitrotyrosine, ortho-tyrosine, and O,O'-dityrosine in brain tissue of 1-methyl-4-phenyl-1,2,3, 6-tetrahydropyridine-treated mice, a model of oxidative stress in Parkinson's disease. J Biol Chem 1999; 274:34621–34628.

132. Przedborski S, Jackson-Lewis V, Yokoyama R, Shibata T, Dawson VL, Dawson TM. Role of neuronal nitric oxide in MPTP (1-methyl-4-phenyl-1,2,3,6-tetrahydropyridine)-induced dopaminergic neurotoxicity. Proc Natl Acad Sci USA 1996; 93:4565–4571.

133. Bredt DS, Glatt CE, Huang PL, Fotuhi M, Dawson TM, Snyder SH. Nitric oxide synthase protein and mRNA are discretely localized in neuronal populations of the mammalian CNS together with NADPH diaphorase. Neuron 1991; 7:615–624.
134. Leonard CS, Kerman I, Blaha G, Taveras E, Taylor B. Interdigitation of nitric oxide synthase-, tyrosine hydroxylase-, and serotonin-containing neurons in and around the laterodorsal and pedunculopontine tegmental nuclei of the guinea pig. J Comp Neurol 1995; 362:411–432.
135. Tieu K, Ischiropoulos H, Przedborski S. Nitric oxide and reactive oxygen species in Parkinson's disease. IUBMB Life 2003; 55:329–335.
136. Mihm MJ, Schanbacher BL, Wallace BL, Wallace LJ, Uretsky NJ, Bauer JA. Free 3-nitro-tyrosine causes striatal neurodegeneration in vivo. J Neurosci 2001; 21:RC149.
137. Ara J, Przedborski S, Naini AB, et al. Inactivation of tyrosine hydroxylase by nitration following exposure to peroxynitrite and 1-methyl-4-phenyl-1,2,3,6-tetrahydropyridine (MPTP). Proc Natl Acad Sci USA 1998; 95:7659–7663.
138. Przedborski S, Chen Q, Vila M, et al. Oxidative post-translational modifications of alpha-synuclein in the 1-methyl-4-phenyl-1,2,3,6-tetrahydropyridine (MPTP) mouse model of Parkinson's disease. J Neurochem 2001; 76:637–640.
139. Chung KK, Dawson TM, Thomas B, et al. S-Nitrosylation of parkin regulates ubiqui-tination and compromises parkin's protective function. Science 2004; 304:1328–1331.
140. Mandavilli BS, Ali SF, Van Houten B. DNA damage in brain mitochondria caused by aging and MPTP treatment. Brain Res 2000; 885:45–52.
141. Mandir AS, Przedborski S, Jackson-Lewis V, et al. Poly (ADP-ribose) polymerase activa-tion mediates MPTP-induced parkinsonism. Proc Natl Acad Sci USA 1999; 96: 5774–5779.
142. Vila M, Przedborski S. Neurological diseases: Targeting programmed cell death in neu-rodegenerative diseases. Nat Rev Neurosci 2003; 4:365–375.
143. Vila M, Jackson-Lewis V, Vukosavic S, et al. Bax ablation prevents dopaminergic neuro-degeneration in the 1-methyl-4-phenyl-1,2,3,6-tetrahydropyridine mouse model of Parkinson's disease. Proc Natl Acad Sci USA 2001; 98:2837–2842.
144. Fannjiang Y, Kim CH, Huganir RL, et al. BAK alters neuronal excitability and can switch from anti- to pro-death function during postnatal development. Developmental Cell 2003; 4:575–585.
145. Yang L, Matthews RT, Schulz JB, et al. 1-Methyl-4-phenyl-1,2,3,6-tetrahydropyride neu-rotoxicity is attenuated in mice overexpressing Bcl-2. J Neurosci 1998; 18:8145–8152.
146. Offen D, Beart PM, Cheung NS, et al. Transgenic mice expressing human Bcl-2 in their neurons are resistant to 6-hydroxydopamine and 1-methyl-4-phenyl-1,2,3,6-tetrahydro-pyridine neurotoxicity. Proc Natl Acad Sci USA 1998; 95:5789–5794.
147. Xu D, Bureau Y, McIntyre DC, et al. Attenuation of ischemia-induced cellular and behavioral deficits by X chromosome-linked inhibitor of apoptosis protein overexpres-sion in the rat hippocampus. J Neurosci 1999; 19:5026–5033.
148. Eberhardt O, Coelln RV, Kugler S, et al. Protection by synergistic effects of adenovirus-mediated X-chromosome-linked inhibitor of apoptosis and glial cell line-derived neurotrophic factor gene transfer in the 1-methyl-4-phenyl-1,2,3,6-tetrahydropyridine model of Parkinson's disease. J Neurosci 2000; 20:9126–9134.
149. Hartmann A, Troadec JD, Hunot S, et al. Caspase-8 is an effector in apoptotic death of dopaminergic neurons in Parkinson's disease, but pathway inhibition results in neuro-nal necrosis. J Neurosci 2001; 21:2247–2255.
150. Viswanath V, Wu Y, Boonplueang R, et al. Caspase-9 activation results in downstream caspase-8 activation and bid cleavage in 1-methyl-4-phenyl-1,2,3,6-tetrahydropyridine-induced Parkinson's disease. J Neurosci 2001; 21:9519–9528.
151. Trimmer PA, Smith TS, Jung AB, Bennett JP Jr. Dopamine neurons from transgenic mice with a knockout of the p53 gene resist MPTP neurotoxicity. Neurodegeneration 1996; 5:233–239.
152. Saporito MS, Brown EM, Miller MS, Carswell S. CEP-1347/KT-7515, an inhibitor of c-jun N-terminal kinase activation, attenuates the 1-methyl-4-phenyl tetrahydropyri-dine-mediated loss of nigrostriatal dopaminergic neurons in vivo. J Pharmacol Exp Ther 1999; 288:421–427.

153. Xia XG, Harding T, Weller M, Bieneman A, Uney JB, Schulz JB. Gene transfer of the JNK interacting protein-1 protects dopaminergic neurons in the MPTP model of Parkinson's disease. Proc Natl Acad Sci USA 2001; 98:10433–10438.
154. Hunot S, Vila M, Teismann P, et al. JNK-mediated induction of cyclooxygenase 2 is required for neurodegeneration in a mouse model of Parkinson's disease. Proc Natl Acad Sci USA 2004; 101:665–670.
155. Mochizuki H, Hayakawa H, Migita M, et al. An AAV-derived Apaf-1 dominant negative inhibitor prevents MPTP toxicity as antiapoptotic gene therapy for Parkinson's disease. Proc Natl Acad Sci USA 2001; 98:10918–10923.
156. Przedborski S, Goldman JE. Pathogenic role of glial cells in Parkinson's disease. In: Hertz L, ed. Non-Neuronal Cells of the Nervous System: Function and Dysfunction. New York: Elsevier, 2004.
157. Liberatore G, Jackson-Lewis V, Vukosavic S, et al. Inducible nitric oxide synthase stimulates dopaminergic neurodegeneration in the MPTP model of Parkinson's disease. Nat Med 1999; 5:1403–1409.
158. Wu DC, Jackson-Lewis V, Vila M, et al. Blockade of microglial activation is neuroprotective in the 1-methyl-4-phenyl-1,2,3,6-tetrahydropyridine mouse model of Parkinson disease. J Neurosci 2002; 22:1763–1771.
159. Du Y, Ma Z, Lin S, et al. Minocycline prevents nigrostriatal dopaminergic neurodegeneration in the MPTP model of Parkinson's disease. Proc Natl Acad Sci USA 2001; 98:14669–14674.
160. Bergman H, Wichmann T, DeLong MR. Reversal of experimental parkinsonism by lesions of the subthalamic nucleus. Science 1990; 249:1436–1438.
161. Limousin P, Krack P, Pollak P, et al. Electrical stimulation of the subthalamic nucleus in advanced Parkinson's disease. N Engl J Med 1998; 339:1105–1111.
162. Gash DM, Zhang ZM, Ovadia A, et al. Functional recovery in parkinsonian monkeys treated with GDNF. Nature 1996; 380:252–255.
163. Kordower JH, Emborg ME, Bloch J, et al. Neurodegeneration prevented by lentiviral vector delivery of GDNF in primate models of Parkinson's disease. Science 2000; 290:767–773.
164. Gill SS, Patel NK, Hotton GR, et al. Direct brain infusion of glial cell line-derived neurotrophic factor in Parkinson disease. Nat Med 2003; 9:589–595.
165. Dauer W, Przedborski S. Parkinson's disease: mechanisms and models. Neuron 2003; 39:889–909.

22 Rotenone Model for Parkinson's Disease

Ranjita Betarbet
Center for Neurodegenerative Diseases, Emory University, Atlanta, Georgia, U.S.A.

J. Timothy Greenamyre
Pittsburgh Institute for Neurodegenerative Diseases, University of Pittsburgh, Pittsburgh, Pennsylvania, U.S.A.

INTRODUCTION

Parkinson's disease (PD) is a late onset, progressive, neurodegenerative, movement disorder affecting more than 2% of the population over the age of 65 years. Clinical symptoms of PD consist of resting tremor, muscular rigidity, bradykinesia, and abnormal postural reflexes (1). The pathologic hallmark of PD is the progressive degeneration of the nigrostriatal pathway and dopaminergic cells of the substantia nigra (2) though recent neuropathologic studies suggest a more extended neuronal degeneration starting in the medulla oblongata that later spreads to the midbrain and cerebral cortex (3). Nevertheless it is the degeneration of the nigrostriatal pathway and subsequent dopamine deficiency in striatum that is believed to underlie many of the clinical manifestations of PD (4–8).

Another important pathologic feature of PD is the presence of fibrillar cytoplasmic inclusions known as Lewy bodies. Lewy bodies contain aggregates of many different proteins including ubiquitin and α-synuclein (9) and are present in the surviving dopaminergic neurons of substantia nigra and in brain regions such as the cerebral cortex and magnocellular basal forebrain nuclei (10). Mutations in α-synuclein gene have been associated with rare familial cases of PD (11). However, Lewy bodies are positive for α-synuclein in the majority of idiopathic PD cases that lack α-synuclein mutations, suggesting a central role for α-synuclein protein in PD pathogenesis (9,12). Additional mutations in two other genes, *PARKIN* (13–15) and ubiquitin carboxy-terminal hydrolase LI (16), have been associated with familial PD and have suggested that dysfunctional protein degradation might be an important factor in the etiology of PD. Proteasomal dysfunction has been reported in sporadic cases of PD (17).

Mitochondrial dysfunction (18–22) and oxidative stress (23) have also been strongly implicated in the pathogenesis of PD. Recent evidence linking recessively inherited mutations in PINK1 (PTEN-induced kinase 1), a putative mitochondrial protein kinase (24), and DJ-1 a protein allegedly associated with oxidative stress (25–27) to familial forms of PD further augment the role of mitochondrial dysfunction and oxidative stress in PD pathogenesis.

Environmental toxins, including pesticides, have also been determined to be risk factors for PD based on epidemiologic observations. Farming, living in rural areas, drinking well water, and exposure to agricultural chemicals are associated with increased risk for PD (28,29).

Today the emerging belief is that a combination of genetic and environmental factors, converging on mitochondrial defects, oxidative stress, and aberrant protein aggregation, account for most cases of PD (30). This review, while discussing the development and characterization of the rotenone model, will emphasize on how a systemic complex I inhibition can result in selective parkinsonian-like pathology and neurodegeneration.

MITOCHONDRIA AND PARKINSON'S DISEASE

Systemic complex I inhibition is one of the key biochemical features of PD that has been virtually ignored, especially in terms of developing an animal model. We proposed that if "systemic complex I inhibition" has a central role in PD pathogenesis then systemic low levels of chronic complex I inhibition would induce selective degeneration of the nigrostriatal pathway. Indeed, continuous low levels of rotenone exposure in rats resulted in selective degeneration of the nigrostriatal pathway. However, before we discuss the rotenone model of PD it would be helpful to describe briefly the role of mitochondria, oxidative phosphorylation, and complex I inhibition.

Mitochondrial Complex I

Mitochondria are cellular organelles that are present in virtually every eukaryotic cell though they differ in shape, size, and number. The central role of mitochondria lies in the production of energy in the form of adenosine triphosphate (ATP) required by the cell via two interrelated sets of reactions: the krebs or the tricarboxylic acid cycle (TCA cycle) and oxidative phosphorylation (31). The TCA cycle takes place in the mitochondria matrix and generates reduced nicotinamide adenine dinucleotide (NADH) and flavin adenine dinucleotide (FADH$_2$). NADH and FADH$_2$ undergo oxidative phosphorylation (oxphos) by donating electrons to the electron transport chain (ETC) and its constituent complex array of enzymes that are located on the inner mitochondrial membrane (Fig. 1). The inner mitochondrial membrane is

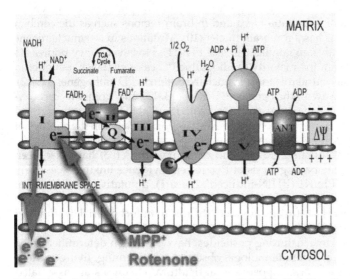

FIGURE 1   Schematic diagram of the mitochondrial ETC. Note the site of complex I inhibition by rotenone and MPP$^+$, electron leakage and ROS production. Abbreviations: ADP, adenosine diphosphate; ATP, adenosine triphosphate; ETC, electron transport chain; FAD, flavin adenine dinucleotide; FADH$_2$, flavin adenine dinucleotide; MPP, 1-methyl-4-phenyl-2,3-dihydropyridinium ion; NADH, nicotinamide dinucleotide; ROS, reactive oxygen species; TCA, trycarboxylic acid.

selectively permeable to ions and the control of its permeability is the key to most mitochondrial functions, including oxphos, intracellular calcium regulation, apoptosis, and cell death. Oxphos consists of two closely coupled processes: electron transport to oxygen and phosphorylation of adenosine diphosphate (ADP). Electrons from NADH enter the ETC via complex I (NADH dehydrogenase or NADH-ubiquinone oxidoreductase). Complex I is composed of 46 subunits, seven of which are mitochondrially encoded. Rotenone and 1-methyl-4-phenyl-2,3-dihydropyridinium ion (MPP$^+$) are known inhibitors (Fig. 1) of this enzyme (32,33). Electrons from complex I are transferred to complex III (ubiquinol-cytochrome c oxidoreductase) via ubiquinone. Ubiquinone also receives electrons from FADH$_2$ most of which is generated by the TCA cycle. From complex III, the electrons are donated to cytochrome c that transfer them to complex IV. Complex IV transfers electrons to molecular oxygen, the final electron acceptor. Complexes I, III, and IV pump protons from the inner mitochondrial matrix to the outer mitochondrial matrix, creating potential energy, stored in the form of an electrochemical gradient. These protons flow back into the matrix through complex V or ATP synthase and provide the energy needed for ATP production (34). Knowledge that human brain contributes 2% of the body weight but produces 20% of ATP confirms the importance of oxphos (35).

As mentioned previously PD has been associated with a systemic but modest complex I inhibition. Schapira and his colleagues first reported selective complex I defects (other complexes were not affected) in substantia nigra of PD patients (20). Later on, reports indicated that the complex I defect is systemic in PD, affecting tissues outside the brain such as platelets, lymphocytes, and muscle (19,21,36–40). The nature of this complex I defect—whether genetic or acquired—remains uncertain. The role of mitochondria in PD has been further accentuated by the observation that MPP$^+$, the active metabolite of 1-methyl-4-phenyl-1,2,3,6-tetrahydropyridine (MPTP) and an inhibitor of complex I of the mitochondrial electron transport chain, causes an acute parkinsonian syndrome (32,41,42).

Mitochondria and Oxidative Stress

Mitochondrial respiration is also a source of reactive oxygen species (ROS). At several locations along the mitochondrial ETC, there are sites of "electron leaks" (Fig. 1). These electrons can combine with molecular oxygen and form reactive oxygen species (43,44), such as superoxide (O$_2$) and hydrogen peroxide (H$_2$O$_2^-$). The ROS can readily react with DNA, lipids, and proteins and cause oxidative damage. Partial complex I inhibition is known to enhance ROS production (44–46). Evidence for the involvement of oxidative stress in PD has also been obtained from PD patients. Increased lipid peroxidation and oxidative damage to DNA and proteins have been observed in substantia nigra of PD patients (23,47–49). Decreased levels of glutathione have also been found in the substantia nigra of PD brains further implicating oxidative stress (50). Oxidative damage in PD may not be selective to substantia nigra, as elevated oxidative protein damage has also been reported throughout PD brain (51).

THE ROTENONE MODEL IN RATS

A naturally occurring compound derived from roots of a plant called *Lonchocarpus* species, rotenone is commonly used as an "organic" insecticide and to kill nuisance fish in lakes. Rotenone is also a classical, high affinity complex I inhibitor, and is typically used to define the specific activity of complex I (52,53). Additionally, rotenone is a lipophilic compound that easily crosses the blood brain barrier. Unlike MPP⁺ rotenone does not require the help of transporters (Uversky, 2004) to cross cellular membranes. Once inside the cell rotenone accumulates in the mitochondria (54), where it impairs oxidative phosphorylation by inhibiting complex I (53).

Rotenone Admistration

To simulate low levels of exposure to a complex I inhibitor during a normal life span, SpragueDawley and Lewis rats were systemically and chronically exposed to low levels of rotenone via an intrajuglar cannula attached to a subcutaneous osmotic minipump (55). Lewis rats developed more consistent lesions and were therefore used exclusively for further studies. At first the doses of rotenone used ranged from 1 to 12 mg/kg/day. At high doses rotenone produced systemic cardiovascular toxicity and nonspecific brain lesions similar to that observed by others (56,57). Downward titration of rotenone dosing resulted in less systemic toxicity and more specific nigrostriatal dopaminergic degeneration. The optimal dose for inducing PD-like pathology was determined to be 2–3 mg/kg/day. It is important to note at this point that even at the "optimal dose," only 30% to 50% of Lewis rats demonstrated PD-like pathology. Nonetheless, systemic, low levels of rotenone administration reproduced pathologic features characteristic of PD (55). Intrajugular cannulation surgeries are however labor-intensive and increases the risk of postsurgical complications. Therefore, an alternative route was developed to administer rotenone. Instead of cannulation and vascular administration rotenone was administered by subcutaneously placed osmotic minipumps that released rotenone into the body cavity (55,58). Subcutaneous administration of rotenone, at 2–3 mg/kg/day in Lewis rats, also produced selective nigrostriatal dopaminergic lesions as previously reported (55). Rotenone, emulsified in sunflower oil, and administered daily by intraperitoneal injections was also able to induce parkinsonian symptoms and degeneration of nigral dopaminergic neurons in Sprague-Dawley rats (59).

Characteristics of Rotenone-Induced Toxicity
Systemic Complex I Inhibition

Consistent with its ability to cross biologic membranes easily, chronic, low doses of systemic rotenone infusion resulted in uniform inhibition of complex I throughout the rat brain. [³H] dihydrorotenone binding to complex I in brain was reduced by approximately 75%. Seventy-five percentage inhibition of specific binding translated to be 20–30 nM of free rotenone in the brain. Rotenone infusion did not have any effect on the enzymatic activities of complexes II and IV, analyzed histochemically (55). This uniform complex I inhibition induced by rotenone was unlike the effects of MPTP, which selectively inhibits complex I in dopaminergic neurons due to the dependence of MPP⁺, the active metabolite of MPTP, on the dopamine transporter.

Selective Nigrostriatal Dopaminergic Degeneration

Interestingly, despite this uniform complex I inhibition, rotenone caused selective degeneration of the nigrostriatal dopaminergic pathway (55,58–60). Immunocytochemistry for tyrosine hydroxylase (TH), a rate limiting enzyme involved in the production of dopamine and a phenotypic marker for dopaminergic neurons, demonstrated absence of dopaminergic innervation in the striatum (Fig. 2). Other dopaminergic markers including dopamine transporter (DAT) and vesicular

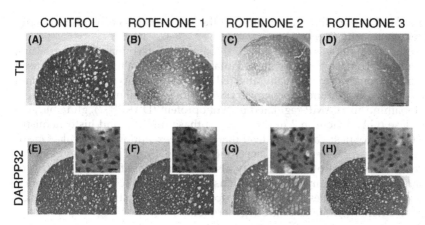

FIGURE 2 Selective degeneration of dopaminergic terminals in the striatum of rotenone-infused rats (2.5–3.0 mg/kg/day). Striatal sections from control (**A, E**) and rotenone-infused rats (**B, C, D, F, G, H**) were stained for TH (**A, B, C, D**) and DARPP32 (**E, F, G, H**) ICC. **B, C,** and **D** represent three different patterns of Striatal lesions following rotenone exposure (3-21 days of rotenone exposure) as determined by TH-ir. Striatal DARPP32-positive neurons were mostly intact following rotenone infusion (**F, H**) despite extensive TH loss, except for a small necroc focal area (**G**) devoid of DARPP32-ir. *Abbreviations*: DARPP32, dopamine and cAMP-regulated phosphoprotein; TH, tyrosine hydroxylase.

monoamine transporter type 2 (VMAT2) confirmed the striatal lesions (60). Staining for neurodegeneration such as silver and fluoro-jade B unambiguously verified that the absence of dopaminergic phenotypic markers in the striatum was due to the degeneration of dopaminergic terminals. The striatal dopaminergic lesions were, either partial or focal, located in the central or dorsolateral region of the anterior striatum or were diffused and spread out to involve most of the motor striatum (Fig. 2). Interestingly, even when the lesion was severe, there was relative sparing of dopaminergic fibers in the medial aspects of the striatum, nucleus accumbens, and olfactory tubercle, areas that are relatively spared in idiopathic PD (55).

Neurodegeneration, at various extents, was also evident in the dopaminergic neurons of the substantia nigra. Animals that had partial striatal lesions had dopaminergic neurons in the substantia nigra that looked relatively normal while animals with extensive striatal lesions had obvious reductions in nigral TH-positive neurons. Silver staining demonstrated clear signs of degenerating nigral neurons with silver deposits in their cell bodies and processes, even in animals that had normal looking TH-positive cells and partial striatal lesions. Rats that had severe striatal lesions exhibited more extensive signs of degeneration in the nigral neurons.

Both TH immunocytochemistry and silver staining demonstrated retrograde degeneration of nigral dopaminergic neurons following rotenone exposure; degeneration began at the terminals in the striatum where the effects were more severe compared to the nigral neurons (55,60,61). Quantitative analysis of dopamine levels has also shown extensive deficiency in the striatum (59), similar to postmortem analysis of brains from PD patients that have shown more extensive loss of striatal dopamine compared to substantia nigra (62). Furthermore, neurons in the lateral and ventral tiers of the substantia nigra appeared to be more vulnerable to systemic rotenone infusion, very similar to the pattern of neuronal vulnerability observed in idiopathic PD. Despite the loss of TH-immunoreactivity in the susbtantia nigra, dopaminergic neurons of the ventral tegmental area (VTA) were spared as in PD.

Also, similar to PD, noradrenergic neurons of the locus ceruleus were also susceptible to rotenone toxicity (55,60,61).

Despite profound loss of presynaptic dopaminergic terminals in the striatum,
the postsynaptic striatal neurons remained intact. In majority of the rotenone infused
rats striatal neurons were minimally affected (Fig. 2) as observed with nissl stain
and NeuN and with immunocytochemistry for various striatal phenotypic markers
such as dopamine and cAMP-regulated phosphoprotein (DARPP32), glutamic acid
decarboxylase (GAD), neuronal nitric oxide synthase (nNOS), and histochemistry
for AchE (acetylcholinesterase). However there was an exception to this rule. One or
two rats with acute focal lesions had a necrotic core (Fig. 2) and showed evidence of
striatal cell loss (60,63). Rotenone toxicity also had minimal effects on neurons of
other brain regions, including globus pallidus and subthalamic nucleus confirmed
with silver staining (58). These data further supported the nigrostriatal dopaminergic
selectivity of rotenone-induced neurodegeneration.

Microglial Activation

PD is characterized by selective activation of nigrostriatal microglial response while
astrocytosis is rarely observed. Selective microglial activation in the striatum and
nigral brain regions was detected in rotenone-infused rats (60,64). Enlarged microglia
with short, stubby processes were detected prior to dopaminergic lesions. Rotenone-
induced microglial activation was less pronounced in the cortex and in rats that did
not develop a striatal lesion. Microglia are the brain's resident immune cells and are
activated in response to immunologic stimuli and/or neuronal injuries. They are
known to produce potentially neurotoxic reactive oxygen species that probably add
to the oxidative stress reported in PD (65,66).

Oxidative Stress

Rotenone-induced complex I inhibition resulted in creased oxidative stress, both
in vitro in neuroblastoma cells (67) and in vivo in rats (68), as implicated by increased
levels of protein carbonyls, a marker for oxidative stress. It was observed that the
toxicity in neuroblastoma cells, chronically exposed to low levels of rotenone, was
mainly due to increased levels of oxidative stress and minimally due to ATP depletion.
Furthermore, rotenone-induced toxicity in cells was attenuated by prior treatment
with α-tocopherol, a known antioxidant, confirming that the toxic action of rotenone
was via oxidative stress (68). Rotenone-infused rats also demonstrated increased
levels of oxidative stress most notably in dopaminergic regions including the
striatum, ventral midbrain, and the olfactory bulb.

Oxidative stress related recessive *DJ-1* mutations are associated with an early-
onset form of parkinsonism in human patients (25). Interestingly, chronic rotenone
exposure, both in vitro and in vivo resulted in oxidative modifications of *DJ-1*
protein by a shift in pI toward a more acidic form and translocating to the outer
mitochondrial membrane from the cytoplasm (69). It is suggested that *DJ-1* is
normally neuroprotective while mutations or oxidative modifications can reduce its
neuroprotective effects (70,71). Thus rotenone-induced toxicity appears to be
strongly associated with oxidative stress, which in turn has been strongly implicated
in PD pathogenesis (23).

α-Synuclein-Positive Cytoplasmic Inclusions

As mentioned previously, α-synuclein-positive cytoplasmic inclusions called Lewy
bodies are characteristic hallmarks of PD pathology, α-synuclein positive inclusions

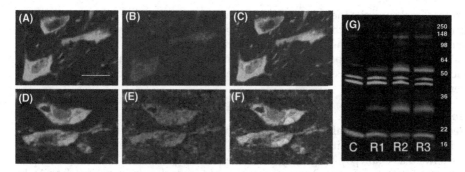

FIGURE 3 α-Synuclein accumulation in dopaminergic nigral neurons. Coronal sections through the substantia nigra from control (**A, B, C**) and rotenone-infused (**D, E, F**) rats were double labeled for TH (**A, D**) and α-synuclein (**B, E**). Note the increased α-synuclein expression in dopaminergic neurons following rotenone exposure. Western immunoblotting (**G**) confirmed the increase in α-synuclein levels (red bands) and accumulation in the ventral midbrain. Note the increased expression and presence of higher molecular weight bands in rotenone exposed rats (R1, R2, R3) as compared to a control rat (**C**). MAPk (green bands) was used as a loading control. *Abbreviations*: MAPK, MAP kinase; TH, tyrosine hydroxylase.

in nigral cells were also detected in rotenone-infused rats (55,58,60). These cytoplasmic inclusions were positive for ubiquitin and appeared as "pale eosinophilic" inclusions with hematoxylin and eosin staining. These inclusions were ultrastructurally similar to Lewy bodies of PD, in that they had a homogenous dense core surrounded by fibrillar elements (55). Biochemical analysis confirmed the accumulation and aggregation of α-synuclein in rotenone-infused rats (Fig. 3). Western immunoblotting demonstrated significant and selective increases in α-synuclein levels in the ventral midbrain regions as well as higher molecular weight bands (~30 and 52 kd) in addition to the 19 kd α-synuclein band (72). In the striatum punctate α-synuclein accumulation was detected in regions that were devoid of TH immunoreactivity (72), very similar to that observed AD/LBD patient (73).

Proteasomal Dysfunction

A dysfunctional ubiquitin proteasome system (UPS) was also a consequence of rotenone-induced complex I inhibition. Ubiquitin independent proteasomal enzymatic activities were significantly and selectively reduced in the ventral midbrain regions in rotenone-infused rats with striatal lesions. Furthermore, ubiquitin conjugated proteins, an indicator of proteins marked for degradation, were markedly increased in ventral midbrain (VMB) suggesting impairment of ubiquitin-dependent proteasome degradation pathway (74).

Impairment of proteasomal function could be due to complex I inhibition-induced changes in bioenergetics such as ATP production and/or complex I inhibition-induced increase in free radicals production resulting in oxidatively damaged proteins. Acute, in vitro studies using ventral mesencephalic primary cultures implied that rotenone-induced impairment of proteasomal function is primarily due to ATP depletion and not from free radical production (75). However chronic exposure to low levels of rotenone, while minimally affecting bioenergetics, significantly increases the levels of oxidative stress, which may have a greater role in neuronal degeneration (67,68). It is possible that increased levels of oxidatively damaged proteins, observed following rotenone-infusion/treatment, could impair proteasomal pathway, by either "clogging-up" the UPS or oxidatively modifying the proteasomal subunits themselves. In fact Shamoto-Nagai et al. (76) have shown that complex I inhibition with rotenone in neuroblastoma SH-SY5Y cells reduced protea-somal activity through increased production of oxidatively modified proteins including oxidative modification of the proteasome itself. Thus it appears that increased oxidative stress could inhibit proteasomal function and eventually lead to neuronal degeneration.

Behavior

Reduced striatal dopaminergic activity is known to cause parkinsonian symptoms in humans such as rigidity and hypokinesia (1). In rats rigidity and akinetic behavior are termed as catalepsy. Catelepsy tests revealed a significant increase in cataleptic behavior in rotenone treated rats as compared to control, vehicle treated rats (1). In addition rotenone-treated rats displayed significant decline in locomotor activities including active sitting, rearing, and line crossing behavior (59). Rigidity and hypo-kinetic behavior as well as flexed posture, similar to the stooped posture of PD patients, were previously reported in rotenone-exposed rats (55,58). Some of the rotenone-infused rats also developed severe rigidity and a few had spontaneously shaking paws that were reminiscent of resting tremor in PD.

The Variability in the Rotenone Model

Since the initial studies with rotenone numerous reports have either confirmed (59,60) or questioned (57,61) the selectivity of rotenone-induced degeneration of the nigros-triatal dopaminergic pathway. These differences could be due to a "small window" for rotenone's action that results in selective neurodegeneration. There exists a threshold for every drug beyond which they have nonspecific or "side effects." For rotenone this threshold appears to be very small—some animals have an acute response while some are not affected by rotenone at all and yet there are some rats that develop very characteristic features of PD. At high doses, as shown by Ferrante et al. (56), rotenone can have nonspecific effects.

The variability observed in rotenone-induced toxicity range from none to nearly complete striatal dopaminergic lesions (55,57,58,60,61) is interesting. This variability clearly demonstrates the individual susceptibility to complex I inhibition in rats which could be due to genetic differences and/or differences in the ability to metabolize environmental toxins (77), similar to individual differences that may determine ones susceptibility to develop PD.

THE ROTENONE MODEL IN MICE

As evident from the studies involving rotenone-infused rats one of the drawbacks of the model appears to be the variability observed in rotenone-induced toxicity especially in terms of using this model for therapeutic investigations. The cause of this variability, as suggested may be due to genetic variability in the out-bred rats used for the study. To circumvent this problem the chronic rotenone studies were carried out in in-bred strain of mice. C57 mice were exposed to various doses of rotenone via subcutaneous osmotic minipumps over a period of one to two weeks. These mice appeared to be relatively resistant to rotenone as compared to the Lewis rats. The doses of rotenone that produced nigral dopaminergic degeneration in mice were 6 and 10 mg/kg/day, more than two to three times the dose that produced nigrostriatal dopaminergic degeneration in rats. Chronic rotenone exposure resulted in significant loss (25–75%) of TH-immunoreactive nigral neurons as determined

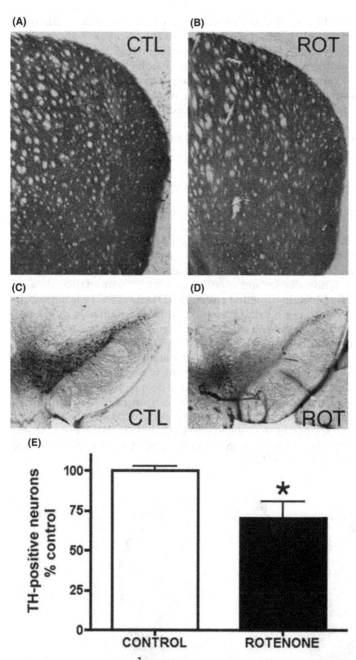

FIGURE 4 Degeneration of nigral dopaminergic neurons in rotenone-infused mice. Coronal sections from both the striatum (**A, B**) and substantia nigra (**C, D**) were stained for stained for TH. Note the loss of TH-positive neurons in the rotenone-exposed substantia nigia (**D**) as compared to the control (**C**). Interestingly, TH-ir was the same in the striatum of control (**A**) and rotenone-exposed (**B**) rats. Stereological analysis (**E**) of TH-positive neurons confirmed the significant loss of dopaminergic neurons following rotenone exposure (10 mg/kg/day; seven days). *Abbreviations*: CTL, control; ROT, rotenone; TH, tyrosine hydroxylase.

by stereologic analysis (Fig. 4). These changes were evident in 50% of the mice exposed to rotenone suggesting that there is more to the variability observed in rotenone-induced toxicity. Interestingly, loss of TH-immunoreactivity in the striatum was not evident in the mice (Fig. 4) that showed massive loss of dopaminergic nigral neurons (>75%). Similar observations have been reported in mice exposed to paraquat (78) and transgenic mice overexpressing mutant α-synuclein (79) were nigral neuronal degeneration does not correlate with dopamine loss in the striatum, suggesting that nigrostriatal dopaminergic degeneration is different in mice as compared to rats where rotenone toxicity appears to be initiated at the terminals and continues in a retrograde manner to the cell bodies.

THE ROTENONE MODEL IN NONHUMAN PRIMATES

Nonhuman primates are closest to humans. Therefore simulating PD in nonhuman primates would be more appropriate to study PD pathogenesis and therapeutic strategies. Two macaques, in two independent laboratories, were administered rotenone via two different routes (80). One monkey received a cumulative dose of 1034 mg/kg rotenone dissolved in corn oil via subcutaneous injections over a period of 19 months while the second monkey received a cumulative dose of 584 mg/kg rotenone dissolved in dimethyl sulfoxide (DMSO):PEG (1:1) via subcutaneous minipumps over a period of 18 months. Both the monkeys developed nigrostriatal degeneration as demonstrated by immunocytochemistry for TH (Fig. 5). Nissl stain, immunocytochemistry for DARPP32, and silver staining demonstrated that selective degeneration of the striatal dopaminergic terminals depended on the dose of rotenone used. The first monkey had a small necrotic core in the striatum while the second monkey did not have degenerating neurons in the striatum. Chronic and systemic rotenone exposure also resulted in increased levels of α-synuclein in nigral neurons as well as in α-synuclein positive cytoplasmic inclusions (Fig. 6) very similar to that observed in human PD (80). Consequently, chronic and systemic rotenone exposure in nonhuman primates recapitulated the characteristic pathologic features of PD.

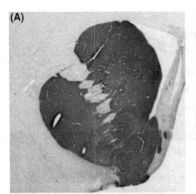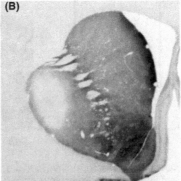

FIGURE 5 Degeneration of dopaminergic terminals in rotenone infused monkey. Coronal sections through the striatum of a normal monkey (**A**) and rotenone-infused monkey (**B**) were processed for TH-immunohistochemistry. Note the reduced TH-ir in both the caudate and putamen, with complete loss of TH-ir in the lateral putamen. *Abbreviation*: TH, tyrosine hydroxylase.

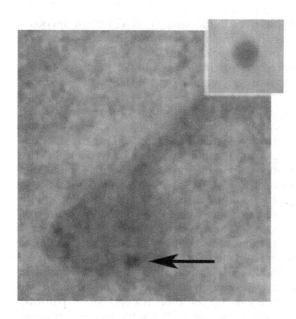

FIGURE 6 α-Synuclein aggregation in a substantia nigra neuron (*arrowhead*), observed in a rotenone-infused monkey, is very similar to that observed in Parkinson's disease patients (inset).

THE ROTENONE MODEL IN FLY

Interestingly, many PD features have been recapitulated in flies, *Drosophila melanogaster* (81). Following several days of sublethal doses of rotenone exposure flies developed locomotor impairments that increased with the dose of rotenone. Immunocytochemistry studies demonstrated a significant and selective loss of dopaminergic neurons in the brain clusters. L-dopa into the feeding medium rescued the behavioral deficits but not neuronal loss implying that locomotor deficits are due to loss of dopaminergic neurons. In contrast, the antioxidant melatonin alleviated both behavioral deficits and neuronal loss suggesting a major role for oxidative stress in neuronal degeneration. The study provides a new model to study PD pathogenesis and to screen therapeutic drugs.

MECHANISMS OF ROTENONE TOXICITY

Rotenone is a specific inhibitor of complex I of the mitochondrial electron transport chain (54). In rats chronic and systemic infusion of rotenone resulted in selective and uniform inhibition of complex I. Based on [3H]dibydrorotenone binding studies (55,82), it was deduced that the free rotenone in the brain of rotenone-infused rats was approximately 20–30 nM. This concentration of rotenone is known to partially inhibit complex I activity.

Oximetry analysis of brain mitochondria indicated that this level of complex I inhibition was inadequate to inhibit glutamate-supported respiration, suggesting that defective ATP production may not be responsible for neurodegeneration. Partial complex I inhibition also stimulates the production of reactive oxygen species (43) as also confirmed in the rotenone-infused rats and in neuroblastoma cells exposed to rotenone; increased levels of carbonyls, a marker for oxidative stress, were detected in dopaminergic brain regions and in cells. DJ-1, an oxidative stress associated protein, underwent oxidative modifications in the same brain regions in rotenone-infused rats (69). Furthermore, α-tocopherol, a known antioxidant, attenuated rotenone-induced toxicity in cells and organotypic slice cultures (68). Thus, studies to understand the mechanisms of rotenone toxicity have indicated that free radical production and subsequent oxidative stress have a pivotal role in rotenone-induced neurodegeneration.

Oxidative damage can also provide partial explanation for rotenone-induced elevations and aggregation of α-synuclein observed selectively in nigral neurons. α-synuclein is known to undergo oxidative modifications in PD brains that can render the protein insoluble leading to aggregation (83). Both in vivo and in vitro studies have demonstrated that rotenone accumulation correlates with upregulation in protein carbonyls suggesting that rotenone can cause oxidative modifications to α-synuclein leading to its aggregation (83,84). Furthermore, prior treatment with α-tocopherol, attenuated rotenone-induced increases in α-synuclein in vitro confirming the association between α-synuclein and oxidative stress.

Rotenone exposure also resulted in proteasomal inhibition, selectively in the ventral midbrain regions in rotenone-infused rats with striatal lesions (74). Proteasomal dysfunction can be attributed to both, increased oxidative stress and increase in α-synuclein levels. Increased oxidative stress can result in generation of oxidatively modified proteins that can ultimately clog up the protein degradation pathway (85,86) or oxidatively modify the proteasomal subunits rendering them dysfunctional (76). Though it is not clear whether α-synuclein gets degraded by the ubiquitin proteasomal pathway (87), increased levels of α-synuclein can inhibit the UPS by interacting with the proteasomal subunits (88). Thus, rotenone-induced oxidative stress and α-synuclein accumulation can inhibit the UPS.

Interestingly, the effects of chronic and systemic rotenone infusion such as uniform complex I inhibition, oxidative stress, α-synuclein aggregation, and proteasomal dysfunction became regionally restricted finally resulting in highly selective nigrostriatal dopaminergic degeneration.

CONCLUSIONS

The rotenone model appears to be an accurate model in that systemic complex I inhibition results in specific, progressive, and chronic degeneration of the nigrostriatal pathway similar to that observed in human PD. It also reproduces oxidative damage, neuronal inclusions and α-synuclein aggregation, and proteasomal dysfunction seen in PD. Thus, the rotenone model recapitulates most of the mechanisms associated with PD pathogenesis. For this reason, neuroprotective drug treatment trials in this model maybe more relevant to PD than other, more acute model systems. The major disadvantage of this model is the variability, with some animals showing lesions while others do not. However, the variability in individual response to rotenone toxicity, provides an opportunity to identify mechanisms involved in selective susceptibility/protection of dopaminergic neurons to complex I inhibition.

SUMMARY

Systemic, chronic, low doses of complex I inhibition with rotenone, in rats, reproduced numerous features of PD including selective nigrostriatal degeneration, formation of synuclein-positive cytoplasmic inclusions, microglial activation, increased oxidative stress, and a dysfunctional UPS. The rotenone model appears to be an accurate model in that systemic complex I inhibition results in selective degeneration of the nigrostriatal pathway similar to that observed in human PD as well as recapitulates most of the mechanisms associated with PD pathogenesis. Furthermore, the variability in individual response to rotenone toxicity provides an opportunity to identify mechanisms involved in selective susceptibility/protection of dopaminergic neurons to complex I inhibition.

ACKNOWLEDGMENTS

This work was supported by NIH grants NS3S899 and ES012068 to JTG.

REFERENCES

1. Klockgether T. Parkinson's disease: clinical aspects. Cell Tissue Res 2004; 318(1):115–120.
2. Wooten GF. Neurochemistry and neuropharmacology of Parkinson's disease. In: Watts RL, Koller, eds. Movement Disorders: Neurologic Principles and Practice. New York: McGraw-Hill, 1997:153–160.
3. Braak H, Ghebremedhin E, Rub U, et al. Stages in the development of Parkinson's disease-related pathology. Cell Tissue Res 2004; 318(1):121–134.
4. Albin RL, Young AB, Penney JB. The functional anatomy of basal ganglia disorders. Trends Neurosci 1989; 12(10):366–375.
5. Crossman AR. Neural mechanisms in disorders of movement. Comp Biochem Physiol A 1989; 93(1):141–149.
6. Klockgether T, Turski L. Excitatory amino acids and the basal ganglia: implications for the therapy of Parkinson's disease. Trends Neurosci 1989; 12(8):285–286.
7. DeLong MR. Primate models of movement disorders of basal ganglia origin. Trends Neurosci 1990; 13(7):281–285.
8. Greenamyre JT. Glutamate-dopamine interactions in the basal ganglia: relationship to Parkinson's disease. J Neural Transm Gen Sect 1993; 91(2–3):255–269.
9. Spillantini MG, Schmidt ML, Lee VM, et al. Alpha-synuclein in Lewy bodies [letter]. Nature. 1997; 388(6645):839–840.
10. Braak H, Braak E, Yilmazer D, et al. Nigral and extranigral pathology in Parkinson's disease. J Neural Transm Suppl 1995; 46:15–31.
11. Polymeropouios MH, Lavedan C, Leroy E, et al. Mutation in the alpha-synuclein gene identified in families with Parkinson's disease [see comments]. Science 1997; 276(5321): 2045–2047.
12. Irizarry MC, Growdon W, Gomez-Isla T, et al. Nigral and cortical Lewy bodies and dystrophic nigral neurites in Parkinson's disease and cortical Lewy body disease contain alpha-synuclein immunoreactivity. J Neuropathol Exp Neurol 1998; 57(4):334–337.
13. Hattori N, Matsumine H, Asakawa S, et al. Point mutations (Thr240Arg and Gln311Stop) [correction of Thr240Arg and Ala311Stop] in the Parkin gene [published erratum appears in Biochem Biophys Res Commun 1998; 251(2):666]. Biochem Biophys Res Commun 1998; 249(3):754–758.
14. Kitada T, Asakawa S, Hattori N, et al. Mutations in the parkin gene cause autosomal recessive juvenile parkinsonism [see comments]. Nature 1998; 392(6676):605–608.
15. Lucking CB, Abbas N, Durr A, et al. Homozygous deletions in parkin gene in European and North African families with autosomal recessive juvenile parkinsonism. The European Consortium on Genetic Susceptibility in Parkinson's Disease and the French Parkinson's Disease Genetics Study Group [letter]. Lancet 1998; 352(9137):1355–1356.
16. Leroy, E, Boyer R, Auburger G, et al. The ubiquitin pathway in Parkinson's disease [letter]. Nature 1998; 395(6701):451–452.
17. McNaught KS, Olanow CW, Halliwell B, et al. Failure of the ubiquitin-proteasome system in Parkinson's disease. Nat Rev Neurosci 2001; 2(8):589–594.
18. Mizuno Y, Ohta S, Tanaka M, et al. Deficiencies in complex I subunits of the respiratory chain in Parkinson's disease. Biochem Biophys Res Commun 1989; 163(3):1450–1455.

19. Parker WD Jr, Boyson SJ, Parks JK. Abnormalities of the electron transport chain in idiopathic Parkinson's disease. Ann Neurol 1989; 26(6):719–723.
20. Schapira AH, Cooper JM, Dexter D, et al. Mitochondrial complex I deficiency in Parkinson's disease [letter] [see comments]. Lancet 1989; 1(8649):1269.
21. Cardellach F, Marti MJ, Fernandez-Sola J, et al. Mitochondrial respiratory chain activity in skeletal muscle from patients with Parkinson's disease [see comments]. Neurology 1993; 43(11):2258–2262.
22. Haas RH, Nasirian F, Nakano K, et al. Low platelet mitochondrial complex I and complex II/III activity in early untreated Parkinson's disease. Ann Neurol 1995; 37(6):714–722.
23. Tenner P. Oxidative mechanisms in nigral cell death in Parkinson's disease. Mov Disord 1998; 13(suppl 1):24–34.
24. Valente EM, Abou-Sleiman PM, Caputo V, et al. Hereditary early-onset Parkinson's disease caused by mutations in PINK1. Science 2004; 304(5674):1158–1160.
25. Bonifati V, Rizzu P, van Baren MJ, et al. Mutations in the DJ-1 gene associated with autosomal recessive early-onset parkinsonism. Science 2003; 299(5604):256–259.
26. Yokata T, Sugawara K, Ito K, et al. Down regulation of DJ-1 enhances cell death by oxidative stress, ER stress and proteasome inhibition. Biochem Biophys Res Commun 2003; 312:1342–1348.
27. Canet-Aviles RM, Wilson MA, Miller DW, et al. The Parkinson's disease protein DJ-1 is neuroprotective due to cysteine-sulfinic acid-driven mitochondrial localization. Proc Natl Acad Sci USA 2004; 101(24):9103–9108.
28. Priyadarshi A, Khuder SA, Schaub EA, et al. A meta-analysis of Parkinson's disease and exposure to pesticides. Neurotoxicology 2000; 21(4):435–440.
29. Priyadarshi A, Khuder SA, Schaub EA, et al. Environmental risk factors and Parkinson's disease: a metaanalysis. Environ Res 2001; 86(2):122–127.
30. Dawson TM, Dawson VL. Molecular pathways of neurodegeneration in Parkinson's disease. Science 2003; 302(5646):819–822.
31. Wallace DC. Diseases of the mitochondrial DNA. Annu Rev Biochem 1992; 61:1175–1212.
32. Nicklas WJ, Vyas I, Heikkila RE. Inhibition of NADH-linked oxidation in brain mitochondria by l-methyl-4-phenyl-pyridine, a metabolite of the neurotoxin, 1-methyM-phenyl-1,2,5,6-tetrahydropyridine. Life Sci 1985; 36(26):2503–2508.
33. Ramsay RR, Krueger MJ, Youngster SK, et al. Interaction of l-methyl-4-phenylpyridinium ion (MPP⁺) and its analogs with the rotenone/piericidin binding site of NADH dehydrogenase. J Neurochem 1991; 56(4):1184–1190.
34. Hatefi Y. The mitochondrial electron transport and oxidative phosphorylation system. Annu Rev Biochem 1985; 54:1015–1069.
35. Greene JG, Greenamyre JT. Bioenergetics and glutamate excitotoxicity. Prog Neurobiol 1996; 48(6):613–634.
36. Bindoff LA, Birch-Machin M, Cartridge NE, et al. Mochondrial function in Parkinson's disease [letter; comment]. Lancet 1989; 2(8653):49.
37. Shoffner JM, Watts RL, Juncos JL, et al. Mitochondrial oxidative phosphoryiation defects in Parkinson's disease [see comments]. Ann Neural 1991; 30(3):332–339.
38. Mann VM, Cooper JM, Krige D, et al. Brain, skeletal muscle and platelet homogenate mitochondrial function in Parkinson's disease. Brain 1992; 115(Pt 2):333–342.
39. Blin O, Desnuelle C, Rascol O, et al. Mitochondrial respiratory failure in skeletal muscle from patients with Parkinson's disease and multiple system atrophy. J Neurol Sci 1994; 125(1):95–101.
40. Mizuno Y, Yoshino H, Ikebe S, et al. Mitochondria! dysfunction in Parkinson's disease. Ann Neural 1998; 44(3 suppl 1):S99–S109.
41. Javitch JA, D'Amato RJ, Strittmatter SM, et al. Parkinsonism-inducmg neurotoxin, N-methyl-4-phenyl-l,2,3,6-tetrahydropyridine: uptake of the metabolite N-methyl-4-phenylpyridine by dopamine neurons explains selective toxicity. Proc Natl Acad Sci USA, 1985; 52(7):2173–2177.
42. Tipton KF, Singer TP. Advances in our understanding of the mechanisms of the neurotoxicity of MPTP and related compounds. J Neurochem 1993; 61(4):1191–1206.
43. Hensley K, Pye QN, Maidt M-L, et al. Interaction of alpha-phenyl-N-tert-butyl nitrone and alternative electron acceptors with complex I indicates a substrate reduction site upstream from the rotenone binding site. J Neurochem 1998; 71(6):2549–2557.

44. Kushnareva Y, Murphy AN, Andreyev A. Complex I-mediated reactive oxygen species generation: modulation by cytochrome c and NAD(P)$^+$ oxidation-reduction state. Biochem J 2002; 368(Pt 2):545–553.
45. Cassarino DS, Fall CP, Swerdlow RH, et al. Elevated reactive oxygen species and antioxidant enzyme activities in animal and cellular models of Parkinson's disease. Biochim Biophys Acta 1997; 1362(1):77–86.
46. Barrientos A, Moraes CT. Titrating the effects of mitochondrial complex I impairment in the cell physiology. J Biol Chem 1999; 274(23):16188–16197.
47. Dexter DT, Carter CJ, Wells FR, et al. Basal lipid peroxidation in substantia nigra is increased in Parkinson's disease. J Neurochem 1989; 52(2):381–389.
48. Yoritaka A, Hattori N, Uchida K, et al. Immunohistochemical detection of 4-hydroxynonenal protein adducts in Parkinson disease. Proc Natl Acad Sci USA 1996; 93(7):2696–2701.
49. Floor E, Wetzel MG. Increased protein oxidation in human substantia nigra pars compact in comparison with basal ganglia and prefrontal cortex measured with an improved dinitrophenylhydrazine assay. J Neurochemistry 1998; 70:268–275.
50. Sian J, Dexter DT, Lees AJ, et al. Alterations in glutathione levels in Parkinson's isease and other neurodegenerative disorders affecting basal ganglia. Ann Neurol 1994; 36(3): 348–355.
51. Alam ZI, Daniel SE, Lees AJ, et al. A generalised increase in protein carbonyls in the brain in Parkinson's but not incidental Lewy body disease. J Neurochem 1997; 69(3):1326–1329.
52. Nicolaou K, Pfefferkorn J-F, Schuler, et al. Combinatorial synthesis of novel and potent inhibitors of NADH: ubiquinone oxidoreductase. Chem Biol 2000; 7(12):979–992.
53. Schuler F, Casida JE. Functional coupling of PSST and KD1 subunits in NADH: ubiquinone oxidoreductase established by photoaffinity labeling. Biochim Biophys Acta 2001; 1506(1):79–87.
54. Talpade DJ, Greene JG, Higgins DS Jr, et al. In vivo labeling of mitochondrial complex I (NADH:ubiquinone oxidoreductase) in rat brain using [(3)H]dihydrorotenone. J Neurochem 2000; 75(6):2611–2621.
55. Betarbet R, Sherer TB, MacKenzie G, et al. Chronic systemic pesticide exposure reproduces features of Parkinson's disease [In Process Citation]. Nat Neurosci 2000; 3(12):1301–1306.
56. Ferrante RJ, Schulz JB, Kowall NW, et al. Systemic administration of rotenone produces selective damage in the striatum and globus pallidus, but not in the substantia nigra. Brain Res 1997; 753(1):157–162.
57. Lapointe N, St-Hilaire M, Martinoli MG, et al. Rotenone induces non-specific central nervous system and systemic toxicity. Faseb J 2004; 18(6):717–719.
58. Sherer TB, Kim JH, Betarbet R, et al. Subcutaneous rotenone exposure causes highly selective dopaminergic degeneration and alpha-synuclein aggregation. Exp Neurol 2003; 179(1):9–16.
59. Alam M, Schmidt WJ. Rotenone destroys dopaminergic neurons and induces parkinsonian symptoms in rats. Behav Brain Res 2002; 136(1):317–324.
60. Zhu C, Vourc'h P, Fernagut PO, et al. Variable effects of chronic subcutaneous administration of rotenone on striatal histology. J Comp Neurol 2004; 478(4):418–426.
61. Hoglinger GU, Feger J, Prigent A, et al. Chronic systemic complex I inhibition induces ahypokinedc multisystem degeneration in rats. J Neurochem 2003; 84(3):491–502.
62. Homykiewicz O. Dopamine (3-hydroxytyramine) and brain function. Pharmacol Rev 1966; 18(2):925–964.
63. Na HM, Betarbet R, Kim JH, et al. Rotenone models of Parkinson's disease selectively destroys striatal dopaminergic terminals and spares postsynaptic striatal neurons. Soc for Neurosci Abstr 2003.
64. Sherer TB, Betarbet R, Kim JH, et al. Selective microglial activation in the rat rotenone model of Parkinson's disease. Neurosci Lett 2003; 341(2):87–90.
65. Liberatore GT, Jackson-Lewis V, Vukosavic S, et al. Inducible nitric oxide synthase stimulates dopaminergic neurodegeneradon in the MPTP model of Parkinson disease. Nat Med 1999; 5(12):1403–1409.
66. Gao HM, Jiang J, Wilson B, et al, Microglial activation-mediated delayed and progressive degeneration of rat nigral dopaminergic neurons: relevance to Parkinson's disease. J Neurochem 2002; 81(6):1285–1297.

67. Sherer TB, Betarbet R, Stout AK, et al. An in vitro model of Parkinson's disease: linking mitochondrial impairment to altered alpha-synuclein metabolism and oxidative damage. J Neurosci 2002; 22(16):7006–7015.
68. Sherer TB, Betarbet R, Testa CM, et al. Mechanism of toxicity in rotenone models of Parkinson's disease. J Neurosci 2003; 23(34):10756–10764.
69. Cookson MR, Canet-Aviles R, Miller D, et al. DJ-I controls neuronal viability in response to mitochondrial damage. Society for Neuroscience Abstr 2004.
70. Mitsumoto A, Nakagawa Y. DJ-1 is an indicator for endogenous reactive oxygen species elicited by endotoxin. Free Radic Res 2001; 35(6):885–893.
71. Mitsumoto A, Nakagawa Y, Takeuchi A, et al. Oxidized forms of peroxicedoxins and DJ-1 on two-dimensional gels increased in response to sublethal levels of paraquat. Free Radic Res 2001; 35(3):301–310.
72. Betarbet R, Sherer TB, Kim J, et al. Rotenone models of Parkinson's disease: altered alpha-synuclein expression following sustained inhibition of complex I. Society for Neuroscience Abstr 2002.
73. Duda JE, Giasson BI, Mabon ME, et al. Novel antibodies to synuclein show abundant striatal pathology in Lewy body diseases. Ann Neurol 2002; 52(2):205–210.
74. Betarbet R, Sherer TB, Lund S, et al. Rotenone models of Parkinson's disease: altered proteasomal activity following sustained inhibition of complex I. Society for Neuroscience Abstr 2003.
75. Hoglinger GU, Canard G, Michel PP, et al. Dysfunction of mitochondrial complex I and the proteasome: interactions between two biochemical deficits in a cellular model of Parkinson's disease. J Neurochem 2003; 86(5):1297–1307.
76. Shamoto-Nagai M, Maruyama W, Kato Y, et al. An inhibitor of mitochondrial complex I, rotenone, inactivates proteasome by oxidative modification and induces aggregation of oxidized proteins in SH-SY5Y cells. J Neurosci Res 2003; 74(4):589–597.
77. Uversky VN. Neurotoxicant-induced animal models of Parkinson's disease: understanding the role of rotenone, maneb and paraquat in neurodegeneration. Cell Tissue Res 2004; 318(1):225–241.
78. McCormack AL, Thiruchelvam M, Manning-Bog AB, et al. Environmental risk factors and Parkinson's disease: selective degeneration of nigral dopaminergic neurons caused by the herbicide paraquat. Neurobiol Dis 2002; 10(2):119–127.
79. West NC, Xu Y, Stirling W, et al. Dopaminergic cell loss in alpha-synuclein transgenic mice. Soc for Neurosci Abstr 2003.
80. Greenamyre JT, Nichols CJ, Na HM, et al. Rotenone-induced parkinsonian pathology in non-human primates. Soc for Neurosci Abstr 2004.
81. Coulom H, Birman S. Chronic exposure to rotenone models sporadic Parkinson's disease in Drosophila melanogaster. J Neurosci 2004; 24(48):10993–10998.
82. Higgins DS Jr, Greenamyre JT. [3H]dihydrorotenone binding to NADH: ubiquinone reductase (complex I) of the electron transport chain: an autoradiographic study. J Neurosci 1996; 16(12):3807–3816.
83. Giasson BI, Duda JE, Murray IV, et al. Oxidative damage linked to neurodegeneration by selective alpha-synuclein nitration in synucleinopathy lesions [In Process Citation]. Science 2000; 290(5493):985–989.
84. Krishnan S, Chi EY, Wood SJ, et al. Oxidative dimer formation is the critical rate-limiting step for Parkinson's disease alpha-synuclein fibrillogenesis. Biochemistry 2003; 42(3):829–837.
85. Reinheckel T, Sitte N, Ullrich O, et al. Comparative resistance of the 20S and 26S proteasome to oxidative stress. Biochem J 1998; 335(Pt 3):637–642.
86. Keller JN, Huang FF, Dimayuga ER, et al. Dopamine induces proteasome inhibition in neural PC12 cell line. Free Radic Biol Med 2000; 29(10):1037–1042.
87. Ciechanover A, Brundin P. The ubiquitin proteasome system in neurodegenerative diseases: sometimes the chicken, sometimes the egg. Neuron 2003; 40(2):427–446.
88. Snyder H, Mensah K, Theisler C, et al. Aggregated and monomeric alpha-synuclein bind to the S6' proteasomal protein and inhibit proteasomal function. J Biol Chem 2003; 278(14):11753–11759.

23 Drug Trials In Animal Models of Parkinson's Disease

Daniel S. Sa and M. Flint Beal

Department of Neurology and Neuroscience, Weill Medical College of Cornell University and New York Presbyterian Hospital, New York, New York, U.S.A.

INTRODUCTION

The previous chapters, from 16 to 22, have focused on the main available animal models of Parkinson's disease (PD), describing its characteristics, reliability, and reproducibility, as well as the ability to produce quantifiable symptoms and pathophysiologic alterations that resemble human PD. It also described its many shortcomings, mostly arising from the fact of studying a different species and our lack of a complete understanding of the true pathophysiologic basis of the disease. Nevertheless, these models provide an opportunity to study potential therapies for PD, not only symptomatic, after the mostly dopaminergic degeneration has taken place but specially in the presymptomatic level, when disease onset can be "predicted" as opposed to human's onset where it usually predates diagnosis and therefore recognition of pathology by many years. It should be recognized that this approach, although providing a better window to evaluate neuroprotection, has many flaws as we are unable to predict the time and means of neurodegeneration onset in humans at least at this point in time.

In this chapter, we will focus on recent drug trials in animal models that either aid in our understanding of neurodegenerative pathways or provide potential therapeutic targets to protect or restore dying neurons, as well as drugs that potentially address other biological processes in PD besides dopaminergic deficits or provide additional symptomatic benefit. Discussion will be limited where trials have reached humans. We will not discuss genetic therapies that have been discussed in detail over the previous chapters pertaining to models based on genetic manipulation.

COENZYME Q10

CoenzymeQ10 (CoQ10) is an important electron transport chain cofactor, serving as antioxidant in mitochondria and lipid membranes. Among a variety of actions, including apoptosis blockade, CoQ10 induces mitochondrial uncoupling which is associated with neuroprotection against 1-methyl-4-phenyl-1,2,3,6-tetrahydropyridine (MPTP) toxicity in primates presumably through reduction of free radicals (1). Further evidence of CoQ10 neuroprotection includes a number of different trials: Beal and his colleagues showed that oral pretreatment with CoQ10 prevented, in a dose-dependent fashion, both ATP depletion and striatal lesions induced by the complex-II inhibitor malonate (2). In a model produced by systemic administration of 3-nitropropionic acid, oral administration of CoQ10 reduced development of striatal lesions, increasing brain mitochondrial concentrations (3). In a C57BL/6 mouse model treated with MPTP, the group that had its diet supplemented with CoQ10 (200 mg/kg/day) had a significant reduction in dopaminergic degeneration compared to the untreated group, as evident by higher striatal dopamine concentration and density of tyrosine hydroxylase immunoreactive (TH-IR) fibers (4).

A phase II trial in humans, double-blind and placebo-controlled in a group of 80 patients who did not require symptomatic treatment showed the drug's safety and tolerability as well as a slowing in the development of disability by 44% at 16 months, as measured by the Unified Parkinson's Disease Rating Scale (UPDRS) in the group treated with 1,200 mg/day (5). This might not have been the optimal dose, as later evidence on a pilot trial in humans attempting multiple different doses (1,200, 1,800, 2,400, 3,000 mg/day) of CoQ10 associated with a stable dose of 1200 IU of vitamin E/day suggested that a higher dosage of 2,400 mg would achieve the highest plasma level without compromising tolerability and therefore could be an adequate dose for future trials; the dose of 3,000 mg/day provided no additional increase in plasma levels (6).

CREATINE

Creatine is the precursor of phosphocreatine, which transfers phosphoryl groups during mitochondrial ATP synthesis. Creatine kinase inhibits opening of the transition pore, which is a step involved in apoptosis, and therefore its modulation could have neuroprotective properties (7). In a study involving MPTP-treated mice, a prior two week creatine supplementation markedly reduced dopaminergic degeneration (8). Based on these observations, a randomized, placebo-controlled clinical trial in untreated PD subjects was initiated with creatine supplements, 5 g BID in a "futility study" design (9).

GLIAL CELL LINE–DERIVED NERVE GROWTH FACTOR

Glial cell line-derived nerve growth factor (GDNF) is a neurotrophic factor for dopaminergic neurons. In the 6-OHDA rodent model, its intrastriatal administration was shown to have neurotrophic effects at the level of the cell bodies and the axon terminals in the striatum, inducing axonal sprouting and regeneration evidenced both biologically and clinically. (10)

Intracerebral injection of GDNF was shown, in an MPTP rhesus monkey model, to increase dopamine levels and fiber density (11). Intraventricular injections also showed good results: on a double-blind study on rhesus monkeys rendered hemiparkinsonian through carotid MPTP injections, there was a clear dose-dependent benefit of GDNF as observed with a standardized behavioral testing (12).

Human trials of GDNF included intraventricular injections, which failed to show any benefit presumably by not reaching its target in the putamen and substantia nigra (13). Delivery through an implanted minipump to the putamen initially showed an improvement in UPDRS scores (14), but later, double-blind, randomized study showed no benefit from the intervention. Furthermore, development of antibodies against GDNF and cerebellar lesions prompted the withdrawal of GDNF from trials by Amgen (15).

ADENOSINE A2A RECEPTOR BLOCKADE

Adenosine receptors have a widespread distribution, except for the A2A receptor that is largely restricted to the striatum (16). This same receptor has been shown to coexpress with dopamine D2 receptors (17), and in 6-OHDA lesioned rats, its blockade potentiated turning behavior induced by dopamine agonists (18). These findings prompted the trial of A2A blockade as a treatment for PD. Kanda et al. showed that

KW-6002 (istradefylline) improved motor function in MPTP common marmosets with little to no induction of the abnormal movements usually generated by dopaminergic agents in these primates (19). Similar results were reported by Grondin and his colleagues, who showed, in an MPTP cynomolgus monkey model, that KW-6002 produced an antiparkinsonian response comparable to levodopa-benserazide with little in the way of dyskinesias; when coadministered with levodopa, the drug potentiated its effects again without a significant increase in involuntary movements (20).

Human data with the same antagonist, istradefylline, studied in a double-blind placebo-controlled fashion over 12 weeks, showed an increase in "on" time subjectively, as measured by patient's diaries but not objectively on the recorded UPDRS measures. "On" time with dyskinesias did increase, although severity of dyskinesias was unchanged (21). In a smaller study involving 15 patients, also double-blind and placebo-controlled, a lower dose of levodopa had its effects potentiated with a comparative reduction in levodopa-induced dyskinesias (LID) (22).

MINOCYCLINE

Minocycline is a member of the tetracycline class of molecules with broad-spectrum antibiotic activity. Its high lipophilicity allows it to diffuse more easily into tissues, including brain (23). It has been shown to inhibit the activity of matrix metalloproteinases (MMPs) (24), decrease microglial activation (25), and inhibit oxidative stress, decreasing ischemic damage in a mouse model by preventing glutamate-induced cell death (26).

In mitochondria isolated suspensions, minocycline was effective in blocking calcium-induced mitochondrial swelling as well as staurosporine-induced cyto-toxicity, and at very high concentrations (100 muM) inhibited complex II/III activity (27). It is also capable of preventing activation of caspases and reducing the activity of inducible nitric oxide synthase, both recognized key aspects in apop-totic cell death (28,29).

In MPTP models of PD, minocycline has been shown to block microglia activation and protect against neurodegeneration (30). Du and his colleagues showed that, when administered within four hours from the acute MPTP insult in a mouse model, nigrostriatal dopaminergic neurodegeneration was prevented as demonstrated by both an increase in tyrosine hydroxylase neurons and stability of dopamine metabolites, possibly through inhibition of 1-methyl-4-pyridinium (MPP(+))-induced glial iNOS expression or direct inhibition of nitric oxide-induced neurotoxicity through inhibition of phosphorylation of p38 mitogen-activated protein kinase (31). Interestingly, additional studies failed to replicate this neuroprotection in MPTP-exposed cynomolgus monkeys, as evidenced clinically by worsening motor scores (including rotarod, pole test, and beam-traversing tasks) and histopathologically by an increased loss of dopaminergic terminals (32). Furthermore, Yang and his colleagues found that microglial activation was blocked, but there was an exacerbation of MPTP-induced damage. This phenomenon is at least in part due to inhibition of dopamine and MPP+ uptake into striatal vesicles by effects of minocycline on the vesicular monoamine transporter (VMAT) (33). It is becoming clear that, as suggested in the 3-NP Huntington's disease (HD) model, minocycline may have variable and possibly detrimental results in different species and models; optimal doses and mode of administration are also not clear (32). Nevertheless, human trials using minocycline are currently under way.

IMMUNOPHILIN LIGANDS

Immunophilin ligands have been shown to have neurotrophic properties in vitro and in vivo. Comparing two different immunophilin ligands, Costantini et al. were able to show that V-10,367 increased the number of tyrosine hydroxylase positive neurites (branching) while FK506 increased the length of tyrosine hydroxylase neurites. Furthermore, oral administration of V-10,367 protected against MPTP-induced loss of striatal axonal density (34).

Further supporting efficacy of FK506, Manakova et al. showed that FK 506 restored reactive oxygen species (ROS) production, inhibited cytochrome C release, increased Bcl-2 protein level, and reduced caspase-3 activation in 6-hydroxy-dopamine (6-OHDA) treated SH-SY5Y cells. However, there was no improvement on ATP levels and p53 and Bax increased. Furthermore, its administration for seven days to 6-OHDA lesioned rats failed to prevent apomorphine-induced circling (35). A phase II clinical trial investigating GPI-1485, another immunophilin ligand that binds to the same proteins that FK506 does started in August 2002 (36).

SONIC HEDGEHOG AGONISTS

The hedgehog family is composed of signaling molecules, including sonic hedgehog is associated with patterning during CNS development. There is also evidence that it promotes survival of dopaminergic neurons, protecting cultures of fetal midbrain dopaminergic neurons from MPP(+). In the adult brain, Bezard et al. showed that sonic hedgehog is reduced in Parkinson's disease, and its injection inhibits electrical activity in the subthalamic nucleus. (37).

Tsuboi and Shults, studying parkinsonian rats, observed that a series of four intrastriatal injections of sonic hedgehog N-terminal fragment (180 ng) on days 1, 3, 5, and 8 (with 6-OHDA being administered on the fourth day) reduced apomorphine-induced rotation and forelimb akinesia, partially preserving dopaminergic axons in the striatum (38). Wyeth Pharmaceutical has a hedgehog agonist under preclinical investigation at this time (39).

MIXED LINEAGE KINASE INHIBITOR

One of the key parts of neuronal cell death pathways during development is the activation of the c-Jun N-terminal kinase (JNK); this step may be of importance in pathologic neurodegeneration as well. As an inhibitor of the mixed lineage kinase (MLK) family of kinases, CEP-1347 has the potential to inhibit the activation of the JNK pathway and therefore cell death in many cell cultures and animal models, maintaining the trophic status of cultured neurons (40). It has also been shown to inhibit microglial inflammation (41).

CEP-1347 and CEP-11004 significantly increased the long-term survival of dopaminergic neurons in primary rat mesencephalon cultures, and after transplantation into the striatum of hemiparkinsonian rats, increased graft size and fiber outgrowth (42). Furthermore, Saporito and his colleagues showed evidence that CEP-1347/KT-7515 was neuroprotective at doses of 0.3 mg/kg/day in an MPTP model, reducing striatal dopaminergic loss by 50% in the low-dose model (20 mg/kg of MPTP) and in the high dose (40 mg/kg of MPTP) model improved dopaminergic cell body loss by 50%, partially preserving striatal dopaminergic terminals. The drug did not inhibit MAO-B or the dopamine transporter, which is consistent with the notion that its putative neuroprotective properties occur downstream of the conversion to MPP+ (43).

Mathiasen and colleagues used CEP-1347 in MPP(+)-induced death of SH-SY5Y cells. They showed that it inhibits MPP(+)-induced cell death and apoptosis, preventing JNK activation (44). The Parkinson Study Group has studied it clinically in a randomized, blinded placebo-controlled study of 30 patients, where its safety and tolerability were shown along with no demonstrable clinical effects on parkinsonian symptoms or levodopa kinetics; these results make the drug suitable for longer studies to address potential neuroprotective properties in humans as the data analysis would likely not be complicated by symptomatic benefits (45). A recent phase III trial was halted due to lack of efficacy.

ALPHA-AMINO-3-HYDROXY-METHYL-4-ISOXAZOLYL-PROPIONIC ACID MODULATION

Amantadine is currently the only documented efficacious treatment option for levodopa-induced dyskinesia (LID); its beneficial effects are thought to be at least in part due to glutamate receptor antagonism (46,47). Calon et al. showed that, in PD patients presenting motor complications, the ^{3}H-[alpha-amino-3-hydroxy-methyl-4-isoxazolyl-propionic acid (AMPA)] binding was increased in the lateral putamen as compared to those without it (48).

In fact, Konitsiotis and colleagues showed that in MPTP-treated monkeys, the AMPA agonist CX516 produced no measurable alteration in motor activity but induced dyskinesia or potentiated LID by up to 52%, while the noncompetitive AMPA antagonist LY300164 (talampanel) in conjunction with low-dose levodopa increased motor activity by up to 86% while decreasing LID by up to 40% (49). IVAX Corp is currently evaluating this drug as an antidyskinetic agent.

Additionally, there are some data suggesting the possibility that this class of drugs could be neuroprotective as well. Erdo and colleagues showed a reduction in infarct size of up to 48.5% in rat models of stroke through one-hour carotid artery occlusions (50). Eisai Co Ltd is currently in phase II tests of an AMPA antagonist, E-2007, as a neuroprotective approach to PD (39)

Another approach to the AMPA receptors has been its potentiation: LY503430, an AMPA receptor potentiator being investigated by Eli Lilly, has been suggested to be neuroprotective in 6-OHDA and MPTP models, where it was also described to exert neurotrophic actions/increase in brain derived neurotrophic factor (BDNF) and increase in growth associated protein-43 (GAP-43) expression (51). These results await independent replication.

OPIOID RECEPTORS

Opioids have been shown to act as modulators, altering the activity of dopamine and gamma-aminobutyric acid (GABA) neurons; within the globus pallidus, enkephalin, and dynorphin can reduce the release of amino acid transmitters, and its synthesis is enhanced in neurons projecting to the pallidal complex in animal models of PD exposed to dopaminergic treatment causing dyskinesias (52).

Furthermore, enadoline, a kappa agonist, was shown to have prokinetic properties in a rat rendered parkinsonian through reserpine-exposure. This effect was synergistic with levodopa (53). Studying PD patients with LID with positron-emission tomography and the opioid receptor ligand [11C]diprenorphine, Piccini et al. observed reduced striatal and thalamic as well as increased prefrontal opioid binding in dyskinetic PD patients as opposed to uncomplicated ones, lending further support to the hypothesis that these receptors are related to either development of LID or the subsequent circuitry rewiring (54).

Cyprodime, a Mu receptor antagonist and naltrindole (delta receptor antagonist) were reported to improve dyskinesias in an MPTP model of PD (52). Conversely, Samadi and his colleagues observed that the use of both naloxone and naltrexone increased the severity of the dyskinesias induced by both levodopa and two different dopamine agonists—SKF 82958, D1 and quinpirole, D2—in the MPTP cynomolgus monkey; they suggested that the possibility of the increased opioid transmission in dyskinesias be a consequence rather than the cause of dyskinesias (55).

Human studies have shown minimal results: naloxone, naltrexone, and spiradoline had little to no effects in some studies, but samples were limited, and, in the case of spiradoline, behavioral side effects limited drug dosing (53,56,57). However, Fox et al. observed an increase in the duration of levodopa effect of 17.5% in a double-blind crossover study of 14 parkinsonian patients with LID treated with naloxone (58). The different results likely reflect the different study designs, as well as limitations of its small samples; nevertheless there is an obvious modulation of dopaminergic transmission in PD by opioid receptors that should be better evaluated to potentially treat wearing-off phenomenon or LID.

ASTROCYTE MODULATION

The calcium binding protein S100B may promote neuronal damage by the activation of various intracellular signaling pathways. Astrocytic activation may increase the production of S100B in the MPTP models of PD, thereby potentiating the neurodegeneration. Arundic acid [(R)-(-)-2-propyloctanoic acid (ONO-2506)] is an agent that inhibits S100B synthesis in cultured astrocytes, which has also been shown to reduce delayed ischemic brain damage in models of cerebral ischemia.

In an MPTP model of PD, Kato and colleagues observed that the ONO-2506 treated mice showed only a 56% loss of tyrosine hydroxylase dopaminergic neurons in the substantia nigra after seven days, as opposed to 87% in the untreated mice; it also induced an earlier appearance of reactive astrocytes and suppressed expression of S-100B, suggesting that the neuroprotective properties were related at least in part to modulation of the astrocytic activation and its production of S-100 protein (59). This drug is currently under phase II trials by its manufacturer, Ono Pharmaceutical Co. Ltd.

GLYCERALDEHYDE-3-PHOSPHATE DEHYDROGENASE INHIBITION

Despite a number of methodologic problems, mostly related to its ability to induce a symptomatic benefit, selegiline, a propargylamine might have mild neuroprotective properties (60). It is unclear whether these putative neuroprotective properties are related to its monoamine oxidase type B (MAO-B) inhibition or additional, unrelated factors. A related analog compound, CGP 3466, that has been developed by Novartis Pharma Research is essentially devoid of MAO-B inhibiting properties but might be neuroprotective. Kragten et al. showed specific binding of the compound to glyceraldehyde-3-phosphate dehydrogenase (GADPH), suggesting that this might be the target related to its neuroprotective properties (61). Furthermore, Carlile et al. reported that CGP3466 reduced apoptosis caused by growth factor withdrawal, binding to GAPDH, converting it from a tetramer to a dimmer, preventing its level increases and nuclear accumulation and decreasing glycolysis (62).

The same group from Novartis also reported that CGP 3466 partially prevented loss of tyrosine hydroxylase-positive cells in the substantia nigra in an MPTP mouse model. In the same paper, they reported an improvement in motor performance on the 6-OHDA rat model when subsequently treated with CGP 3466 although a symptomatic benefit cannot be completely excluded despite their claims (63). A group from the Netherlands reported similar findings in a double-hit monkey MPTP model, where CGP 3466 systemic injection between the two MPTP doses prevented most of the motor worsening. (64). Initial human clinical trials in PD and amyotrophic lateral sclerosis (ALS) were disappointing and this compound is no longer under development (Waldmeier P, personal communication).

COX-2 INHIBITORS

Cyclooxygenase (COX) is an enzyme that participates in the synthesis of the family of prostanoids, which includes prostaglandins, prostacyclin, and thromboxanes. It exists in two isoforms: COX-2 is the inducible isoform, expressed in response to a variety of molecules including growth factors and cytokines. In the brain, it has been associated with proinflammatory activities and, possibly, neurodegeneration, although it is also known to contribute to a variety of normal brain functions such as synaptic activity, memory consolidation, and functional hyperemia (65).

In COX-2 knockout mice, the extent of MPTP-induced neurodegeneration as measured by the number of tyrosine hydroxylase immunoreactive neurons in the substantia nigra pars compacta was greatly reduced as compared to the wild type mice, suggesting a role of COX-2 in neurodegeneration as well as a potential role for neuroprotection through its inhibition (66). Similar results were shown by Przedborski's group in an MPTP model, where inhibition of COX-2 also markedly reduced nigrostriatal degeneration (67).

Hunot and his colleagues have also showed that COX-2 is a target of JNK2 and JNK3 activation and likely indispensable to MPTP-induced dopaminergic degeneration in mice, suggesting that this may be a very important neurodegeneration pathway in PD (68). Conversely, Przybylkowski et al., in a mice MPTP model, found that rofecoxib in a dose of 10 mg/kg started on the first day after MPTP administration failed to provide any neuroprotection, observing as well that the COX-2 expression increase correlated with the recovery phase as opposed to the acute phase (69). In our studies, administration of rofecoxib exerted significant protection against MPTP-induced depletion of dopamine and loss of dopaminergic neurons (70). The results are still somewhat contradictory, and the real role of COX-2 as well as the neuroprotective capabilities of its inhibition remains controversial.

DOPAMINE D3 RECEPTOR AGONIST

The expression of D3 receptors is decreased in MPTP monkeys; however, its expression has been shown to increase in PD patients with LID. Interestingly, Bezard and his colleagues showed that D3 receptor-selective agonists can improve LID in MPTP treated macaques without changing symptomatic efficiency of levodopa; D3 antagonists also attenuated dyskinesias, but to the expense of worsening motor function (71). The same group, however, showed a different response in squirrel monkeys submitted to MPTP followed by levodopa therapy, BP897 significantly reduced LIDs but associated with an overall reduction in levodopa efficacy (72). These results not only suggest that the efficacy of this drug could be less than anticipated in PD patients, but also remind us of the inherent species differences and the limitations of animal studies as predictive of results in humans.

CONCLUSION

The multitude of treatment options and disease pathways currently under investigation shows us that PD is obviously far beyond a dopaminergic deficit; the research suggests multiple transmitter deficits and disease pathways that should be addressed both individually and together in attempts to provide better symptomatic relief and ways to slow and even reverse disease. The current models provide windows into disease processes and pathophysiologic alterations and also provide means of studying disease-modifying approaches and their safety before they are tried in humans.

However, the adequacy of our models has been questioned by recent failures when some drugs were studied in humans following promising results in animal models. Most of these had been studied in 6-OHDA and MPTP models, raising questions not only about the models but the hypotheses, designs, and tools used to evaluate disease in these models, as compared to markers of disease progression in humans (73). One obvious example is the GDNF trial that had remarkable results in MPTP monkeys but no response in a double-blind trial (12,15). Additional examples of remarkable differences in results between animals and man include ifenprodil, remacemide, and CEP-1347 (74,–76).

Nonetheless, the models continue to advance our understanding of disease and provide a means to execute initial experiments without exposing human subjects to unnecessary risks. It is likely that future developments improving the current models or developing additional ones with a closer resemblance to the likely pathogenesis of PD, that is, a slow, continuous environmental effect acting on a genetic predisposition, will improve our chances of accurately and more directly translating animal data into human clinical practice. In this respect, the development of a slowly induced MPTP model using pumps, which leads to Lewy body–like inclusions is promising (77). Ideally, however, one would like to develop a transgenic mouse model of PD in order to test therapies. Initial results using mice overexpressing α-synuclein or with knockouts of *PARKIN* or *DJ-1* have been disappointing. However, PINK knockout mice and mice with LRRK2 mutations are under development and may provide improved models for testing of novel therapeutics.

REFERENCES

1. Horvath TL, Diano S, Leranth C, et al. Coenzyme Q induces nigral mitochondrial uncoupling and prevents dopamine cell loss in a primate model of Parkinson's disease. Endocrinology 2003; 144:2757–2760.
2. Beal MF, Henshaw R, Jenkins BJ, et al. Coenzyme Q10 and nicotinamide blocktriatal lesions produced by the mitochondrial toxin malonate. Ann Neurol 1994; 36:882–888.
3. Matthews RT, Yang L, Browne S, et al. Coenzyme Q10 administration increases brain mitochondrial concentrations and exerts neuroprotective effects. Proc Natl Acad Sci USA 1998; 95:8892–8897.
4. Beal MF, Matthews RT, Tieleman A, et al. Coenzyme Q10 attenuates the 1-methyl-4-phenyl-1,2,3,tetrahydropyridine (MPTP) induced loss of striatal dopamine and dopaminergic axons in aged mice. Brain Res 1998; 2;783:109–114.

5. Shults CW, Oakes D, Kieburtz K, et al. Parkinson Study Group. Effects of coenzyme Q10 in early Parkinson's disease: evidence of slowing of the functional decline. Arch Neurol 2002; 59:1541–1550.

6. Shults CW, Beal MF, Song D, et al. Pilot trial of high dosages of coenzyme Q10 in patients with Parkinson's disease. Exp Neurol 2004; 188:491–494.

7. Tarnopolsky MA, Beal MF. Potential for creatine and other therapies targeting cellular energy dysfunction in neurological disorders. Ann Neurol 2001; 49:561–574.

8. Matthews RT, Ferrante RJ, Klivenyi P, et al. Creatine and cyclocreatine attenuate MPTP neurotoxicity. Exp Neurol 1999; 157:142–149.

9. LeWitt P. Clinical trials of neuroprotection for Parkinson's disease. Neurology 2004; 63 (7 Suppl 2):S23–S31.

10. Bjorklund A, Rosenblad C, Winkler C, et al. Studies on neuroprotective and regenerative effects of GDNF in a partial lesion model of Parkinson's disease. Neurobiol Dis 1997; 4:186–200.

11. Gash DM, Zhang Z, Ovadia A, et al. Functional recovery in parkinsonian monkeys treated with GDNF. Nature 1996; 380:252–255.

12. Zhang Z, Miyoshi Y, Lapchak PA, et al. Dose response to intraventricular glial cell line-derived neurotrophic factor administration in parkinsonian monkeys. J Pharmacol Exp Ther 1997; 282:1396–1401.

13. Nutt JG, Burchiel KJ, Comella CL, et al. The ICV GDNF Study Group. Randomized, double-blind trial of glial cell line-derived neurotrophic factor (GDNF) in PD. Neurology 2003; 60:69–73.

14. Gill SS, Patel NK, Hotton GR, et al. Direct brain infusion of glial cell line-derived neurotrophic factor in Parkinson's disease. Nat Med 2003; 9:589–595.

15. Lang AE, Gill S, Brooks D, et al. Multicenter, double-blind, randomized, placebo-controlled, parallel group trial of liatermin (rmetHuGDNF) administered by bilateral intraputaminal (IPu) infusion to subjects with idiopathic Parkinson's disease. 129th Annual Meeting of the American Neurological Association. Platform presentation WIP 1.

16. Svenningsson P, Le Moine C, Fisone G, et al. Distribution, biochemistry and function of striatal adenosine A2A receptors. Prog Neurobiol 1999; 59:355–396.

17. Svenningsson P, Lindskog M, Rognoni F, et al. Activation of adenosine A2A receptor and dopamine D1 receptors stimulates cyclic AMP-dependent phosphorylation of DARPP-32 in distinct population of striatal projection neurons. Neuroscience 1998; 84:223–228.

18. Pinna A, di Chiara G, Wardas J, et al. Blockade of A2a adenosine receptors positively modulates turning behaviour and c-Fos expression induced by D1 agonists in dopamine-denervated rats. Eur J Neurosci 1996; 8:1176–1181.

19. Kanda T, Jackson MJ, Smith LA, et al. Adenosine A2A antagonist: a novel antiparkinsonian agent that does not provoke dyskinesia in parkinsonian monkeys. Ann Neurol 1998; 43:507–513.

20. Grondin R, Bedard PJ, Hadj Tahar A, et al. Antiparkinsonian effect of a new selective adenosine A2A receptor antagonist in MPTP-treated monkeys. Neurology 1999; 52:1673–1677.

21. Hauser RA, Hubble JP, Truong DD. Istradefylline US-001 Study Group. Randomized trial of the adenosine A(2A) receptor antagonist istradefylline in advanced PD. Neurology 2003; 61:297–303.

22. Bara-Jimenez W, Sherzai A, Dimitrova T, et al. Adenosine A(2A) receptor antagonist treatment of Parkinson's disease. Neurology. 2003; 61:293–296.

23. Klein NC, Cunha BA, Tetracyclines. Med Clin North Am 1995; 79:789–801.

24. Power C, Henry S, Del Bigio MR, et al. Intracerebral hemorrhage induces macrophage activation and matrix metalloproteinases. Ann Neurol 2003; 53:731–742.

25. Yrjanheikki J, Keinanen R, Pellikka M, et al. Tetracyclines inhibit microglial activation and are neuroprotective in global brain ischemia. Proc Natl Acad Sci USA 1998; 95:15769–15774.

26. Morimoto N, Shimazawa M, Yamashima T, et al. Minocycline inhibits oxidative stress and decreases in vitro and in vivo ischemic neuronal damage. Brain Res 2005; 1044:8–15.

27. Fernandez-Gomez FJ, Galindo MF, Gomez-Lazaro M, et al. Involvement of mitochondrial potential and calcium buffering capacity in minocycline cytoprotective actions. Neuroscience 2005; 133:959–967.

28. Arvin KL, Han BH, Du Y, et al. Minocycline markedly protects the neonatal brain against hypoxic-ischemic injury. Ann Neurol 2002; 52:54–61.
29. Chen M, Ona VO, Li M, et al. Minocycline inhibits caspase-1 and caspase-3 expression and delays mortality in a transgenic mouse model of Huntington disease. Nat Med 2000; 6:797–801.
30. Thomas M, Le WD. Minocycline: neuroprotective mechanisms in Parkinson's disease. Curr Pharm Des 2004; 10(6):679–686.
31. Du Y, Ma Z, Lin S, et al. Minocycline prevents nigrostriatal dopaminergic neurodegeneration in the MPTP model of Parkinson's disease. Proc Natl Acad Sci USA 2001; 98:14669–14674.
32. Diguet E, Fernagut PO, Wei X, et al. Deleterious effects of minocycline in animal models of Parkinson's disease and Huntington's disease. Eur J Neurosci 2004; 19:3266–3276.
33. Yang L, Sugama S, Chirichigno JW, et al. Minocycline enhances MPTP toxicity to dopaminergic neurons. J Neurosci Res 2003; 74:278–285.
34. Costantini LC, Chaturvedi P, Armistead DM, et al. A novel immunophilin ligand: distinct branching effects on dopaminergic neurons in culture and neurotrophic actions after oral administration in an animal model of Parkinson's disease. Neurobiol Dis 1998; 5:97–106.
35. Manakova S, Singh A, Kaariainen T, et al. Failure of FK506 (tacrolimus) to alleviate apomorphine-induced circling in rat Parkinson model in spite of some cytoprotective effects in SH-SY5Y dopaminergic cells. Brain Res 2005; 1038:83–91.
36. Marshall VL, Grosset DG. GPI-1485 (Guilford). Curr Opin Investig Drugs 2004; 5:107–112.
37. Bezard E, Baufreton J, Owens G, et al. Sonic hedgehog is a neuromodulator in the adult subthalamic nucleus. FASEB J 2003; 17:2337–2338.
38. Tsuboi K, Shults CW. Intrastriatal injection of sonic hedgehog reduces behavioral impairment in a rat model of Parkinson's disease. Exp Neurol 2002; 173:95–104.
39. Johnston TH, Brotchie JM. Drugs in development for Parkinson's disease. Curr Opin Investig Drugs 2004; 5:720–726.
40. Wang LH, Besirli CG, Johnson EM Jr. Mixed-lineage kinases: a target for the prevention of neurodegeneration. Annu Rev Pharmacol Toxicol 2004; 44:451–474.
41. Lund S, Porzgen P, Mortensen AL, et al. Inhibition of microglial inflammation by the MLK inhibitor CEP-1347. J Neurochem 2005; 92:1439–1451.
42. Boll JB, Geist MA, Kaminski Schierle GS, et al. Improvement of embryonic dopaminergic neurone survival in culture and after grafting into the striatum of hemiparkinsonian rats by CEP-1347. J Neurochem 2004; 88:698–707.
43. Saporito MS, Brown EM, Miller MS, et al. CEP-1347/KT-7515, an inhibitor of c-jun N-terminal kinase activation, attenuates the 1-methyl-4-phenyl tetrahydropyridine-mediated loss of nigrostriatal dopaminergic neurons in vivo. J Pharmacol Exp Ther 1999; 288:421–427.
44. Mathiasen JR, McKenna BA, Saporito MS, et al. Inhibition of mixed lineage kinase 3 attenuates MPP+-induced neurotoxicity in SH-SY5Y cells. Brain Res 2004; 1003:86–97.
45. Parkinson Study Group. The safety and tolerability of a mixed lineage kinase inhibitor (CEP-1347) in PD. Neurology 2004; 62:330–332.
46. Blanchet PJ, Metman LV, Chase TN. Renaissance of amantadine in the treatment of Parkinson's disease. Adv Neurol 2003; 91:251–257.
47. Chase TN, Oh JD. Striatal mechanisms and pathogenesis of parkinsonian signs and motor complications. Ann Neurol 200; 47(suppl):S122–S130.
48. Calon F, Rajput AH, Hornykiewicz O, et al. Levodopa-induced motor complications are associated with alterations of glutamate receptors in Parkinson's disease. Neurobiol Dis 2003; 14:404–416.
49. Konitsiotis S, Blanchet PJ, Verhagen L, et al. AMPA receptor blockade improves levodopa-induced dyskinesia in MPTP monkeys. Neurology 2000; 54:1589–95.
50. Erdo F, Berzsenyi P, Andrasi F. The AMPA-antagonist talampanel is neuroprotective in rodent models of focal cerebral ischemia. Brain Res Bull 2005; 66:43–49.
51. O'Neill MJ, Murray TK, Clay MP, et al. LY503430: pharmacology, pharmacokinetics, and effects in rodent models of Parkinson's disease. CNS Drug Rev 2005; 11:77–96.
52. Henry B, Brotchie JM. Potential of opioid antagonists in the treatment of levodopa-induced dyskinesias in Parkinson's disease. Drugs Aging 1996; 9:149–158.

53. Hughes NR, McKnight AT, Woodruff GN, et al. Kappa-opioid receptor agonists increase locomotor activity in the monoamine-depleted rat model of parkinsonism. Mov Disord 1998; 13:228–233.
54. Piccini P, Weeks RA, Brooks DJ. Alterations in opioid receptor binding in Parkinson's disease patients with levodopa-induced dyskinesias. Ann Neurol 1997; 42:720–726.
55. Samadi P, Gregoire L, Bedard PJ. Opioid antagonists increase the dyskinetic response to dopaminergic agents in parkinsonian monkeys: interaction between dopamine and opioid systems. Neuropharmacology 2003; 45:954–963.
56. Sandyk R, Snider SR. Naloxone treatment of L-dopa-induced dyskinesias in Parkinson's disease. Am J Psychiatry 1986; 143:118.
57. Manson AJ, Katzenschlager R, Hobart J, et al. High dose naltrexone for dyskinesias induced by levodopa. J Neurol Neurosurg Psychiatry 2001; 70:554–556.
58. Fox S, Silverdale M, Kellett M, et al. Non-subtype-selective opioid receptor antagonism in treatment of levodopa-induced motor complications in Parkinson's disease. Mov Disord 2004; 19:554–560.
59. Kato H, Kurosaki R, Oki C, et al. Arundic acid, an astrocyte-modulating agent, protects dopaminergic neurons against MPTP neurotoxicity in mice. Brain Res 2004; 1030:66–73.
60. Stocchi F, Olanow W. Neuroprotection in Parkinson's disease: clinical trials. Ann Neurol 2003; 53(suppl 3):S87–S97.
61. Kragten E, Lalande I, Zimmerman R, et al. Glyceraldehyde-3-phosphate dehydrogenase, the putative target of the antiapoptotic compounds CGP 3466 and R-(-)-deprenyl. J Biol Chem 1998; 273:5821–5828.
62. Carlile GW, Chalmesr-Redman RM, Tatton NA, et al. Reduced apoptosis after nerve growth factor and serum withdrawal: conversion of tetrameric glyceraldehyde-3-phosphate dehydrogenase to a dimer. Mol Pharmacol 2000; 57:2–12.
63. Waldmeier PC, Spooren WP, Hengerer B. CGP 3466 protects dopaminergic neurons in lesion models of Parkinson's disease. Naunyn Schmiedebergs Arch Pharmacol 2000; 362:526–537.
64. Andringa G, Cools AR. The neuroprotective effects of CGP 3466B in the best in vivo model of Parkinson's disease, the bilaterally MPTP-treated rhesus monkey. J Neural Transm Suppl 2000; 60:215–225.
65. Minghetti L. Cyclooxygenase-2 (COX-2) in inflammatory and degenerative brain diseases. J Neuropathol Exp Neurol 2004; 63:901–910.
66. Feng Z, Li D, Fung PC, et al. COX-2-deficient mice are less prone to MPTP-neurotoxicity than wild-type mice. Neuroreport 2003; 14:1927–1929.
67. Teismann P, Vila M, Choi DK, et al. COX-2 and neurodegeneration in Parkinson's disease. Ann N Y Acad Sci 2003; 991:272–277.
68. Hunot S, Vila M, Teismann P, et al. JNK-mediated induction of cyclooxygenase 2 is required for neurodegeneration in a mouse model of Parkinson's disease. Proc Natl Acad Sci USA 2004; 101:665–670.
69. Przybylkowski A, Kurkowska-Jastrzebska I, Joniec I, et al. Cyclooxygenases mRNA and protein expression in striata in the experimental mouse model of Parkinson's disease induced by 1-methyl-4-phenyl-1,2,3,6-tetrahydropyridine administration to mouse. Brain Res 2004; 1019:144–151.
70. Klivenyi P, Gardian G, Calingasan NY, et al. Additive neuroprotective effects of creatine and a cyclooxygenase 2 inhibitor against dopamine depletion in the 1-methyl-4-phenyl-1,2,3,6-tetrahydropyridine (MPTP) mouse model of Parkinson's disease. J Mol Neurosci 2003; 21:191–198.
71. Bezard E, Ferry S, Mach U, et al. Attenuation of levodopa-induced dyskinesia by normalizing dopamine D3 receptor function. Nat Med 2003;9:762–767.
72. Hsu A, Togasaki DM, Bezard E, et al. Effect of the D3 dopamine receptor partial agonist BP897 [N-[4-(4-(2-methoxyphenyl)piperazinyl)butyl]-2-naphthamide] on L-3,4-dihydroxyphenylalanine-induced dyskinesias and parkinsonism in squirrel monkeys. J Pharmacol Exp Ther 2004; 311:770–777.
73. Linazasoro G. recent failures of new potential symptomatic treatments for Parkinson's Disease: causes and solutions. Mov Disord 2004; 19:743–754.
74. Montastruc JL, Rascol O, Senard JM, et al. A pilot study of N-methyl-D-aspartate (NMDA) antagonist in Parkinson's disease. J Neurol Neurosurg Psychiatry 1992; 55:630–631.

75. Greenamyre JT, Eller RV, Zhang Z, et al. Antiparkinsonian effects of remacemide hydrochloride, a glutamate antagonist, in rodent and primate models of Parkinson's disease. Ann Neurol 1994; 35:655–661.

76. Parkinson Study group. A randomized, controlled trial of remacemide for motor fluctuations in Parkinson's disease. Neurology 2001; 56:455–462.

77. Fornai F, Schluter OM, Lenzi P, et al. Parkinson-like syndrome induced by continuous MPTP infusion: convergent roles of the ubiquitin-proteasome system and alpha-synuclein. Proc Natl Acad Sci USA 2005; 102:3413–3418.

Index